2012
YEAR BOOK OF
CARDIOLOGY®

The 2012 Year Book Series

Year Book of Anesthesiology and Pain Management™: Drs Chestnut, Abram, Black, Gravlee, Lien, Mathru, and Roizen

Year Book of Cardiology®: Drs Gersh, Cheitlin, Elliott, Gold, Graham, and Thourani

Year Book of Critical Care Medicine®: Drs Dries, Zanotti-Cavazzoni, Latenser, Martinez, Rincon, and Zwank

Year Book of Dermatology and Dermatologic Surgery™: Dr Del Rosso

Year Book of Diagnostic Radiology®: Drs Elster, Abbara, Oestreich, Offiah, Rosado de Christenson, Stephens, and Strickland

Year Book of Emergency Medicine®: Drs Hamilton, Bruno, Handly, Minczak, Mullin, Quintana, and Ramoska

Year Book of Endocrinology®: Drs Schott, Apovian, Clarke, Eugster, Ludlam, Meikle, Oetgen, Ovalle, Schteingart, and Toth

Year Book of Gastroenterology™: Drs Talley, DeVault, Harnois, Murray, Pearson, Philcox, Picco, and Smith

Year Book of Hand and Upper Limb Surgery®: Drs Yao, Adams, Isaacs, Lee, and Rizzo

Year Book of Medicine®: Drs Barker, Garrick, Gersh, Khardori, LeRoith, Panush, Talley, and Thigpen

Year Book of Neonatal and Perinatal Medicine®: Drs Fanaroff, Benitz, Donn, Neu, Papile, Polin, and Van Marter

Year Book of Neurology and Neurosurgery®: Drs Klimo, Minagar, Gandhi, House, Liu, Mazia, Panagariya, Ragel, Riesenburger, Robottom, Schwendimann, Shafazand, Uhm, and Yang

Year Book of Obstetrics, Gynecology, and Women's Health®: Drs Dungan and Shulman

Year Book of Oncology®: Drs Arceci, Bauer, Chiorean, Gordon, Lawton, Murphy, Thigpen, and Tsao

Year Book of Ophthalmology®: Drs Rapuano, Cohen, Flanders, Hammersmith, Milman, Myers, Nagra, Nelson, Penne, Pyfer, Sergott, Shields, Talekar, and Vander

Year Book of Orthopedics®: Drs Morrey, Huddleston, Rose, Swiontkowski, and Trigg

Year Book of Otolaryngology-Head and Neck Surgery®: Drs Sindwani, Balough, Franco, Gapany, and Mitchell

Year Book of Pathology and Laboratory Medicine®: Drs Raab and Bissell

Year Book of Pediatrics®: Dr Stockman

2012

The Year Book of CARDIOLOGY®

Editor in Chief
Bernard J. Gersh, MB, ChB, DPhil, FRCP
Professor of Medicine, Mayo Clinic College of Medicine; Consultant, Division of Cardiovascular Diseases, Mayo Clinic, Rochester, Minnesota

Editors
Melvin D. Cheitlin, MD, MACC
Emeritus Professor of Medicine, University of California, San Francisco; Former Chief of Cardiology, San Francisco General Hospital, San Francisco, California

William J. Elliott, MD, PhD
Professor of Preventive Medicine, Internal Medicine, and Pharmacology, Head, Division of Pharmacology, Pacific Northwest University of Health Sciences, Yakima, Washington

Michael R. Gold, MD, PhD
Michael E. Assey Professor of Medicine; Director of Cardiology, Medical University of South Carolina, Charleston, South Carolina

Thomas P. Graham, MD
Professor Emeritus of Pediatrics, Vanderbilt University School of Medicine; Division of Cardiology, Vanderbilt Children's Hospital, Nashville, Tennessee

Vinod H. Thourani, MD
Associate Professor of Cardiothoracic Surgery, Associate Director, Structural Heart Center, Associate Director, CT Surgery Clinical Research Unit, Associate Director, Residency Program, Emory University Hospital Midtown, Cardiac Surgery, Atlanta, Georgia

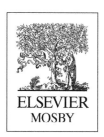

ELSEVIER
MOSBY

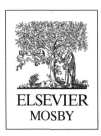

ELSEVIER MOSBY

Vice President, Continuity: Kimberly Murphy
Developmental Editor: Katie Hartner
Production Supervisor, Electronic Year Books: Donna M. Skelton
Electronic Article Manager: Emily Ogle
Illustrations and Permissions Coordinator: Dawn A. Vohsen

2012 EDITION

Printed and bound by CPI Group (UK) Ltd, Croydon, CR0 4YY
Transferred to Digital Print 2012

Editorial Office:
Elsevier
1600 John F. Kennedy Blvd.
Suite 1800
Philadelphia, PA 19103-2899

International Standard Serial Number: 0145-4145
International Standard Book Number: 978-0-323-08874-9

Contributing Editors

Michael L. Bernard, MD, PhD
Clinical Instructor, Division of Cardiology, Medical University of South Carolina, Charleston, South Carolina

William W. Brabham, MD
Clinical Instructor, Division of Cardiology, Medical University of South Carolina, Charleston, South Carolina

Frank A. Cuoco, Jr, MD, MBA
Assistant Professor, Department of Medicine, Medical University of South Carolina, Charleston, South Carolina

Azeem R. Khan, MD
Chief Resident, Cardiothoracic Surgery, Emory University School of Medicine, Atlanta, Georgia

Soumya R. Neravetla, MD
Structural Heart and Transcatheter Valve Fellow, Emory University School of Medicine, Atlanta, Georgia

Robert B. Leman, MD, FACC, FACP
Professor of Medicine, Medical University of South Carolina, Charleston, South Carolina

Peter Netzler, MD
Fellow, Division of Cardiology, Medical University of South Carolina, Charleston, South Carolina

Christopher P. Rowley, MD
Fellow, Division of Cardiology, Medical University of South Carolina, Charleston, South Carolina

Vinod H. Thourani, MD
Associate Professor of Cardiothoracic Surgery, Associate Director, Structural Heart and Transcatheter Valve Program, Associate Director, Cardiothoracic Surgery Residency Program, Associate Director, Cardiothoracic Surgery Clinical Research Unit, Emory University School of Medicine, Atlanta, Georgia

J. Lacy Sturdivant, MD
Assistant Professor, Department of Medicine, Medical University of South Carolina, Charleston, South Carolina

J. Marcus Warton, MD
Frank Tourville Professor of Medicine, Chief of Electrophysiology, Medical University of South Carolina, Charleston, South Carolina

Table of Contents

JOURNALS REPRESENTED   xi

INTRODUCTION   xiii

1. Hypertension   1
   Guidelines and Overviews   1
   Epidemiological Studies   31
   Hypertension and Cardiovascular Risk   47
   Miscellaneous.   57
   Clinical Trials.   87
2. Pediatric Cardiovascular Disease   111
   Tetralogy of Fallot   111
   Transposition of the Great Arteries   117
   Fontan Operation.   119
   Hypoplastic Left Heart Syndrome   126
   Pulmonary Atresia/Intact Ventricular Septum   132
   Surgical Therapy   135
   Follow-up and Outcome Studies   138
   Coarctation, Interrupted Arch   141
   Miscellaneous.   143
3. Cardiac Surgery   155
   Coronary Artery Disease   155
   Valve Disease   164
   Transplantation/Ventricular Assist Devices.   169
   Outcomes and Quality Assessment   171
   Miscellaneous.   174
4. Coronary Heart Disease   181
   Acute ST-Segment Elevation Myocardial Infarction   181
   Chronic Coronary Artery Disease   210
   Coronary Bypass Surgery and Percutaneous Coronary
     Intervention   216
   Epidemiology   245
   Miscellaneous.   261
   Non-ST Elevation Acute Coronary Syndromes   284

5. Non-Coronary Heart Disease in Adults   291
   Congestive Heart Failure Therapy and Technology   291
   Medical Treatment of Congestive Heart Failure   321
   Pathogenesis and Prognosis   345
   Myocarditis and Cardiomyopathy   358
   Valvular Heart Disease and Infective Endocarditis.   375
   Miscellaneous.   407

6. Cardiac Arrhythmias, Conduction Disturbances, and
   Electrophysiology   427
   Atrial Fibrillation   427
   Devices.   452
   Sudden Cardiac Death   474
   Miscellaneous.   484

   ARTICLE INDEX   493

   AUTHOR INDEX   505

Journals Represented

Journals represented in this YEAR BOOK are listed below.

American Heart Journal
American Journal of Cardiology
American Journal of Medicine
Annals of Internal Medicine
Annals of Thoracic Surgery
Archives of Internal Medicine
British Medical Journal
Circulation
Circulation Cardiovascular Quality and Outcomes
Circulation Research
Europace
European Heart Journal
European Journal of Echocardiography
European Journal of Internal Medicine
Heart
Heart Rhythm
Hypertension
International Journal of Cardiology
Journal of Cardiac Failure
Journal of Heart and Lung Transplantation
Journal of Hypertension
Journal of the American College of Cardiology
Journal of the American College of Cardiology Cardiovascular Imaging
Journal of the American College of Cardiology Cardiovascular Interventions
Journal of the American Medical Association
Journal of the American Society of Echocardiography
Journal of Thoracic and Cardiovascular Surgery
Lancet
Lancet Oncology
Nature
Neurology
New England Journal of Medicine
Pediatric Radiology
Surgery
Thrombosis Research
Transplantation
United Kingdom National Health Service

STANDARD ABBREVIATIONS

The following terms are abbreviated in this edition: acquired immunodeficiency syndrome (AIDS), cardiopulmonary resuscitation (CPR), central nervous system (CNS), cerebrospinal fluid (CSF), computed tomography (CT), deoxyribonucleic acid (DNA), electrocardiography (ECG), health maintenance organization (HMO), human immunodeficiency virus (HIV), intensive care unit (ICU), intramuscular (IM), intravenous (IV), magnetic resonance (MR) imaging (MRI), ribonucleic acid (RNA), and ultrasound (US).

NOTE

The YEAR BOOK OF CARDIOLOGY is a literature survey service providing abstracts of articles published in the professional literature. Every effort is made to assure the accuracy of the information presented in these pages. Neither the editors nor the publisher of the YEAR BOOK OF CARDIOLOGY can be responsible for errors in the original materials. The editors' comments are their own opinions. Mention of specific products within this publication does not constitute endorsement.

To facilitate the use of the YEAR BOOK OF CARDIOLOGY as a reference tool, all illustrations and tables included in this publication are now identified as they appear in the original article. This change is meant to help the reader recognize that any illustration or table appearing in the YEAR BOOK OF CARDIOLOGY may be only one of many in the original article. For this reason, figure and table numbers will often appear to be out of sequence within the YEAR BOOK OF CARDIOLOGY.

Introduction

It was another slow year for the field of hypertension in 2011. The expected date of release of the new and updated US hypertension guidelines, The Eighth Report of the Joint National Committee on Prevention, Detection, Evaluation, and Treatment of High Blood Pressure (JNC 8) was pushed back yet again. Great Britain's National Institute for Health and Clinical Excellence released their new guidelines in April 2011; one of the major changes was the recommendation that ambulatory blood pressure monitoring be performed for every person initially suspected of having hypertension. Separate articles comparing methods of diagnosing hypertension and an economic analysis that supported initial ambulatory blood pressure monitoring were later published separately in *BMJ* and *The Lancet*, respectively. The American College of Cardiology Foundation and the American Heart Association released a set of hypertension guidelines for elderly patients. More controversial were new meta-analyses suggesting that the recommended target blood pressure for patients with chronic kidney disease (< 130/80 mm Hg) was not well supported by clinical trial evidence. Although a similar conclusion was reached about patients with diabetes in a controversial article in 2010, a meta-analysis of more than 73 000 diabetic patients in clinical trials suggested that more intensive antihypertensive treatment was in fact beneficial. This was also the case for "high-risk" (but not hypertensive) patients who had their cardiovascular risk reduced when given antihypertensive drug therapy in 25 clinical trials. The Blood Pressure Lowering Treatment Trialists' Collaboration published the results of their meta-regression analyses that indicated that antihypertensive drug therapy is effective across all levels of blood pressure and is not dependent on the baseline blood pressure. This conclusion fit well with a review from the Global Burden of Disease Group at the World Health Organization, who looked at global trends in systolic blood pressure and predicted this will become a major serious public health problem for developing nations in just a decade or so.

Angiotensin receptor blockers (ARBs) were exonerated in two meta-analyses; one refuted the hypothesis that these drugs don't prevent myocardial infarction, and the other rebutted last year's allegation that they cause cancer. A second meta-analysis involving more than 324 000 clinical trial subjects also concluded that there was no significant increase in cancer associated with the use of any or all antihypertensive drugs. A meta-analysis showed a significant risk of stroke associated with prehypertension. A systematic review of the cost-effectiveness of dietary sodium restriction suggested this would be a low-cost, high-reward, and cost-saving intervention for most populations. The antihypertensive efficacy of low-dose (12.5 mg/d) hydrochlorothiazide was questioned in a meta-analysis of ambulatory blood pressure monitoring studies. The addition of a renin-angiotensin system inhibitor was shown to reduce the incidence and severity of dihydropyridine calcium channel blocker-associated pedal edema, although most of the data were obtained with angiotensin converting-enzyme (ACE) inhibitors.

Several epidemiological studies published in 2011 estimated the prevalence of resistant hypertension. Two separate analyses of the US National Health and Nutrition Examination Surveys (NHANES) came to similar conclusions about its prevalence ($\sim 13\%$ of the treated hypertensive population) and risk factors. Resistant hypertension was diagnosed in 12.2% of 68 045 Spanish patients with hypertension, but 38% were found to have the "white-coat phenomenon" by ambulatory blood pressure monitoring. The clinical characteristics of patients with resistant hypertension were similar in US surveys, the Spanish cohort, and in those who developed it after enrollment in the Anglo-Scandinavian Cardiac Outcomes Trial (ASCOT). The issue of dietary sodium consumption and cardiovascular risk was again controversial, with a 2-phase prospective cohort study (European Project on Genes in Hypertension, EPOGH) suggesting an inverse relationship, but a J-shaped relationship was seen in a post-hoc analysis of the ONgoing Telmisartan Alone or in combination with Ramipril Global Endpoints Trial (ONTARGET). A new method of estimating sodium and potassium intake from dietary recall questionnaires showed a direct and near-linear relationship of sodium intake and mortality and of sodium/potassium ratio and cardiovascular events in the Third NHANES data set. An analysis of the "Pay for Performance" strategy for implementing goal-oriented primary care (of hypertension and other chronic conditions) in Great Britain showed that performance improved even before the program was started and had less effect than many American authorities would have predicted. Among patients with diabetes in the Framingham Heart Study, hypertension was responsible for 30% of the population-attributable risk for death and for 25% for cardiovascular events. Analysis of a large pharmacy claims database in Italy showed wide variability in long-term persistence with specific antihypertensive agents within a pharmacological class, suggesting that guidelines should discuss individual agents rather than broad pharmacological classes. Two reports about ACE-inhibitors contradicted prior knowledge: ACE-inhibitor use during the first trimester of pregnancy was not associated with an increased risk of birth defects in a Californian cohort of 465 754 mothers and babies, and a high proportion (48%) of individuals who suffered angioedema during treatment with an ACE-inhibitor had a recurrent episode, even after stopping the drug.

A number of articles further explored the relationship between hypertension and cardiovascular risk. Two used the database from the Multiple Risk Factor Intervention Trial (MRFIT) and compared cardiovascular events or electrocardiographic signs of left ventricular hypertrophy in patients in the Stepped Care arm who received either chlorthalidone or hydrochlorothiazide. In both cases, chlorthalidone was associated with better outcomes. A single measurement of blood pressure was found inadequate for assessing control of hypertension in an individual patient, whether performed in the office or at home, yet it did significantly correlate with long-term mortality in 18-year-old Swedish men. A post-hoc analysis of the Prevention Regimen for Effectively Avoiding Second Strokes (PRoFESS) trial showed that the mean of 2 blood pressure measurements before randomization was significantly related to the risk of recurrent stroke, with an increased risk in those with "very low" systolic blood pressures (< 120 mm Hg), similar to the J-shaped curve seen for systolic blood pressure and recurrent myocardial infarction. A post-hoc analysis of the ONTARGET data set showed that more frequent achievement of currently recommended blood pressure targets was associated with a lower risk of stroke and renal events, but not coronary heart disease events, again consistent with the J-shaped curve for myocardial infarction. In patients with chronic kidney disease, ambulatory blood pressure (particularly nighttime blood pressure) was a significant predictor of renal and cardiovascular risk, but office blood pressure was unrelated to either. A large Italian study was able to show that better adherence to antihypertensive therapy was associated with improved prognosis, compared with those who consumed less than 25% of their prescribed pills. And lastly, a 4.5-year treatment with chlorthalidone-based antihypertensive drugs prolonged life over the next 22 years better than placebo, with about 1 day of increased survival for every month of treated hypertension.

There was relatively little emphasis this year on "causes of hypertension." Perhaps the most important article on this topic was a report of the genome-wide association discovery of polymorphisms related to hypertension and cardiovascular risk; although not available to the general public as of yet, this has important implications for future work. Perhaps the oldest technique of assessing systolic blood pressure, palpation of the pulse (and the method of Riva-Rocci) was found to still be relevant today, although a "fudge factor" of 6 mm Hg has to be added to the palpated measurement. A population-based cohort study from Finland used home blood pressure monitoring to identify risk factors for "masked hypertension" and found that the only psychological characteristic of such patients is a higher risk of hypochondriasis.

Compared with previous years, 2011 saw fewer reports of important clinical trials that are likely to change clinical practice. Perhaps the most disappointing was the finding that an ARB was not successful in reducing either cardiovascular risk or functional status in hypertensive patients with an acute stroke less than 30 hours after onset of symptoms. Decreased dietary sodium intake was found to be more effective in lowering blood pressure and proteinuria than adding an ARB to chronic kidney disease patients who were already taking an ACE-inhibitor. Compared with eplerenone, spironolactone was more effective in lowering blood pressure in hypertensive patients with hyperaldosteronism. A post-hoc analysis of the Felodipine EVent Reduction (FEVER) trial provided evidence that the traditional target systolic blood pressure of < 140 mm Hg was associated with reduced risks of stroke, cardiovascular events, and death. Lower rates of cardiovascular complications, retinopathy, and neuropathy were seen in patients with diabetes randomized to a combination of a calcium antagonist and ACE-inhibitor compared with placebo (whose blood pressures were controlled with other therapies), but the primary endpoint, decline in glomerular filtration rate, was not significantly different. A Japanese trial of second-line therapies (ARB, β-blocker, or thiazide) after inadequate blood pressure control with a dihydropyridine calcium antagonist showed no significant differences in blood pressures or cardiovascular events (although the number of patients with events was about half of what was expected). The initial combination of the direct renin inhibitor, aliskiren and amlodipine, was more successful in reducing blood pressure than either drug alone; at the end of 2011, it was announced that a trial of aliskiren plus a renin-angiotensin system blocker in diabetic patients with chronic kidney disease was stopped prematurely because of adverse effects of the combination, so promotion of aliskiren plus valsartan ceased. A clinical trial showed that automated (versus healthcare provider-determined) office blood pressure measurements reduced the "white-coat effect" and had higher-quality readings. A complex randomized trial showed better short-term office blood pressure control in hypertensive US veterans who performed home blood pressure monitoring, with transtelephonic relaying of data to healthcare professionals who could provide feedback about it. Similarly, a randomized trial of providing digital video discs that contained videoclips of patients from the community who successfully dealt with their hypertension significantly improved blood pressures in African Americans with uncontrolled hypertension in a "safety-net clinic"; no significant change was seen in those with controlled blood pressures at randomization.

One can hope that 2011 was "the calm before the storm" in hypertension, as 2012 appears to be filled with many exciting developments, including JNC 8 and other important, federally approved treatment guidelines.

William J. Elliott, MD, PhD

1 Hypertension

Guidelines and Overviews

NICE clinical guideline 127: Hypertension: Clinical management of primary hypertension in adults

Williams B, for The Guideline Development Groups, National Collaborating Centres, and NICE Project Team. United Kingdom National Health Service: National Institute for Health and Clinical Excellence (Univ of Leicester and Univ Hosps of Leicester NHS Trust, London, UK)

United Kingdom Natl Health Serv 1-36, 2011

Objectives and Targets.—This guidance updates and replaces the United Kingdom's National Institute for Health and Clinical Excellence (NICE) hypertension guidelines issued in 2004 and 2006. It is intended to provide advice about patient-centered care for persons with elevated blood pressure, but no other conditions for which NICE guidance has already been offered.

Major New Points.—Diagnosis: 24-hour ambulatory blood pressure monitoring (with at least 14 measurements/day) should be offered for every newly-diagnosed person with hypertension. Home blood pressure monitoring can be used to confirm a diagnosis of hypertension if two consecutive measurements are taken at least 1 minute apart, morning and evening, for at least 4, but preferably 7 days. Drug therapy: Drug treatment should be offered to all people with stage 2 hypertension, and all people with stage 1 hypertension younger than 80 years of age with target organ damage, established cardiovascular disease, renal disease, diabetes, or a 10-year risk of cardiovascular disease > 20%. Seek specialist advice for people with stage 1 hypertension younger than 40 years for assessment of target organ damage and secondary causes of hypertension. Monitoring and target blood pressures: For people who display the "white-coat effect," consider using home or ambulatory blood pressures as an adjunct to office measurements. Step 1 antihypertensive treatment for people over age 55 or blacks should be a calcium antagonist, with either chlorthalidone or indapamide as an alternative. Otherwise an ACE-inhibitor (or an angiotensin receptor blocker, if cough or angioedema) should be offered. For people with resistant hypertension (already taking a calcium antagonist, ACE-inhibitor, and thiazide-like diuretic), consider low-dose spironolactone or higher-dose chlorthalidone

1

or indapamide, depending on the serum potassium. Target blood pressures should be <140/90 mm Hg for people less than 80 years of age, and <150/90 mm Hg otherwise.

Rationale.—The NICE Economics Team has performed incremental cost-utility analyses, typically based on meta-analyses of clinical trial data, to formulate each of these recommendations, using national data and recent costs of interventions (including drug therapy) to the National Health Service. Most of these are (or soon will be) available either on the NICE website, or published in the medical literature.

Conclusions.—These recommendations are for primary care of people with raised blood pressure. Other NICE guidances provide advice about appropriate treatments for complicated hypertension, including type 2 diabetes (CG 87), heart failure (CG 108), pregnancy (CG 107), chronic kidney disease (CG 73), stroke (CG 68), secondary prevention of myocardial infarction (CG 48), etc.

▶ There is new pervasive emphasis among guideline writers to require that all recommendations be very evidence based, using clinical trials or meta-analyses of clinical trials as the highest-ranking evidence.[1] The United Kingdom National Institute for Health and Clinical Excellence (NICE) guidelines have taken these new paradigms 1 step further, however, because their Economics Group performed cost-utility analyses, informed by the clinical trial results, and populated by nationwide costs to the National Health Service (NHS) of all procedures and drugs. It is remarkable, for example, that the cost of amlodipine to the UK NHS is about 10- to 50-fold lower than the average wholesale price of the very same medication in the United States. This makes translation of the NICE guidelines across the Atlantic Ocean very challenging.

The NICE hypertension guidelines are also clearly meant to apply ONLY to people with raised blood pressure—no further complications or other diseases that might reasonably influence treatment. On first reading, therefore, there appears to be no lower blood pressure target for diabetics or people with chronic kidney disease, which is consistent with several recent meta-analyses. However, the NICE Clinical Guideline 127 makes specific reference to earlier NICE guidelines about each of these conditions. Only after accessing other guidelines, for example, does one learn that a blood pressure target of less than 130/80 mm Hg is recommended for diabetics with chronic kidney disease, nondiabetics with chronic kidney disease, and greater than 1 gm/d of proteinuria[2] or diabetics with kidney, eye, or cerebrovascular damage.[3]

The new NICE recommendations to routinely use 24-hour ambulatory blood pressure monitoring for the initial diagnosis of hypertension are a departure from previous NICE guidelines,[4,5] but the economic and clinical advantages of using it to rule out "white-coat hypertension" have been published nearly 15 years ago and have recently been published in detail.[6] Because of its huge purchasing power, the UK NHS has obtained a very low price for the technology, approximately 25% to 33% of current US prices. The NICE recommendations about antihypertensive drug therapy are little changed from the 2006 recommendations, relegating β-blockers to step 4 therapy and recommending amlodipine as initial therapy for all but white people less than 55 years of age. This is presumably based on the results of the Anglo-Scandinavian Cardiac Outcomes Trial, in which the amlodipine-based regimen was superior in some secondary endpoints over an atenolol-based regimen.[7] The new NICE guidelines recommend spironolactone as fourth-line therapy (again as used in ASCOT[8]), which is now becoming more common in many centers across the world.

Many of these NICE recommendations are implementable in health care systems other than the UK NHS, but one wonders if the unique acquisition costs for many of the recommended procedures and agents will make them cost prohibitive elsewhere. This is especially likely to be true in low-income countries.[9]

W. J. Elliott, MD, PhD

References

1. Sackett DL, Rosenberg WM, Gray JA, Haynes RB, Richardson WS. Evidence based medicine: what it is and what it isn't. *BMJ.* 1996;312:71-72.
2. National Institute for Health and Clinical Excellence. CG 73 Chronic kidney disease: Early identification and management of chronic kidney disease in adults in primary and secondary care: NICE guideline. http://www.nice.org.uk/nicemedia/live/12069/42117/42117.pdf. Accessed October 31, 2011.
3. National Institute for Health and Clinical Excellence. CG 87 Type 2 diabetes— Newer agents (a partial update of CG 66): NICE guideline. http://guidance.nice.org.uk/CG87/NICEGuidance/Pdf/English. Accessed October 31, 2011.
4. National Institute for Health and Clinical Excellence. CG 34 Hypertension: Management of hypertension in adults in primary care: NICE guideline. http://www.nice.org.uk/CG034. Accessed October 31, 2011.
5. Essential Hypertension: Managing Adult Patients in Primary Care. 2004. NICE Clinical Guideline 18. http://www.nice.org.uk/nicemedia/live/10986/30118/30118.pdf. Accessed June 03, 2011.
6. Lovibond K, Jowett S, Barton P, et al. Cost-effectiveness of options for the diagnosis of high blood pressure in primary care: a modelling study. *Lancet.* 2011; 378:1219-1230.
7. Dahlöf B, Sever PS, Poulter NR, et al. Prevention of cardiovascular events with an antihypertensive regimen of amlodipine adding perindopril as required versus atenolol adding bendroflumethiazide as required, in the Anglo-Scandinavian Cardiac Outcomes Trial-Blood Pressure Lowering Arm (ASCOT-BPLA): a multicentre randomised controlled trial. *Lancet.* 2005;366:895-906.
8. Chapman N, Dobson J, Wilson S, et al; Anglo-Scandinavian Cardiac Outcomes Trial Investigators. Effect of spironolactone on blood pressure in subjects with resistant hypertension. *Hypertension.* 2007;49:839-845.
9. Danaei G, Finucane MM, Lin JK, et al; Global Burden of Metabolic Risk Factors of Chronic Diseases Collaborating Group (Blood Pressure). National, regional, and global trends in systolic blood pressure since 1980: systematic analysis of health examination surveys and epidemiological studies with 786 country-years and 5·4 million participants. *Lancet.* 2011;377:568-577.

Relative effectiveness of clinic and home blood pressure monitoring compared with ambulatory blood pressure monitoring in diagnosis of hypertension: systematic review

Hodgkinson J, Mant J, Martin U, et al (Univ of Birmingham, Edgbaston; Univ of Cambridge, UK; et al)
BMJ 342:d3621, 2011

Objective.—To determine the relative accuracy of clinic measurements and home blood pressure monitoring compared with ambulatory blood pressure monitoring as a reference standard for the diagnosis of hypertension.

Design.—Systematic review with meta-analysis with hierarchical summary receiver operating characteristic models. Methodological quality was appraised, including evidence of validation of blood pressure measurement equipment.

Data Sources.—Medline (from 1966), Embase (from 1980), Cochrane Database of Systematic Reviews, DARE, Medion, ARIF, and TRIP up to May 2010.

Eligibility Criteria for Selecting Studies.—Eligible studies examined diagnosis of hypertension in adults of all ages using home and/or clinic blood pressure measurement compared with those made using ambulatory monitoring that clearly defined thresholds to diagnose hypertension.

Results.—The 20 eligible studies used various thresholds for the diagnosis of hypertension, and only seven studies (clinic) and three studies (home) could be directly compared with ambulatory monitoring. Compared with ambulatory monitoring thresholds of 135/85 mm Hg, clinic measurements over 140/90 mm Hg had mean sensitivity and specificity of 74.6% (95% confidence interval 60.7% to 84.8%) and 74.6% (47.9% to 90.4%), respectively, whereas home measurements over 135/85 mm Hg had mean sensitivity and specificity of 85.7% (78.0% to 91.0%) and 62.4% (48.0% to 75.0%).

Conclusions.—Neither clinic nor home measurement had sufficient sensitivity or specificity to be recommended as a single diagnostic test. If ambulatory monitoring is taken as the reference standard, then treatment decisions based on clinic or home blood pressure alone might result in substantial overdiagnosis. Ambulatory monitoring before the start of lifelong drug treatment might lead to more appropriate targeting of treatment, particularly around the diagnostic threshold.

▶ Many different methods of obtaining blood pressure measurements have been developed, which have advantages and disadvantages for many patients. Office blood pressure readings have been the gold standard for research for more than a century, but few medical offices routinely take the standardized approach that takes time, effort, and testing and retraining of observers.[1] Automated office blood pressures have recently been advanced as a reasonably accurate alternative for busy primary care settings.[2] Home readings reduce the risk of the "white-coat response," and correlate better with target-organ damage, but can have their own disadvantages for some patients.[3] Twenty-four—hour ambulatory blood pressure monitoring has recently been recommended by the recently issued British hypertension guidelines for people suspected of having hypertension,[4] because the procedure is cost effective in their National Health Service.[5]

These authors therefore performed a systematic review and meta-analysis of the diagnostic characteristics of office versus home blood pressure measurements, using the 24-hour ambulatory blood pressure monitoring results as the gold standard. Perhaps because this is a very hot topic and has been addressed by well-done, widely cited studies in many countries, the authors' main conclusions are not surprising, as they reflect the conclusions of the summarized studies. The contentious and rather subjective issue is whether office or home reading is sufficiently insensitive and nonspecific for diagnosing hypertension to recommend the more technically challenging 24-hour blood pressure monitoring, especially if it must be performed more than annually. The economics of 24-hour blood pressure monitoring differ in the United Kingdom and the United States, which is likely why their respective governmental health care authorities have nearly diametrically opposite policies regarding implementation and reimbursement for the procedure.

The authors believe that their analysis has several limitations, including the lack of a quality score for the included studies, lack of direct comparisons across the methods, variability of diagnostic thresholds for hypertension, variability in the number of measurements used for each technique, and major differences in the demographic characteristics of the studied populations. It is nonetheless likely that when 24-hour ambulatory blood pressure monitoring is not available, home readings would be wise in selected patients to supplement information from traditional office readings. Unfortunately, in the United States, interpretation of home readings is not currently reimbursed, although it has been recommended.[6]

W. J. Elliott, MD, PhD

References

1. Pickering TG, Hall JE, Appel LJ, et al; Subcommittee of Professional and Public Education of the American Heart Association Council on High Blood Pressure Research. Recommendations for blood pressure measurement in humans and experimental animals: Part 1: blood pressure measurement in humans: a statement for professionals from the Subcommittee of Professional and Public Education of the American Heart Association Council on High Blood Pressure Research. *Hypertension.* 2005;45:142-161.
2. Myers MG, Godwin M, Dawes M, et al. Conventional versus automated measurement of blood pressure in primary care patients with systolic hypertension: randomised parallel design controlled trial. *BMJ.* 2011;342:d286.
3. Bray EP, Holder R, Mant J, McManus RJ. Does self-monitoring reduce blood pressure? Meta-analysis with meta-regression of randomized controlled trials. *Ann Med.* 2010;42:371-386.
4. Williams B, Williams H, Northedge J, et al; for The Guideline Development Groups, National Collaborating Centres, and NICE Project Team. NICE Clinical Guideline 127: Hypertension: Clinical Management of Primary Hypertension in Adults. United Kingdom National Health Service: National Institute for Health and Clinical Excellence. http://www.nice.org.uk/CG127. Accessed August 24, 2011.
5. Lovibond K, Jowett S, Barton P, et al. Cost-effectiveness of options for the diagnosis of high blood pressure in primary care: a modelling study. *Lancet.* 2011; 378:1219-1230.
6. Pickering TG, Miller NH, Ogedegbe G, Krakoff LR, Artinian NT, Goff D; American Heart Association, American Society of Hypertension, Preventive Cardiovascular

Nurses Association. Call to action on use and reimbursement for home blood pressure monitoring: executive summary. A joint scientific statement from the American Heart Association, American Society of Hypertension, and Preventive Cardiovascular Nurses Association. *Hypertension.* 2008;52:1-9.

ACCF/AHA 2011 Expert Consensus Document on Hypertension in the Elderly: A Report of the American College of Cardiology Foundation Task Force on Clinical Expert Consensus Documents Developed in Collaboration With the American Academy of Neurology, American Geriatrics Society, American Society for Preventive Cardiology, American Society of Hypertension, American Society of Nephrology, Association of Black Cardiologists, and European Society of Hypertension

Aronow WS, Fleg JL, Pepine CJ, et al (National Heart, Lung, and Blood Institute, USA)
J Am Coll Cardiol 57:2037-2114, 2011

Background.—Hypertension is common in persons age 65 years or older, so these individuals are more likely to suffer organ damage or clinical cardiovascular disease (CVD). Because the Hypertension in the Very Elderly Trial (HYVET) has documented the benefits of antihypertensive treatment for persons even age 80 years or older, it is important to understand the issues relevant to hypertension management in older patients.

Physical Findings and Diagnosis.—Age-associated increases in the prevalence of hypertension result from changes in arterial structure and function. With age, vessel distensibility diminishes, pulse wave velocity increases, late systolic blood pressure (SBP) is augmented, myocardial oxygen demand rises, and organ perfusion is limited. Adding coronary stenosis or a drug-induced excessive reduction in diastolic blood pressure (DBP) enhances these adverse conditions. Other causes of hypertension include renal artery stenosis, obstructive sleep apnea, primary aldosteronism, and thyroid disorders. Contributing factors are lifestyle, substance use, and medication effects. Elderly persons with poor BP control can suffer cerebrovascular disease, coronary artery disease, disorders of left ventricular (LV) structure and function, cardiac rhythm disorders, aortic and peripheral arterial disease, chronic kidney disease, ophthalmologic disorders, and quality of life deterioration.

The diagnosis of hypertension is based on at least three BP measurements done on at least two separate office visits. Patients should be seated comfortably for at least 5 minutes with the feet on the floor, the back supported, the arm supported horizontally, and the BP cuff at heart level. Findings should consider possible pseudohypertension (falsely increased SBP caused by sclerotic arteries) and white-coat hypertension, which must be ruled out. Besides accurately determining that the patient's BP is elevated, the clinician must identify reversible and/or treatable causes, evaluate for organ damage, assess for other CVD risk factors and/or comorbid conditions, and identify barriers to treatment compliance. Clinicians conduct a thorough history, physical examination, and laboratory testing, which should focus on urinalysis to detect renal damage, blood chemistries, cholesterol and triglyceride status, fasting blood sugar levels, and electro-cardiographic results. Certain patients may benefit from two-dimensional electrocardiography to detect LV hypertrophy and LV dysfunction. Quality of life and cognitive function should also be determined.

Management.—Evidence-based guidelines are currently unavailable, so the management of hypertension relies on expert opinion. Lifestyle modi-fication can be sufficient for milder forms of hypertension. Drug therapy is begun at the lowest dose and gradually increased based on BP responses until one reaches the maximum tolerated dose. If BP response is insuffi-cient with a single agent, a second drug from another class is added, with adjustments to ensure tolerance and effectiveness. If BP response is insufficient with two agents at full dose levels, a third drug from another class is added. Treatment must be individualized in elderly patients, with evaluation of possible reasons for inadequate BP response conducted before adding new antihypertensive drugs. Elderly patients take an average of at least six prescription drugs so the clinician must be concerned about polypharmacy, nonadherence, and potential drug interactions.

The principal drug classes used to manage hypertension are thiazide diuretics, often the initial agent given; non-thiazide diuretics such as indapa-mide, furosemide, mineralocorticoid antagonists, epithelial sodium transport channel antagonists, beta blockers, calcium antagonists, and angiotensin-converting enzyme inhibitors (ACEIs); direct renin inhibitors such as aliski-ren; and nonspecific vasodilators, which have unfavorable side effects and should be used only in combination therapy. Combination therapy is effica-cious, avoids adverse effects, is convenient, and facilitates compliance. Some combinations of ACEIs, angiotensin receptor blockers, and calcium antagonists provide even greater protection for the cardiovascular system. Most elderly patients will need at least two drugs. If the initial BP is over 20/10 mm Hg above the goal, initiation of therapy may be best accomplished with two drugs. Patients with complicated hypertension are given multiple agents based on their comorbid conditions. Special recommendations are also applicable to elderly black individuals, octogenarians, and persons with resistant hypertension.

Conclusions.—Current recommendations recognize that elderly patients with hypertension can benefit from nonpharmacologic interventions but should receive drug therapy if they remain hypertensive. SBP values of <140 mm Hg are an appropriate goal for most patients 79 years of age or younger. The goal for patients 80 years or older is 140 to 145 mm Hg, if toler-ated. Further research is needed to define the pathogenesis of increased vascular and LV stiffness, set appropriate treatment thresholds and goals, compare the effectiveness of various treatment strategies, and assess the relative safety and efficacy of various approaches in preventing mortality and morbidity.

▶ These guidelines were assembled using old-fashioned methods, rather than by the "new paradigm," which involves gathering all the available evidence, ranking it by study design, performing rigorous meta-analyses of trials that addressed a similar question, and deciding that there is no significant benefit to any more intensive or more expensive intervention.[1,2] It is anticipated, for example, that the Eighth Report of the Joint National Committee on Prevention, Detection, Evaluation, and Treatment of High Blood Pressure is using this new paradigm. Instead, these authors gathered expert opinion about many important questions and synthesized these opinions to form recommendations that many would argue are not very "evidence-based."

Perhaps not surprisingly, these guidelines differ only in small ways from the Seventh Report of the Joint National Committee on Prevention, Detection, Evaluation, and Treatment of High Blood Pressure.[3] Many of these authors served on that committee, and their opinions have generally changed very little. One surprising omission from this set of guidelines is the recommendation to achieve a blood pressure of less than 130/80 mm Hg for patients with established heart disease, and less than 125/75 mm Hg in those with heart failure.[4] There was little overlap between these authors and the authors of that Scientific Statement from the American Heart Association in 2007, which may be part of the reason why these specific recommendations were not accepted for older patients. It does appear, however, from the long discussion (and the 740 references) in this document that there is more concern about lowering blood pressure "too far" by this expert panel than in many others, which may be perfectly appropriate for a guideline written about elderly patients.

Although these guidelines are interesting, they differ little from national guidelines about hypertension in general published more than 8 years ago,[3] they do not use the "evidence-based approach," and they do not break much new ground.[5,6] These features make it less likely that these will be widely discussed or implemented, particularly because the Joint National Committee will likely update these guidelines soon.

W. J. Elliott, MD, PhD

References

1. NICE clinical guideline 127: Hypertension: Clinical management of primary hypertension in adults. http://www.nice.org.uk/CG127. Accessed August 24, 2011.
2. Smith SC Jr, Benjamin EJ, Bonow RO, et al. AHA/ACCF secondary prevention and risk reduction therapy for patients with coronary and other atherosclerotic vascular disease: 2011 update: a guideline from the American Heart Association and American College of Cardiology Foundation. *Circulation*. 2011;124:2458-2473.
3. Chobanian AV, Bakris GL, Black HR, et al; Joint National Committee on Prevention, Detection, Evaluation, and Treatment of High Blood Pressure; National High Blood Pressure Education Program Coordinating Committee. Seventh Report of the Joint National Committee on Prevention, Detection, Evaluation, and Treatment of High Blood Pressure. *Hypertension*. 2003;42:1206-1252.
4. Rosendorff C, Black HR, Cannon CP, et al; American Heart Association Council for High Blood Pressure Research; American Heart Association Council on Clinical Cardiology; American Heart Association Council on Epidemiology and Prevention. Treatment of hypertension in the prevention and management of ischemic heart disease: a Scientific Statement from the American Heart Association Council for High Blood Pressure Research and the Councils on Clinical Cardiology and Epidemiology and Prevention. *Circulation*. 2007;115:2761-2788.
5. Elliott WJ. What should be the blood pressure target for diabetic patients? *Curr Opin Cardiol*. 2011;26:308-313.

6. Upadhyay A, Earley A, Haynes SM, Uhlig K. Systematic review: blood pressure target in chronic kidney disease and proteinuria as an effect modifier. *Ann Intern Med.* 2011;154:541-548.

Systematic Review: Blood Pressure Target in Chronic Kidney Disease and Proteinuria as an Effect Modifier

Upadhyay A, Earley A, Haynes SM, et al (Tufts Univ School of Medicine, Boston, MA)

Ann Intern Med 154:541-548, 2011

Background.—The optimal blood pressure target in patients with chronic kidney disease (CKD) is unclear.

Purpose.—To summarize trials comparing lower versus higher blood pressure targets in adult patients with CKD and focus on proteinuria as an effect modifier.

Data Sources.—MEDLINE and the Cochrane Central Register of Controlled Trials (July 2001 through January 2011) were searched for reports from randomized, controlled trials with no language restriction.

Study Selection.—Authors screened abstracts to identify reports from trials comparing blood pressure targets in adults with CKD that had more than 50 participants per group; at least 1-year follow-up; and outcomes of death, kidney failure, cardiovascular events, change in kidney function, number of antihypertensive agents, and adverse events.

Data Extraction.—Reviewers extracted data on study design, methods, sample characteristics, interventions, comparators, outcomes, number of medications, and adverse events and rated study quality and quality of analyses for proteinuria subgroups.

Data Synthesis.—Three trials with a total of 2272 participants were included. Overall, trials did not show that a blood pressure target of less than 125/75 to 130/80 mm Hg is more beneficial than a target of less than 140/90 mm Hg. Lower-quality evidence suggests that a low target may be beneficial in subgroups with proteinuria greater than 300 to 1000 mg/d. Participants in the low target groups needed more antihypertensive medications and had a slightly higher rate of adverse events.

Limitations.—No study included patients with diabetes. Trial duration may have been too short to detect differences in clinically important outcomes, such as death and kidney failure. Ascertainment and reporting of adverse events was not uniform.

Conclusion.—Available evidence is inconclusive but does not prove that a blood pressure target of less than 130/80 mm Hg improves clinical outcomes more than a target of less than 140/90 mm Hg in adults with CKD. Whether a lower target benefits patients with proteinuria greater than 300 to 1000 mg/d requires further study.

► Recent US[1,2] and international[3] hypertension guidelines have consistently recommended a blood pressure target of less than 130/80 mm Hg for patients with chronic kidney disease (CKD), but even more recent guidelines from the United Kingdom's National Institute for Health and Clinical Excellence (NICE) may have rescinded this target,[3] based on their collection and interpretation of clinical trial evidence. The authors therefore performed their own systematic review and meta-analysis of the lower blood pressure target for patients with CKD, even before the draft NICE guidelines were made public.

They found and analyzed only 3 trials that met their stringent entry criteria: the Modification of Diet in Renal Disease (MDRD) study,[4] the African American Study of Kidney (AASK) disease and hypertension trial,[5] and the second Renoprotection In Non-diabetic (REIN-2) renal disease trial.[6] Each of these trials has its own challenges: the MDRD (median follow-up: 2.2 years) oversampled patients with polycystic kidney disease, for which blood pressure reduction is one of several modalities that has not shown benefit in many epidemiological and longitudinal studies. The AASK trial (median follow-up: 3.8 years) did achieve a nice blood pressure separation between the randomized groups but was confounded by another randomization (to amlodipine, which was stopped early, metoprolol, or ramipril) and by the selected endpoint of the change in renal function between 3 months and 3 years after randomization. The REIN-2 trial, which enrolled only 338 subjects (compared with 1094 in AASK and 890 in MDRD, and followed them for only 1.9 years of median follow-up) tested the lower blood pressure target by simply adding a dihydropyridine calcium antagonist or placebo to a low-dose ACE inhibitor, and did not prespecify a blood pressure target.

It is perhaps not surprising, therefore, that the systematic review of these trials concluded that there is no proven benefit of a lower blood pressure target for patients with CKD. Perhaps because of inherent differences in baseline characteristics, treatment regimens, and endpoints across trials, however, the authors did not report a meta-analysis or other estimate of the effectiveness of a lower blood pressure goal for preventing progression of renal disease. They simply concluded that the 3 trials "failed to show a benefit of a lower-than-usual blood pressure goal." An Appendix (available from the Annals of Internal Medicine's online site, and discussed in the article) showed a benefit of the lower blood pressure in 7 of 11 subgroup analyses that dichotomized patients according to baseline protein excretion rates. They therefore hold out the possibility that some future research study might be able to prove that a lower blood pressure goal could potentially show a benefit in patients with CKD and major proteinuria (e.g., >1000 mg/d). Some would say that there is little reason to do such a study, since the majority of subgroup analyses have already proven it and it would perhaps be unethical to deny patients this already demonstrated benefit. The lack of therapeutic equipoise in patients with proteinuria will likely sustain the blood pressure target for all patients with CKD at less than 140/90 mm Hg, rather than less than 130/80 mm Hg. This will make life easier for physicians and patients but likely lead to much higher Medicare expenditures through its new "Pay-for-Performance" plans.[7]

W. J. Elliott, MD, PhD

References

1. Chobanian AV, Bakris GL, Black HR, et al; Joint National Committee on Prevention, Detection, Evaluation, and Treatment of High Blood Pressure. National Heart, Lung, and Blood Institute; National High Blood Pressure Education Program Coordinating Committee. Seventh Report of the Joint National Committee on Prevention, Detection, Evaluation, and Treatment of High Blood Pressure. *Hypertension.* 2003;42:1206-1252.
2. Kidney Disease Outcomes Quality Initiative (K/DOQI). K/DOQI clinical practice guidelines on hypertension and antihypertensive agents in chronic kidney disease. *Am J Kidney Dis.* 2004;43:S1-S290.
3. NICE clinical guideline 127: Hypertension: Clinical management of primary hypertension in adults. http://www.nice.org.uk/CG127. Accessed August 24, 2011.
4. Sarnak MJ, Greene T, Wang X, et al. The effect of a lower target blood pressure on the progression of kidney disease: long-term follow-up of the Modification of Diet in Renal Disease study. *Ann Intern Med.* 2005;142:342-351.
5. Appel LJ, Wright JT Jr, Greene T, et al; AASK Collaborative Research Group. Intensive blood-pressure control in hypertensive chronic kidney disease. *N Engl J Med.* 2010;363:918-929.
6. Ruggenenti P, Perna A, Loriga G, et al; REIN-2 Study Group. Blood-pressure control for renoprotection in patients with non-diabetic chronic renal disease (REIN-2): multicentre, randomised controlled trial. *Lancet.* 2005;365:939-946.
7. Tanenbaum SJ. Pay for performance in Medicare: evidentiary irony and the politics of value. *J Health Polit Policy Law.* 2009;34:717-746.

Antihypertensive Treatment and Secondary Prevention of Cardiovascular Disease Events Among Persons Without Hypertension: A Meta-Analysis

Thompson AM, Hu T, Eshelbrenner CL, et al (Tulane Univ School of Public Health and Tropical Medicine, New Orleans, LA; Tulane Univ School of Medicine, New Orleans, LA; et al)

JAMA 305:913-922, 2011

Context.—Cardiovascular disease (CVD) risk increases beginning at systolic blood pressure levels of 115 mm Hg. Use of antihypertensive medications among patients with a history of CVD or diabetes and without hypertension has been debated.

Objective.—To evaluate the effect of antihypertensive treatment on secondary prevention of CVD events and all-cause mortality among persons without clinically defined hypertension.

Data Sources.—Meta-analysis with systematic search of MEDLINE (1950 to week 3 of January 2011), EMBASE, and the Cochrane Collaboration Central Register of Controlled Clinical Trials and manual examination of references in selected articles and studies.

Study Selection.—From 874 potentially relevant publications, 25 trials that fulfilled the predetermined inclusion and exclusion criteria were included in the meta-analysis.

Data Extraction.—Information on participant characteristics, trial design and duration, treatment drug, dose, control, and clinical events were extracted using a standardized protocol. Outcomes included stroke, myocardial infarction (MI), congestive heart failure (CHF), composite CVD outcomes, CVD mortality, and all-cause mortality.

Results.—Compared with controls, participants receiving antihypertensive medications had a pooled relative risk of 0.77 (95% confidence interval [CI], 0.61 to 0.98) for stroke, 0.80 (95% CI, 0.69 to 0.93) for MI, 0.71 (95% CI, 0.65 to 0.77) for CHF, 0.85 (95% CI, 0.80 to 0.90) for composite CVD events, 0.83 (95% CI, 0.69 to 0.99) for CVD mortality, and 0.87 (95% CI, 0.80 to 0.95) for all-cause mortality from random-effects models. The corresponding absolute risk reductions per 1000 persons were −7.7 (95% CI, −15.2 to −0.3) for stroke, −13.3 (95% CI, −28.4 to 1.7) for MI, −43.6 (95% CI, −65.2 to −22.0) for CHF events, −27.1 (95% CI, −40.3 to −13.9) for composite CVD events, −15.4 (95% CI, −32.5 to 1.7) for CVD mortality, and −13.7 (95% CI, −24.6 to −2.8) for all-cause mortality. Results did not differ according to trial characteristics or subgroups defined by clinical history.

Conclusions.—Among patients with clinical history of CVD but without hypertension, antihypertensive treatment was associated with decreased risk of stroke, CHF, composite CVD events, and all-cause mortality. Additional randomized trial data are necessary to assess these outcomes in patients without CVD clinical recommendations.

▶ One of the more controversial recent proposals was the development and promulgation of the "PolyPill™," which contains 3 antihypertensive and 2 other drugs, which has been hypothesized to be able to reduce cardiovascular disease by 80%.[1] The inventors of this strategy further recommended that we "stop routinely measuring blood pressure, and start routinely lowering it," as the PolyPill would be taken by all high-risk patients, not just those with hypertension.[2]

Although the authors of this meta-analysis do not specifically cite the above idea, they collected all the nonhypertensive subgroups of clinical trials involving any or all antihypertensive medications to determine if such therapy would reduce the risk of cardiovascular events compared with placebo. Some of the trials had already published the results in the nonhypertensive subgroups, but the authors had to request outcomes data from the original authors of several trials. They reported the results of random effects models because several of their endpoints showed significant inhomogeneity across the 25 selected trials. The heterogeneity of the study designs and baseline characteristics of the patients across studies was likely the major reason for these differences.

Four of their 6 selected endpoints showed a significant benefit, but myocardial infarction and cardiovascular death showed only nonsignificant trends in the beneficial direction. Because few trials reported results for subgroups categorized by baseline blood pressures, it was not possible to examine differences across blood pressures, either baseline or achieved. A meta-regression analysis plotting the difference in systolic blood pressures between randomized groups and the odds ratio for the endpoints for their 25 trials would be very helpful in solidifying their hypothesis.

Because many of their 25 trials were performed in heart failure (in which inhibitors of the renin-angiotensin-aldosterone system are highly beneficial, presumably "independent of blood pressures") or after myocardial infarction (in which beta-blockers have a salutary effect, independent of blood pressure), there is concern that antihypertensive drugs (or their combinations[3]) may not have significant benefits in nonhypertensive patients without these 2 conditions. It is likely, however, that the advocates of the PolyPill will use this meta-analysis as confirmation of their hypotheses.[2] It is unlikely, however, that antihypertensive drug therapy will be recommended for all nonhypertensive people in either the upcoming Eighth Report of the Joint National Committee on Prevention, Detection, Evaluation, and Treatment of High Blood Pressure or the US Food and Drug Administration.

W. J. Elliott, MD, PhD

References

1. Wald NJ, Law MR. A strategy to reduce cardiovascular disease by more than 80%. *BMJ*. 2003;326:1419.
2. Law MR, Morris JK, Wald NJ. Use of blood pressure lowering drugs in the prevention of cardiovascular disease: meta-analysis of 147 randomised trials in the context of expectations from prospective epidemiological studies. *BMJ*. 2009; 338:b1665.
3. Wald DS, Law M, Morris JK, Bestwick JP, Wald NJ. Combination therapy versus monotherapy in reducing blood pressure: meta-analysis on 11,000 participants from 42 trials. *Am J Med*. 2009;122:290-300.

The effects of blood pressure reduction and of different blood pressure-lowering regimens on major cardiovascular events according to baseline blood pressure: meta-analysis of randomized trials
Czernichow S, on behalf of the Blood Pressure Lowering Treatment Trialists' Collaboration (The George Inst, Sydney, Australia; et al)
J Hypertens 29:4-16, 2011

Background.—The benefits of reducing blood pressure are well established, but there remains uncertainty about whether the magnitude of the effect varies with the initial blood pressure level. The objective was to compare the risk reductions achieved by different blood pressure-lowering regimens among individuals with different baseline blood pressures.

Methods.—Thirty-two randomized controlled trials were included and seven comparisons between different types of treatments were made. For each comparison, the primary prespecified analysis included calculation of summary estimates of effect using random-effects meta-analysis for major cardiovascular events in four groups defined by baseline SBP (<140, 140–159, 160–179, and ≥180 mmHg).

Results.—There were 201 566 participants among whom 20 079 primary outcome events were observed. There was no evidence of differences in the proportionate risk reductions achieved with different blood pressure-lowering regimens across groups defined according to higher or lower levels of baseline SBP (all *P* for trend >0.17). This finding was broadly consistent for comparisons of different regimens, for DBP categories, and for commonly used blood pressure cut-points.

Conclusion.—It appears unlikely that the effectiveness of blood pressure-lowering treatments depends substantively upon starting blood pressure level. As the majority of patients in the trials contributing to these overviews had a history of hypertension or were receiving background blood pressure-lowering therapy, the findings suggest that additional blood pressure reduction in hypertensive patients meeting initial blood pressure targets will produce further benefits. More broadly, the data are supportive of the utilization of blood pressure-lowering regimens in high-risk patients with and without hypertension.

▶ It is a well-known fact that the degree of blood pressure decreases with any therapy depends primarily on the baseline measurement, as in the first law of forestry, "The bigger they come, the harder they fall." In early hypertension trials, for example, it didn't take long for major benefits to be observed among the patients with initial diastolic blood pressures between 115 and 129 mm Hg (even after 6 days of bed rest in the hospital[1] on a low-salt diet) compared with those whose initial diastolic blood pressures were 90 to 114 mm Hg.[2] Some have been concerned that it is becoming more and more difficult to show benefits of drug treatment in clinical trials, not only because so many other effective preventive therapies are taken concomitantly, but also because the baseline blood pressures are lower in recent trials compared with those conducted in the 1970s and 1980s, for example. This phenomenon is difficult, if not impossible, to address by analyzing individual trials, because randomization makes it more likely that the baseline blood pressures between groups will be quite similar. Only in meta-analyses and meta-regression analyses of large numbers of trials can one perform statistical adjustments for baseline blood pressure across many trials to see if this makes any difference.

These authors have access to a great deal of information about hypertension clinical trials, having contracted with the lead investigators of most hypertension trials done after 1992 to make their data available for their series of prospectively collected meta-analyses. They were therefore able to perform many analyses that other investigators could not. The simple message of their analyses is that the proportional reduction in cardiovascular risk across more than 20 000 endpoints did not vary significantly according to the baseline blood pressure levels. This is reassuring to many who wondered about this issue but had no way to answer the question. The authors point out that the exclusion criteria for many trials prohibited enrollment of subjects with very elevated blood pressures, perhaps diluting the beneficial effects of antihypertensive treatment. They also express concern that many trials, especially some more recent ones,[3-7] added randomized antihypertensive drug treatment to other antihypertensive treatments, which also dilutes their ability to discern the cardiovascular benefits of the randomized treatment.

The authors' conclusions are broadly consistent with similar analyses (using much smaller numbers of outcomes, which presents a potential problem with statistical power) undertaken by the PROGRESS investigators, who asserted that the benefits observed in their trial were seen at all levels of baseline blood pressure.[8]

W. J. Elliott, MD, PhD

References

1. Effects of treatment on morbidity in hypertension. Results in patients with diastolic blood pressures averaging 115 through 129 mm Hg. *JAMA*. 1967;202:1028-1034.
2. Effects of treatment on morbidity in hypertension. II. Results in patients with diastolic blood pressure averaging 90 through 114 mm Hg. *JAMA*. 1970;213:1143-1152.
3. Yusuf S, Sleight P, Pogue J, Bosch J, Davies R, Dagenais G. Effects of an angiotensin-converting-enzyme inhibitor, ramipril, on cardiovascular events in high-risk patients. The Heart Outcomes Prevention Evaluation Study Investigators. *N Engl J Med*. 2000;342:145-153.
4. Patel A, MacMahon S, Chalmers J, et al; ADVANCE Collaborative Group. Effects of a fixed combination of perindopril and indapamide on macrovascular and microvascular outcomes in patients with type 2 diabetes mellitus (the ADVANCE trial): a randomised controlled trial. *Lancet*. 2007;370:829-840.
5. Yusuf S, Teo KK, Pogue J, et al; ONTARGET Investigators. Telmisartan, ramipril, or both in patients at high risk for vascular events. *N Engl J Med*. 2008;358: 1547-1559.
6. Yusuf S, Teo K, Anderson C, et al; Telmisartan Randomised AssessmeNt Study in ACE iNtolerant subjects with cardiovascular Disease (TRANSCEND) Investigators. Effects of the angiotensin-receptor blocker telmisartan on cardiovascular events in high-risk patients intolerant to angiotensin-converting enzyme inhibitors: a randomised controlled trial. *Lancet*. 2008;371:1174-1183.
7. Yusuf S, Diener HC, Sacco RL, et al; PRoFESS Study Group. Telmisartan to prevent recurrent stroke and cardiovascular events. *N Engl J Med*. 2008;359: 1225-1237.
8. PROGRESS Collaborative Group. Randomised trial of a perindopril-based blood-pressure-lowering regimen among 6,105 individuals with previous stroke or transient ischaemic attack. *Lancet*. 2001;358:1033-1041.

National, regional, and global trends in systolic blood pressure since 1980: systematic analysis of health examination surveys and epidemiological studies with 786 country-years and 5·4 million participants
Danaei G, on behalf of the Global Burden of Metabolic Risk Factors of Chronic Diseases Collaborating Group (Blood Pressure) (Harvard School of Public Health, Boston, MA; et al)
Lancet 377:568-577, 2011

Background.—Data for trends in blood pressure are needed to understand the effects of its dietary, lifestyle, and pharmacological determinants; set intervention priorities; and evaluate national programmes. However, few worldwide analyses of trends in blood pressure have been done. We estimated worldwide trends in population mean systolic blood pressure (SBP).

Methods.—We estimated trends and their uncertainties in mean SBP for adults 25 years and older in 199 countries and territories. We obtained data from published and unpublished health examination surveys and epidemiological studies (786 country-years and 5·4 million participants). For each sex, we used a Bayesian hierarchical model to estimate mean SBP by age, country, and year, accounting for whether a study was nationally representative.

Findings.—In 2008, age-standardised mean SBP worldwide was 128·1 mm Hg (95% uncertainty interval 126·7—129·4) in men and 124·4 mm Hg (123·0—125·9) in women. Globally, between 1980 and 2008, SBP decreased by 0·8 mm Hg per decade (−0·4 to 2·2, posterior probability of being a true decline=0·90) in men and 1·0 mm Hg per decade (−0·3 to 2·3, posterior probability=0·93) in women. Female SBP decreased by 3·5 mm Hg or more per decade in western Europe and Australasia (posterior probabilities ≥0·999). Male SBP fell most in high-income North America, by 2·8 mm Hg per decade (1·3—4·5, posterior probability >0·999), followed by Australasia and western Europe where it decreased by more than 2·0 mm Hg per decade (posterior probabilities >0·98). SBP rose in Oceania, east Africa, and south and southeast Asia for both sexes, and in west Africa for women, with the increases ranging 0·8—1·6 mm Hg per decade in men (posterior probabilities 0·72—0·91) and 1·0—2·7 mm Hg per decade for women (posterior probabilities 0·75—0·98). Female SBP was highest in some east and west African countries, with means of 135 mm Hg or greater. Male SBP was highest in Baltic and east and west African countries, where mean SBP reached 138 mm Hg or more. Men and women in western Europe had the highest SBP in high-income regions.

Interpretation.—On average, global population SBP decreased slightly since 1980, but trends varied significantly across regions and countries. SBP is currently highest in low-income and middle-income countries. Effective population-based and personal interventions should be targeted towards low-income and middle-income countries.

▶ This is 1 of 3 back-to-back-to-back papers in *The Lancet* from the Global Burden of Disease Group about the state of cardiovascular risk factors (eg, body-mass index and serum cholesterol) around the world.[1,2] The researchers gathered all the published and unpublished data they could find from epidemiological studies and cross-sectional surveys, segregating the countries by income status and the populations by gender. Because there were major uncertainties about these data, particularly in low-income countries, they ended up estimating systolic blood pressures for many low-income countries using a generalized linear model and then used a Bayesian hierarchical model to estimate mean systolic blood pressure for each gender-age, country, and year. This methodology has the virtue of not being dependent on precise estimates in every segment modeled but often results in estimates ("posterior probabilities") that are less precise than might be obtained using other, more traditional methods.

Despite the large number of actual and imputed data, their major conclusions are not surprising. High-income countries (especially those in North America, Australasia, and Western Europe) saw a fall in mean systolic blood pressure (after adjustment for age) in both men and women since 1980, but low-income countries saw an increase (especially in East and West Africa). As with many previous summaries of high-quality country-specific data,[3] men and women from Western Europe had the highest systolic blood pressures among high-income countries.

The implications of these findings for the global burden of cardiovascular disease are consistent with many other publications from this very productive group[4,5] and others.[6,7] In the next few years to decades, it is likely that cardiovascular disease will overtake infectious diseases as the foremost cause of death and disability worldwide, even in low-income countries. The fact that people living in these countries currently have the highest blood pressures makes them a suitable target primarily for lifestyle modifications (especially weight control), because even what are perceived as "inexpensive" antihypertensive drug therapies in high-income countries are beyond the economic means of many people in low-income countries.[8,9] This is also part of the reason for the development of 1 or more forms of "the Polypill" which presumably can be manufactured and distributed at very low cost.[10]

W. J. Elliott, MD, PhD

References

1. Finucane MM, Stevens GA, Cowan MJ, et al; Global Burden of Metabolic Risk Factors of Chronic Diseases Collaborating Group (Body Mass Index). National, regional, and global trends in body-mass index since 1980: systematic analysis of health examination surveys and epidemiological studies with 960 country-years and 9·1 million participants. *Lancet.* 2011;377:557-567.
2. Farzadfar F, Finucane MM, Danaei G, et al; Global Burden of Cardiovascular Risk Factors of Chronic Disease Collaborating Group (Cholesterol). National, regional, and global trends in total serum cholesterol since 1980: systematic analysis of health examination surveys and epidemiological studies with 321 country-years and 3.0 million participants. *Lancet.* 2011;377:578-588.
3. Wolf-Maier K, Cooper RS, Kramer H, et al. Hypertension treatment and control in five European countries, Canada, and the United States. *Hypertension.* 2004; 43:10-17.
4. Murray CJ, Lopez AD. Mortality by cause for eight regions of the world: Global Burden of Disease Study. *Lancet.* 1997;349:1269-1276.
5. Ezzati M, Lopez AD, Rodgers A, Vander Hoorn S, Murray CJ; Comparative Risk Assessment Collaborating Group. Selected major risk factors and global and regional burden of disease. *Lancet.* 2002;360:1347-1360.
6. Kearney PM, Whelton M, Reynolds K, Muntner P, Whelton PK, He J. Global burden of hypertension: analysis of worldwide data. *Lancet.* 2005;365:217-223.
7. Lawes CM, Vander Hoorn S, Rodgers A; International Society of Hypertension. Global burden of blood-pressure-related disease, 2001. *Lancet.* 2008;371: 1513-1518.
8. Alwan A, Maclean DR, Riley LM, et al. Monitoring and surveillance of chronic non-communicable diseases: progress and capacity in high-burden countries. *Lancet.* 2010;376:1861-1868.
9. Anand SS, Yusuf S. Stemming the global tsunami of cardiovascular disease [Editorial]. *Lancet.* 2011;377:529-532.
10. Gaziano TA, Opie LH, Weinstein MC. Cardiovascular disease prevention with a multidrug regimen in the developing world: a cost-effectiveness analysis. *Lancet.* 2006;368:679-686.

Effects of telmisartan, irbesartan, valsartan, candesartan, and losartan on cancers in 15 trials enrolling 138 769 individuals

The ARB Trialists Collaboration (McMaster Univ, Hamilton, Canada; Univ of Gothenburg, Sweden; et al)
J Hypertens 29:623-635, 2011

Background.—Angiotensin-converting enzyme inhibitors (ACEi) and angiotensin II receptor blockers (ARBs) reduce cardiovascular disease (CVD) events, but a recent meta-analysis of selected studies suggested that ARBs may increase cancer risks.

Objective.—Candesartan, irbesartan, telmisartan, valsartan, and losartan were assessed for incident cancers in 15 large parallel long-term multicenter double-blind clinical trials of these agents involving 138 769 participants.

Patients and Methods.—Individuals at high CVD risk were randomized to telmisartan (three trials, $n = 51\,878$), irbesartan (three trials, $n = 14\,859$), valsartan (four trials, $n = 44\,264$), candesartan (four trials, $n = 18\,566$), and losartan (one trial, $n = 9193$) and followed for 23–60 months. Incident cancer cases were compared in patients randomized to ARBs versus controls. In five trials ($n = 42\,403$), the ARBs were compared to ACEi and in 11 trials ($n = 63\,313$) to controls without ACEi. In addition, in seven trials ($n = 47\,020$), the effect of ARBs with ACEi was compared to ACEi alone and in two trials ARBs with ACEi versus ARB alone ($n = 25\,712$).

Results.—Overall, there was no excess of cancer incidence with ARB therapy compared to controls in the 15 trials [4549 (6.16%) cases of 73 808 allocated to ARB versus 3856 (6.31%) of 61 106 assigned to non-ARB controls; odds ratio (OR) 1.00, 95% confidence interval (CI) 0.95–1.04] overall or when individual ARBs were examined. ORs comparing combination therapy with ARB along with ACEi versus ACEi was 1.01 (95% CI 0.94–1.10), combination versus ARB alone 1.02 (95% CI 0.91–1.13), ARB alone versus ACEi alone 1.06 (95% CI 0.97–1.16) and ARB versus placebo/control without ACEi 0.97 (95% CI 0.91–1.04). There was no excess of lung, prostate or breast cancer, or overall cancer deaths associated with ARB treatment.

Conclusion.—There was no significant increase in the overall or site-specific cancer risk from ARBs compared to controls.

▶ This article was likely generated in response to the very provocative and controversial meta-analysis published last year that concluded that angiotensin receptor blockers (ARBs) significantly increase the risk of any and all cancers by an unknown mechanism.[1] Although this was disputed nearly immediately by investigators whose trials with an ARB were not included in the report,[2] and a more sophisticated set of meta-analyses did not confirm the significantly increased risk of cancer (but left open the possibility that the combination of an angiotensin-converting enzyme (ACE) inhibitor and ARB might still be associated with more cancers),[3] these authors obviously felt compelled to pool their data and have the definitive, patient-level meta-analysis performed by an institution separate from the sponsors of the trials (the Population Health Research Institute of McMaster University). Contrarians will point out that at least 4 of the senior members of this Institute (Professors Teo, Gao, Yusuf, and Connolly) served in high-ranking positions on the investigative teams of several of these trials, which were supported by pharmaceutical companies and therefore might not have been as "independent" of conflicts of interest as some might prefer.

These authors not only showed that the odds ratio for incident cancer in ARB trials was nearly exactly 1.00 (as would be expected with no association), but also that lung cancer (which was reportedly elevated in the 5 trials included in the initial meta-analysis[1]) was not significantly increased, nor was any specific site more commonly affected by cancer. These authors attribute the significant result found in the original meta-analysis to be likely due to chance, and an inverse bias that results from publishing data that might be worrisome in the interest of full disclosure. Their data are consistent with those of 2 previous meta-analyses showing no significant association of antihypertensive drugs and subsequent cancers.[3,4] Yet they admit that their comprehensive meta-analysis has some limitations, especially because of the limited follow-up duration in most of the included trials. The increased risk of cancer in the ACE inhibitor + ARB arm of the ONgoing Telmisartan Alone and in combination with Ramipril Global Endpoint Trial (ONTARGET)[5] was nearly exactly opposite to data from the VALsartan In Acute myocardial iNfarcTion (VALIANT) trial,[6] suggesting that both results were likely due to chance.

These results, as well as others,[3,4] should reassure physicians, patients, and investigative reporters specializing in health care that ARBs are unlikely to be associated with incident cancer. Unfortunately, these data received less than 1% of the exposure in the lay press than the original, now-refuted meta-analysis. It seems difficult to generate good news about health care today.

W. J. Elliott, MD, PhD

References

1. Sipahi I, Debanne SM, Rowland DY, Simon DI, Fang JC. Angiotensin-receptor blockade and risk of cancer: meta-analysis of randomised controlled trials. *Lancet Oncol.* 2010;11:627-636.
2. Goldstein MR, Mascitelli L, Pezzetta F, et al. Angiotensin-receptor blockade, cancer, and concerns. *Lancet Oncol.* 2010;11:817-818.
3. Bangalore S, Kumar S, Kjeldsen SE, et al. Antihypertensive drugs and risk of cancer: network meta-analyses and trial sequential analyses of 324,168 participants from randomized trials. *Lancet Oncol.* 2010;12:65-82.
4. Coleman CI, Baker WL, Kluger J, White CM. Antihypertensive medication and their impact on cancer incidence: a mixed treatment comparison meta-analysis of randomized controlled trials. *J Hypertens.* 2008;26:622-629.
5. ONTARGET Investigators, Yusuf S, Teo KK, Pogue J, et al. Telmisartan, ramipril, or both in patients at high risk for vascular events. *N Engl J Med.* 2008;358: 1547-1559.
6. Pfeffer MA, McMurray JJ, Velazquez EJ, et al; VALIANT Investigators. Valsartan, captopril, or both in myocardial infarction complicated by heart failure, left ventricular dysfunction, or both. *N Engl J Med.* 2003;349:1893-1906.

Angiotensin receptor blockers and risk of myocardial infarction: meta-analyses and trial sequential analyses of 147 020 patients from randomised trials
Bangalore S, Kumar S, Wetterslev J, et al (New York Univ School of Medicine, NY; Univ of Nebraska, Omaha; et al)
BMJ 342:d2234, 2011

Objectives.—To evaluate the cardiovascular outcomes and other outcomes associated with angiotensin receptor blockers.

Design.—Systematic review of randomised controlled trials with meta-analysis and trial sequential analysis (TSA).

Data Sources and Study Selection.—Pubmed, Embase, and CENTRAL searches for randomised clinical trials, until August 2010, of angiotensin receptor blockers compared with controls (placebo/active treatment) that enrolled at least 100 participants and had a follow-up of at least one year.

Data Extraction.—Myocardial infarction, death, cardiovascular death, angina pectoris, stroke, heart failure, and new onset diabetes.

Results.—37 randomised clinical trials included 147 020 participants and had a total follow-up of 485 166 patient years. When compared with controls (placebo/active treatment), placebo, or active treatment, angiotensin receptor blockers were not associated with an increase in the risk of myocardial infarction (relative risk 0.99, 95% confidence interval 0.92 to 1.07), death, cardiovascular death, or angina pectoris. Compared with controls, angiotensin receptor blockers were associated with a reduction in the risk of stroke (0.90, 0.84 to 0.98), heart failure (0.87, 0.81 to 0.93), and new onset diabetes (0.85, 0.78 to 0.93), with similar results when compared with placebo or with active treatment. Based on trial sequential analysis, there is no evidence even for an average 5.0-7.5% (upper confidence interval 5-11%) relative increase in myocardial infarction (absolute increase of 0.3%), death, or cardiovascular death with firm evidence for relative risk reduction of stroke (at least 1%, average 10%) (compared with placebo only), heart failure (at least 5%, average 10%), and new onset diabetes (at least 4%, average 10%) with angiotensin receptor blockers compared with controls.

Conclusions.—This large and comprehensive analysis produced firm evidence to refute the hypothesis that angiotensin receptor blockers increase the risk of myocardial infarction (ruling out even a 0.3% absolute increase). Compared with controls, angiotensin receptor blockers reduce the risk of stroke, heart failure, and new onset diabetes.

▶ The question of whether angiotensin receptor blockers (ARBs) prevent coronary heart disease as well as other antihypertensive therapies has been quite controversial. The Valsartan Antihypertensive Long-term Use Evaluation (VALUE) trial found amlodipine to be significantly more effective than valsartan in preventing myocardial infarction (a prespecified secondary endpoint), but this did not account for a rather large difference between randomized groups in systolic blood pressure.[1] A provocative Letter to the Editor of the *British Medical*

Journal by Verma and Strauss performed a selective review of ARB trials and concluded that they "may increase myocardial infarction—and patients may need to be told," which generated many letters of rebuttal.[2] A preliminary report of network meta-analyses also concluded that the difference in coronary heart disease risk between ARBs and placebo in trials reported through 2008 was not significant, perhaps because the numbers of afflicted patients was smaller than many other comparisons.[3]

These authors collected all the data from outcome trials involving ARBs through 2010 and performed random effects meta-analyses of mortality, cardiovascular mortality, myocardial infarction, angina pectoris, stroke, heart failure, and new-onset diabetes, comparing ARBs with any and all other treatment strategies ("control"), which were stratified as placebo/no treatment or other antihypertensive agent comparator. Their major conclusions were that ARBs were not significantly worse than control in coronary heart disease, angina pectoris, death, or cardiovascular death and were significantly better than control for stroke, heart failure, and new-onset diabetes. While this is reassuring news for many physicians and patients, fixed effects meta-analyses of combined data (ie, both placebo and active comparator) showed near significant inhomogeneity for myocardial infarction ($P = .055$) and cardiovascular mortality ($P = .09$) and highly significant inhomogeneity for angina pectoris ($P < .001$), stroke ($P < .007$), heart failure ($P < .001$), and new-onset diabetes ($P < .003$). There is little doubt that some of this is due to mixing of the effects of placebo and several active treatments, which are likely to have different effects on the chosen endpoint (eg, diuretics or beta-blockers increasing the risk of new-onset diabetes, whereas ACE-inhibitors have no significant difference from ARBs on this endpoint).[4]

Although these data are helpful in understanding that ARBs are unlikely to significantly increase the risk of myocardial infarction and other manifestations of coronary heart disease in clinical trials, there is still doubt that they may not decrease these risks as well as other antihypertensive agents, particularly if they don't lower blood pressure as much (eg, as in VALUE).[1] This is likely to be a controversy that will continue for many years, since statistical techniques that allow adjustment of summary odds ratios from Bayesian or network meta-analyses for different levels of achieved blood pressures are not available.

W. J. Elliott, MD, PhD

References

1. Julius S, Kjeldsen SE, Weber M, et al; VALUE trial group. Outcomes in hypertensive patients at high cardiovascular risk treated with regimens based on valsartan or amlodipine: the VALUE randomised trial. *Lancet.* 2004;363:2022-2031.
2. Verma S, Strauss M. Angiotensin receptor blockers and myocardial infarction [Letter]. *BMJ.* 2004;329:1248-1249.
3. Elliott WJ, Basu S, Meyer PM. Initial drugs for coronary heart disease prevention in hypertensive patients: network and Bayesian meta-analyses of clinical trial data [abstract]. *J Clin Hypertens (Greenwich).* 2009;11:A7.
4. Elliott WJ, Meyer PM. Incident diabetes in clinical trials of antihypertensive drugs: a network meta-analysis. *Lancet.* 2007;369:201-207.

Antihypertensive drugs and risk of cancer: network meta-analyses and trial sequential analyses of 324 168 participants from randomised trials

Bangalore S, Kumar S, Kjeldsen SE, et al (New York Univ School of Medicine; Univ of Nebraska Med Ctr, Omaha; Univ of Oslo, Norway; et al)

Lancet Oncol 12:65-82, 2011

Background.—The risk of cancer from antihypertensive drugs has been much debated, with a recent analysis showing increased risk with angiotensin-receptor blockers (ARBs). We assessed the association between antihypertensive drugs and cancer risk in a comprehensive analysis of data from randomised clinical trials.

Methods.—We undertook traditional direct comparison meta-analyses, multiple comparisons (network) meta-analyses, and trial sequential analyses. We searched PubMed, Embase, and the Cochrane Central Register of Controlled Trials from 1950, to August, 2010, for randomised clinical trials of antihypertensive therapy (ARBs, angiotensin-converting enzyme inhibitors [ACEi], β blockers, calcium-channel blockers [CCBs], or diuretics) with follow-up of at least 1 year. Our primary outcomes were cancer and cancer-related deaths.

Findings.—We identified 70 randomised controlled trials (148 comparator groups) with 324 168 participants. In the network meta-analysis (fixed-effect model), we recorded no difference in the risk of cancer with ARBs (proportion with cancer 2·04%; odds ratio 1·01, 95% CI 0·93−1·09), ACEi (2·03%; 1·00, 0·92−1·09), β blockers (1·97%; 0·97, 0·88−1·07), CCBs (2·11%; 1·05, 0·96−1·13), diuretics (2·02%; 1·00, 0·90−1·11), or other controls (1·95%, 0·97, 0·74−1·24) versus placebo (2·02%). There was an increased risk with the combination of ACEi plus ARBs (2·30%, 1·14, 1·02−1·28); however, this risk was not apparent in the random-effects model (odds ratio 1·15, 95% CI 0·92−1·38). No differences were detected in cancer-related mortality for ARBs (death rate 1·33%; odds ratio 1·00, 95% CI 0·87−1·15), ACEi (1·25%; 0·95, 0·81−1·10), β blockers (1·23%; 0·93, 0·80−1·08), CCBs (1·27%; 0·96, 0·82−1·11), diuretics (1·30%; 0·98, 0·84−1·13), other controls (1·43%; 1·08, 0·78−1·46), and ACEi plus ARBs (1·45%; 1·10, 0·90−1·32). In direct comparison meta-analyses, similar results were recorded for all antihypertensive classes, except for an increased risk of cancer with ACEi and ARB combination (OR 1·14, 95% CI 1·04−1·24; p=0·004) and with CCBs (1·06, 1·01−1·12; p=0·02). However, we noted no significant differences in cancer-related mortality. On the basis of trial sequential analysis, our results suggest no evidence of even a 5−10% relative risk (RR) increase of cancer and cancer-related deaths with any individual class of antihypertensive drugs studied. However, for the ACEi and ARB combination, the cumulative Z curve crossed the trial sequential monitoring boundary, suggesting firm evidence for at least a 10% RR increase in cancer risk.

Interpretation.—Our analysis refutes a 5·0−10·0% relative increase in the risk of cancer or cancer-related death with the use of ARBs, ACEi, β blockers, diuretics, and CCBs. However, increased risk of cancer with the combination of ACEi and ARBs cannot be ruled out.

▶ The literature contains many publications suggesting that antihypertensive agents increase the risk of cancer; some of these hypotheses implicate specific drug classes and specific cancers (eg, reserpine and breast cancer[1]), sometimes with a plausible pathophysiological connection (eg, diuretics and renal cell cancer).[2] Other mechanisms, such as inhibition of apoptosis, have been proposed for other agents (eg, calcium antagonists, which have been postulated to cause any and all kinds of cancer,[3] or perhaps mainly breast cancer[4]). Only angiotensin converting enzyme inhibitors have been suggested to protect against cancer in 1 single-center, retrospective study.[5] In a controversial, recent meta-analysis, angiotensin receptor blockers (ARBs) were found to be associated with a significant increase in all-cause cancer,[6] but when data that were not available to these authors were garnered from another trial, the meta-analytic increase in risk was reduced to nearly nothing.[7]

These authors therefore collected all the data from outcome trials involving the major current classes of antihypertensive drugs through 2010 and performed several types of meta-analyses regarding the outcomes of cancer and cancer mortality. Their "network meta-analyses" were actually performed using Bayesian techniques (via WINBUGS, which does not provide a measure of "incoherence," as does the original network methodology technique advanced by Lumley[8]). Their major conclusions were that ARBs were not significantly different from other antihypertensive drugs, although the numbers of afflicted patients for each drug class were small. Indeed, the fact that no "signal" was seen for any single class of antihypertensive drugs makes one wonder about the statistical power of these analyses, including the cancer mortality comparisons (which have even lower statistical power). The counterargument to this is the finding that the combination of an ACE inhibitor and an ARB was associated with a significantly higher risk of cancer (but not cancer mortality); the significant difference was largely (∼93%) driven by 1 trial, the ONgoing Telmisartan And Ramipril Global outcomes Evaluation Trial (ONTARGET),[9] which was also seen in trial-sequential analyses. The authors suggest that the ONTARGET results were not biologically plausible, because the short duration of the study is insufficient time for the complex processes that generate clinical cancers. It would also be helpful to know some details about the statistical power of the authors' calculations and how their results differ if other methodologies (eg, the network meta-analyses of Lumley[8]) were to be used.

These data refute the allegation that ARBs significantly increase the risk of cancer but leave open the possibility that their combination with ACE inhibitors may do so. There seem to be, however, other reasons to avoid using this combination in hypertensive patients, although the benefits in heart failure due to diminished left ventricular function have been demonstrated.[10,11] It should be noted that these data also speak against the prior allegations by the last and senior author of this investigative group that diuretics increase the risk of cancer,[12] although renal cell carcinoma was not specifically analyzed. On June 2, 2011, the US Food and Drug Administration announced that it had also concluded, based on a trial-level meta-analysis of 31 trials that included 155 816 patients, that there was no clear and substantial evidence that ARBs increase the risk of cancer.[13]

W. J. Elliott, MD, PhD

References

1. The Boston Collaborative Drug Surveillance Project. Reserpine and breast cancer. *Lancet.* 1974;304:669-671.
2. Heath CW Jr, Lally CA, Calle EE, McLaughlin JK, Thum MJ. Hypertension, diuretics, and antihypertensive medication as possible risk factors for renal cell cancer. *Am J Epidemiol.* 1997;145:607-613.
3. Pahor M, Guralnik JM, Ferrucci L, et al. Calcium-channel blockade and incidence of cancer in aged populations. *Lancet.* 1996;348:493-497.
4. Fitzpatrick AL, Daling JR, Furberg CD, Kronmal RA, Weissfeld JL. Use of calcium channel blockers and breast carcinoma risk in postmenopausal women. *Cancer.* 1997;80:1438-1447.
5. Lever AF, Hole DJ, Gillis CR, et al. Do inhibitors of angiotensin-I-converting enzyme protect against risk of cancer? *Lancet.* 1998;352:179-184.
6. Sipahi I, Debanne SM, Rowland DY, Simon DI, Fang JC. Angiotensin-receptor blockade and risk of cancer: meta-analysis of randomised controlled trials. *Lancet Oncol.* 2010;11:627-636.
7. Julius S, Kjeldsen SE, Weber MA. Angiotensin-receptor blockade, cancer, and concerns. *Lancet Oncol.* 2010;11:821-822.
8. Lumley T. Network meta-analysis for indirect treatment comparisons. *Stat Med.* 2002;21:2313-2324.
9. Yusuf S, Teo KK, Pogue J, et al; for the ONTARGET Investigators. Telmisartan, ramipril, or both in patients at high risk for vascular events. *Lancet.* 2008;358:1547-1559.
10. Cohn JN, Tognoni G; for the Val-HeFT Investigators. A randomized trial of the angiotensin-receptor blocker valsartan in chronic heart failure. *N Engl J Med.* 2001;345:1667-1675.
11. McMurray JJV, Ostergren J, Swedberg K, et al; CHARM Investigators and Committees. Effects of candesartan in patients with chronic heart failure and reduced left-ventricular systolic function taking angiotensin-converting-enzyme inhibitors: the CHARM-Added trial. *Lancet.* 2003;362:767-771.
12. Grossman E, Messerli FH, Goldbourt U. Does diuretic therapy increase the risk of renal cell carcinoma? *Am J Cardiol.* 1999;83:1090-1093.
13. FDA Drug Safety Communication: No increase in risk of cancer with certain blood pressure drugs—Angiotensin receptor blockers (ARBs). http://www.fda.gov/Drugs/DrugSafety/ucm257516.htm. Accessed 03 June 2011.

The cost-effectiveness of interventions designed to reduce sodium intake
Wang G, Labarthe D (Ctrs for Disease Control and Prevention (CDC), Atlanta, GA)
J Hypertens 29:1693-1699, 2011

Background.—To guide resource allocation, policy makers need evidence of the cost-effectiveness of interventions. We summarized such evidence on selected interventions to reduce sodium intake that would be intended as population wide approaches to control hypertension.

Methods.—We conducted a comprehensive literature review of journal articles published in English from January 2000 to May 2010 by searching the databases of *PubMed, EMBASE, MEDLINE,* and *EconLit.* We selected original research articles for abstracting the evidence on cost-effectiveness of interventions, cost savings and the costs of intervention implementation.

Results.—From the 53 references obtained from the literature search, we identified 11 original research articles that provided relevant information on the medical cost savings, implementation costs, or cost-effectiveness of interventions to reduce sodium intake. The interventions were low in cost, e.g., one study showed that the cost ranged from US $0.03 to 0.32 per person per year for awareness campaign through mass media outlets and government regulations on food products in low and middle-income countries. Population-wide interventions for salt reduction are very cost-effective such as only ARS$ 151 per disability-adjusted life-year (DALY) saved in Argentina, whereas statin therapy to lower high cholesterol was $ 70 994 per DALY saved. Another study showed that sodium reduction could save US$ 18 billion in annual US healthcare costs by reducing sodium intake to 2300 mg/day.

Conclusion.—The literature provided economic evidence that was in favor of population-wide interventions designed to reduce sodium intake. Reducing the intake of sodium through such initiatives might be one of the best buys in public health. However, the small body of literature and hypothetical scenarios in most studies might limit policy implications of the findings.

▶ In 2009, the US Congress charged the Centers for Disease Control and Prevention with the task of devising a plan to reduce dietary sodium consumption in the United States,[1] but exactly how that might be accomplished is unclear. Two major articles were published last year that examined the cost-effectiveness of dietary sodium restriction in the United States, and both reported very impressive economic benefits, primarily as health care costs avoided due to reductions in hospitalization for cardiovascular diseases.[2,3] Despite the current US federal budget crisis, implementation of a "salt tax" was projected to be less effective and provide a lower savings rate than a voluntary program, spearheaded by food manufacturers.[3]

Although these investigators conclude with the usual disclaimer that this article does not reflect the official viewpoints of the Centers for Disease Control and Prevention or of the US federal government, they provide a nice overview of economic analyses of dietary sodium restriction in both developed and developing nations. All 11 selected articles conclude that a nationwide, population-based program of dietary sodium restriction involves low cost, provides major reductions in cardiovascular disease events, and is overall quite cost-saving. These conclusions should assuage at least some critics of the proposed new programs in the United States who think that the overall results would be different in this country, compared with the successes already seen in the United Kingdom and Finland, for example.

The authors conclude with several politically correct limitations of their review that will provide useful rebuttal for those who believe that such a dietary sodium reduction program in the United States is unnecessary and an infringement on American citizens' personal freedoms. They note that no specific intervention strategies have been demonstrated in the United States. All US cost data from the studies are imprecise, and the costs of implementing any intervention are unknown. Even in other parts of the world, data on health and medical costs have been largely extrapolated and therefore are imprecise. They further point out that "publication bias" may have limited their review, so that they could find only positive studies; they searched only 4 citation databases (and excluded the "gray literature"). The studies they included did not analyze health care systems (aside from the dichotomy of developed and developing nations), did not have firm data about the costs of implementing any specific strategy, and were all simulation studies, rather than those based on proper, prospective, randomized clinical trials. These concerns are likely to limit the enthusiasm of elected officials to implement unproven methods that theoretically would improve the public health and greatly reduce health care costs.

W. J. Elliott, MD, PhD

References

1. Frieden TR, Briss PA. We can reduce dietary sodium, save money and save lives [Editorial]. *Ann Intern Med.* 2010;152:526-527.
2. Bibbins-Domingo K, Chertow GM, Coxson PG, et al. Projected effect of dietary salt reductions on future cardiovascular disease. *N Engl J Med.* 2010;363:590-599.
3. Smith-Spangler CM, Juusola JL, Enns EA, Owens DK, Garber AM. Population strategies to decrease sodium intake and the burden of cardiovascular disease: a cost-effectiveness analysis. *Ann Intern Med.* 2010;152:481-487.

Antihypertensive Efficacy of Hydrochlorothiazide as Evaluated by Ambulatory Blood Pressure Monitoring: A Meta-Analysis of Randomized Trials
Messerli FH, Makani H, Benjo A, et al (Columbia Univ College of Physicians and Surgeons, NY)
J Am Coll Cardiol 57:590-600, 2011

Objectives.—The purpose of this study was to evaluate the antihypertensive efficacy of hydrochlorothiazide (HCTZ) by ambulatory blood pressure (BP) monitoring.

Background.—HCTZ is the most commonly prescribed antihypertensive drug worldwide. More than 97% of all HCTZ prescriptions are for 12.5 to 25 mg per day. The antihypertensive efficacy of HCTZ by ambulatory BP monitoring is less well defined.

Methods.—A systematic review was made using Medline, Cochrane, and Embase for all the randomized trials that assessed 24-h BP with HCTZ in comparison with other antihypertensive drugs.

Results.—Fourteen studies of HCTZ dose 12.5 to 25 mg with 1,234 patients and 5 studies of HCTZ dose 50 mg with 229 patients fulfilled the inclusion criteria. The decrease in 24-h BP with HCTZ dose 12.5 to 25 mg was systolic 6.5 mm Hg (95% confidence interval: 5.3 to 7.7

mm Hg) and diastolic 4.5 mm Hg (95% confidence interval: 3.1 to 6.0 mm Hg) and was inferior compared with the 24-h BP reduction of angiotensin-converting enzyme inhibitors (mean BP reduction 12.9/7.7 mm Hg; p < 0.003), angiotensin-receptor blockers (mean BP reduction 13.3/7.8 mm Hg; p < 0.001), beta-blockers (mean BP reduction 11.2/8.5 mm Hg; p < 0.00001), and calcium antagonists (mean BP reduction 11.0/8.1 mm Hg; p < 0.05). There was no significant difference in both systolic (p = 0.30) and diastolic (p = 0.15) 24-h BP reduction between HCTZ 12.5 mg (5.7/3.3 mm Hg) and HCTZ 25 mg (7.6/5.4 mm Hg). However, with HCTZ 50 mg, the reduction in 24-h BP was significantly higher (12.0/5.4 mm Hg) and was comparable to that of other agents.

Conclusions.—The antihypertensive efficacy of HCTZ in its daily dose of 12.5 to 25 mg as measured in head-to-head studies by ambulatory BP measurement is consistently inferior to that of all other drug classes. Because outcome data at this dose are lacking, HCTZ is an inappropriate first-line drug for the treatment of hypertension.

▶ According to the authors, in 2008, hydrochlorothiazide (HCTZ) was the most commonly prescribed antihypertensive drug in the United States, with about 134 million prescriptions, far ahead of second-place atenolol at 44 million. Approximately a third of the prescriptions were for monotherapy and about two-thirds as combination therapy (typically with an angiotensin converting enzyme inhibitor, angiotensin receptor blocker, a potassium-sparing diuretic, or a beta-blocker). By 2010, an estimated 104 million prescriptions containing HCTZ were dispensed, 55% of which were as single-pill combinations,[1,2] typically for doses in the 12.5 to 25 mg/day range. Unfortunately, the few successful clinical trials using HCTZ as initial antihypertensive therapy all used higher doses (typically 25—200 mg/day),[3-6] and no trials have used these high doses since the Multiple Risk Factor Intervention Trial determined that initial chlorthalidone should be preferred over HCTZ for hypertension,[7,8] which forever removed HCTZ from consideration as the initial diuretic for National Institutes of Health—sponsored trials.

These authors therefore collected all the published and unpublished ambulatory blood pressure monitoring data comparing the currently favored "low doses" of HCTZ with other antihypertensive drugs. Although the data speak for themselves, the first author has been widely quoted in news reports, chastising the pharmaceutical industry and physicians for nearly always selecting HCTZ as the thiazide diuretic to combine with other antihypertensive agents, or to prescribe, rather than chlorthalidone or indapamide. The conclusions of this article regarding the relative inferiority of HCTZ are reasonably well supported by other meta-analyses that used blood pressure changes as the primary endpoint,[9,10] but not so clearly supported by other meta-analyses that use cardiovascular events as the relevant endpoints.[11,12] The recent British National Institute for Health and Clinical Excellence guidelines also expressed a preference for chlorthalidone or indapamide, over HCTZ or bendroflumethiazide.[13]

Taken together, these data suggest that low-dose HCTZ should be increased for patients with resistant hypertension because the 50 mg/day dose is at least not statistically significantly inferior to moderate doses of other antihypertensive agents. It is doubtful that the many single-pill combinations that currently contain 12.5 to 25 mg doses of HCTZ will be reformulated either to contain a larger dose or to replace HCTZ with a "more potent" thiazide-like diuretic, as the authors recommend.

W. J. Elliott, MD, PhD

References

1. *2010 Top 200 Branded Drugs by Total Prescriptions. Drug Topics.* http://www.drugtopics.modernmedicine.com/drugtopics/data/articlestandard//drugtopics/252011/727256/article.pdf. June 2011. Accessed October 29, 2011.
2. *2010 Top 200 Generic Drugs by Total Prescriptions. Drug Topics.* http://www.drugtopics.modernmedicine.com/drugtopics/data/articlestandard//drugtopics/252011/727243/article.pdf. June 2011. Accessed October 29, 2011.
3. Effects of treatment on morbidity in hypertension. Results in patients with diastolic blood pressures averaging 115 through 129 mm Hg. *JAMA.* 1967;202:1028-1034.
4. Effects of treatment on morbidity in hypertension. II. Results in patients with diastolic blood pressure averaging 90 through 114 mm Hg. *JAMA.* 1970;213:1143-1152.
5. Helgeland A. Treatment of mild hypertension: a five year controlled drug trial. The Oslo study. *Am J Med.* 1980;69:725-732.
6. Amery A, Birkenhäger W, Brixko P, et al. Mortality and morbidity results from the European Working Party on High Blood Pressure in the Elderly Trial. *Lancet.* 1985;1:1349-1354.
7. Mortality after 10 1/2 years for hypertensive participants in the Multiple Risk Factor Intervention Trial. *Circulation.* 1990;82:1616-1628.
8. Dorsch MP, Gillespie BW, Erickson SR, Bleske BE, Weder AB. Chlorthalidone reduces cardiovascular events compared with hydrochlorothiazide: a retrospective cohort analysis. *Hypertension.* 2011;57:689-694.
9. Carter BL, Ernst ME, Cohen JD. Hydrochlorothiazide versus chlorthalidone: evidence supporting their interchangeability. *Hypertension.* 2004;43:4-9.
10. Ernst ME, Carter BL, Zheng S, Grimm RH Jr. Meta-analysis of dose-response characteristics of hydrochlorothiazide and chlorthalidone: effects on systolic blood pressure and potassium. *Am J Hypertens.* 2010;23:440-446.
11. Psaty BM, Lumley T, Furberg CD. Meta-analysis of health outcomes of chlorthalidone-based vs nonchlorthalidone-based low-dose diuretic therapies. *JAMA.* 2004;292:43-44.
12. Elliott WJ, Basu S, Meyer PM. Network meta-analysis of heart failure prevention by antihypertensive drugs [Letter]. *Arch Intern Med.* 2011;171:472-473.
13. NICE clinical guideline 127: Hypertension: Clinical management of primary hypertension in adults. http://www.nice.org.uk/CG127. Accessed August 24, 2011.

Effect of Renin-Angiotensin System Blockade on Calcium Channel Blocker-Associated Peripheral Edema

Makani H, Bangalore S, Romero J, et al (St Luke's Roosevelt Hosp, NY; New York Univ School of Medicine)
Am J Med 124:128-135, 2011

Background.—Peripheral edema is a common adverse effect of calcium channel blockers. The addition of a renin-angiotensin system blocker, either an angiotensin-converting enzyme inhibitor or an ARB, has been shown to reduce peripheral edema in a dose-dependent way.

Methods.—We performed a MEDLINE/COCHRANE search for all prospective randomized controlled trials in patients with hypertension, comparing calcium channel blocker monotherapy with calcium channel blocker/renin-angiotensin system blocker combination from 1980 to the present. Trials reporting the incidence of peripheral edema or withdrawal of patients because of edema and total sample size more than 100 were included in this analysis.

Results.—We analyzed 25 randomized controlled trials with 17,206 patients (mean age 56 years, 55% were men) and a mean duration of 9.2 weeks. The incidence of peripheral edema with calcium channel blocker/renin-angiotensin system blocker combination was 38% lower than that with calcium channel blocker monotherapy ($P < .00001$) (relative risk [RR] 0.62; 95% confidence interval [CI], 0.53-0.74). Similarly, the risk of withdrawal due to peripheral edema was 62% lower with calcium channel blocker/renin-angiotensin system blocker combination compared with calcium channel blocker monotherapy ($P = .002$) (RR 0.38; 95% CI, 0.22-0.66). ACE inhibitors were significantly more efficacious than ARBs in reducing the incidence of peripheral edema ($P < .0001$) (ratio of RR 0.74; 95% CI, 0.64-0.84) (indirect comparison).

Conclusion.—In patients with hypertension, the calcium channel blocker/ renin-angiotensin system blocker combination reduces the risk of calcium channel blocker-associated peripheral edema when compared with calcium channel blocker monotherapy. ACE inhibitor seems to be more efficacious than ARB in reducing calcium channel blocker-associated peripheral edema, but head-to-head comparison studies are needed to prove this.

▶ In the United Kingdom's new guidelines from their National Institute for Health and Clinical Excellence,[1] calcium channel blockers are recommended first-line therapy for blacks and patients older than 55 years, but they have had a checkered past in the United States.[2-5] Even in the Antihypertensive and Lipid-Lowering to Prevent Heart Attack Trial (ALLHAT), the most popular dihydropyridine calcium antagonist, amlodipine, was not superior to chlorthalidone in preventing myocardial infarction and was inferior in preventing heart failure.[6] In the 2010 prescription data, amlodipine accounted for approximately 73% of the dispensed drugs in the calcium channel blocker class.[7,8] The most common adverse effect of amlodipine, as with other dihydropyridine calcium antagonists, is pedal edema,[9] which is also the most common cause of its discontinuation.[10] The combination of an angiotensin-converting enzyme (ACE)-inhibitor and a dihydropyridine calcium antagonist not only reduces the severity and incidence of pedal edema, but also was superior to the combination of an ACE-inhibitor and hydrochlorothiazide in one trial.[11] Because the effects of angiotensin receptor blockers (ARBs) are similar but have not been studied head to head with ACE-inhibitors, these authors performed a systematic review to examine the incidence and discontinuation rates of dihydropyridine calcium antagonists, used alone or in combination with an ACE-inhibitor or an ARB.

The authors were careful to attempt to control for the potent confounder of dose of dihydropyridine calcium antagonist, for which the FDA-approved product information (for amlodipine) shows a strong graded or dose-response relationship: 1.8% with 2.5 mg/d, 3% with 5 mg/d, and 10.8% with 10 mg/d. Sex is also a known confounder (with women suffering much higher rates of pedal edema) and is handled here only by respecting the randomization within each trial and not performing sex-specific meta-analyses.

The authors couch their conclusions in terms of the relative risk of pedal edema, which certainly looks more impressive than the corresponding absolute risk estimates: 6% versus 3.2% for incidence (combination vs monotherapy), and 2% versus 0.6% for discontinuation. The absolute risk estimates are helpful in determining the number needed to treat with the combination to prevent an event, which is about 36 for incidence and 72 for discontinuation of the calcium antagonist.

The authors' calculations of the relative effectiveness of ACE-inhibitors and ARBs in preventing pedal edema make it clearer why no head-to-head study of this endpoint using these 2 drug classes have been performed: the indirect comparison shows a significantly better effect of the older, generically available ACE-inhibitors. Only 1 published trial so far has reported edema rates with the direct renin inhibitor aliskiren, and the results were not significantly better than with amlodipine alone. The authors conclude with a nice discussion of the pathophysiology of pedal edema and why venodilation with a renin-angiotensin-system inhibitor should unload the increased capillary pressure caused by the arterial dilation from the calcium antagonist. But it is disturbing that no comments are made about the relative effectiveness of ACE-inhibitors, ARBs, and renin inhibitors in restoring capillary pressure, which is presumably the mechanism behind the effect.

W. J. Elliott, MD, PhD

References

1. NICE clinical guideline 127: Hypertension: Clinical management of primary hypertension in adults. http://www.nice.org.uk/CG127. Accessed 24 August 2011.
2. Psaty BM, Heckbert SR, Koepsell TD, et al. The risk of myocardial infarction associated with antihypertensive drug therapies. *JAMA*. 1995;274:620-625.
3. Furberg CD, Psaty BM, Meyer JV. Nifedipine. Dose-related increase in mortality in patients with coronary heart disease. *Circulation*. 1995;92:1326-1331.
4. Psaty BM, Smith NL, Siscovick DS, et al. Health outcomes associated with antihypertensive therapies used as first-line agents. A systematic review and meta-analysis. *JAMA*. 1997;277:739-745.
5. Wassertheil-Smoller S, Psaty B, Greenland P, et al. Association between cardiovascular outcomes and antihypertensive drug treatment in older women. *JAMA*. 2004; 292:2849-2859.
6. ALLHAT Officers and Coordinators for the ALLHAT Collaborative Research Group, The Antihypertensive and Lipid-Lowering Treatment to Prevent Heart Attack Trial. Major outcomes in high-risk hypertensive patients randomized to angiotensin-converting enzyme inhibitor or calcium channel blocker vs diuretic: the Antihypertensive and Lipid-Lowering Treatment to Prevent Heart Attack Trial (ALLHAT). *JAMA*. 2002;288:2981-2997.
7. *2010 Top 200 Branded Drugs By Total Prescriptions. Drug Topics*. http://www.drugtopics.modernmedicine.com/drugtopics/data/articlestandard//drugtopics/252011/727256/article.pdf; June 2011. Accessed October 29, 2011.

8. *2010 Top 200 generic drugs by total prescriptions. Drug Topics.* http://www. drugtopics.modernmedicine.com/drugtopics/data/articlestandard//drugtopics/ 252011/727243/article.pdf; June 2011. Accessed October 29, 2011.
9. Law M, Wald N, Morris J. Lowering blood pressure to prevent myocardial infarctions and strokes: a new preventive strategy. *Health Technol Assess.* 2003;7:1-94.
10. Brown MJ, Palmer CR, Castaigne A, et al. Morbidity and mortality in patients randomised to double-blind treatment with a long-acting calcium-channel blocker or diuretic in the International Nifedipine GITS study: Intervention as a Goal in Hypertension Treatment (INSIGHT). *Lancet.* 2000;356:366-372.
11. Jamerson K, Weber MA, Bakris GL, et al; ACCOMPLISH Trial Investigators. Benazepril plus amlodipine or hydrochlorothiazide for hypertension in high-risk patients. *N Engl J Med.* 2008;359:2417-2428.

Epidemiological Studies

Presence of baseline prehypertension and risk of incident stroke: A meta-analysis

Lee M, Saver JL, Chang B, et al (Univ of California, Los Angeles; Univ of California, San Diego; et al)

Neurology 77:1330-1337, 2011

Objective.—To qualitatively and quantitatively assess the association of prehypertension with incident stroke through a meta-analysis of prospective cohort studies.

Methods.—We searched Medline, Embase, the Cochrane Library, and bibliographies of retrieved articles. Prospective cohort studies were included if they reported multivariate-adjusted relative risks (RRs) and corresponding 95% confidence intervals (CI) of stroke with respect to baseline prehypertension.

Results.—Twelve studies with 518,520 participants were included. Prehypertension was associated with risk of stroke (RR 1.55, 95% CI 1.35−1.79; $p < 0.001$). Seven studies further distinguished a low prehypertensive population (systolic blood pressure [SBP] 120−129 mm Hg or diastolic blood pressure [DBP] 80−84 mm Hg) and a high prehypertensive population (SBP 130−139 mm Hg or DBP 85−89 mm Hg). Among persons with lower-range prehypertension, stroke risk was not significantly increased (RR 1.22, 0.95−1.57). However, for persons with higher values within the prehypertensive range, stroke risk was substantially increased (RR 1.79, 95% CI 1.49−2.16).

Conclusions.—Prehypertension is associated with a higher risk of incident stroke. This risk is largely driven by higher values within the prehypertensive range and is especially relevant in nonelderly persons. Randomized trials to evaluate the efficacy of blood pressure reduction in persons with this designation are warranted.

▶ Meta-analyses of epidemiological and clinical trial data suggest that stroke is the cardiovascular outcome that is most dependent on blood pressure. The Seventh Report of the Joint National Committee on Prevention, Detection, Evaluation, and Treatment of High Blood Pressure simplified the classification of blood pressure in the United States[1] by categorizing individuals with blood pressure in the 120 to 139/80 to 89 mm Hg range as "prehypertensives." Most analyses of stroke risk in population-based samples of prehypertensive subjects, however, have been suggestive, but not overwhelmingly persuasive, presumably because they lack sufficient statistical power, usually because the number of stroke outcomes is small (due to a lower risk than hypertension, a short follow-up interval, or the transition of many prehypertensives to treated hypertensive persons). This is exactly the situation for which a meta-analysis is well suited, so the authors gathered all the data they could find on the topic and directly addressed the issue.

Their major conclusions are, as might be expected, that prehypertension does significantly increase the risk of stroke, compared with those who have "normal blood pressure," and that this increase in risk is present even in younger individuals. This alone would have major public health implications. They dug a little deeper into the data, however, and discovered that the majority of the increased risk occurs in what was formerly called "high-normal blood pressure" (eg, in the Sixth Report of the Joint National Committee on Prevention, Detection, Evaluation, and Treatment of High Blood Pressure[2]). This was precisely the blood pressure range targeted for inclusion in the Trial of Prevention of Hypertension (TROPHY) study,[3] which demonstrated that it was feasible to prevent hypertension with a moderate dose of candesartan, which also reduced the number of hospitalizations from 6 to 1 during the 2-year treatment phase.

The authors admit to 3 major limitations of their data. The baseline blood pressures for nearly all of their included studies were determined only once. They express concern about possible "publication bias" and attempted to limit this by surveying all available databases; they did not, however, include the traditional "funnel plots" that examine this possibility. Lastly, they found significant inhomogeneity across all 12 studies, which they attempted to investigate by subgroup analysis, rather than using a random-effects model (which is a more traditional way of overcoming this challenge).

Some have suggested that by pointing out the excess cardiovascular risk of prehypertension and the trials suggesting cardiovascular benefit of lowering blood pressure in prehypertensive patients, public health authorities are being pressured to reduce the threshold for treatment to greater than 120/80 mm Hg. Some have even implicated the pharmaceutical industry (and their agents) in this process that might increase prescriptions and profits, but most expert panels have instead recommended only lifestyle modifications, rather than drug therapy, for prehypertensive patients. Whether cost-effectiveness analyses will show an overall economic benefit of drug treatment of prehypertension is uncertain, but the recent British National Institute for Health and Clinical Excellence guidelines did not include such a recommendation,[4] suggesting that, at least in the United Kingdom, such treatment is probably not cost-saving, as was, for example, the case for drug therapy of hypertension, which saved both lives, life-years, and money.

W. J. Elliott, MD, PhD

References

1. Chobanian AV, Bakris GL, Black HR, et al; Joint National Committee on Prevention, Detection, Evaluation, and Treatment of High Blood Pressure. National Heart, Lung, and Blood Institute; National High Blood Pressure Education Program Coordinating Committee. Seventh report of the Joint National Committee on prevention, detection, evaluation, and treatment of high blood pressure. *Hypertension.* 2003;42: 1206-1252.
2. The sixth report of the Joint National Committee on Prevention, Detection, Evaluation, and Treatment of High Blood Pressure. *Arch Intern Med.* 1997;157: 2413-2446.
3. Julius S, Nesbitt SD, Egan B, et al. Feasibility of treating prehypertension with an angiotensin-receptor blocker. *N Engl J Med.* 2006;354:1685-1697.
4. Williams B, Williams H, Northedge J, et al; for The Guideline Development Groups. National Collaborating Centres; NICE Project Team. United Kingdom National Health Service: National Institute for Health and Clinical Excellence. NICE clinical guideline 127: Hypertension: Clinical management of primary hypertension in adults. http://www.nice.org.uk/CG127. Accessed August 24, 2011.

Baseline predictors of resistant hypertension in the Anglo-Scandinavian Cardiac Outcome Trial (ASCOT): a risk score to identify those at high-risk
Gupta AK, on behalf of the ASCOT investigators (Imperial College London, UK; et al)
J Hypertens 29:2004-2013, 2011

Background.—Resistant hypertension is a well recognized clinical entity, which has been inadequately researched to date.

Methods.—A multivariable Cox model was developed to identify baseline predictors of developing resistant hypertension among 3666 previously untreated Anglo-Scandinavian Cardiac Outcome Trial (ASCOT) patients and construct a risk score to identify those at high risk. Secondary analyses included evaluations among all 19 257 randomized patients.

Results.—One-third (1258) of previously untreated, and one-half (9333) of all randomized patients (incidence rates 75.2 and 129.7 per 1000 person-years, respectively) developed resistant hypertension during a median follow-up of 5.3 and 4.8 years, respectively. Increasing strata of baseline SBP (151−160, 161−170, 171−180, and >180 mm Hg) were associated with increased risk of developing resistant hypertension [hazard ratio 1.24 (95% confidence interval, CI 0.81−1.88), 1.50 (1.03−2.20), 2.15 (1.47−3.16), and 4.43 (3.04−6.45), respectively]. Diabetes, left ventricular hypertrophy, male sex, and raised BMI, fasting glucose, and alcohol intake were other significant determinants of resistant hypertension. Randomization to amlodipine ± perindopril vs. atenolol ± thiazide [0.57 (0.50−0.60)], previous use of aspirin [0.78 (0.62−0.98)], and randomization to atorvastatin vs. placebo [0.87 (0.76−1.00)] significantly reduced the risk of resistant hypertension. Secondary analysis results were similar. The risk score developed allows accurate risk allocation (Harrell's C-statistic 0.71), with excellent calibration (Hosmer−Lemeshow χ^2

statistics, $P = 0.99$). A 12-fold (8.4–17.4) increased risk among those in the highest vs. lowest risk deciles was apparent.

Conclusion.—Baseline SBP and choice of subsequent antihypertensive therapy were the two most important determinants of resistant hypertension in the ASCOT population. Individuals at high risk of developing resistant hypertension can be easily identified using an integer-based risk score.

▶ The Anglo-Scandinavian Cardiac Outcomes Trial (ASCOT)[1] has served in Great Britain as a template for optimal hypertension treatment, much as the Antihypertensive and Lipid-Lowering to prevent Heart Attack Trial (ALLHAT)[2] has in the United States. The 2 studies differed, however, in many ways, including the proportion of enrolled subjects who were not taking antihypertensive drug therapy at randomization (19% vs 10%, respectively), and the effectiveness of the lipid-lowering intervention (early termination of placebo arm vs nonsignificant benefit, respectively). The ALLHAT Research Group has not published its experience in subjects with resistant hypertension, perhaps because most randomized subjects would have not received a diuretic, by protocol. In contrast, the ASCOT trial has contributed an important article about the efficacy of spironolactone (as fourth-line therapy to lower blood pressure) in their subjects with resistant hypertension.[3] This article describes their efforts to identify risk factors for resistant hypertension in their subjects.

Their conclusions are not very surprising: the biggest predictor of resistant hypertension was a very elevated baseline blood pressure. The other risk factors were those clinical characteristics that have been seen in other studies,[4,5] particularly in population-based samples:[6,7] diabetes, left ventricular hypertrophy, male gender, obesity, and alcohol intake. It is also not surprising that randomization to the drug regimen that more effectively lowered blood pressure (ie, amlodipine ± perindopril, rather than atenolol ± bendroflumethiazide) should decrease the risk of resistant hypertension (although the ASCOT investigators defined this as uncontrolled blood pressure despite[3] antihypertensive medications, rather than insisting that the "ideal" treatment regimen should include a diuretic, as did a recent American Heart Association Scientific Statement[8]). Why aspirin use at baseline or randomization to atorvastatin should reduce the risk of resistant hypertension is unclear and not discussed by the authors.

The authors admit to several limitations of their data and analyses. One was the need for a "competing risks analysis" that lumped death or development of resistant hypertension as a composite endpoint because of the observation that older patients with higher blood pressures might have died before 3-drug therapy could be evaluated. They express concern that their study population may not be representative of all hypertensive patients since it was predominantly white, with 3 or more traditional cardiovascular risk factors at baseline, and the trial design that compared only two 2-drug combinations. They have published (as a supplementary appendix) a simple, integer-based algorithm to calculate a 5-year risk of resistant hypertension based on easily measured baseline characteristics, which will likely become a useful tool for British hypertensives, but it was not included in the most recent British hypertension guidelines.[9] It would be quite useful if this (or a similar) algorithm could be used to predict the 5-year risk of cardiovascular outcomes in this population.

W. J. Elliott, MD, PhD

References

1. Dahlöf B, Sever PS, Poulter NR, et al; ASCOT Investigators. Prevention of cardiovascular events with an antihypertensive regimen of amlodipine adding perindopril as required versus atenolol adding bendroflumethiazide as required, in the Anglo-Scandinavian Cardiac Outcomes Trial-Blood Pressure Lowering Arm (ASCOT-BPLA): a multicentre randomised controlled trial. *Lancet.* 2005;366:895-906.
2. ALLHAT Officers and Coordinators for the ALLHAT Collaborative Research Group. The Antihypertensive and Lipid-Lowering Treatment to Prevent Heart Attack Trial. Major outcomes in high-risk hypertensive patients randomized to angiotensin-converting enzyme inhibitor or calcium channel blocker vs diuretic: the Antihypertensive and Lipid-Lowering Treatment to Prevent Heart Attack Trial (ALLHAT). *JAMA.* 2002;288:2981-2997.
3. Chapman N, Dobson J, Wilson S, et al; Anglo-Scandinavian Cardiac Outcomes Trial Investigators. Effect of spironolactone on blood pressure in subjects with resistant hypertension. *Hypertension.* 2007;49:839-845.
4. McAdam-Marx C, Ye X, Sung JC, Brixner DI, Kahler KH. Results of a retrospective, observational pilot study using electronic medical records to assess the prevalence and characteristics of patients with resistant hypertension in an ambulatory care setting. *Clin Ther.* 2009;31:1116-1123.
5. de la Sierra A, Segura J, Banegas JR, et al. Clinical features of 8295 patients with resistant hypertension classified on the basis of ambulatory blood pressure monitoring. *Hypertension.* 2011;57:898-902.
6. Persell SD. Prevalence of resistant hypertension in the United States, 2003-2008. *Hypertension.* 2011;57:1076-1080.
7. Egan BM, Zhao Y, Axon RN, Brzezinski WA, Ferdinand KC. Uncontrolled and apparent treatment resistant hypertension in the United States, 1988 to 2008. *Circulation.* 2011;124:1046-1058.
8. Calhoun DA, Jones D, Textor S, et al. Resistant hypertension: diagnosis, evaluation, and treatment. A Scientific Statement from the American Heart Association Professional Education Committee of the Council for High Blood Pressure Research. *Hypertension.* 2008;51:1403-1419.
9. Williams B, Williams H, Northedge J, et al; for The Guideline Development Groups, National Collaborating Centres, and NICE Project Team. NICE Clinical Guideline 127: Hypertension: Clinical Management of Primary Hypertension in Adults. United Kingdom National Health Service: National Institute for Health and Clinical Excellence. http://www.nice.org.uk/CG127. Accessed August 24, 2011.

Fatal and Nonfatal Outcomes, Incidence of Hypertension, and Blood Pressure Changes in Relation to Urinary Sodium Excretion

Stolarz-Skrzypek K, for the European Project on Genes in Hypertension (EPOGH) Investigators (Univ of Leuven, Belgium; et al)
JAMA 305:1777-1785, 2011

Context.—Extrapolations from observational studies and short-term intervention trials suggest that population-wide moderation of salt intake might reduce cardiovascular events.

Objective.—To assess whether 24-hour urinary sodium excretion predicts blood pressure (BP) and health outcomes.

Design, Setting, and Participants.—Prospective population study, involving 3681 participants without cardiovascular disease (CVD) who are members of families that were randomly enrolled in the Flemish Study on Genes, Environment, and Health Outcomes (1985-2004) or in the European Project on Genes in Hypertension (1999-2001). Of 3681 participants without CVD, 2096 were normotensive at baseline and 1499 had BP and sodium excretion measured at baseline and last follow-up (2005-2008).

Main Outcome Measures.—Incidence of mortality and morbidity and association between changes in BP and sodium excretion. Multivariable-adjusted hazard ratios (HRs) express the risk in tertiles of sodium excretion relative to average risk in the whole study population.

Results.—Among 3681 participants followed up for a median 7.9 years, CVD deaths decreased across increasing tertiles of 24-hour sodium excretion, from 50 deaths in the low (mean, 107 mmol), 24 in the medium (mean, 168 mmol), and 10 in the high excretion group (mean, 260 mmol; $P<.001$), resulting in respective death rates of 4.1% (95% confidence interval [CI], 3.5%-4.7%), 1.9% (95% CI, 1.5%-2.3%), and 0.8% (95% CI, 0.5%-1.1%). In multivariable-adjusted analyses, this inverse association retained significance ($P=.02$): the HR in the low tertile was 1.56 (95% CI, 1.02-2.36; $P=.04$). Baseline sodium excretion predicted neither total mortality ($P=.10$) nor fatal combined with nonfatal CVD events ($P=.55$). Among 2096 participants followed up for 6.5 years, the risk of hypertension did not increase across increasing tertiles ($P=.93$). Incident hypertension was 187 (27.0%; HR, 1.00; 95% CI, 0.87-1.16) in the low, 190 (26.6%; HR, 1.02; 95% CI, 0.89-1.16) in the medium, and 175 (25.4%; HR, 0.98; 95% CI, 0.86-1.12) in the high sodium excretion group. In 1499 participants followed up for 6.1 years, systolic blood pressure increased by 0.37 mm Hg per year ($P<.001$), whereas sodium excretion did not change (-0.45 mmol per year, $P=.15$). However, in multivariable-adjusted analyses, a 100-mmol increase in sodium excretion was associated with 1.71 mm Hg increase in systolic blood pressure ($P<.001$) but no change in diastolic BP.

Conclusions.—In this population-based cohort, systolic blood pressure, but not diastolic pressure, changes over time aligned with change in sodium excretion, but this association did not translate into a higher risk of hypertension or CVD complications. Lower sodium excretion was associated with higher CVD mortality.

▶ The association between increased dietary sodium intake and incident hypertension is more widely accepted than the further association with cardiovascular disease events and mortality.[1] A prominent critic of the latter link has produced several analyses of epidemiological data sets showing no significant relationship,[2,3] as well as the theory that increasing dietary sodium lowers plasma renin activity, higher levels of which have been linked (at least in his analyses) to an increased risk of cardiovascular events.[4] These investigators therefore gathered data on these issues from their original population-based sample of 3360

Flemish subjects, to which were added another 1187 subjects from the Czech Republic, Italy, Poland, and Russia about 10 years later. They assessed sodium intake by 24-hour urinary collections, which have their own validity challenges (as evidenced in this population by 19% and 14% whose collections were deemed inadequate), but are believed, in general, to be more reliable than 24-hour dietary recall estimates. This resulted in a recruited population (approximately 66% of those invited to participate) with a baseline median age of 40.9 years, that was 53% female, 28% smokers, 12% with drug-treated hypertension, median body-mass index of 25.2 kg/m^2, and a sodium excretion rate of 178 mmol/24 hours.

The authors' major conclusions were that, over approximately 6 years of follow-up, sodium excretion did not predict incident hypertension but was significantly associated only with a longitudinal rise in systolic blood pressure (only in the larger Flemish cohort). Perhaps more important, over approximately 8 years of follow-up, individuals in the lowest tertile of urinary sodium excretion had a significantly higher risk of cardiovascular mortality ($P < .001$) and events ($P < .02$) using unadjusted Kaplan-Meier survival statistics, but this was barely significant ($P < .04$, with no adjustment made for multiple comparisons) after adjustment for baseline differences across the groups.

Despite a number of strengths of their data and analyses, the authors acknowledge several limitations. They collected only one 24-hour urine sample from each participant, which may not have been representative of the chronic intake of sodium. Their study population was relatively young, so few participants had cardiovascular events (232 of 3681, or 6.3%) or death (219 of 3681, or 5.9%); in fact, far more subjects were lost to follow-up than had outcomes. Their population was exclusively white Europeans, who were not tested for salt sensitivity. There were no analyses performed regarding sodium/potassium ratios, which was recently shown to be a better predictor of cardiovascular mortality in the US population.[1] They make a large point that their subjects were not instructed about the putative link among salt consumption, hypertension, or cardiovascular events before collecting the index 24-hour urine, but one wonders whether their statistical adjustments and sensitivity analyses that omitted events occurring at different times after enrollment were sufficient to rule out the possibility that hypertensive subjects (who had higher cardiovascular risk overall) routinely ingested less dietary sodium at baseline than their nonhypertensive counterparts.

These data and the authors' conclusions generated much interest in the popular press, as well as editors' correspondence.[5] The authors feel that their new data contradict decades of epidemiological and clinical trial data, as well as a recent meta-analysis, supporting population-wide sodium restriction as a means to lower blood pressure and reduce cardiovascular risk.[6] It is doubtful that many public health authorities in Finland or England, where a population-based reduction in sodium intake has reduced rates of cardiovascular events, would agree with the authors' assessments.[7] Recent cost-effectiveness analyses have suggested major benefits of such a nationwide program in the United States.[8,9]

W. J. Elliott, MD, PhD

References

1. Yang Q, Liu T, Kuklina EV, et al. Sodium and potassium intake and mortality among US adults: prospective data from the Third National Health and Nutrition Examination Survey. *Arch Intern Med.* 2011;171:1183-1191.
2. Alderman MH, Cohen H, Madhavan S. Dietary sodium intake and mortality: the National Health and Nutrition Examination Survey (NHANES I). *Lancet.* 1998; 351:781-785.
3. Cohen HW, Hailpern SM, Alderman MH. Sodium intake and mortality follow-up in the Third National Health and Nutrition Examination Survey (NHANES III). *J Gen Intern Med.* 2008;23:1297-1302.
4. Alderman MH, Madhavan S, Ooi WL, Cohen H, Sealey JE, Laragh JH. Association of the renin-sodium profile with the risk of myocardial infarction in patients with hypertension. *N Engl J Med.* 1991;324:1098-1104.
5. Aleksandrova K, Pischon T, Weikert C, et al. Urinary sodium excretion and cardiovascular disease mortality. *JAMA.* 2011;306:1083-1088 [Letters].
6. Strazzullo P, D'Elia L, Kandala NB, Cappuccio FP. Salt intake, stroke, and cardiovascular disease: meta-analysis of prospective studies. *BMJ.* 2009;339:b4567.
7. He FJ, MacGregor GA. A comprehensive review on salt and health and current experience of worldwide salt reduction programmes. *J Hum Hypertens.* 2009; 23:363-384.
8. Bibbins-Domingo K, Chertow GM, Coxson PG, et al. Projected effect of dietary salt reductions on future cardiovascular disease. *N Engl J Med.* 2010;362:590-599.
9. Smith-Spangler CM, Juusola JL, Enns EA, Owens DK, Garber AM. Population strategies to decrease sodium intake and the burden of cardiovascular disease: a cost-effectiveness analysis. *Ann Intern Med.* 2010;152:481-487.

Sodium and Potassium Intake and Mortality Among US Adults: Prospective Data From the Third National Health and Nutrition Examination Survey

Yang Q, Liu T, Kuklina EV, et al (Emory Univ Atlanta, GA; et al)
Arch Intern Med 171:1183-1191, 2011

Background.—Several epidemiologic studies suggested that higher sodium and lower potassium intakes were associated with increased risk of cardiovascular diseases (CVD). Few studies have examined joint effects of dietary sodium and potassium intake on risk of mortality.

Methods.—To investigate estimated usual intakes of sodium and potassium as well as their ratio in relation to risk of all cause and CVD mortality, the Third National Health and Nutrition Examination Survey Linked Mortality File (1988-2006), a prospective cohort study of a nationally representative sample of 12 267 US adults, studied all-cause, cardiovascular, and ischemic heart (IHD) diseases mortality.

Results.—During a mean follow-up period of 14.8 years, we documented a total of 2270 deaths, including 825 CVD deaths and 443 IHD deaths. After multivariable adjustment, higher sodium intake was associated with increased all-cause mortality (hazard ratio [HR], 1.20; 95% confidence interval [CI], 1.03-1.41 per 1000 mg/d), whereas higher potassium intake was associated with lower mortality risk (HR, 0.80; 95% CI, 0.67-0.94 per 1000 mg/d). For sodium-potassium ratio, the adjusted HRs comparing the highest quartile with the lowest quartile were HR, 1.46 (95% CI, 1.27-1.67) for all-cause mortality; HR, 1.46 (95% CI, 1.11-1.92) for CVD mortality; and HR, 2.15 (95% CI, 1.48-3.12) for IHD mortality. These findings did not differ significantly by sex, race/ethnicity, body mass index, hypertension status, education levels, or physical activity.

Conclusion.—Our findings suggest that a higher sodium potassium ratio is associated with significantly increased risk of CVD and all-cause mortality, and higher sodium intake is associated with increased total mortality in the general US population.

▶ Although higher reported intake of dietary sodium has been strongly and consistently linked to incident hypertension, many epidemiological studies have been unable to show a significant further link to increased risk of cardiovascular disease events (or mortality), and some have actually suggested an inverse association.[1] For example, in a previous analysis of this very same Third National Health and Nutrition Examination Survey (NHANES III), there was no significant relationship between dietary sodium intake (assessed by a 1-day dietary recall) and subsequent cardiovascular mortality.[2] Because this earlier report had only a 3.5-year average follow-up, better methods of estimating dietary intake of sodium and potassium have been developed[3] and recent research has suggested that the ratio of dietary sodium/potassium is a better predictor of cardiovascular events than sodium intake,[4] these authors reexamined this nationally representative data set of 12 267 US adults, now with 14.8 years of follow-up, for evidence of a significant relationship between dietary sodium or sodium/potassium ratio and cardiovascular events and mortality.

Perhaps the most important methodological advantage used in this article was the National Cancer Institute's mixed effects modeling of sodium and potassium intake, which depended greatly on validating the single-day dietary recall in more than 12 000 subjects, with a subsequent second attempt (on a different workday) in 912 of these individuals. Although it seems odd that the validity of an estimate can be greatly improved by corroborating the initial value in such a small subset of people, this method at least captures some of the intraindividual variability that is known to occur with single-day recalls. It would have been interesting to see how the authors' conclusions might have been changed had they not used this novel method of estimating dietary intake of sodium and potassium. Based on their report of the nonsignificant association of dietary sodium (alone) and either cardiovascular mortality or ischemic heart disease mortality (as seen previously[2]), it is likely that using this new method to estimate dietary intake was not all that important. Instead, their finding of a highly significant association of the dietary sodium/potassium ratio with all-cause, cardiovascular, and ischemic heart disease mortality is the more important predictor.

Despite a number of strengths of their data and analyses, the authors acknowledge several limitations. For the vast majority of their subjects (>92%), no follow-up dietary data were available, which increases concern about the validity and variability of the dietary recall information, which was not corroborated by a 24-hour urinary collection. No quantitative data about the use of table salt were available from the NHANES III data set, so this covariate was not used in "adjusted models." Lastly, the authors worry that their conclusions may have been confounded by other dietary variables, which is difficult to adjust for in multivariate models.

These data did not address the issue of whether it might be better to restrict dietary sodium (as is currently being done, both in the US and overseas, after having been found to be cost-effective in 2 recent nationwide modeling studies in the US[5,6]), or to increase dietary potassium. The latter is of special concern for people with chronic kidney disease or those who use blockers of the renin-angiotensin-aldosterone system. However, the editorialists for this article recommended plant-based diets,[7] especially fruits and vegetables, as a good and safe source of dietary potassium for most US adults. Further research on the potential benefits of such programs seems warranted.

W. J. Elliott, MD, PhD

References

1. Stolarz-Skrzypek K, Kuznetsova T, Thijs L, et al. Fatal and nonfatal outcomes, incidence of hypertension, and blood pressure changes in relation to urinary sodium excretion. *JAMA*. 2011;305:1777-1785.
2. Cohen HW, Hailpern SM, Alderman MH. Sodium intake and mortality follow-up in the Third National Health and Nutrition Examination Survey (NHANES III). *J Gen Intern Med*. 2008;23:1297-1302.
3. Tooze JA, Kipnis V, Buckman DW, et al. A mixed-effects model approach for estimating the distribution of usual intake of nutrients: the NCI method. *Stat Med*. 2010;29:2857-2868.
4. Adrogué HJ, Madias NE. Shared primacy of sodium and potassium on cardiovascular risk. *Am J Kidney Dis*. 2009;54:598-601.
5. Bibbins-Domingo K, Chertow GM, Coxson PG, et al. Projected effect of dietary salt reductions on future cardiovascular disease. *N Engl J Med*. 2010;362:590-599.
6. Smith-Spangler CM, Juusola JL, Enns EA, Owens DK, Garber AM. Population strategies to decrease sodium intake and the burden of cardiovascular disease: a cost-effectiveness analysis. *Ann Intern Med*. 2010;152:481-487.
7. Silver LD, Farley TA. Sodium and potassium intake: mortality effects and policy implications: comment on "Sodium and potassium intake and mortality among US adults" [Editorial]. *Arch Intern Med*. 2011;171:1191-1192.

Effect of pay for performance on the management and outcomes of hypertension in the United Kingdom: interrupted time series study
Serumaga B, Ross-Degnan D, Avery AJ, et al (Harvard Med School and Harvard Pilgrim Health Care Inst, Boston, MA; Univ of Nottingham Med School, UK; et al)
BMJ 342:d108, 2011

Objective.—To assess the impact of a pay for performance incentive on quality of care and outcomes among UK patients with hypertension in primary care.

Design.—Interrupted time series.

Setting.—The Health Improvement Network (THIN) database, United Kingdom.

Participants.—470 725 patients with hypertension diagnosed between January 2000 and August 2007.

Intervention.—The UK pay for performance incentive (the Quality and Outcomes Framework), which was implemented in April 2004 and included specific targets for general practitioners to show high quality care for patients with hypertension (and other diseases).

Main Outcome Measures.—Centiles of systolic and diastolic blood pressures over time, rates of blood pressure monitoring, blood pressure control, and treatment intensity at monthly intervals for baseline (48 months) and 36 months after the implementation of pay for performance. Cumulative incidence of major hypertension related outcomes and all cause mortality for subgroups of newly treated (treatment started six months before pay for performance) and treatment experienced (started treatment in year before January 2001) patients to examine different stages of illness.

Results.—After accounting for secular trends, no changes in blood pressure monitoring (level change 0.85, 95% confidence interval −3.04 to 4.74, P=0.669 and trend change −0.01, −0.24 to 0.21, P=0.615), control (−1.19, −2.06 to 1.09, P=0.109 and −0.01, −0.06 to 0.03, P=0.569), or treatment intensity (0.67, −1.27 to 2.81, P=0.412 and 0.02, −0.23 to 0.19, P=0.706) were attributable to pay for performance. Pay for performance had no effect on the cumulative incidence of stroke, myocardial infarction, renal failure, heart failure, or all cause mortality in both treatment experienced and newly treated subgroups.

Conclusions.—Good quality of care for hypertension was stable or improving before pay for performance was introduced. Pay for performance had no discernible effects on processes of care or on hypertension related clinical outcomes. Generous financial incentives, as designed in the UK pay for performance policy, may not be sufficient to improve quality of care and outcomes for hypertension and other common chronic conditions.

▶ Many have decried the suboptimal blood pressure control rates in most parts of the world,[1] including the United States and the United Kingdom.[2,3] Both countries have now implemented financial incentives for physicians to achieve better nationwide blood pressure control, which in the United Kingdom had the potential to increase a physician's pay from their National Health Service by as much as 50%.[4]

Sadly, there have been few efforts to assess whether these financial incentives actually perform as intended, or, as others have suggested, may have adverse effects, such as excluding persons with severe illnesses from routine care.[5] These authors therefore accessed The Health Improvement Network database, which contains primary care medical records of about 6.2 million patient-years from 158 general practices in the United Kingdom. They used time-series modeling to assess whether blood pressure control (using a relatively large number of metrics) improved in their study population after April 2004, which was the implementation date for the financial incentives. Only 5 of the 136 "quality indicators" that were addressed by the Pay-for-Performance financial incentives involved blood pressure, but apparently 20% of the health care resources from these practices were directed to improving blood pressure control (to < 150/90 mm Hg, which is higher than the targets traditionally recommended in the United States). Their major conclusion was that blood pressure control rates (and several related parameters) increased prior to the April 2004 date and continued thereafter at roughly the same incremental rate. They also found no significant improvement in hypertension-related outcomes (stroke, myocardial infarction, renal failure, heart failure, or all cause mortality) after the institution of financial incentives. Interestingly, they detected no "gaming of the system" to achieve higher reimbursement (eg, selectively increasing treatment intensity for patients who were close to goal).

These data differ substantially from those gathered in Canada, where a health education program directed at health care professionals and the public has had a clear, substantial, significant, and important impact on prescribing of antihypertensive drugs, blood pressure control, and cardiovascular events.[6]

The authors note several limitations of their data. No concomitant control group was studied, because all practices had the Pay-for-Performance implemented simultaneously. The generalizability of their findings to other primary care settings—for example, those without a single-payor system—is unknown. They conclude that the "bonuses" paid to physicians have had no significant impact on quality of care. They hypothesize that these monies might be better spent in the future on other effective modalities, such as case management or comanagement of hypertension by nurses[7] and pharmacists,[8] and simplification of the "multiple messages" (from 136 quality measures) to a smaller number of selected outcomes. Whether the US Center for Medicare and Medicaid Services will gather data from the current US effort to reward physicians for achieving goals set by current treatment guidelines and modify how it pays physicians based on such results remains to be seen.

W. J. Elliott, MD, PhD

References

1. Danaei G, Finucane MM, Lin JK, et al. National, regional, and global trends in systolic blood pressure since 1980: systematic analysis of health examination surveys and epidemiological studies with 786 country-years and 5·4 million participants. *Lancet.* 2011;377:568-577.
2. Fang J, Alderman MH, Keenan NL, Ayala C, Croft JB. Hypertension control at physicians' offices in the United States. *Am J Hypertens.* 2008;21:136-142.
3. Wang YR, Alexander GC, Stafford RS. Outpatient hypertension treatment, treatment intensification, and control in Western Europe and the United States. *Arch Intern Med.* 2007;167:141-147.
4. Roland M. Linking physicians' pay to the quality of care—a major experiment in the United Kingdom. *N Engl J Med.* 2004;351:1448-1454.
5. Tanenbaum SJ. Pay for performance in Medicare: evidentiary irony and the politics of value. *J Health Polit Policy Law.* 2009;34:717-746.
6. Campbell NR, Brant R, Johansen H, et al; Canadian Hypertension Education Program Outcomes Research Task Force. Increases in antihypertensive prescriptions and reductions in cardiovascular events in Canada. *Hypertension.* 2009;53:128-134.
7. Clark CE, Smith LF, Taylor RS, Campbell JL. Nurse led interventions to improve control of blood pressure in people with hypertension: systematic review and meta-analysis. *BMJ.* 2010;341:c3995.

Chapter 1—Hypertension / **43**

8. Weber CA, Ernst ME, Sezate GS, Zheng S, Carter BL. Pharmacist-physician comanagement of hypertension and reduction in 24-hour ambulatory blood pressures. *Arch Intern Med.* 2010;170:1634-1639.

Maternal exposure to angiotensin converting enzyme inhibitors in the first trimester and risk of malformations in offspring: a retrospective cohort study
Li D-K, Yang C, Andrade S, et al (Kaiser Foundation Res Inst, Oakland, CA; Meyers Primary Care Inst, Worcester, MA)
BMJ 343:d5931, 2011

Objective.—To examine a reported association between use of angiotensin converting enzyme (ACE) inhibitors during the first trimester and risk of malformations in offspring.

Design.—A population based, retrospective cohort study linking automated clinical and pharmacy databases including comprehensive electronic medical records.

Participants.—Pregnant women and their live born offspring (465 754 mother-infant pairs) in the Kaiser Permanente Northern California region from 1995 to 2008.

Main Outcome Measure.—Congenital malformation in live births.

Results.—The prevalence of ACE inhibitor use in the first trimester only was 0.9/1000, and the use of other antihypertensive medications was 2.4/1000. After adjustment for maternal age, ethnicity, parity, and obesity, use of ACE inhibitors during the first trimester only seemed to be associated with increased risk of congenital heart defects in offspring compared with normal controls (those with neither hypertension nor use of any antihypertensives during pregnancy) (15/381 (3.9%) v 6232/400 021 (1.6%) cases, odds ratio 1.54 (95% confidence interval 0.90 to 2.62)). A similar association was observed for use of other antihypertensives (28/1090 (2.6%) cases of congenital heart defects, odds ratio 1.52 (1.04 to 2.21)). However, compared with hypertension controls (those with a diagnosis of hypertension but without use of antihypertensives) (708/29 735 (2.4%) cases of congenital heart defects), neither use of ACE inhibitors or of other antihypertensives in the first trimester was associated with increased congenital heart defects risk (odds ratios 1.14 (0.65 to 1.98) and 1.12 (0.76 to 1.64) respectively).

Conclusions.—Maternal use of ACE inhibitors in the first trimester has a risk profile similar to the use of other antihypertensives regarding malformations in live born offspring. The apparent increased risk of malformations associated with use of ACE inhibitors (and other antihypertensives) in the first trimester is likely due to the underlying hypertension rather than the medications.

▶ Fetotoxicity of antihypertensive agents that interfere directly with the renin-angiotensin-aldosterone system results in craniofacial abnormalities, renal agenesis, and other malformations, which has been better documented when they are administered during the second and third trimesters of pregnancy.[1,2] A widely cited 2006 article from the Tennessee Medicaid Database concluded that congenital heart defects were also significantly more common when angiotensin-converting enzyme (ACE)-inhibitors were taken during the first trimester (compared with other antihypertensive drugs)[3] and raised fears that any exposure to ACE-inhibitors during pregnancy was risky and unwise. In retrospect, the increase in risk was largely caused by atrial septal defects, which are typically considered less serious or life threatening than the malformations seen after exposure during the second and third trimesters. Two large subsequent studies found no difference in risk between ACE-inhibitors or other antihypertensive drugs taken during the first trimester,[4,5] making it more likely that the birth defects could more properly be attributed to hypertension and not ACE-inhibitors themselves.

These authors therefore collected data from the Northern California Kaiser Permanente database from 1995 to 2008, containing nearly half a million infants who were examined for birth defects and whose mothers had pharmacy dispensing records that provided the data for fetal exposure to antihypertensive drugs. They also collected data about maternal history of overweight and diabetes mellitus, which they used as covariates in their analyses, since both of these conditions can be confounders for the association between congenital heart defects and antihypertensive drug use. The prevalence of ACE-inhibitor use during the first trimester was tiny (381 of 465 754 mothers), even compared with use of other antihypertensive drugs (1090), but that was higher than the number of mothers with hypertension that did not receive antihypertensive drugs (708). These small numbers limit the precision of the estimated risk of congenital heart defects in the infants, widen the confidence intervals, and could possibly lead to a type 2 statistical error when comparing the rates for ACE-inhibitor versus other antihypertensive drug use.

The authors claim that their population sample is likely to be more sensitive to identify birth defects in mothers who took antihypertensive drugs during pregnancy, as their sample size is 15 times larger than that of the cohort from Tennessee. However, the number of women who took ACE-inhibitors (the most important determinant of risk for rare outcomes) was less than 2-fold higher (381 vs 209), perhaps because the Tennessee cohort was assembled earlier (from 1985–2000), when the risks of first-trimester ACE-inhibitor treatment were thought to be lower, or perhaps because Tennessee physicians had not been repeatedly warned about the potential risks.

While it is reassuring that this dataset, like 2 before it, did not confirm the original report of increased risk of congenital heart defects in infants whose mothers took ACE-inhibitors during the first trimester of pregnancy, it seems unlikely that we should change the current practice, developed after the Tennessee report, to routinely prescribe ACE-inhibitors only to women who are not pregnant, not at risk for pregnancy, and not actively trying to become pregnant.

W. J. Elliott, MD, PhD

References

1. From the Centers for Disease Control and Prevention. Postmarketing surveillance for angiotensin-converting enzyme inhibitor use during the first trimester of

pregnancy—United States, Canada and Israel, 1987-1995. *JAMA.* 1997;277: 1193-1194.
2. Ratnapalan S, Koren G. Taking ACE inhibitors during pregnancy. Is it safe? *Can Fam Physician.* 2002;48:1047-1049.
3. Cooper WO, Hernandez-Diaz S, Arbogast PG, et al. Major congenital malformations after first-trimester exposure to ACE inhibitors. *N Engl J Med.* 2006;354: 2443-2451.
4. Caton AR, Bell EM, Druschel CM, et al. Antihypertensive medication use during pregnancy and the risk of cardiovascular malformations. *Hypertension.* 2009;54: 63-72.
5. Lennestål R, Otterblad OP, Kännén B. Maternal use of antihypertensive drugs in early pregnancy and delivery outcome, notably the presence of congenital heart defects in the infants. *Eur J Clin Pharmacol.* 2009;65:615-625.

Long-term follow-up of 111 patients with angiotensin-converting enzyme inhibitor-related angioedema
Beltrami L, Zanichelli A, Zingale L, et al (IRCCS, Milan, Italy; Luigi Sacco Hospital, Milan, Italy; et al)
J Hypertens 29:2273-2277, 2011

Objective.—To investigate, for the first time, the frequency of recurrences of angiotensin-converting enzyme inhibitor (ACE-I)-related angioedema after the discontinuation of ACE-I.

Methods.—This retrospective study was conducted in an outpatient tertiary-level centre for a total period of 173 months (about 14 years). Consecutive patients with recurrent angioedema symptoms, initiated during treatment with an ACE-I, who had been followed for at least 12 months after discontinuation of the drug were eligible. The primary study variable was the incidence of recurrences of angioedema after ACE-I discontinuation. Angioedema location, type of ACE-I and indication for this treatment and the drugs prescribed after the discontinuation of ACE-I were also evaluated.

Results.—In total, 111 patients were followed; 54 of them (49%) were on enalapril. After discontinuation from ACE-I, 51 patients (46%) had further recurrences of angioedema; in 18 relapsers (16% of the total), the frequency of angioedema recurrences remained unchanged when compared with that reported during ACE-I treatment. The large majority of relapsers (88%) had the first recurrence of angioedema within the first month since ACE-I discontinuation. The switch to a different antihypertensive therapy did not seem associated with a reduction in the frequency of angioedema attacks.

Conclusion.—Even with all the limitations on any observational analysis, this long-term study suggests for the first time that patients with angioedema started while on ACE-I treatment seem to have a condition predisposing to angioedema that is elicited by the treatment with these drugs. Further studies in this field appear advocated due to the potential severity of angioedema attacks.

▶ Angioedema is an acute, serious disorder, typically involving the face (85%) and tongue (40%), but allegedly 10% of patients experience laryngeal involvement, which may compromise the airway and become life-threatening.[1] Angiotensin converting enzyme (ACE) inhibitors are currently the most common reversible cause of this disorder, which is thought to result from these drugs' action on kininase II, which is responsible for the metabolism of bradykinin.[1] Estimates of the incidence of ACE-inhibitor-associated angioedema range from 0.2%[2] in a large database from the Department of Veterans Affairs to 0.7% in the only clinical trial to use angioedema as a primary outcome measure.[3] This was an approximately 3-fold lower incidence higher incidence than that seen with omapatrilat,[4] which resulted in discontinuation of nearly all development of vasopeptidase inhibitors. In Europe, an intravenous bradykinin receptor antagonist, icatibant, is approved for emergency treatment of ACE-inhibitor-associated angioedema, but the drug missed achieving statistical significance in its US trials, so it is now available in the US only as a treatment option for hereditary angioedema.[5] Perhaps because angioedema can occur with any drug, it has been difficult to prospectively enroll subjects who have suffered angioedema in a trial to see if it recurs. As a result, a prospective observational study such as this one provides the most useful information about the risk of angioedema recurrence and its risk factors.

These authors collected baseline and outcome data from 111 consecutive patients with ACE-inhibitor-associated angioedema. A full 46% had recurrent episodes of angioedema, 88% within the first month, despite stopping the ACE inhibitor. In patients with recurrences, the attack rate was not different after stopping the ACE inhibitor, and there was no specific class of antihypertensive agent that was associated with an increased risk of recurrence.

These data suggest but do not prove (as a randomized clinical trial might) that ACE inhibitors "uncover" a propensity to angioedema in those who experience the problem. Unfortunately, their experience suggests that the severity of the attacks increases if the ACE inhibitor is not discontinued, which appears to be the wisest treatment plan. Perhaps the most amazing thing about this article is that the authors admit that their longer-term data contradict their short-term conclusion that switching to an ARB after ACE-inhibitor-associated angioedema increased the risk of recurrence.[6] It would be nice to have a mechanism to annotate this earlier report (eg, as in a published Erratum) to indicate that longer-term follow-up results in a different conclusion. Perhaps the most evidence-based data about this are those from CHARM-Alternative, in which candesartan had only 1 case of recurrent angioedema in 39 subjects, compared with 0 in placebo-treated patients.[7] Although unlikely to be upheld or cited in a court of law, the worldwide experience now suggests that an angiotensin receptor blocker (ARB) is no more likely to cause recurrent angioedema after an ACE inhibitor than any other antihypertensive drug class. Both physicians and patients may now have a greater sense of safety using an ARB in this setting, although such risk still exists.

W. J. Elliott, MD, PhD

References

1. Hoover T, Lippmann M, Grouzmann E, Marceau F, Herscu P. Angiotensin converting enzyme inhibitor induced angio-oedema: a review of the pathophysiology and risk factors. *Clin Exp Allergy.* 2010;40:50-61.

2. Miller DR, Oliveria SA, Berlowitz DR, Fincke BG, Stang P, Lillienfeld DE. Angioedema incidence in US veterans initiating angiotensin-converting enzyme inhibitors. *Hypertension.* 2008;51:1624-1630.
3. Kostis JB, Kim HJ, Rusnak J, et al. Incidence and characteristics of angioedema associated with enalapril. *Arch Intern Med.* 2005;165:1637-1642.
4. Kostis JB, Packer M, Black HR, Schmieder R, Henry D, Levy E. Omapatrilat and enalapril in patients with hypertension: the Omapatrilat Cardiovascular Treatment vs. Enalapril (OCTAVE) trial. *Am J Hypertens.* 2004;17:103-111.
5. Cicardi M, Banerji A, Bracho F, et al. Icatibant, a new bradykinin-receptor antagonist, in hereditary angioedema. *N Engl J Med.* 2010;363:532-541.
6. Cicardi M, Zingale LC, Bergamaschini L, Agostoni A. Angioedema associated with angiotensin-converting enzyme inhibitor use: outcome after switching to a different treatment. *Arch Intern Med.* 2004;164:910-913.
7. Granger CB, McMurray JJ, Yusuf S, et al; CHARM Investigators and Committees. Effects of candesartan in patients with chronic heart failure and reduced left-ventricular systolic function intolerant to angiotensin-converting-enzyme inhibitors: the CHARM-Alternative trial. *Lancet.* 2003;362:772-776.

Hypertension and Cardiovascular Risk

Chlorthalidone Reduces Cardiovascular Events Compared With Hydrochlorothiazide: A Retrospective Cohort Analysis

Dorsch MP, Gillespie BW, Erickson SR, et al (Univ of Michigan Health System, Ann Arbor; Univ of Michigan, Ann Arbor)
Hypertension 57:689-694, 2011

There is significant controversy around whether chlorthalidone (CTD) is superior to hydrochlorothiazide (HCTZ) in hypertension management. The objective of this analysis was to evaluate the effects of CTD compared with HCTZ on cardiovascular event (CVE) rates. We performed a retrospective observational cohort study from the Multiple Risk Factor Intervention Trial data set from the National Heart, Lung, and Blood Institute. The Multiple Risk Factor Intervention Trial was a cardiovascular primary prevention trial where participants were men 35 to 57 years of age enrolled and followed beginning in 1973. CVEs were measured yearly, and time to event was assessed by Cox regression. Systolic blood pressure, total cholesterol, low-density lipoprotein cholesterol, high-density lipoprotein cholesterol, triglyceride, potassium, glucose, and uric acid were measured yearly. The difference between groups was evaluated by repeated-measures mixed modeling, and each model was adjusted for predictors of each variable. CVEs were significantly lower in those on CTD (adjusted hazard ratio: 0.51 [95% CI: 0.43 to 0.61]; $P<0.0001$) and on HCTZ (adjusted hazard ratio: 0.65 [95% CI: 0.55 to 0.75]; $P<0.0001$) compared with those who took neither drug. When comparing the 2 drugs, CTD had significantly fewer CVEs compared with HCTZ ($P<0.0016$). CTD displayed significantly lower SBP ($P<0.0001$), lower total cholesterol ($P=0.0001$), lower low-density lipoprotein cholesterol ($P=0.0009$), lower potassium ($P=0.0003$), and higher uric acid ($P<0.0001$) over time compared with HCTZ. In conclusion, both HCTZ and CTD reduce CVEs compared with neither drug. When comparing both drugs, CTD reduces CVEs more than HCTZ, suggesting that CTD may be the preferred thiazide-type diuretic for hypertension in patients at high risk of CVEs.

▶ Hydrochlorothiazide is by far the most prescribed thiazide or thiazide-like diuretic in the United States and has been formulated into many single-pill combination products and accounted for about 134 million prescriptions in 2010.[1] Nonetheless, the National Institutes of Health has mandated that its funded clinical trials (eg, the Systolic Hypertension in the Elderly Program[2] and its pilot study,[3] the Antihypertensive and Lipid-Lowering to prevent Heart Attack Trial[4]) be performed instead with chlorthalidone since about 1989. A detailed rationale for this decision by the National Institutes of Health has never been revealed, but careful reading of several articles regarding the Multiple Risk Factor Intervention Trial (MRFIT) provide some hints about the process and outcomes.[5,6] The decision to mandate (at about 5.5 years of follow-up) that all centers use chlorthalidone was initially based on an interim analysis that demonstrated better prevention of death and cardiac morbidity with chlorthalidone (compared with the "Referred-Care" controls), and a simultaneous increase in mortality and cardiac morbidity for subjects treated with hydrochlorothiazide (compared with those centers' Referred-Care controls). Perhaps more importantly, after the switch from hydrochlorothiazide to chlorthalidone, there was a near-significant improvement in mortality and cardiac morbidity in these centers' Stepped Care participants, compared with their Referred-Care controls.[7,8] This article presents an analysis of data obtained from the MRFIT trial via the Freedom of Information Act and provides the most detailed analysis so far about the only trial that has outcomes data with chlorthalidone and hydrochlorothiazide, although it was not a head-to-head randomized comparison.

These authors also chose to analyze the data in a modified intent-to-treat analysis, by separating individuals who reported not taking the prescribed antihypertensive therapy (an initial diuretic in all Stepped-Care centers). This was presumably necessary because so many subjects (~75%) did not persist with their originally assigned treatment. More traditional analyses would have simply compared event rates in the 4 groups: Stepped-Care (hydrochlorothiazide or chlorthalidone) or Referred-Care (hydrochlorothiazide or chlorthalidone) and probably would have reported the numbers of subjects afflicted with each of the observed endpoints. These authors report only hazard ratios and the fact that 1244 subjects suffered cardiovascular events during the 7 years of follow-up.

These data are nonetheless interesting, despite the lapse of more than 20 years after their collection. They do suggest that, at the higher doses used (compared with those today), chlorthalidone was superior to hydrochlorothiazide in lowering blood pressure, with less effect on total and low-density lipoprotein cholesterol and glucose levels (consistent with a recent meta-analysis based on randomized trials[9]) and, most importantly, prevention of cardiovascular events. It is extremely unlikely that we will ever have outcomes data comparing 2 initial diuretics for hypertension; these MRFIT analyses may be the best indirect comparison ever.

W. J. Elliott, MD, PhD

References

1. Messerli FH, Makani H, Benjo A, Romero J, Alviar C, Bangalore S. Antihypertensive efficacy of hydrochlorothiazide as evaluated by ambulatory blood pressure monitoring: a meta-analysis of randomized trials. *J Am Coll Cardiol.* 2011;57: 590-600.
2. Prevention of stroke by antihypertensive drug treatment in older persons with isolated systolic hypertension. Final results of the Systolic Hypertension in the Elderly Program (SHEP). SHEP Cooperative Research Group. *JAMA.* 1991;265:3255-3264.
3. Perry HM Jr, Smith WM, McDonald RH, et al. Morbidity and mortality in the Systolic Hypertension in the Elderly Program (SHEP) pilot study. *Stroke.* 1989; 20:4-13.
4. ALLHAT Officers and Coordinators for the ALLHAT Collaborative Research Group, The Antihypertensive and Lipid-Lowering Treatment to Prevent Heart Attack Trial. Major outcomes in high-risk hypertensive patients randomized to angiotensin-converting enzyme inhibitor or calcium channel blocker vs diuretic: the Antihypertensive and Lipid-Lowering Treatment to Prevent Heart Attack Trial (ALLHAT). *JAMA.* 2002;288:2981-2997.
5. Kolata G. Heart study produces a surprise result. *Science.* 1982;218:31-32.
6. Bartsch G, Broste S, Grandits G, et al. Hydrochlorothiazide, chlorthalidone and mortality in the Multiple Risk Factor Intervention Trial [abstract]. *Circulation.* 1984;70:1438.
7. Mortality after 10 1/2 years for hypertensive participants in the Multiple Risk Factor Intervention Trial. *Circulation.* 1990;82:1616-1628.
8. Elliott WJ, Grimm RH Jr. Using diuretics in practice—one opinion. *J Clin Hypertens (Greenwich).* 2008;10:856-862.
9. Elliott WJ, Meyer PM. Incident diabetes in clinical trials of antihypertensive drugs: a network meta-analysis. *Lancet.* 2007;369:201-207.

Long-Term Effects of Chlorthalidone Versus Hydrochlorothiazide on Electrocardiographic Left Ventricular Hypertrophy in the Multiple Risk Factor Intervention Trial

Ernst ME, for the Multiple Risk Factor Intervention Trial Research Group (Univ of Iowa; et al)
Hypertension 58:1001-1007, 2011

Chlorthalidone (CTD) reduces 24-hour blood pressure more effectively than hydrochlorothiazide (HCTZ), but whether this influences electrocardiographic left ventricular hypertrophy is uncertain. One source of comparative data is the Multiple Risk Factor Intervention Trial, which randomly assigned 8012 hypertensive men to special intervention (SI) or usual care. SI participants could use CTD or HCTZ initially; previous analyses have grouped clinics by their main diuretic used (C-clinics: CTD; H-clinics: HCTZ). After 48 months, SI participants receiving HCTZ were recommended to switch to CTD, in part because higher mortality was observed for SI compared with usual care participants in H-clinics, whereas the opposite was found in C-clinics. In this analysis, we examined change in continuous measures of electrocardiographic left ventricular hypertrophy using both an ecological analysis by previously reported C- or H-clinic groupings and an individual participant analysis where use of CTD or HCTZ by SI participants was considered and updated annually. Through 48 months, differences between SI and usual care in left ventricular hypertrophy were larger for C-clinics compared with H-clinics (Sokolow-Lyon: -93.9 versus -54.9 μV, $P=0.049$; Cornell voltage: -68.1 versus -35.9 μV, $P=0.019$; Cornell voltage product: -4.6 versus -2.2 μV/ms, $P=0.071$; left ventricular mass: -4.4 versus -2.8 g, $P=0.002$). At the individual participant level, Sokolow-Lyon and left ventricular mass were significantly lower for SI men receiving CTD compared with HCTZ through 48 months and 84 months of follow-up. Our findings on left ventricular hypertrophy support the idea that greater blood pressure reduction with CTD than HCTZ may have led to differences in mortality observed in the Multiple Risk Factor Intervention Trial.

▶ The majority of the prescriptions for nonloop diuretics in the United States are for hydrochlorothiazide (HCTZ), which is also a common component of single-pill combination products. Yet chlorthalidone is the thiazidelike diuretic that has been used in clinical trials sponsored by the US National Institutes of Health since the early 1980s. The rationale for the decision to use chlorthalidone over hydrochlorothiazide received very little publicity at the time.[1,2] Differences between the 2 drugs have recently been highlighted by the disparate results of ALLHAT, which showed superiority of chlorthalidone[3] compared with either ANBP-2[4] or ACCOMPLISH[5] (both of which showed inferior results with hydrochlorothiazide). Some of these authors directly compared the 2 agents' effects on blood pressure,[6] another group has formally analyzed the outcomes in the Multiple Risk Factor Intervention Trial (MRFIT) and demonstrated what the MRFIT Steering Committee observed, which led to the switching from HCTZ to chlorthalidone of all subjects in that trial who were originally taking HCTZ.[7]

To assess whether there were differences in target-organ damage during MRFIT that could be attributed to the different diuretics, these authors dusted off a great deal of old data and examined the serial changes in electrocardiographic voltage (or other criteria for left ventricular hypertrophy) in the 2 treated groups. They were rewarded by finding that greater longitudinal reductions in several parameters related to electrocardiographic manifestations of hypertension in the group given chlorthalidone than in the group given HCTZ. This is consistent with the hypothesis that chlorthalidone provided better blood pressure control, which might be the reason regression of left ventricular hypertrophy and cardiac morbidity and mortality were better in the chlorthalidone-treated group.

As always, these decades-old data leave room for doubt. The selection of diuretic was not randomized in the study, and there were many "cross-overs" and "dropouts" that tend to bias the result toward the null. The doses of diuretics used in MRFIT were much higher than those used today; some have criticized the 12.5-mg/d dose of hydrochlorothiazide as being too low to provide comparable blood pressure reductions to other antihypertensive drugs.[8] These authors used the extant electrocardiographic criteria for left ventricular hypertrophy in the 1980s rather than more sensitive echocardiographic or magnetic resonance imaging techniques that are more widely used today. Finally, there were some inconsistencies in their results, particularly when the data were analyzed using the more specific "Cornell voltage-duration" criteria for left ventricular hypertrophy. It is nonetheless interesting that data from more than 30 years ago are still useful in addressing unresolved questions about drugs that were approved by the US Food and Drug Administration in the late 1960s!

W. J. Elliott, MD, PhD

References

1. Kolata G. Heart study produces a surprise result. *Science.* 1982;218:31-32.
2. Mortality after 10 1/2 years for hypertensive participants in the Multiple Risk Factor Intervention Trial. *Circulation.* 1990;82:1616-1628.
3. ALLHAT Officers and Coordinators for the ALLHAT Collaborative Research Group. The Antihypertensive and Lipid-Lowering Treatment to Prevent Heart Attack Trial. Major outcomes in high-risk hypertensive patients randomized to angiotensin-converting enzyme inhibitor or calcium channel blocker vs diuretic: the Antihypertensive and Lipid-Lowering Treatment to Prevent Heart Attack Trial (ALLHAT). *JAMA.* 2002;288:2981-2997.
4. Wing LM, Reid CM, Ryan P, et al; Second Australian National Blood Pressure Study Group. A comparison of outcomes with angiotensin-converting—enzyme inhibitors and diuretics for hypertension in the elderly. *N Engl J Med.* 2003;348:583-592.
5. Jamerson K, Weber MA, Bakris GL, et al; ACCOMPLISH Trial Investigators; Benazepril plus amlodipine or hydrochlorothiazide for hypertension in high-risk patients. *N Engl J Med.* 2008;359:2417-2428.
6. Ernst ME, Carter BL, Goerdt CJ, et al. Comparative antihypertensive effects of hydrochlorothiazide and chlorthalidone on ambulatory and office blood pressure. *Hypertension.* 2006;47:352-358.
7. Dorsch MP, Gillespie BW, Erickson SR, Bleske BE, Weder AB. Chlorthalidone reduces cardiovascular events compared with hydrochlorothiazide: a retrospective cohort analysis. *Hypertension.* 2011;57:689-694.
8. Messerli FH, Makani H, Benjo A, Romero J, Alviar C, Bangalore S. Antihypertensive efficacy of hydrochlorothiazide as evaluated by ambulatory blood pressure monitoring: a meta-analysis of randomized trials. *J Am Coll Cardiol.* 2011;57:590-600.

Association of blood pressure in late adolescence with subsequent mortality: cohort study of Swedish male conscripts
Sundström J, Neovius M, Tynelius P, et al (Uppsala Univ, Sweden; Karolinska Institutet, Stockholm, Sweden)
BMJ 342:d643, 2011

Objective.—To investigate the nature and magnitude of relations of systolic and diastolic blood pressures in late adolescence to mortality.

Design.—Nationwide cohort study.

Setting.—General community in Sweden.

Participants.—Swedish men (n=1 207 141) who had military conscription examinations between 1969 and 1995 at a mean age of 18.4 years, followed up for a median of 24 (range 0-37) years.

Main Outcome Measures.—Total mortality, cardiovascular mortality, and non-cardiovascular mortality.

Results.—During follow-up, 28 934 (2.4%) men died. The relation of systolic blood pressure to total mortality was U shaped, with the lowest risk at a systolic blood pressure of about 130 mm Hg. This pattern was driven by the relation to non-cardiovascular mortality, whereas the relation to cardiovascular mortality was monotonically increasing (higher risk with higher blood pressure). The relation of diastolic blood pressure to mortality risk was monotonically increasing and stronger than that of systolic blood pressure, in terms of both relative risk and population attributable fraction (deaths that could be avoided if blood pressure was in the optimal range). Relations to cardiovascular and non-cardiovascular mortality were similar, with an apparent risk threshold at a diastolic blood pressure of about 90 mm Hg, below which diastolic blood pressure and mortality were unrelated, and above which risk increased steeply with higher diastolic blood pressures.

Conclusions.—In adolescent men, the relation of diastolic blood pressure to mortality was more consistent than that of systolic blood pressure. Considering current efforts for earlier detection and prevention of risk, these observations emphasise the risk associated with high diastolic blood pressure in young adulthood.

▶ Blood pressure is a potent risk factor for cardiovascular morbidity and mortality,[1] but the focus changes from diastolic blood pressure in younger people to systolic blood pressure past 50 years of age.[2] Some have suggested that because the absolute risk of cardiovascular events is small in younger people, a more focused approach solely on systolic blood pressure is warranted.[3] This study was therefore undertaken to compare the predictive value of systolic and diastolic blood pressures in a large cohort of male Swedes who were examined before joining the armed services at around age 18 and were then followed prospectively for more than 24 years.

The methods used to measure blood pressure in the Swedish military conscription service differ from current US guidelines and practice.[4] A single blood pressure reading was taken after 5 to 10 minutes of quiet rest in the supine position and was repeated (and replaced) if it was either high or low. The authors used standard techniques for the remainder of their methodologies and, amazingly, lost no subjects to follow-up; they even knew which men emigrated and when. The finding that is most difficult to explain was the J- or U-shaped curve for diastolic blood pressure, because the military conscription service routinely excluded young men with disabilities and chronic diseases, so the likelihood of "reverse causality" is remote. The authors discuss a number of other possibilities, including chronic cerebral hypoperfusion and ischemia (perhaps related to accidental death), suicide, and other options, but none seems a clear favorite.

These data are consistent with many other data sets in even larger cohorts of older people,[1] but these are perhaps the most useful population-based data from a white, northern European cohort. The obvious limitations of including no women, minorities, or non-Swedes do not lessen their impact. They remind us of the importance of measuring blood pressure in adolescent men, despite the fact that most of them have many decades before cardiovascular events occur.

W. J. Elliott, MD, PhD

References

1. Lewington S, Clarke R, Qizilbash N, Peto R, Collins R; Prospective Studies Collaboration. Age-specific relevance of usual blood pressure to vascular mortality: a meta-analysis of individual data for one million adults in 61 prospective studies. *Lancet.* 2002;360:1903-1913.
2. Burt VL, Cutler JA, Higgins M, et al. Trends in the prevalence, awareness, treatment, and control of hypertension in the adult US population. Data from the health examination surveys, 1960 to 1991. *Hypertension.* 1995;26:60-69.
3. Izzo JL Jr, Levy D, Black HR. Clinical advisory statement. Importance of systolic blood pressure in older Americans. *Hypertension.* 2000;35:1021-1024.
4. Pickering TG, Hall JE, Appel LJ, et al; Subcommittee of Professional and Public Education of the American Heart Association Council on High Blood Pressure Research. Recommendations for blood pressure measurement in humans and experimental animals: Part 1: blood pressure measurement in humans: a statement for professionals from the Subcommittee of Professional and Public Education of the American Heart Association Council on High Blood Pressure Research. *Hypertension.* 2005;45: 142-161.

Blood Pressure Targets Recommended by Guidelines and Incidence of Cardiovascular and Renal Events in the Ongoing Telmisartan Alone and in Combination With Ramipril Global Endpoint Trial (ONTARGET)

Mancia G, Schumacher H, Redon J, et al (Università Milano-Bicocca, Monza, Milano, Italy; Boehringer-Ingelheim, Germany; Carlos III, Hospital Clinico Universitario, Valencia, Spain; et al)
Circulation 124:1727-1736, 2011

Background.—Hypertension treatment guidelines recommend that blood pressure (BP) be lowered to <140/90 mm Hg, but that a reduction to <130/80 mm Hg be adopted in patients at high cardiovascular (CV) risk. We investigated the CV and renal benefits associated with these BP targets in the high-CV-risk population of the Ongoing Telmisartan Alone and in Combination With Ramipril Global End Point Trial (ONTARGET).

Methods and Results.—Patients were divided into 4 groups according to the proportion of in-treatment visits before the occurrence of an event (<25%—>75%) in which BP was reduced to <140/90 or <130/80 mm Hg. After adjustment for demographic and clinical variables, a progressive increase in the proportion of visits in which BP was reduced to <140/90 or <130/80 mm Hg was associated with a progressive reduction in the risk of stroke, new onset of microalbuminuria or macroalbuminuria, and return to normoalbuminuria in albuminuric patients. An increased frequency of BP control to either target did not have any consistent effect on the adjusted risk of myocardial infarction and heart failure. The adjusted risk of CV events was reduced by increasing the frequency of BP control to <140/90 mm Hg, but not to <130/80 mm Hg. Similar findings were obtained for the achievement of the BP target in the visit preceding a CV event.

Conclusion.—The more frequent achievement of the BP targets recommended by guidelines led to cerebrovascular and renal protection, but did not increase cardiac protection. Overall, CV protection was favorably affected by the less tight but not by the tighter BP target.

Clinical Trial Registration.—URL: http://www.clinicaltrials.gov. Unique identifier: NCT00153101.

▶ One of the more contentious controversies in hypertension today is the proper target blood pressure for high-risk patients. Traditional principles of preventive medicine suggest that higher-risk patients should have lower therapeutic targets, such as the various levels of low-density lipoprotein cholesterol recommended for different risk groups in the most recent updates from the National Cholesterol Education Program.[1] This concept was endorsed, without much good clinical trial evidence for it, in US National Hypertension guidelines in Joint National Committee (JNC) 6[2] and JNC 7[3] for diabetics and those with chronic kidney disease; an American Heart Association Scientific Statement added patients with established heart disease to those for whom a blood pressure target of less than 130/80 mm Hg was recommended,[4] based primarily on a posthoc analysis of progression of plaque by ultrasound scan. Disciples of evidence-based medicine have assailed these recommendations, and it is likely that some, if not all, recommendations to achieve the less-than 130/80 mm Hg target will soon be abandoned in the United States, as has been done in other recent guidelines.[5,6]

These authors have access to data from more than 25 000 high-risk patients who were randomly assigned to different antihypertensive drug regimens that showed no outcome differences across the randomized groups. They therefore had the capacity to analyze their data *post hoc* to see if more or less frequent achievement of in-treatment blood pressure targets was associated with a graded degree of cardiovascular risk. Their data are interesting, although obviously confounded by *post-hoc* assumptions[7] as well as other issues. They suggest that the blood pressure target of less than 140/90 mm Hg seems to be reasonably well supported by their data for essentially all endpoints. The target of less than 130/80 mm Hg was seemingly effective in reducing stroke and progression of renal disease (pretty much irrespective of how that endpoint was defined: end-stage renal disease, doubling of serum creatinine, or multiple cutpoints for albuminuria).

The authors' conclusions are consistent with similar analyses done in other trials, either as a primary analysis (eg, Action to Control Cardiovascular Outcomes in Diabetes[8]) or in *post-hoc* analyses (eg, International Verapamil-Trandolapril Study[9]) that suggest that stroke is more sensitive to lowered blood pressure than most other endpoints and that lowering blood pressure too far may increase cardiac events. It will be difficult to sort out these important ideas without more trials that specifically randomize and successfully treat patients to different blood pressure targets, as was attempted in the Hypertension Optimal Treatment Study.[10]

W. J. Elliott, MD, PhD

References

1. Grundy SM, Cleeman JI, Merz CNB, et al; National Heart, Lung, and Blood Institute; American College of Cardiology Foundation; American Heart Association.

Implications of recent clinical trials for the National Cholesterol Education Program Adult Treatment Panel III Guidelines. *Circulation.* 2004;110:227-239.

2. The Sixth Report of the Joint National Committee on Prevention, Detection, Evaluation, and Treatment of High Blood Pressure. *Arch Intern Med.* 1997;157:2413-2446.
3. Chobanian AV, Bakris GL, Black HR, et al; Joint National Committee on Prevention, Detection, Evaluation, and Treatment of High Blood Pressure. National Heart, Lung, and Blood Institute; National High Blood Pressure Education Program Coordinating Committee. Seventh report of the Joint National Committee on Prevention, Detection, Evaluation, and Treatment of High Blood Pressure. *Hypertension.* 2003;42:1206-1252.
4. Rosendorff C, Black HR, Cannon CP, et al; American Heart Association Council for High Blood Pressure Research; American Heart Association Council on Clinical Cardiology; American Heart Association Council on Epidemiology and Prevention. Treatment of hypertension in the prevention and management of ischemic heart disease: a scientific statement from the American Heart Association Council for High Blood Pressure Research and the Councils on Clinical Cardiology and Epidemiology and Prevention. *Circulation.* 2007;115:2761-2788.
5. Mancia G, Laurent S, Agabiti-Rosei E, et al. Reappraisal of European guidelines on hypertension management: a European Society of Hypertension Task Force document. *J Hypertens.* 2009;27:2121-2158.
6. Williams B, Williams H, Northedge J, et al; Guideline Development Groups, National Collaborating Centres, and NICE Project Team. NICE Clinical Guideline 127: Hypertension: Clinical Management of Primary Hypertension in Adults. United Kingdom National Health Service: National Institute for Health and Clinical Excellence. http://www.nice.org.uk/CG127. Accessed August 24, 2011.
7. Davis EM, Appel LJ, Wang X, et al; African American Study of Kidney Disease and Hypertension Research Collaborative Group. Limitations of analyses based on achieved blood pressure: lessons from the African American study of kidney disease and hypertension trial. *Hypertension.* 2011;57:1061-1068.
8. ACCORD Study Group, Cushman WC, Evans GW, Byington RP, et al. Effects of intensive blood-pressure control in type 2 diabetes mellitus. *N Engl J Med.* 2010; 362:1575-1585.
9. Messerli FH, Mancia G, Conti CR, et al. Dogma disputed: can aggressively lowering blood pressure in hypertensive patients with coronary artery disease be dangerous? *Ann Intern Med.* 2006;144:884-893.
10. Hansson L, Zanchetti A, Carruthers SG, et al. Effects of intensive blood-pressure lowering and low-dose aspirin in patients with hypertension: principal results of the Hypertension Optimal Treatment (HOT) randomised trial. HOT Study Group. *Lancet.* 1998;351:1755-1762.

Better compliance to antihypertensive medications reduces cardiovascular risk

Corrao G, Parodi A, Nicotra F, et al (Univ of Milano-Bicocca, Italy)
J Hypertens 29:610-618, 2011

Objective.—The effect of compliance with antihypertensive medications on the risk of cardiovascular outcomes in a population without a known history of cardiovascular disease has been addressed by a large population-based prospective, cohort study carried out by linking Italian administrative databases.

Methods.—The cohort of 242 594 patients aged 18 years or older, residents in the Italian Lombardy Region, who were newly treated for hypertension during 2000—2001, was followed from index prescription until 2007.

During this period patients who experienced a hospitalization for coronary or cerebrovascular disease were identified (outcome). Exposure to antihypertensive drugs from index prescription until the date of hospitalization or censoring was assessed. Proportional hazards models were fitted to assess the association between persistence on and adherence with antihypertensive drug therapy and outcome. Data were adjusted for several covariates.

Results.—During an average follow-up of 6 years, 12 016 members of the cohort experienced the outcome. Compared with patients who experienced at least one episode of treatment discontinuation, those who continued treatment had a 37% reduced risk of cardiovascular outcomes (95% confidence interval 34—40%). Compared with patients who had very low drug coverage (proportion of days covered ≤25%), those at intermediate (from 51 to 75%) and high coverage (>75%) had risk reductions of 20% (16—24%) and 25% (20—29%), respectively. Similar effects were observed when coronary and cerebrovascular events were considered separately.

Conclusions.—In the real life setting, fulfillment compliance with antihypertensive medications is effective in the primary prevention of cardiovascular outcomes.

▶ Although hypertension can be treated by a variety of blood pressure—lowering medications, the observed reductions in cardiovascular events are generally lower than those predicted from epidemiologic studies. Many believe that this occurs primarily because many patients discontinue their antihypertensive medications over time for one of many possible reasons.[1] This phenomenon is common to many chronic conditions,[2] for which 1-year persistence rates average about 50% across the world.[3] It is impossible to demonstrate that long-term adherence to antihypertensive drug therapy improves prognosis in clinical trials, because nonpersistent subjects in these trials are routinely exhorted to restart their medications, which typically are provided free of charge. Disciples of evidence-based medicine would argue that large cohort studies that have suggested improved persistence reduces cardiovascular risk are, by their very nature unconvincing, because this study design ranks lower on the hierarchy of medical evidence.[4] These authors therefore took advantage of their large, government-funded pharmacy claims database in Lombardy, Italy, to see whether individuals who were more persistent with their prescription antihypertensive medications had fewer adverse cardiovascular events.

These authors used somewhat different cutpoints for their definitions of high, medium, or low adherence than are typically used in the literature.[1-3,5] Many authorities have suggested that 80% adherence is good, and less than 50% is poor.[5] These cutoffs are easier to justify than measures of persistence, simply because many patients consume antihypertensive and other medications inconsistently, and stopping for a week or a month does not correlate in large populations with complete discontinuation of medications forever. Furthermore, the authors' use of individuals who were less than 25% adherent to therapy as controls (who made up about a quarter of their sample, a much higher proportion than is seen in many other health care systems!)[2,3,6-8] may have inflated the benefits of persistent treatment in their study. There are a number of strengths to the authors' methodologies, however. They included only patients who had neither cardiovascular prescriptions (including antihypertensive agents) nor hospitalizations in the previous 3 years and included essentially everyone who started antihypertensive therapy in their large population.

The authors' conclusions are broadly consistent with similar data from other locales (most often with smaller numbers of subjects with events)[5,9-11] and support the hypothesis that taking antihypertensive medications as prescribed reduces the risk of future cardiovascular events.

W. J. Elliott, MD, PhD

References

1. Elliott WJ. Improving outcomes in hypertensive patients: focus on adherence and persistence with antihypertensive therapy. *J Clin Hypertens (Greenwich)*. 2009; 11:376-382.
2. Briesacher BA, Andrade SE, Fouayzi H, Chan KA. Comparison of drug adherence rates among patients with seven different medical conditions. *Pharmacotherapy*. 2008;28:437-443.
3. Osterberg L, Blaschke T. Adherence to medication. *N Engl J Med*. 2005;353: 487-497.
4. Sackett DL, Rosenberg WMC, Gray JA, Haynes RB, Richardson WS. Evidence Based Medicine: what it is and what it isn't [Editorial]. *BMJ*. 1996;312:71-72.
5. Mazzaglia G, Ambrosioni E, Alacqua M, et al. Adherence to antihypertensive medications and cardiovascular morbidity among newly diagnosed hypertensive patients. *Circulation*. 2009;120:1598-1605.
6. Caro JJ, Salas M, Speckman JL, Raggio G, Jackson JD. Persistence with treatment for hypertension in actual practice. *CMAJ*. 1999;160:31-37.
7. Siegel D, Lopez J, Meier J. Antihypertensive medication adherence in the Department of Veterans Affairs. *Am J Med*. 2007;120:26-32.
8. Elliott WJ, Plauschinat CA, Skrepnek GH, Gause D. Persistence, adherence, and risk of discontinuation associated with commonly prescribed antihypertensive drug monotherapies. *J Am Board Fam Med*. 2007;20:72-80.
9. Ho PM, Magid DJ, Shetterly SM, et al. Importance of therapy intensification and medication nonadherence for blood pressure control in patients with coronary heart disease. *Arch Intern Med*. 2008;168:271-276.
10. Sokol MC, McGuigan KA, Verbrugge RR, Epstein RS. Impact of medication adherence on hospitalization risk and healthcare cost. *Med Care*. 2005;43:521-530.
11. Liu PH, Hu FC, Wang JD. Differential risks of stroke in pharmacotherapy on uncomplicated hypertensive patients? *J Hypertens*. 2009;27:174-180.

Miscellaneous

Effects of intensive blood pressure reduction on myocardial infarction and stroke in diabetes: a meta-analysis in 73913 patients

Reboldi G, Gentile G, Angeli F, et al (Univ of Perugia, Italy; Hosp 'Santa Maria della Misericordia', Italy; et al)
J Hypertens 29:1253-1269, 2011

Objective.—Guidelines generally recommend intensive lowering of blood pressure (BP) in patients with type 2 diabetes. There is uncertainty about the impact of this strategy on case-specific events. Thus, we generated estimates of the effects of BP reduction on the risk of myocardial infarction (MI) and stroke in diabetic patients.

Methods.—We selected studies which compared different BP-lowering agents and different BP intervention strategies in patients with diabetes. Outcome measures were MI and stroke. We abstracted information about study design, intervention, population, outcomes, and methodological quality for a total of 73 913 patients with diabetes (295 652 patient-years of exposure) randomized in 31 intervention trials.

Results.—Overall, experimental treatment reduced the risk of stroke by 9% ($P = 0.0059$), and that of MI by 11% ($P = 0.0015$). Allocation to more-tight, compared with less-tight, BP control reduced the risk of stroke by 31% [relative risk (RR) 0.61, 95% confidence interval (CI) 0.48−0.79], whereas the reduction in the risk of MI approached, but did not achieve, significance [odds ratio (OR) 0.87, 95% CI 0.74−1.02]. In a meta-regression analysis, the risk of stroke decreased by 13% (95% CI 5−20, $P = 0.002$) for each 5-mmHg reduction in SBP, and by 11.5% (95% CI 5−17, $P < 0.001$) for each 2-mmHg reduction in DBP. In contrast, the risk of MI did not show any association with the extent of BP reduction (SBP: $P = 0.793$; DBP: $P = 0.832$).

Conclusion.—In patients with diabetes, protection from stroke increases with the magnitude of BP reduction. We were unable to detect such a relation for MI.

▶ The lower-than-usual blood pressure goal recommended for diabetics in recent US[1,2] and international[3] hypertension guidelines have been challenged by a Cochrane Collaboration meta-analysis[4] and rejected by the even more recent guidelines from the United Kingdom's National Institute for Health and Clinical Excellence (NICE).[5] The authors, therefore, performed their own systematic review and meta-analysis of the lower blood pressure target for patients with diabetes, even before the draft NICE guidelines were made public.

These authors accepted 31 clinical trials that examined outcomes in diabetic hypertensives, but only a small subset of these trials specifically tested the hypothesis that a lower-than-usual blood pressure target might prevent cardiovascular events. A more selective and more recent systematic review and meta-analysis identified only 5 trials to answer this question[6] and concluded (as did these authors) that there was a benefit of the lower blood pressure target on stroke and major cardiovascular events but not myocardial infarction, cardiovascular death, death, or heart failure. These were also the conclusions of the 2005 meta-analysis of the Blood Pressure Lowering Trialists' Collaboration.[7]

It is perhaps not surprising that stroke should be more sensitive to blood pressure manipulation than myocardial infarction, as hypertension's population-based attributable risk for stroke is about 50% but for myocardial infarction is only perhaps 25% to 33%. This difference has been seen in many trials and many meta-regression analyses.

The more difficult question is whether the decrease in stroke risk associated with a lower blood pressure target can or should be considered sufficient to continue to recommend less than 130/80 mm Hg for diabetics. The large Action to Control Cardiovascular Risk in Diabetes (ACCORD)[8] trial has already concluded that the correct answer is "No!" It is doubtful that the upcoming

Eighth Report of the (US) Joint National Committee on Prevention, Detection, Evaluation, and Treatment of High Blood Pressure will be dissuaded from the ACCORD conclusion by this (or any other) meta-analysis.

W. J. Elliott, MD, PhD

References

1. Chobanian AV, Bakris GL, Black HR, et al; National High Blood Pressure Education Program Coordinating Committee. Seventh report of the Joint National Committee on Prevention, Detection, Evaluation and Treatment of High Blood Pressure. *Hypertension.* 2003;42:1206-1252.
2. American Diabetes Association. Standards of medical care in diabetes—2011. *Diabetes Care.* 2011;34:S11-S61.
3. Mancia G, Laurent S, Agabiti-Rosei E, et al. Reappraisal of European guidelines on hypertension management: a European Society of Hypertension Task Force document. *J Hypertens.* 2009;27:2121-2158.
4. Arguedas JA, Perez MI, Wright JM. Treatment blood pressure targets for hypertension. *Cochrane Database Syst Rev.* 2009;(3): CD004349.
5. NICE clinical guideline 127: Hypertension: Clinical management of primary hypertension in adults. http://www.nice.org.uk/CG127. Accessed August 24, 2011.
6. Elliott WJ. What should be the blood pressure target for diabetics? *Curr Opin Cardiol.* 2011;26:308-313.
7. Turnbull F, Neal B, Algert C, et al; for the Blood Pressure Lowering Treatment Trialists' Collaboration. Effects of different blood pressure-lowering regimens on major cardiovascular events in individuals with and without diabetes mellitus: results of prospectively designed overviews of randomized trials. *Arch Intern Med.* 2005;165:1410-1419.
8. Cushman WC, Evans GW, Byington RP, et al; on behalf of The Action to Control Cardiovascular Risk in Diabetes (ACCORD) Study Group. Effects of intensive blood-pressure control in type 2 diabetes mellitus. *N Engl J Med.* 2010;362: 1575-1585.

Prevalence of Resistant Hypertension in the United States, 2003—2008
Persell SD (Northwestern Univ, Chicago, IL)
Hypertension 57:1076-1080, 2011

The prevalence of resistant hypertension is unknown. Much previous knowledge comes from referral populations or clinical trial participants. Using data from the National Health and Nutrition Examination Survey from 2003 through 2008, nonpregnant adults with hypertension were classified as resistant if their blood pressure was $\geq 140/90$ mm Hg and they reported using antihypertensive medications from 3 different drug classes or drugs from ≥ 4 antihypertensive drug classes regardless of blood pressure. Among US adults with hypertension, 8.9% (SE: 0.6%) met criteria for resistant hypertension. This represented 12.8% (SE: 0.9%) of the antihypertensive drug-treated population. Of all drug-treated adults whose hypertension was uncontrolled, 72.4% (SE: 1.6%) were taking drugs from <3 classes. Compared with those with controlled hypertension using 1 to 3 medication classes, adults with resistant hypertension were more likely to be older, to be non-Hispanic black, and to have higher body mass index (all $P<0.001$).

They were more likely to have albuminuria, reduced renal function, and self-reported medical histories of coronary heart disease, heart failure, stroke, and diabetes mellitus ($P<0.001$). Most (85.6% [SE: 2.4%]) individuals with resistant hypertension used a diuretic. Of this group, 64.4% (SE: 3.2%) used the relatively weak thiazide diuretic hydrochlorothiazide. Although not rare, resistant hypertension is currently found in only a modest proportion of the hypertensive population. Among those classified here as resistant, inadequate diuretic therapy may be a modifiable therapeutic target. Cardiovascular diseases, diabetes mellitus, obesity, and renal dysfunction were all common in this population.

▶ "Resistant hypertension" has been variously defined, but a recent Scientific Statement from the American Heart Association accepts any patient whose blood pressure is ≥140/90 mm Hg, despite prescription of 3 drugs, or any patient who takes ≥4 antihypertensive agents per day.[1] Accurate estimates of the prevalence of this condition are difficult to obtain.[1] Some useful data come from clinical trials, the recruitment process of which seldom accounts for the biases of referral and volunteerism.[2,3] Other estimates come from centers that specialize in treating this problem[4,5]; only a few reports come from population-based surveys or registries.[6] The author therefore studied the National Health and Nutrition Examination Surveys (NHANES), which attempt to attain a representative sample of noninstitutionalized, civilian adult Americans from 2003 to 2008.

The sample size for the 3 surveys was 15 968 nonpregnant adults, of whom 898 had no blood pressure readings and were therefore excluded. Medication use was assessed by reference to pill bottles in 89.8% of subjects and reflected the 30 days prior to the examination (which eliminated another 2% of the subjects). NHANES methodology typically oversamples minority and older populations, but it is unclear how these data were adjusted in these analyses. Other data, for example, indicate that the overall prevalence of hypertension has remained relatively constant in the United States since about 1994 at approximately 29%[7]; data from this article suggest a higher prevalence of 35.4% (5230/[15 070*0.98]).

The author correctly identifies several limitations of these data, including the lack of information about adherence and "white-coat hypertension," (which was noted in about 38% of Spanish "resistant" hypertensives[6]), and one-time or occasional use of a drug (eg, furosemide) versus usual daily use. The author also notes (as have others[8]) that few individuals used chlorthalidone or a loop diuretic and that resistant hypertension was significantly more common among older people, blacks, diabetics, and those with pre-existing cardiovascular or renal disease. Thus, this estimate of the prevalence of resistant hypertension at about 9% of hypertensives, although lower than others,[1-9] is probably one of the more valid determinations in a nationwide, population-based, cross-sectional study.

W. J. Elliott, MD, PhD

References

1. Calhoun DA, Jones D, Textor S, et al. Resistant hypertension: diagnosis, evaluation, and treatment. A scientific statement from the American Heart Association

Professional Education Committee of the Council for High Blood Pressure Research. *Hypertension.* 2008;51:1403-1419.

2. Cushman WC, Ford CE, Cutler JA, et al. Success and predictors of blood pressure control in diverse North American settings: the antihypertensive and lipid-lowering treatment to prevent heart attack trial (ALLHAT). *J Clin Hypertens (Greenwich).* 2002;4:393-404.

3. Chapman N, Dobson J, Wilson S, et al; Anglo-Scandinavian Cardiac Outcomes Trial Investigators. Effect of spironolactone on blood pressure in subjects with resistant hypertension. *Hypertension.* 2007;49:839-845.

4. Garg JP, Elliott WJ, Folker A, Izhar M, Black HR; RUSH University Hypertension Service. Resistant hypertension revisited: a comparison of two university-based cohorts. *Am J Hypertens.* 2005;18:619-626.

5. Taler SJ, Textor SC, Augustine JE. Resistant hypertension: comparing hemodynamic management to specialist care. *Hypertension.* 2002;39:982-988.

6. de la Sierra A, Segura J, Banegas JR, et al. Clinical features of 8295 patients with resistant hypertension classified on the basis of ambulatory blood pressure monitoring. *Hypertension.* 2011;57:898-902.

7. Egan BM, Zhao Y, Axon RN. US trends in prevalence, awareness, treatment and control of hypertension: 1998-2008. *JAMA.* 2010;303:2043-2050.

8. De Nicola L, Borrelli S, Gabbai FB, et al. Burden of resistant hypertension in hypertensive patients with non-dialysis chronic kidney disease. *Kidney Blood Press Res.* 2011;34:58-67.

9. McAdam-Marx C, Ye X, Sung JC, Brixner DI, Kahler KH. Results of a retrospective, observational pilot study using electronic medical records to assess the prevalence and characteristics of patients with resistant hypertension in an ambulatory care setting. *Clin Ther.* 2009;31:1116-1123.

Uncontrolled and Apparent Treatment Resistant Hypertension in the United States, 1988 to 2008

Egan BM, Zhao Y, Axon RN, et al (Med Univ of South Carolina, Charleston; et al)

Circulation 124:1046-1058, 2011

Background.—Despite progress, many hypertensive patients remain uncontrolled. Defining characteristics of uncontrolled hypertensives may facilitate efforts to improve blood pressure control.

Methods and Results.—Subjects included 13 375 hypertensive adults from National Health and Nutrition Examination Surveys (NHANESs) subdivided into 1988 to 1994, 1999 to 2004, and 2005 to 2008. Uncontrolled hypertension was defined as blood pressure $\geq 140/\geq 90$ mm Hg and apparent treatment-resistant hypertension (aTRH) when subjects reported taking ≥ 3 antihypertensive medications. Framingham 10-year coronary risk was calculated. Multivariable logistic regression was used to identify clinical characteristics associated with untreated, treated uncontrolled on 1 to 2 blood pressure medications, and aTRH across all 3 survey periods. More than half of uncontrolled hypertensives were untreated across surveys, including 52.2% in 2005 to 2008. Clinical factors linked with untreated hypertension included male sex, infrequent healthcare visits (0 to 1 per year), body mass index <25 kg/m^2, absence of chronic kidney disease, and Framingham 10-year coronary risk $<10\%$ ($P<0.01$). Most treated uncontrolled patients reported taking 1 to 2 blood pressure medications, a proxy for therapeutic inertia. This group was older, had higher Framingham 10-year coronary risk than patients controlled on 1 to 2 medications ($P<0.01$), and comprised 34.4% of all uncontrolled and 72.0% of treated uncontrolled patients in 2005 to 2008. We found that aTRH increased from 15.9% (1998–2004) to 28.0% (2005–2008) of treated patients ($P<0.001$). Clinical characteristics associated with aTRH included ≥4 visits per year, obesity, chronic kidney disease, and Framingham 10-year coronary risk >20% ($P<0.01$).

Conclusion.—Untreated, undertreated, and aTRH patients have consistent characteristics that could inform strategies to improve blood pressure control by decreasing untreated hypertension, reducing therapeutic inertia in undertreated patients, and enhancing therapeutic efficiency in aTRH.

▶ The prevalence of resistant hypertension in the United States is difficult to estimate precisely, although a recent Scientific Statement from the American Heart Association[1] codified the definition as "hypertension treated with 4 antihypertensive medications or a blood pressure ≥140/90 mm Hg despite 3 drugs." Because the prevalence of hypertension in US adults has been relatively constant at about 29% from 1994 to 2008,[2] and the number of people taking multiple antihypertensive medications is small, the National Health and Nutrition Examination Surveys (NHANES) from 2003 to 2008 had to be pooled to provide a reasonably precise estimate of the prevalence of resistant hypertension, which was 9% of hypertensives, or 12.8% of treated hypertensives.[3] These data from a representative sample of the US population are lower than estimates from a US managed care organization (12.4%),[4] or in Spain (12.2%).[5]

These authors used a slightly different approach to overcome the relatively small numbers of people with resistant hypertension surveyed in NHANES. They expanded the number of surveys to match their previous work[2] and calculated the proportion of "uncontrolled hypertensives" that were treated with ≥3 drugs as well as "apparent treatment-resistant hypertensives" who were treated with ≥3 drugs. Overall, from 1988 to 2008, the proportion of controlled hypertensives improved (ie, declined) over time, but the proportion of "apparent treatment-resistant hypertension" increased from 15.9% (from 1998 to 2004) to 28.0% (2005 to 2008). They found that untreated hypertensives were more likely to be men, obese, and infrequent visitors to medical offices and have no chronic kidney disease. Like other authors,[3,5] they found that "apparent treatment-resistant hypertensives" were also more likely to be obese, male, and frequent visitors to medical offices or clinics and have high cardiovascular risk and chronic kidney disease. Surprisingly, they did not identify diabetes mellitus as a risk factor for either problem, perhaps because they used the less-than 140/90 mm Hg cutoff, rather than the less-than 130/80 mm Hg recommended by 2007-11 US hypertension treatment guidelines.[6,7]

The authors' conclusions are broadly consistent with a separate analysis of the same dataset[3] and support the hypothesis that targeting obese men with high cardiovascular risk who take few antihypertensive medications despite fairly frequent visits to health care providers might improve blood pressure control in the United States even further.

W. J. Elliott, MD, PhD

References

1. Calhoun DA, Jones D, Textor S, et al. Resistant hypertension: diagnosis, evaluation, and treatment. A scientific statement from the American Heart Association Professional Education Committee of the Council for High Blood Pressure Research. *Hypertension.* 2008;51:1403-1419.
2. Egan BM, Zhao Y, Axon RN. US trends in prevalence, awareness, treatment, and control of hypertension, 1988−2008. *JAMA.* 2010;303:2043-2050.
3. Persell SD. Prevalence of resistant hypertension in the United States, 2003−2008. *Hypertension.* 2011;57:1076-1080.
4. McAdam-Marx C, Ye X, Sung JC, Brixner DI, Kahler KH. Results of a retrospective, observational pilot study using electronic medical records to assess the prevalence and characteristics of patients with resistant hypertension in an ambulatory care setting. *Clin Ther.* 2009;31:1116-1123.
5. de la Sierra A, Segura J, Banegas JR, et al. Clinical features of 8295 patients with resistant hypertension classified on the basis of ambulatory blood pressure monitoring. *Hypertension.* 2011;57:898-902.
6. Chobanian AV, Bakris GL, Black HR, et al; Joint National Committee on Prevention, Detection, Evaluation, and Treatment of High Blood Pressure. National Heart, Lung, and Blood Institute; National High Blood Pressure Education Program Coordinating Committee. Seventh report of the Joint National Committee on Prevention, Detection, Evaluation, and Treatment of High Blood Pressure. *Hypertension.* 2003; 42:1206-1252.
7. Basevi V, Di Mario S, Morciano C, Nonino F, Magrini N. Comment on: American Diabetes Association. Standards of medical care in diabetes—2011. Diabetes Care 2011;34(Suppl. 1):S11-S61. *Diabetes Care.* 2011;34:e53.

Clinical features of 8295 patients with resistant hypertension classified on the basis of ambulatory blood pressure monitoring

de la Sierra A, Segura J, Banegas JR, et al (Univ of Barcelona, Terrassa, Spain; Hosp 12 de Octubre, Madrid, Spain; Autonomous Univ, Madrid, Spain; et al)
Hypertension 57:898-902, 2011

We aimed to estimate the prevalence of resistant hypertension through both office and ambulatory blood pressure monitoring in a large cohort of treated hypertensive patients from the Spanish Ambulatory Blood Pressure Monitoring Registry. In addition, we also compared clinical features of patients with true or white-coat-resistant hypertension. In December 2009, we identified 68 045 treated patients with complete information for this analysis. Among them, 8295 (12.2% of the database) had resistant hypertension (office blood pressure $\geq$140 and/or 90 mm Hg while being treated with $\geq$3 antihypertensive drugs, 1 of them being a diuretic). After ambulatory blood pressure monitoring, 62.5% of patients were classified as true resistant hypertensives, the remaining 37.5% having white-coat resistance. The former group was younger, more frequently men, with a longer duration of hypertension and a worse cardiovascular risk profile. The group included larger proportions of smokers, diabetics, target organ damage (including left ventricular hypertrophy, impaired renal function, and microalbuminuria), and documented cardiovascular disease. Moreover, true resistant hypertensives exhibited in a greater proportion a riser pattern (22% versus 18%; $P<0.001$). In conclusion, this study first reports the prevalence of resistant hypertension in a large cohort of patients in usual daily practice. Resistant hypertension is present in 12% of the treated hypertensive population, but among them more than one third have normal ambulatory blood pressure. A worse risk profile is associated with true resistant hypertension, but this association is weak, thus making it necessary to assess ambulatory blood pressure monitoring for a correct diagnosis and management.

▶ "Resistant hypertension" has been difficult to define, both diagnostically and etiologically. A recent Scientific Statement from the American Heart Association accepts "any patient whose blood pressure is ≥140/90 mm Hg, despite prescription of 3 drugs, or any patient who takes ≥4 antihypertensive agents/day."[1] The differential diagnosis for this condition includes a wide variety of options, including "white-coat hypertension." The prevalence of resistant hypertension was thought to be approximately 15% to 20% of hypertensives, but more recent data suggest a lower number (9%–14%).[2,3] Estimates of the true prevalence of "white-coat hypertension" have also been imprecise, but identification of patients with resistant hypertension who have white-coat hypertension is of great public health importance, because these have a better prognosis than "true" resistant hypertension.[4]

These data are interesting from a number of perspectives. They estimate that, in Spain, 12.2% of hypertensives have resistant hypertension, as defined by the American Heart Association's Scientific Statement.[1] Perhaps more important, 37.5% of patients with resistant hypertension displayed white-coat hypertension on ambulatory blood pressure monitoring. These data support the recent update of British hypertension guidelines that suggest a wider role for ambulatory blood pressure monitoring for achieving a proper diagnosis in a person thought to have hypertension.[5] These authors also found that those who displayed the "white-coat effect" were significantly older and had a significantly lower prevalence of every cardiovascular risk factor that was examined. Perhaps more interestingly, those with white-coat resistant hypertension were significantly less likely to show the "early morning surge" in blood pressure that has been linked epidemiologically to higher rates of cardiovascular events.

One wonders how applicable these data are to American and northern European populations. Some reports suggest that Spanish and Italian hypertensives are more likely to display the white-coat effect; indeed, the initial report of the phenomenon came from Milan. However, these data do remind us that ambulatory blood pressure monitoring can help distinguish between "true" and "white-coat" resistant hypertension, the latter of which has a lower risk of future cardiovascular events.

*Disclosure: I wrote the invited editorial for reference.[6]

W. J. Elliott, MD, PhD

References

1. Calhoun DA, Jones D, Textor S, et al. Resistant hypertension: diagnosis, evaluation, and treatment. A scientific statement from the American Heart Association Professional Education Committee of the Council for High Blood Pressure Research. *Hypertension.* 2008;51:1403-1419.
2. McAdam-Marx C, Ye X, Sung JC, Brixner DI, Kahler KH. Results of a retrospective, observational pilot study using electronic medical records to assess the prevalence and characteristics of patients with resistant hypertension in an ambulatory care setting. *Clin Ther.* 2009;31:1116-1123.
3. Persell SD. Prevalence of resistant hypertension in the United States, 2003–2008. *Hypertension.* 2011;57:1076-1080.
4. Fagard RH, Cornelissen VA. Incidence of cardiovascular events in white-coat, masked and sustained hypertension versus true normotension: a meta-analysis. *J Hypertens.* 2007;25:2193-2198.
5. Williams B, Williams H, Northedge J, et al; Guideline Development Groups, National Collaborating Centres, and NICE Project Team. NICE Clinical Guideline 127: Hypertension: Clinical Management of Primary Hypertension in Adults. United Kingdom National Health Service: National Institute for Health and Clinical Excellence. http://www.nice.org.uk/CG127. Accessed August 24, 2011.
6. Elliott WJ. High prevalence of white-coat hypertension in Spanish resistant hypertensive patients [Editorial Commentary]. *Hypertension.* 2011;57:889-890.

Urinary Sodium and Potassium Excretion and Risk of Cardiovascular Events

O'Donnell MJ, Yusuf S, Mente A, et al (McMaster Univ, Hamilton, Ontario, Canada; et al)
JAMA 306:2229-2238, 2011

Context.—The precise relationship between sodium and potassium intake and cardiovascular (CV) risk remains uncertain, especially in patients with CV disease.

Objective.—To determine the association between estimated urinary sodium and potassium excretion (surrogates for intake) and CV events in patients with established CV disease or diabetes mellitus.

Design, Setting, and Patients.—Observational analyses of 2 cohorts (N=28 880) included in the ONTARGET and TRANSCEND trials (November 2001-March 2008 from initial recruitment to final follow-up). We estimated 24-hour urinary sodium and potassium excretion from a morning fasting urine sample (Kawasaki formula). We used restricted cubic spline plots to describe the association between sodium and potassium excretion and CV events and mortality, and to identify reference categories for sodium and potassium excretion. We used Cox proportional hazards multivariable models to determine the association of urinary sodium and potassium with CV events and mortality.

Main Outcome Measures.—CV death, myocardial infarction (MI), stroke, and hospitalization for congestive heart failure (CHF).

Results.—At baseline, the mean (SD) estimated 24-hour excretion for sodium was 4.77 g (1.61); and for potassium was 2.19 g (0.57). After a median follow-up of 56 months, the composite outcome occurred in 4729 (16.4%) participants, including 2057 CV deaths, 1412 with MI, 1282 with stroke, and 1213 with hospitalization for CHF. Compared with the reference group with estimated baseline sodium excretion of 4 to 5.99 g per day (n=14 156; 6.3% participants with CV death, 4.6% with MI, 4.2% with stroke, and 3.8% admitted to hospital with CHF), higher baseline sodium excretion was associated with an increased risk of CV death (9.7% for 7-8 g/day; hazard ratio [HR], 1.53; 95% CI, 1.26-1.86; and 11.2% for >8 g/day; HR, 1.66; 95% CI, 1.31-2.10), MI (6.8%; HR, 1.48; 95% CI, 1.11-1.98 for >8 g/day), stroke (6.6%; HR, 1.48; 95% CI, 1.09-2.01 for >8 g/day), and hospitalization for CHF (6.5%; HR, 1.51; 1.12-2.05 for >8 g/day). Lower sodium excretion was associated with an increased risk of CV death (8.6%; HR, 1.19; 95% CI, 1.02-1.39 for 2-2.99 g/day; 10.6%; HR, 1.37; 95% CI, 1.09-1.73 for <2 g/day), and hospitalization for CHF (5.2%; HR, 1.23; 95% CI, 1.01-1.49 for 2-2.99 g/day) on multivariable analysis. Compared with an estimated potassium excretion of less than 1.5 g per day (n=2194; 6.2% with stroke), higher potassium excretion was associated with a reduced risk of stroke (4.7% [HR, 0.77; 95% CI, 0.63-0.94] for 1.5-1.99 g/day; 4.3% [HR, 0.73; 95% CI, 0.59-0.90] for 2-2.49 g/day; 3.9% [HR, 0.71; 95% CI, 0.56-0.91] for 2.5-3 g/day; and 3.5% [HR, 0.68; 95% CI, 0.49-0.92] for >3 g/day) on multivariable analysis.

Conclusions.—The association between estimated sodium excretion and CV events was J-shaped. Compared with baseline sodium excretion of 4 to 5.99 g per day, sodium excretion of greater than 7 g per day was associated with an increased risk of all CV events, and a sodium excretion of less than 3 g per day was associated with increased risk of CV mortality and hospitalization for CHF. Higher estimated potassium excretion was associated with a reduced risk of stroke.

▶ This post-hoc analysis of data from 2 related clinical trials attempts to address the important and controversial issue of dietary cation consumption (very roughly estimated at 1 point in time) and subsequent risk of cardiovascular events over about 56 months in patients at high risk for these events. Although some have expressed concern that reduction of dietary sodium may increase cardiovascular risk in the general population or in hypertensive individuals,[1,2] recent meta-analyses[3] and a recent US population-based cohort study[4] have both suggested that moderate dietary sodium restriction would be a good strategy to reduce blood pressure and cardiovascular risk. This conclusion agrees with official governmental opinions,[5] recent cost-effectiveness calculations,[6,7] and recent experience in Finland and the United Kingdom. One possible way of integrating all these data is to hypothesize a "J-shaped curve" for dietary sodium consumption and cardiovascular risk, which is in accord with these authors' data and conclusions. The caveat is the population-attributable risk of the low-sodium diet group; in this cohort, only 3% of the total patient population had an estimated 24-hour sodium excretion rate of < 2 g/d (which is currently recommended in the United States),[5] and only 29% had their rates in the next lowest category (2.0–3.99 g/d).

There are many challenges with the authors' methods of data collection, most especially the estimation of daily sodium intake based on a urinary sample collected in the morning.[8] About 70% of their study population was hypertensive, and about 29% were treated with diuretics, so a substantial proportion should have received advice about a low-sodium diet as part of their long-term treatment; the fact that only 3% had an estimated 24-hour sodium excretion of < 2 g/d is, therefore, quite surprising. If one ignores this small subset (which is admittedly one of the primary conclusions of the study), the authors' conclusions are remarkably similar to another recent analysis of population-based data from NHANES that used somewhat more sophisticated techniques of estimating urinary sodium excretion.[4]

All in all, these data are consistent with the majority of the world's literature that suggests that most people in western societies consume too much sodium. Whether a barely significant increase in risk for the 3% with the lowest estimated sodium consumption (uncorrected for multiple comparisons) should overrule the highly significant graded increase in risk for the 68% whose estimated sodium consumption was ≥4 g/d is a question for public policymakers. Further confirmation in a randomized clinical trial (not another cohort study[9]) of the excess risk among those with estimated sodium consumption in the currently recommended range should be required as well before this guideline is abandoned.

W. J. Elliott, MD, PhD

References

1. Cohen HW, Hailpern SM, Alderman MH. Sodium intake and mortality follow-up in the Third National Health and Nutrition Examination Survey (NHANES III). *J Gen Intern Med.* 2008;23:1297-1302.
2. Alderman MH. Reducing dietary sodium: the case for caution. *JAMA.* 2010;303: 448-449.
3. He FJ, MacGregor GA. Effect of modest salt reduction on blood pressure: a meta-analysis of randomized trials. Implications for public health. *J Hum Hypertens.* 2002;16:761-770.
4. Yang Q, Liu T, Kuklina EV, et al. Sodium and potassium intake and mortality among US adults: prospective data from the Third National Health and Nutrition Examination Survey. *Arch Intern Med.* 2011;171:1183-1191.
5. US Department of Health and Human Services and US Department of Agriculture. *Dietary Guidelines for Americans, 2010.* 7th ed. Washington, DC: US Government Printing Office; 2011.
6. Bibbins-Domingo K, Chertow GM, Coxson PG, et al. Projected effect of dietary salt reductions on future cardiovascular disease. *N Engl J Med.* 2010;363:590-599.
7. Smith-Spangler CM, Juusola JL, Enns EA, Owens DK, Garber AM. Population strategies to decrease sodium intake and the burden of cardiovascular disease: a cost-effectiveness analysis. *Ann Intern Med.* 2010;152:481-487.
8. Whelton PK. Urinary sodium and cardiovascular disease risk: informing guidelines for sodium consumption. *JAMA.* 2011;306:2262-2264.
9. Stolarz-Skrzypek K, Kuznetsova T, Thijs L, et al. Fatal and nonfatal outcomes, incidence of hypertension, and blood pressure changes in relation to urinary sodium excretion. *JAMA.* 2011;305:1777-1785.

Cardiovascular Outcomes in Framingham Participants With Diabetes: The Importance of Blood Pressure

Chen G, McAlister FA, Walker RL, et al (Univ of Calgary, Alberta, Canada; Univ of Alberta, Edmonton, Canada)
Hypertension 57:891-897, 2011

We designed this study to explore to what extent the excess risk of cardiovascular events in diabetic individuals is attributable to hypertension. We retrospectively analyzed prospectively collected data from the Framingham original and offspring cohorts. Of the 1145 Framingham subjects newly diagnosed with diabetes mellitus who did not have a previous history of cardiovascular events, 663 (58%) had hypertension at the time that diabetes mellitus was diagnosed. During 4154 person-years of follow-up, 125 died, and 204 experienced a cardiovascular event. Framingham participants with hypertension at the time of diabetes mellitus diagnosis exhibited higher rates of all-cause mortality (32 versus 20 per 1000 person-years; $P<0.001$) and cardiovascular events (52 versus 31 per 1000 person-years; $P<0.001$) compared with normotensive subjects with diabetes mellitus. After adjustment for demographic and clinical covariates, hypertension was associated with a 72% increase in the risk of all-cause death and a 57% increase in the risk of any cardiovascular event in individuals with diabetes mellitus. The population-attributable risk from hypertension in individuals with diabetes mellitus was 30% for all-cause death and 25% for any cardiovascular event (increasing to 44% and 41%, respectively, if the 110 normotensive subjects who developed hypertension during follow-up were excluded from the analysis). In comparison, after adjustment for concurrent hypertension, the population-attributable risk from diabetes mellitus in Framingham subjects was 7% for all-cause mortality and 9% for any cardiovascular disease event. Although diabetes mellitus is associated with increased risks of death and cardiovascular events in Framingham subjects, much of this excess risk is attributable to coexistent hypertension.

▶ Hypertension and diabetes often travel together in large populations; diabetics have a higher prevalence of hypertension than nondiabetics, and hypertensives have a higher prevalence of diabetes than nonhypertensives.[1,2] Furthermore, the risk of cardiovascular events is about 2-fold higher for patients with both hypertension and diabetes, compared with the risk of diabetic nonhypertensive patients or nondiabetic hypertensive patients.[3,4] For these reasons, it is difficult to sort out the population-attributable risk for cardiovascular disease of diabetes and hypertension. One method of attempting this is to analyze outcomes data from a closed cohort of patients in which the dates of onset of hypertension and diabetes are known, such as the Framingham Heart Study, which is what these authors did.

Assembly of the cohort was an interesting process: they used data from the original Framingham cohort (1968–1996) and the Framingham offspring cohort (1971–2001), excluded those who were originally younger than 35 years of age, from which 482 individuals were found who were normotensive when diabetes was diagnosed and 663 who were hypertensive when diabetes was first diagnosed. They then followed these individuals forward over time for the occurrence of cardiovascular events. Their major result was that hypertensive patients (at the onset of diabetes) had a significantly higher risk of both death and cardiovascular events compared with normotensives. The population-attributable risk of hypertension for death among new diabetics was 30% and 25% for cardiovascular events. These estimates were quite a bit higher than the population-attributable risk for diabetes in the same population. Their conclusion was that hypertension is a big contributor to the risk of death and cardiovascular events in diabetics.

The authors acknowledge a number of limitations to their data and conclusions. They had far better data on the date of onset of diabetes than hypertension, which makes it difficult to perform the reverse association of existing diabetes on new-onset hypertension. This is particularly important because follow-up blood pressures were generally lower (because of the institution of antihypertensive therapy) than at diagnosis, which was not the case for serum glucose measurements (which some say are more difficult to control than blood pressures). Similarly, they had no data on albuminuria, left ventricular hypertrophy, or other target organ damage from hypertension and could not use these covariates in their adjusted analyses.

These data nonetheless suggest that the presence of hypertension greatly influences prognosis in newly diagnosed diabetics. Whether these data from Framingham can be extrapolated to other populations, especially minority, in the United States (or overseas) is still an open question.

W. J. Elliott, MD, PhD

References

1. Hypertension in Diabetes Study (HDS): II. Increased risk of cardiovascular complications in hypertensive type 2 diabetic patients. *J Hypertens*. 1993;11:319-325.
2. Holman RR, Paul SK, Bethel MA, Neil HA, Matthews DR. Long-term follow-up after tight control of blood pressure in type 2 diabetes. *N Engl J Med*. 2008;359: 1565-1576.
3. Turnbull F, Neal B, Algert C, et al; Blood Pressure Lowering Treatment Trialists' Collaboration. Effects of different blood pressure-lowering regimens on major cardiovascular events in individuals with and without diabetes mellitus: results of prospectively designed overviews of randomized trials. *Arch Intern Med*. 2005;165:1410-1419.
4. Almgren T, Wilhelmsen L, Samuelsson O, Himmelmann A, Rosengren A, Andersson OK. Diabetes in treated hypertension is common and carries a high cardiovascular risk: results from a 28-year follow-up. *J Hypertens*. 2007;25:1311-1317.

Heterogeneity in antihypertensive treatment discontinuation between drugs belonging to the same class

Mancia G, Parodi A, Merlino L, et al (Univ of Milano-Bicocca, Milan, Italy)
J Hypertens 29:1012-1018, 2011

Objectives.—Discontinuation of antihypertensive treatment is known to be different for different classes of antihypertensive drugs. No information is available on whether this phenomenon differs for drugs belonging to the same class. This is clinically relevant because treatment discontinuation is mainly responsible for poor blood pressure control in the antihypertensive population.

Methods.—We studied a large (n = 131,472) cohort of patients aged 40-80 years who lived in Lombardy (Italy) and received their first antihypertensive drug prescription during 2005. Discontinuation was defined by the absence of any antihypertensive drug prescription during the 90-day period following the end of the latest prescription. Class-related and drug-related discontinuation rates were standardized according to the demographic and therapeutic structure of the entire cohort and expressed as number of patients who experienced discontinuation every 100 person-months.

Results.—Standardized rates of discontinuation ranged from 6.2 to 24.4 events every 100 person-months for patients who started monotherapy with an angiotensin receptor antagonist and a diuretic, respectively. However, there was a significant heterogeneity between treatment discontinuation rates within each class and the heterogeneity differed between classes. The highest discontinuation rate was 13.9-fold for channel blockers, but only 1.7-fold for angiotensin receptor antagonists. Within this class, losartan showed a discontinuation rate significantly greater than that of the other angiotensin receptor antagonists whose discontinuation rate was similar. A significant heterogeneity also characterized initial treatment with fixed-dose combinations of different angiotensin-converting enzyme inhibitors or angiotensin receptor antagonists with a diuretic.

Conclusion.—Comparison of treatment discontinuation between antihypertensive drug classes masks the fact that this phenomenon is heterogeneous within any given class. This is relevant to calculations of the cost-benefit of treatment, which, thus, should be drug-based rather than class-based.

▶ While many reports have indicated that different pharmacologic classes of antihypertensive drugs are associated with different rates of persistence (ie, long-term adherence to medication),[1-5] there are only a few that have suggested that some specific drugs have higher persistence rates than others in the same pharmacologic class.[6] In many cases, this phenomenon is observed because one medication is taken more often each day (eg, 4 times daily) than another (eg, once daily), and reflects an ease of administration or convenience advantage for the drug with better persistence. In the United States, the preferences of some formularies drive persistence, because the nonpreferred drug is often replaced, for economic reasons, by a drug that can be obtained at a lower acquisition cost (either out-of-pocket copayment on the part of the patient or through a lower-priced contract to the managed care organization with a manufacturer or distributor).

The medical care and pharmacy system is quite different in Italy, as all antihypertensive medications are deemed "life saving" and are all paid for by the National Health Insurance plan. This provides an excellent setting to study patients' persistence with antihypertensive medications, without the usual economic confounders found in the United States and some other countries.

There are several interesting observations that one can make about the authors' data. The first is that angiotensin-converting enzyme (ACE)-inhibitors were the most frequently prescribed monotherapy (26.2%), followed by β-blockers (14.5%), calcium antagonists (13.1%), and angiotensin receptor blockers (12.4%). The most commonly prescribed combinations were an ACE-inhibitor + diuretic (8.9%), or 2 diuretics (eg, a thiazide and triamterene, 8.1%). These proportions are somewhat different than recent data from the United States.[7] The overall discontinuation rate was 11.6 discontinuations per 100 patient-months, or 139 per 100 patient-years. This is higher than the world's average (an estimated 50% of patients stop their initial medication in a year)[8] but consistent with other pharmacy claims data from Italy,[2,3] where the persistence rates are lower than in other countries and health care systems.[1,4-6] One wonders if the authors should have adjusted their data for the length of time the medications were available for prescribing, as newer drugs had less time on the market and therefore were least likely to have been discontinued. This phenomenon was, in fact, significant for all drug classes.

Most of the in-class persistence differences that the authors observed can be easily explained, either from differences in antihypertensive efficacy (eg, losartan) or from frequency of administration (eg, captopril). The fact that 3-times-daily nicardipine was less likely to be taken persistently than once-daily dihydropyridine calcium antagonists is similarly not surprising. Older patients appear to be less persistent with verapamil (presumably due to higher rates of constipation) than with amlodipine, and in these Italian patients, fourth-generation dihydropyridine calcium antagonists (eg, lercanidipine or manidipine) had better persistence than older dihydropyridine calcium antagonists, perhaps because they cause less pedal edema. Most pharmacologists would agree with the authors that cost-benefit calculations, as well as treatment guidelines, that lump all agents of the same pharmacologic class are probably not very useful or realistic, as they ignore in-class differences (in cost and persistence) across specific agents.

W. J. Elliott, MD, PhD

References

1. Caro JJ, Salas M, Speckman JL, Raggio G, Jackson JD. Persistence with treatment for hypertension in actual practice. *CMAJ*. 1999;160:31-37.
2. Degli Esposti L, Degli Esposti E, Valpiani G, et al. A retrospective, population-based analysis of persistence with antihypertensive drug therapy in primary care practice in Italy. *Clin Ther*. 2002;24:1347-1357.
3. Mazzaglia G, Mantovani LG, Sturkenboom MC, et al. Patterns of persistence with antihypertensive medications in newly diagnosed hypertensive patients in Italy: a retrospective cohort study in primary care. *J Hypertens*. 2005;23:2093-2100.
4. Siegel D, Lopez J, Meier J. Antihypertensive medication adherence in the Department of Veterans Affairs. *Am J Med*. 2007;120:26-32.
5. Elliott WJ, Plauschinat CA, Skrepnek GH, Gause D. Persistence, adherence, and risk of discontinuation associated with commonly prescribed antihypertensive drug monotherapies. *J Am Board Fam Med*. 2007;20:72-80.
6. Hasford J, Mimran A, Simons WR. A population-based European cohort study of persistence in newly diagnosed hypertensive patients. *J Hum Hypertens*. 2002;16:569-575.
7. Fang J, Alderman MH, Keenan NL, Ayala C, Croft JB. Hypertension control at physicians' offices in the United States. *Am J Hypertens*. 2008;21:136-142.
8. Elliott WJ. Improving outcomes in hypertensive patients: focus on adherence and persistence with antihypertensive therapy. *J Clin Hypertens (Greenwich)*. 2009;11:376-382.

Measuring blood pressure for decision making and quality reporting: where and how many measures?

Powers BJ, Olsen MK, Smith VA, et al (Duke Univ, Durham, NC)
Ann Intern Med 154:781-788, 2011

Background.—The optimal setting and number of blood pressure (BP) measurements that should be used for clinical decision making and quality reporting are uncertain.

Objective.—To compare strategies for home or clinic BP measurement and their effect on classifying patients as having BP that was in or out of control.

Design.—Secondary analysis of a randomized, controlled trial of strategies to improve hypertension management. (ClinicalTrials.gov registration number: NCT00237692).

Setting.—Primary care clinics affiliated with the Durham Veterans Affairs Medical Center.

Participants.—444 veterans with hypertension followed for 18 months.

Measurements.—Blood pressure was measured repeatedly by using 3 methods: standardized research BP measurements at 6-month intervals; clinic BP measurements obtained during outpatient visits; and home BP measurements using a monitor that transmitted measurements electronically.

Results.—Patients provided 111,181 systolic BP (SBP) measurements (3218 research, 7121 clinic, and 100,842 home measurements) over 18 months. Systolic BP control rates at baseline (mean SBP < 140 mm Hg for clinic or research measurement; <135 mm Hg for home measurement) varied substantially, with 28% classified as in control by clinic measurement, 47% by home measurement, and 68% by research measurement. Short-term variability was large and similar across all 3 methods of measurement, with a mean within-patient coefficient of variation of 10% (range, 1% to 24%). Patients could not be classified as having BP that was in or out of control with 80% certainty on the basis of a single clinic SBP measurement from 120 mm Hg to 157 mm Hg. The effect of within-patient variability could be greatly reduced by averaging several measurements, with most benefit accrued at 5 to 6 measurements.

Limitations.—The sample was mostly men with a long-standing history of hypertension and was selected on the basis of previous poor BP control.

Conclusion.—Physicians who want to have 80% or more certainty that they are correctly classifying patients' BP control should use the average of several measurements. Hypertension quality metrics based on a single clinic measurement potentially misclassify a large proportion of patients.

▶ Blood pressures can be estimated using various techniques in several settings, but the method that corresponds best to "controlled blood pressure" or predicts long-term prognosis and therefore should be used for monitoring and reimbursement is unclear. These authors used a prospectively collected set of data from 3 settings in 444 hypertensive patients (done as a post hoc analysis of a clinical trial[1]) to investigate the minimum number of readings in the medical office, a research setting, or at home to determine whether blood pressure was "adequately controlled."

Most research shows that the best diagnostic modality and best predictor of outcomes is 24-hour ambulatory blood pressure monitoring,[2] but reimbursement for this procedure by the Center for Medicare and Medicaid Services is limited to individuals who have clear and convincing evidence for "white-coat hypertension." As a result, this procedure has been largely limited to research settings and is not routinely used in clinical practice.[3] Traditionally in the United States, office blood pressures are measured in a series of 3 consecutive readings in the seated position after 5 minutes of quiet rest.[4] In 2007, the National Committee on Quality Assurance (NCQA) ruled that the lowest systolic and lowest diastolic readings can be considered the "blood pressure for this visit" even if they were not measured simultaneously. Approximately 45% of American hypertensive patients now perform home blood pressure readings, but these are currently not recognized by NCQA or the Healthcare Effectiveness Data Information Set criteria and are not reimbursed.[5]

These authors' data suggest that the standardized blood pressure measurements mandated by research protocols (which nearly always involve multiple readings at a given visit) provide better estimates of controlled blood pressure, compared with either home readings or a single office reading. Although this seems intrinsically obvious,[6] multiple readings are unfortunately not implemented in clinical practice as often as they probably should be. Perhaps it would help to disseminate the authors' conclusion that a single reading provides only 80% confidence that the systolic blood pressure in a given patient is actually between 120 and 157 mm Hg! This conclusion is consistent with another recent article that recommends a series of 5 automated office blood pressure measurements for routine office blood pressure determination.[7]

W. J. Elliott, MD, PhD

References

1. Bosworth HB, Powers BJ, Olsen MK, et al. Home blood pressure management and improved blood pressure control: results from a randomized controlled trial. *Arch Intern Med.* 2011;171:1173-1180.
2. Hodgkinson J, Mant J, Martin U, et al. Relative effectiveness of clinic and home blood pressure monitoring compared with ambulatory blood pressure monitoring in diagnosis of hypertension: systematic review. *BMJ.* 2011;342:d3621.
3. Giles TD, Egan P. Pay (adequately) for what works: the economic undervaluation of office and ambulatory blood pressure recordings. *J Clin Hypertens (Greenwich).* 2008;10:257-259.
4. Pickering TG, Hall JE, Appel LJ, et al; Subcommittee of Professional and Public Education of the American Heart Association Council on High Blood Pressure Research. Recommendations for blood pressure measurement in humans and experimental animals: Part 1: blood pressure measurement in humans: a statement for professionals from the Subcommittee of Professional and Public Education of the American Heart Association Council on High Blood Pressure Research. *Hypertension.* 2005;45:142-161.
5. Pickering TG, Miller NH, Ogedegbe G, Krakoff LR, Artinian NT, Goff D; American Heart Association; American Society of Hypertension; Preventive Cardiovascular Nurses Association. Call to action on use and reimbursement for home blood pressure monitoring: executive summary: a joint Scientific Statement from the American

Heart Association, American Society of Hypertension, and Preventive Cardiovascular Nurses Association. *Hypertension.* 2008;52:1-9.

6. Myers MG, Valdivieso M, Kiss A. Optimum frequency of office blood pressure measurement using an automated sphygmomanometer. *Blood Press Monit.* 2008; 13:333-338.

7. Myers MG, Godwin M, Dawes M, et al. Conventional versus automated measurement of blood pressure in primary care patients with systolic hypertension: randomised parallel design controlled trial. *BMJ.* 2011;342:d286.

Level of Systolic Blood Pressure Within the Normal Range and Risk of Recurrent Stroke

Ovbiagele B, for the PROFESS Investigators (Univ of California, San Diego; et al)
JAMA 306:2137-2144, 2011

Context.—Recurrent stroke prevention guidelines suggest that larger reductions in systolic blood pressure (SBP) are positively associated with a greater reduction in the risk of recurrent stroke and define an SBP level of less than 120 mm Hg as normal. However, the association of SBP maintained at such levels with risk of vascular events after a recent ischemic stroke is unclear.

Objective.—To assess the association of maintaining low-normal vs high-normal SBP levels with risk of recurrent stroke.

Design, Setting, and Patients.—Post hoc observational analysis of a multicenter trial involving 20 330 patients (age ≥50 years) with recent non–cardioembolic ischemic stroke; patients were recruited from 695 centers in 35 countries from September 2003 through July 2006 and followed up for 2.5 years (follow-up ended on February 8, 2008). Patients were categorized based on their mean SBP level: very low–normal (<120 mm Hg), low-normal (120-<130 mm Hg), high-normal (130-<140 mm Hg), high (140-<150 mm Hg), and very high (≥150 mm Hg).

Main Outcome Measures.—The primary outcome was first recurrence of stroke of any type and the secondary outcome was a composite of stroke, myocardial infarction, or death from vascular causes.

Results.—The recurrent stroke rates were 8.0% (95% CI, 6.8%-9.2%) for the very low–normal SBP level group, 7.2% (95% CI, 6.4%-8.0%) for the low-normal SBP group, 6.8% (95% CI, 6.1%-7.4%) for the high-normal SBP group, 8.7% (95% CI, 7.9%-9.5%) for the high SBP group, and 14.1% (95% CI, 13.0%-15.2%) for the very high SBP group. Compared with patients in the high-normal SBP group, the risk of the primary outcome was higher for patients in the very low–normal SBP group (adjusted hazard ratio [AHR], 1.29; 95% CI, 1.07-1.56), in the high SBP group (AHR, 1.23; 95% CI, 1.07-1.41), and in the very high SBP group (AHR, 2.08; 95% CI, 1.83-2.37). Compared with patients in the high-normal SBP group, the risk of secondary outcome was higher for patients in the very low–normal SBP group (AHR, 1.31; 95% CI, 1.13-1.52), in the low-normal SBP group (AHR, 1.16; 95% CI, 1.03-1.31), in the high SBP group (AHR, 1.24; 95% CI, 1.11-1.39), and in the very high SBP group (AHR, 1.94; 95% CI, 1.74-2.16).

Conclusion.—Among patients with recent non—cardioembolic ischemic stroke, SBP levels during follow-up in the very low—normal (<120 mm Hg), high (140-<150 mm Hg), or very high (≥150 mm Hg) range were associated with increased risk of recurrent stroke.

Trial Registration.—clinicaltrials.gov Identifier: NCT00153062 (Table 4).

▶ Elevated blood pressure is a well-recognized and eminently treatable risk factor for recurrent stroke in patients with established cerebrovascular disease.[1,2] Controversy still exists, however, regarding the most appropriate pharmacologic intervention(s), as well as the target blood pressure to be obtained.[2,3] Many post hoc analyses of clinical trials and other large databases have suggested the existence of a "J-shaped curve" (increased risk with very low diastolic blood pressures), especially for patients with coronary heart disease,[4] but most recent analyses have not observed a significant increase in risk for stroke among patients with the lowest achieved systolic or diastolic blood pressures,[4-6] irrespective of whether they had preexisting heart or cerebrovascular disease.

These authors therefore analyzed the large data set from the Prevention Regimen for Effectively Avoiding Second Strokes (PROFESS) trial, involving more than 20 000 subjects with a noncardioembolic stroke in the previous 120 days, followed for a mean of 2.5 years. The 2 × 2 factorial design of the trial did not find a significant benefit of the randomized treatments on recurrent stroke (although a meta-analysis that included the PROFESS and TRANSCEND patients did show a significant benefit, as published in the original TRANSCEND report[7]).

Their major conclusion was that both higher and lower systolic blood pressures after randomization were associated with an increased risk of recurrent

TABLE 4.—Adjusted Risk of Clinical Outcomes by Mean Systolic Blood Pressure Level in 20 330 Patients With a Recent Ischemic Stroke

| | Mean Systolic Blood Pressure Level, mm Hg | | | | |
	High-Normal (130-<140; n = 6004)	Very Low—Normal (<120; n = 1919)	Low-Normal (120-<130; n = 3982)	High (140-<150; n = 4520)	Very High (≥150; n = 3905)
AHR (95% CI)					
Stroke[a]	1 [Reference]	1.29 (1.07-1.56)	1.10 (0.95-1.28)	1.23 (1.07-1.41)	2.08 (1.83-2.37)
Stroke, MI, or vascular death[b]	1 [Reference]	1.31 (1.13-1.52)	1.16 (1.03-1.31)	1.24 (1.11-1.39)	1.94 (1.74-2.16)
Fatal stroke[c]	1 [Reference]	0.63 (0.26-1.49)	1.01 (0.64-1.89)	1.50 (0.94-2.40)	2.51 (1.62-3.09)

Abbreviations: AHR, adjusted hazard ratio; MI, myocardial infarction.

[a]Adjusted for age, sex, previous stroke, congestive heart failure, diabetes, MI, hypertension, current smoking status, baseline National Institutes of Health Stroke Scale score, qualifying stroke due to small vessel disease, previous transient ischemic attack, and Asian ethnicity.

[b]Adjusted for age, sex, previous stroke, congestive heart failure, diabetes, MI, hyperlipidemia, coronary artery disease, current smoking status, antihypertensive medication use at baseline, baseline National Institutes of Health Stroke Scale score, qualifying stroke due to small vessel disease, body mass index (calculated as weight in kilograms divided by height in meters squared), black race, white race, previous transient ischemic attack, and Asian ethnicity.

[c]Adjusted for age, sex, previous stroke, congestive heart failure, diabetes, MI, treatment with angiotensin receptor blocker, antiplatelet treatment at baseline, baseline National Institutes of Health Stroke Scale score, body mass index (calculated as weight in kilograms divided by height in meters squared), and previous transient ischemic attack.

stroke (as well as with the composite of stroke, myocardial infarction, or cardiovascular death), compared with the "reference standard" of 130 to 139 mm Hg. Their analyses also show that the group with the lowest achieved systolic blood pressures had the greatest average falls in systolic blood pressure, which is consistent with the hypothesis that overaggressive blood pressure lowering can increase cardiovascular risk. They also mention that their conclusions were independent of baseline blood pressures, but the adjusted risk of clinical outcomes in Table 4 do not include an adjustment for baseline blood pressures (which may, in fact, lead to overadjustment of the 1790 subjects with recurrent stroke observed in the trial). Their conclusion that blood pressure lowering, especially in the first few months after stroke, should be limited to a target systolic blood pressure of 130 to 139 mm Hg is based on a post hoc analysis and therefore is more hypothesis-generating than strong evidence that might change the next set of clinical guidelines.[3]

W. J. Elliott, MD, PhD

References

1. Rashid P, Leonardi-Bee J, Bath P. Blood pressure reduction and secondary prevention of stroke and other vascular events: a systematic review. *Stroke*. 2003;34: 2741-2748.
2. Elliott WJ. Treatment of hypertension with cerebrovascular disease: what is the evidence?. Chapter 13. In: Weir MR, ed. *Evidence-Based Management of Hypertension*. Abdon, Shropshire, UK: TFM Publishing, Ltd; 2010:171-186.
3. Furie KL, Kasner SE, Adams RJ, et al. Guidelines for the prevention of stroke in patients with stroke or transient ischemic attack: a guideline for healthcare professionals from the American Heart Association/American Stroke Association. *Stroke*. 2011;42:227-276.
4. Messerli FH, Mancia G, Conti CR, et al. Dogma disputed: can aggressively lowering blood pressure in hypertensive patients with coronary artery disease be dangerous? *Ann Intern Med*. 2006;144:884-893.
5. Chrysant SG, Chrysant GS. Effectiveness of lowering blood pressure to prevent stroke versus to prevent coronary events. *Am J Cardiol*. 2010;106:825-829.
6. Arima H, Chalmers J, Woodward M, et al; PROGRESS Collaborative Group. Lower target blood pressures are safe and effective for the prevention of recurrent stroke: the PROGRESS Trial. *J Hypertens*. 2006;24:1201-1208.
7. Telmisartan Randomised AssessmeNt Study in ACE iNtolerant subjects with cardiovascular Disease (TRANSCEND) Investigators, Yusuf S, Teo K, Anderson C, et al. Effects of the angiotensin-receptor blocker telmisartan on cardiovascular events in high-risk patients intolerant to angiotensin-converting enzyme inhibitors: a randomised controlled trial. *Lancet*. 2008;372:1174-1183.

Prognostic role of ambulatory blood pressure measurement in patients with nondialysis chronic kidney disease
Minutolo R, Agarwal R, Borrelli S, et al (Second Univ of Naples, Italy; Indiana Univ School of Medicine, Indianapolis; et al)
Arch Intern Med 171:1090-1098, 2011

Background.—Ambulatory blood pressure (BP) measurement allows a better risk stratification in essential hypertension compared with office blood pressure measurement, but its prognostic role in nondialysis chronic kidney disease has been poorly investigated.

Methods.—The prognostic role of daytime and nighttime systolic BP (SBP) and diastolic BP (DBP) in comparison with office measurements was evaluated in 436 consecutive patients with chronic kidney disease. Primary end points were time to renal death (end-stage renal disease or death) and time to fatal and nonfatal cardiovascular events. Quintiles of BP were used to classify patients.

Results.—The mean (SD) age of the patients was 65.1 (13.6) years, and the glomerular filtration rate was 42.9 (19.7) mL/min/1.73 m^2; 41.7% of the participants were women, 36.5% had diabetes, and 30.5% had cardiovascular disease. Office-measured SBP/DBP values were 146 (19)/82 (12) mm Hg; daytime SBP/DBP was 131 (17)/75 (11) mm Hg, and nighttime SBP/DBP was 122 (20)/66 (10) mm Hg. During follow-up (median, 4.2 years), 155 and 103 patients reached the renal and cardiovascular end points, respectively. Compared with a daytime SBP of 126 to 135 mm Hg, patients with an SBP of 136 to 146 mm Hg and those with an SBP higher than 146 mm Hg had an increased adjusted risk of the cardiovascular end point (hazard ratio [HR], 2.23; 95% confidence interval [CI], 1.13-4.41 and 3.07; 1.54-6.09) and renal death (1.72; 1.02-2.89 and 1.85; 1.11-3.08). Nighttime SBPs of 125 to 137 mm Hg and higher than 137 mm Hg also increased the risk of the cardiovascular end point (HR, 2.52; 95% CI, 1.11-5.71 and 4.00; 1.77-9.02) and renal end point (1.87; 1.03-3.43 and 2.54; 1.41-4.57) with respect to the reference SBP value of 106-114 mm Hg. Office measurement of BP did not predict the risk of the renal or cardiovascular end point. Patients who were nondippers and those who were reverse dippers had a greater risk of both end points.

Conclusion.—In chronic kidney disease, ambulatory BP measurement and, in particular, nighttime BP measurement, allows more accurate prediction of renal and cardiovascular risk; office measurement of BP does not predict any outcome.

▶ Office blood pressure targets for patients with chronic kidney disease are controversial, because most guidelines rely on data from observational studies and post-hoc analyses of clinical trials to justify the goal of less than 130/80 mm Hg, rather than the limited data from randomized clinical trials.[1] Office blood pressures are typically confounded by the "white-coat effect" and the presence of "masked hypertension"; as a result, the recent British National Institute for Health and Clinical Excellence guidelines recommend 24-hour ambulatory blood pressure monitoring for people suspected of having hypertension,[2] which is cost effective in the United Kingdom.[3] The utility of ambulatory blood pressure monitoring to predict prognosis in patients with chronic kidney disease is less well studied. Cohort studies of US veterans showed better prediction of cardiovascular and renal morbidity and mortality with ambulatory than office blood pressures, but the difference did not persist after statistical adjustment for baseline covariates.[4,5] This paradox led this team of Italian nephrologists to collaborate with the investigator who headed the US veterans' cohort study, so that data from their Italian cohort of 436 consecutive patients could be analyzed in a similar fashion.

Despite some very large and potentially important differences between the Italian and US veterans' cohorts, the analyses provide very similar conclusions. Office blood pressures did not correlate with the risk of cardiovascular or renal endpoints, but ambulatory measurements were very strong predictors of both. As with previous experience in patients without impaired renal function, nocturnal blood pressures were important additional predictors of cardiovascular events.

The authors worry that their all-white Italian cohort had few diabetics, underwent ambulatory blood pressure monitoring only once, and excluded normotensive patients from their analysis. Despite these concerns, their conclusions are strikingly similar to those drawn from the US veterans' cohort. In fact, they conform to Sir Austin Bradford Hill's criteria for strengthening the link between a risk factor and an outcome, as the same findings are now reproduced in a quite different population.

W. J. Elliott, MD, PhD

References

1. Upadhyay A, Earley A, Haynes SM, Uhlig K. Systematic review: blood pressure target in chronic kidney disease and proteinuria as an effect modifier. *Ann Intern Med.* 2011;154:541-548.
2. Williams B, Williams H, Northedge J, et al; Guideline Development Groups, National Collaborating Centres, and NICE Project Team. NICE clinical guideline 127: Hypertension: Clinical management of primary hypertension in adults. United Kingdom National Health Service: National Institute for Health and Clinical Excellence. http://www.nice.org.uk/CG127. Accessed August 24, 2011.
3. Lovibond K, Jowett S, Barton P, et al. Cost-effectiveness of options for the diagnosis of high blood pressure in primary care: a modelling study. *Lancet.* 2011; 378:1219-1230.
4. Agarwal R, Andersen MJ. Prognostic importance of ambulatory blood pressure recordings in patients with chronic kidney disease. *Kidney Int.* 2006;69:1175-1180.
5. Agarwal R, Andersen MJ. Blood pressure recordings within and outside the clinic and cardiovascular events in chronic kidney disease. *Am J Nephrol.* 2006;26: 503-510.

Association Between Chlorthalidone Treatment of Systolic Hypertension and Long-term Survival

Kostis JB, Cabrera J, Cheng JQ, et al (UMDNJ-Robert Wood Johnson Med School, New Brunswick, NJ; Rutgers Univ, Piscataway, NJ; et al)
JAMA 306:2588-2593, 2011

Context.—In the Systolic Hypertension in the Elderly Program (SHEP) trial, conducted between 1985 and 1990, antihypertensive therapy with chlorthalidone-based stepped-care therapy resulted in a lower rate of cardiovascular events than placebo but effects on mortality were not significant.

Objective.—To study the gain in life expectancy of participants randomized to active therapy at the 22-year follow-up.

Design, Setting, and Participants.—A National Death Index ascertainment of death in the long-term follow-up of a randomized, placebo-controlled, clinical trial (SHEP) of patients aged 60 years or older with isolated systolic hypertension. Recruitment was between March 1, 1985, and January 15, 1988. After the end of a 4.5-year randomized phase of the SHEP trial, all participants were advised to receive active therapy. The time interval between the beginning of recruitment and the ascertainment of death by National Death Index (December 31, 2006) was approximately 22 years (21 years 10 months).

Main Outcome Measures.—Cardiovascular death and all-cause mortality.

Results.—At the 22-year follow-up, life expectancy gain, expressed as the area between active (n = 2365) and placebo (n = 2371) survival curves, was 105 days (95% CI, −39 to 242; $P = .07$) for all-cause mortality and 158 days (95% CI, 36-287; $P = .009$) for cardiovascular death. Each month of active treatment was therefore associated with approximately 1 day extension in life expectancy. The active treatment group had higher survival free from cardiovascular death vs the placebo group (hazard ratio [HR], 0.89; 95% CI, 0.80-0.99; $P = .03$) but similar survival for all-cause mortality (HR, 0.97; 95% CI, 0.90-1.04; $P = .42$). There were 1416 deaths (59.9%) in the active treatment group and 1435 deaths (60.5%) in the placebo group (log-rank $P = .38$, Wilcoxon $P = .24$). Cardiovascular death was lower in the active treatment group (669 deaths [28.3%]) vs the placebo group (735 deaths [31.0%]; log-rank $P = .03$, Wilcoxon $P = .02$). Time to 70th percentile survival was 0.56 years (95% CI, −0.14 to 1.23) longer in the active treatment group vs the placebo group (11.53 vs 10.98 years; $P = .03$) for all-cause mortality and 1.41 years (95% CI, 0.34-2.61; 17.81 vs 16.39 years; $P = .01$) for survival free from cardiovascular death.

Conclusion.—In the SHEP trial, treatment of isolated systolic hypertension with chlorthalidone stepped-care therapy for 4.5 years was associated with longer life expectancy at 22 years of follow-up.

▶ The Systolic Hypertension in the Elderly Program (SHEP) was a landmark trial in hypertension, showing for the first time a major, significant reduction in stroke[1] (primary endpoint) as well as coronary heart disease events[1] (one of the secondary endpoints) and heart failure[2] (part of a composite secondary endpoint) in the group randomized to active antihypertensive drug therapy (chlorthalidone, followed by atenolol, if required). SHEP was followed by studies in Europe[3] and China[4] that used different antihypertensive regimens but basically showed very similar results; some believe these trials were unethical, because SHEP had already proved the benefits of drug treatment. However, SHEP was not powered to compare mortality during the planned 4.5 years of follow-up, and some have claimed (particularly on the basis of a meta-analysis from the last millennium[5]) that antihypertensive drugs increase mortality in older hypertensive patients. So this subgroup of the original SHEP investigators used the National Death Index to assess whether a 4.5-year period of active antihypertensive therapy would have a persistent effect on long-term mortality, even after all subjects in the

SHEP trial were recommended to receive active antihypertensive therapy from their nonstudy physicians.

It is unfortunately not known how many of the group randomized to placebo followed this advice, but the original SHEP report indicates that 44% had already begun taking antihypertensive therapy during the 4.5 years of follow-up. It is likely that this high degree of "crossover" would bias the results of long-term mortality follow-up toward the null. The authors also have no information about nonfatal events in the SHEP participants because they were prohibited by the Health Information Portability and Accountability Act (and other considerations) from collecting such data. Some would argue that the granting of a Waiver of Consent by the University of Texas Institutional Review Board for this follow-up study was in violation of the spirit of this law, which mandated that all personal health information in all research records be expunged on or before April 13, 2003.

The authors do not specify how many of their study subjects could not be matched with National Death Index information, which is a common concern about such searches, particularly for women (who are more likely than men to change last names in governmental files). The authors also do not correct for "multiple comparisons" because they assessed both all-cause and cardiovascular mortality in their study. Some would argue that because of this twin primary endpoint, they should have used an acceptable P value of $< .025$, rather than $< .05$, which would have sadly not been met.

Nonetheless, these SHEP data join with similar data from the Systolic Hypertension in Europe trial (which had only a 1.9-year average duration of placebo treatment),[6] as well as several other studies in hypertension,[7] dyslipidemia,[8] and diabetes,[9] suggesting that early treatment may have major beneficial effects in the long-term. Such benefits have not, however, been seen in all such studies.[10] The "major marketing take-home message" from these data, that each extra month of treatment prolongs life by a day, may or may not be exact, but it is catchy and likely to be something that is easy for both physicians and patients to remember about antihypertensive drug therapy.

W. J. Elliott, MD, PhD

References

1. Prevention of stroke by antihypertensive drug treatment in older persons with isolated systolic hypertension. Final results of the Systolic Hypertension in the Elderly Program (SHEP). SHEP Cooperative Research Group. *JAMA*. 1991;265:3255-3264.
2. Kostis JB, Davis BR, Cutler J, et al. Prevention of heart failure by antihypertensive drug treatment in older persons with isolated systolic hypertension. SHEP Cooperative Research Group. *JAMA*. 1997;278:212-216.
3. Staessen JA, Fagard R, Thijs L, et al; Systolic Hypertension in Europe (Syst-EUR) Trial Investigators. Morbidity and mortality in the placebo-controlled European Trial on Isolated Systolic Hypertension in the Elderly. *Lancet*. 1997;360:757-764.
4. Liu L, Wang JG, Gong L, Liu G, Staessen JA. Comparison of active treatment and placebo in older Chinese patients with isolated systolic hypertension. Systolic Hypertension in China (Syst-China) Collaborative Group. *J Hypertens*. 1998; 16:1823-1829.
5. Gueyffier F, Bulpitt C, Boissel JP, et al. Antihypertensive drugs in very old people: a subgroup meta-analysis of randomised controlled trials. INDANA Group. *Lancet*. 1999;353:793-796.

6. Staessen JA, Thijisq L, Fagard R, et al; Systolic Hypertension in Europe (Syst-Eur) Trial Investigators. Effects of immediate versus delayed antihypertensive therapy on outcome in the Systolic Hypertension in Europe Trial. *J Hypertens.* 2004;22: 847-857.
7. Kostis WJ, Thijs L, Richart T, Kostis JB, Staessen JA. Persistence of mortality reduction after the end of randomized therapy in clinical trials of blood pressure-lowering medications. *Hypertension.* 2010;56:1060-1068.
8. Kostis WJ, Moreyra AE, Cheng JQ, Dobrzynski JM, Kostis JB. Continuation of mortality reduction after the end of randomized therapy in clinical trials of lipid-lowering therapy. *J Clin Lipidol.* 2011;5:97-104.
9. Gaede P, Lund-Andersen H, Parving HH, Pedersen O. Effect of a multifactorial intervention on mortality in type 2 diabetes. *N Engl J Med.* 2008;358:580-591.
10. Holman RR, Paul SK, Bethel MA, Neil HA, Matthews DR. Long-term follow-up after tight control of blood pressure in type 2 diabetes. *N Engl J Med.* 2008;359: 1565-1576.

Genetic variants in novel pathways influence blood pressure and cardiovascular disease risk

The International Consortium for Blood Pressure Genome-Wide Association Studies (Johns Hopkins Univ School of Medicine, Baltimore, MD; Queen Mary Univ of London, UK; Univ of Washington, Seattle; et al)
Nature 478:103-109, 2011

Blood pressure is a heritable trait influenced by several biological pathways and responsive to environmental stimuli. Over one billion people worldwide have hypertension (≥ 140 mm Hg systolic blood pressure or ≥ 90 mm Hg diastolic blood pressure). Even small increments in blood pressure are associated with an increased risk of cardiovascular events. This genome-wide association study of systolic and diastolic blood pressure, which used a multi-stage design in 200,000 individuals of European descent, identified sixteen novel loci: six of these loci contain genes previously known or suspected to regulate blood pressure (*GUCY1A3–GUCY1B3, NPR3–C5orf23, ADM, FURIN–FES, GOSR2, GNAS–EDN3*); the other ten provide new clues to blood pressure physiology. A genetic risk score based on 29 genome-wide significant variants was associated with hypertension, left ventricular wall thickness, stroke and coronary artery disease, but not kidney disease or kidney function. We also observed associations with blood pressure in East Asian, South Asian and African ancestry individuals. Our findings provide new insights into the genetics and biology of blood pressure, and suggest potential novel therapeutic pathways for cardiovascular disease prevention.

▶ Two years ago, several of these authors published 2 important genome-wise association studies involving more than 25 000 people of European ancestry, which identified 13 genetic loci associated with both systolic and diastolic blood pressures and the presence of hypertension.[1,2] This work is a meta-analysis of those and other genome-wide association studies with staged follow-up genotyping that identified new blood pressure—related genetic loci.

Most of the methodology reported in this article will not be very familiar to practicing physicians who are not well versed in modern medical genetics. Probably the most impressive and easily understood detail is the very small threshold P-value for the reported associations. This is common in genetics, especially in genome-wide association studies, because of the hundreds of thousands of single-nucleotide polymorphisms that are examined in these studies, resulting in millions of comparisons.

This article takes these concepts a step further and proposes a risk calculator for hypertension, left ventricular hypertrophy, stroke, and heart disease that is based solely on the presence or absence of these genetic loci. Interestingly, no simple prediction was possible for kidney disease, perhaps because dialysis is less commonly undertaken outside the United States. The authors indicate that much more work is needed to investigate most of the new genetic loci, which might lead to a better understanding of their role in health and disease. There may well come a time, perhaps in the distant future,[3] when genotyping of an individual will provide useful information about blood pressure—related prognosis.

W. J. Elliott, MD, PhD

References

1. Newton-Cheh C, Johnson T, Gateva V, et al. Genome-wide association study identifies eight loci associated with blood pressure. *Nat Genet.* 2009;41:666-676.
2. Levy D, Ehret GB, Rice K, et al. Genome-wide association study of blood pressure and hypertension. *Nat Genet.* 2009;41:677-687.
3. Arnett DK, Claas SA, Lynch AI. Has pharmacogenetics brought us closer to 'personalized medicine' for initial drug treatment of hypertension? *Curr Opin Cardiol.* 2009;24:333-339.

Reliability of palpation of the radial artery compared with auscultation of the brachial artery in measuring SBP

van der Hoeven NV, van den Born B-JH, van Montfrans GA (Academic Med Ctr, Amsterdam, The Netherlands)
J Hypertens 29:51-55, 2011

Background.—Systolic blood pressure contributes more to cardiovascular disease than DBP, especially in elderly persons. Palpation of the radial artery to assess SBP — Riva-Rocci's technique — may be an attractive alternative for auscultatory SBP in these patients. Therefore, we investigated the difference between SBP determined by palpation of the radial artery (pSBP) and SBP assessed by auscultation of the brachial artery (aSBP).

Methods.—Patients were included from the waiting room of a hypertension outpatient clinic. In each patient eight simultaneous pSBP and aSBP measurements were assessed by two observers in the same arm. After every two readings the observers switched between pSBP and aSBP.

Results.—Forty patients were included, 25 men (62.5%), mean age 55.3 years (range 24—78). From a total of 320 measurements, mean difference between pSBP and aSBP was −5.2 mm Hg (range −12—26 mm Hg)

(*P*<0.01). This difference correlated significantly with BMI (*r*=0.51, *P*< 0.01), but not with age (*r*=0.15, *P*=0.35), pulse rate (*r*=0.29, *P*=0.09) or mean SBP (*r*=0.03, *P*=0.85). After averaging the first three comparisons, reproducibility did not improve when increasing the number of comparisons. When correcting for the underestimation of 6 mm Hg over the first three comparisons, Riva-Rocci's technique estimates SBP with an acceptable accuracy.

Conclusion.—In clinical practice, Riva-Rocci's palpatory technique offers an acceptable alternative for auscultatory SBP measurement. It is recommended to take three measurements and then correct for the average underestimation of 6 mm Hg.

▶ Sometimes, what's old is what's new, and sometimes what's old becomes "classic." Perhaps that is the message of this article, which compared 2 century-old methods of estimating systolic blood pressure in a convenience sample of 40 consecutive subjects attending a hypertension center in Holland. The rationale for this comparison is reasonably compelling: A Clinical Advisory Statement from the American Heart Association more than 10 years ago suggested that systolic is the most important, single blood pressure compared with diastolic or pulse pressure[1]; this conclusion was subsequently corroborated by an analysis from the Prospective Studies Collaboration.[2] The authors of this article assert that a proper comparison of the palpatory method of Riva-Rocci and the ausculatory method of Korotkoff has never been published, but it seems likely that such comparisons were done sometime during the last millennium and simply not deemed worthy of completing the manuscript. Modern statistical methods and Bland-Altman plots make it more likely that the finding of no significant difference between the 2 methods would be more likely to be publishable today.

The most important point of this article is that the 2 methods provide very similar information that is highly correlated. The unfortunate aspect is that there seems to be a systematic underestimation of the systolic pressure by 6 mm Hg using the Riva-Rocci method, which might be very difficult to explain from first principles. There is a hint in the "pseudo" Bland-Altman plot (Fig 2, which uses the mean of the palpated and auscultated systolic blood pressures on the x-axis) of the article, which indicates that systolic blood pressure was underestimated by about 22 mm Hg in 2 subjects and by more than 20 mm Hg in 5 (of 40!) subjects, using the palpatory method. The authors discuss the history and possible reasons for this discrepancy, noting that Korotkoff observed a systolic blood pressure higher than 10 to 12 mm Hg using his auscultatory method compared with the palpatory method.[3-6] The rationale is that the palpatory method takes about 3 heartbeats before the pulse is detected, compared with the auscultatory method, which would average about a 6 mm Hg difference with a heart rate of 60 per minute.

The authors admit to some limitations of their study, including the fact that a small number of subjects were studied, and all were recruited from a waiting room of a hypertension center. This provided a wide range of measured systolic blood pressures (about 105—230 mm Hg, according to Fig 2) but may not be representative of the broader population. They recommend that the Riva-Rocci

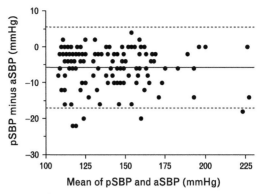

FIGURE 2.—Comparison of the first three SBP measurements assessed by palpation and the first three SBP measurements assessed by auscultation for all patients ($n = 120$). On the horizontal axis of the Bland–Altman plot the mean palpatory SBP (pSBP) and auscultatory SBP (aSBP) measurement is shown. The vertical axis shows the difference between pSBP and aSBP. The solid line represents the mean at −5.7 mmHg. The dashed lines represent 1.96 times the SD above and below the mean at 5.6mmHg and −17.0 mmHg, respectively. pSBP, SBP assessed by palpation; aSBP, SBP assessed by auscultation. (Reprinted from van der Hoeven NV, van den Born BJ, van Montfrans GA. Reliability of palpation of the radial artery compared with auscultation of the brachial artery in measuring SBP. *J Hypertens*. 2011;29:51-55, © Lippincott Williams & Wilkins.)

method not be forgotten but used in addition to, and possibly instead of, the Korotkoff method, at least for determining the "peak inflation level" before applying the stethoscope.[7]

W. J. Elliott, MD, PhD

References

1. Izzo JL Jr, Levy D, Black HR. Clinical advisory statement. Importance of systolic blood pressure in older Americans. *Hypertension*. 2000;35:1021-1024.
2. Lewington S, Clarke R, Qizilbash N, Peto R, Collins R; Prospective Studies Collaboration. Age-specific relevance of usual blood pressure to vascular mortality: a meta-analysis of individual data for one million adults in 61 prospective studies. *Lancet*. 2002;360:1903-1913.
3. Korotkoff NC. To the question of methods of determining the blood pressure (from the clinic of Professor CP Federoff). *Rep Imperial Mil Acad [in Russian]*. 1905;11:365-367.
4. Dock W. Korotkoff's sounds. *N Engl J Med*. 1980;302:1264-1267.
5. Korotkov NS. Concerning the problem of the methods of blood pressure measurement. *J Hypertens*. 2005;23:5.
6. Paskalev D, Kircheva A, Krivoshiev S. A centenary of auscultatory blood pressure measurement: a tribute to Nikolai Korotkoff. *Kidney Blood Press Res*. 2005;28:259-263.
7. Pickering TG, Hall JE, Appel LJ, et al; Subcommittee of Professional and Public Education of the American Heart Association Council on High Blood Pressure Research. Recommendations for blood pressure measurement in humans and experimental animals: Part 1: blood pressure measurement in humans: a statement for professionals from the Subcommittee of Professional and Public Education of the American Heart Association Council on High Blood Pressure Research. *Hypertension*. 2005;45:142-161.

Determinants of masked hypertension in the general population: the Finn-Home study

Hänninen M-RA, Niiranen TJ, Puukka PJ, et al (Natl Inst for Health and Welfare, Turku, Finland; et al)
J Hypertens 29:1880-1888, 2011

Introduction.—Home blood pressure (BP) measurement has allowed the identification of individuals with normal office and elevated out-of-office BP (masked hypertension). It is, however, not feasible to measure home BP on all office normotensive individuals. The objective of the present study was to identify demographic, lifestyle, clinical and psychological characteristics suggestive of masked hypertension.

Methods.—Study population was drawn from the participants of a multidisciplinary epidemiological survey, the Health 2000 Study. The untreated nationwide population sample ($n = 1459$, age 45—74 years) underwent office (duplicate measurements on one visit) and home (duplicate measurements on 7 days) BP measurements and risk factor evaluation. Psychometric tests assessed psychological distress, hypochondriasis, depression and alexithymia. Masked hypertension was defined as normal office BP (<140/90 mmHg) with elevated home BP (≥135/85 mmHg).

Results.—The prevalence of masked hypertension was 8.1% in the untreated Finnish adult population. The cardiovascular risk profile of masked hypertensive patients resembled that of sustained hypertensive patients. High-normal systolic and diastolic office BP, older age, greater BMI, current smoking, excessive alcohol consumption, diabetes and electrocardiographic left-ventricular hypertrophy were independent determinants of masked hypertension in multivariate logistic regression analysis. Masked hypertension was also independently associated with hypochondria.

Conclusion.—Masked hypertension is a common phenomenon in an untreated adult population. Physicians should consider home BP measurement if a patient has high-normal office BP, diabetes, left-ventricular hypertrophy, or several other conventional cardiovascular risk factors.

▶ "Masked hypertension" is the term given to the condition in which people have "normal" blood pressures when measured in the medical office but elevated readings outside it. It is often considered the "reverse" of "white-coat hypertension" and is most reliably detected using ambulatory blood pressure monitoring. Recent estimates put the prevalence of masked hypertension at approximately 7% to 17% of the general population.[1] Although originally thought to be found more in individuals with a stressful life who find acute peace and tranquility in a health care environment, it has since been found to be associated with an increased risk of cardiovascular events not significantly different from individuals with sustained hypertension.[2] People with the condition are traditionally not prescribed antihypertensive medications because their blood pressures are (by definition) at or below goal in the medical office setting. Concern about masked hypertension was one of the reasons that the recent British National Institute of Health and Clinical Excellence guidelines recommended ambulatory blood pressure monitoring for all who are suspected of having a blood pressure problem, because masked hypertension cannot be detected by office visits.[3]

These investigators approached the problem of masked hypertension with a slightly different focus than many others have. They assessed the prevalence of the condition in a population-based survey of 1459 untreated Finns who were 45 to 74 years of age, measured their office blood pressures on 1 office visit and twice daily for a week at home, and subjected them to a broad array of psychological questionnaires. This was done because only 2 previous studies have been performed in this area, and 1 found lower type-A personality scores and fewer depressive symptoms in subjects with masked hypertension[4]; the other showed no such differences (but the population studied included only controlled hypertensives).[5] The results of their survey showed an 8% prevalence of masked hypertension in the untreated Finnish population, about the same as other reports using home blood pressure readings to detect the elevated out-of-office blood pressures. As with all threshold-based diagnoses, the higher the office blood pressures (albeit < 140/90 mm Hg), the greater was the risk of masked hypertension. Finally, as in other studies,[5-9] risk factors for masked hypertension included male gender, older age, obesity, cigarette smoking, alcohol consumption, diabetes, and electrocardiographic left ventricular hypertrophy. Of all the psychological characteristics, only hypochondriasis was independently associated with masked hypertension.

The authors concluded that home blood pressure monitoring is most appropriate for patients with normal in-office blood pressures with other risk factors for masked hypertension. Whether hypochondriasis should be a consideration in this decision is uncertain, but hypochondriacs would probably be more likely to accept the recommendation to perform home blood pressure monitoring because it would feed their hypothesis that they are really "sicker" than their physicians understand.

W. J. Elliott, MD, PhD

References

1. Bobrie G, Clerson P, Ménard J, Postel-Vinay N, Chatellier G, Plouin PF. Masked hypertension: a systematic review. *J Hypertens.* 2008;26:1715-1725.
2. Fagard RH, Cornelissen VA. Incidence of cardiovascular events in white-coat, masked and sustained hypertension versus true normotension: a meta-analysis. *J Hypertens.* 2007;25:2193-2198.
3. Williams B, Williams H, Northedge J, et al; for The Guideline Development Groups, National Collaborating Centres, and NICE Project Team. United Kingdom National Health Service: National Institute for Health and Clinical Excellence. NICE clinical guideline 127: Hypertension: Clinical management of primary hypertension in adults. http://www.nice.org.uk/CG127. Accessed August 24, 2011.
4. Konstantopoulou AS, Konstantopoulou PS, Papargyriou IK, Liatis ST, Stergiou GS, Papadogiannis DE. Masked, white coat and sustained hypertension: comparison of target organ damage and psychometric parameters. *J Hum Hypertens.* 2010;24: 151-157.
5. Mallion JM, Clerson P, Bobrie G, Genes N, Vaisse B, Chatellier G. Predictive factors for masked hypertension within a population of controlled hypertensives. *J Hypertens.* 2006;24:2365-2370.
6. Ungar A, Pepe G, Monami M, et al. Isolated ambulatory hypertension is common in outpatients referred to a hypertension centre. *J Hum Hypertens.* 2004;18: 897-903.

7. Lee HY, Park JB. Prevalence and risk factors of masked hypertension identified by multiple self-blood pressure measurement [Letter]. *Hypertension.* 2008;52: e137-e138.
8. Wang GL, Li Y, Staessen JA, Lu L, Wang JG. Anthropometric and lifestyle factors associated with white-coat, masked and sustained hypertension in a Chinese population. *J Hypertens.* 2007;25:2398-2405.
9. Makris TK, Thomopoulos C, Papadopoulos DP, et al. Association of passive smoking with masked hypertension in clinically normotensive nonsmokers. *Am J Hypertens.* 2009;22:853-859.

Clinical Trials

Cost-effectiveness of options for the diagnosis of high blood pressure in primary care: a modelling study
Lovibond K, Jowett S, Barton P, et al (Royal College of Physicians, London, UK; Univ of Birmingham, UK; et al)
Lancet 378:1219-1230, 2011

Background.—The diagnosis of hypertension has traditionally been based on blood-pressure measurements in the clinic, but home and ambulatory measurements better correlate with cardiovascular outcome, and ambulatory monitoring is more accurate than both clinic and home monitoring in diagnosing hypertension. We aimed to compare the cost-effectiveness of different diagnostic strategies for hypertension.

Methods.—We did a Markov model-based probabilistic cost-effectiveness analysis. We used a hypothetical primary-care population aged 40 years or older with a screening blood-pressure measurement greater than 140/90 mm Hg and risk-factor prevalence equivalent to the general population. We compared three diagnostic strategies—further blood pressure measurement in the clinic, at home, and with an ambulatory monitor—in terms of lifetime costs, quality-adjusted life years, and cost-effectiveness.

Findings.—Ambulatory monitoring was the most cost-effective strategy for the diagnosis of hypertension for men and women of all ages. It was cost-saving for all groups (from −£56 [95% CI −105 to −10] in men aged 75 years to −£323 [−389 to −222] in women aged 40 years) and resulted in more quality-adjusted life years for men and women older than 50 years (from 0·006 [0·000 to 0·015] for women aged 60 years to 0·022 [0·012 to 0·035] for men aged 70 years). This finding was robust when assessed with a wide range of deterministic sensitivity analyses around the base case, but was sensitive if home monitoring was judged to have equal test performance to ambulatory monitoring or if treatment was judged effective irrespective of whether an individual was hypertensive.

Interpretation.—Ambulatory monitoring as a diagnostic strategy for hypertension after an initial raised reading in the clinic would reduce misdiagnosis and save costs. Additional costs from ambulatory monitoring are counterbalanced by cost savings from better targeted treatment.

Ambulatory monitoring is recommended for most patients before the start of antihypertensive drugs.

▶ This is the detailed cost-effectiveness analysis that supports the new recommendation from the 2011 British national hypertension guidelines (issued by the National Institute for health and Clinical Excellence [NICE])[1] that a 24-hour ambulatory blood pressure monitoring (ABPM) session be performed before the diagnosis of hypertension is established. These authors had previously published a systematic review and meta-analysis of the world's literature comparing the efficacy of office, home, and ABPM in diagnosing hypertension, which confirms that ABPM is the most accurate diagnostic technique and the best predictor of target-organ damage and future cardiovascular events.[2]

The fact that ABPM is cost-saving, because it can properly diagnose pure "white-coat hypertension," is not new. Several articles published in the 20th century demonstrated that ABPM can save the long-term costs of follow-up and (unneeded) medication for the roughly 18% to 33% of people with elevated office blood pressures.[3-5] This was presumably the reason that the US Health Care Financing Administration decided to reimburse physicians (albeit with a very low payment) for ABPM in 2001,[6] but if and only if a number of preconditions were met (including a lack of target-organ damage, at least 2 in-office readings above 140/90 mm Hg, and at least 3 readings outside the office with "substantially lower blood pressures"), and the ABPM clearly demonstrated white-coat hypertension. This set of conditions makes it risky for American physicians to order an ABPM (much less purchase the expensive equipment), because only after the ABPM is performed can a determination be made as to whether payment will be made.

In the United Kingdom, however, the NICE guidelines (and the recommendation to uniformly perform ABPM before diagnosing hypertension) pertain only to patients with "pure uncomplicated hypertension," which is rare in the United States. Presumably (but not explicitly stated in this report or in the NICE guidelines themselves), the presence of target-organ damage would make an ABPM unnecessary. The cost of the ABPM equipment used in these analyses ($1016) does not include the required computer, software, and ancillary equipment (multiple cuffs, etc). The cost in Britain is much lower than current manufacturers' suggested retail prices in the United States ($2999 for the Spacelabs 90 217, $2695 for the Suntech Oscar 2) presumably because the National Health Service (NHS) Supply Chain catalogue has negotiated a reasonable price for the technology, which is illegal in the United States. Furthermore, it is likely that the NHS will receive a "quantity discount" for the ABPM equipment, because this diagnostic technique will now become far more common in primary care medical homes and outpatient diagnostic testing facilities, compared with before the new NICE hypertension guideline was issued.

Several other issues are raised by the editorialist.[7] The cost-savings disappear if the ABPM is done more frequently than once every 5 years, which is probably too infrequent for people at high risk of requiring treatment for hypertension. There is also some concern about differing thresholds for treatment in the United Kingdom compared with the United States, where diabetics and patients with chronic kidney disease (not to mention those with established heart disease) have been recommended by US national guidelines to attain and maintain blood pressures under 130/80 mm Hg. The NICE group does not consider these "uncomplicated hypertensives," so they fall beyond the scope of Clinical Guideline 127. They also presumably ought to have an ABPM before initiating antihypertensive therapy because the prevalence of white-coat hypertension is similar in these groups as in the general hypertensive population.

These cost-effectiveness calculations have changed public policy in the United Kingdom, but it is unlikely that they will do so in the United States because the costs of antihypertensive therapy and ABPM technology are much greater, which presents a formidable barrier for recommending routine ABPM before drug treatment of hypertension.

W. J. Elliott, MD, PhD

References

1. NICE clinical guideline 127: Hypertension: Clinical management of primary hypertension in adults. http://www.nice.org.uk/CG127. Accessed August 24, 2011.
2. Hodgkinson J, Mant J, Martin U, et al. Relative effectiveness of clinic and home blood pressure monitoring compared with ambulatory blood pressure monitoring in diagnosis of hypertension: systematic review. *BMJ*. 2011;342:d3621.
3. Krakoff LR, Schechter C, Fahs M, Andre M. Ambulatory blood pressure monitoring: is it cost-effective? *J Hypertens*. 1991;9:S28-S30.
4. Krakoff LR. Ambulatory blood pressure monitoring can improve cost-effective management of hypertension. *Am J Hypertens*. 1993;6:220S-224S.
5. Yarows SA, Khoury S, Sowers JR. Cost effectiveness of 24-hour ambulatory blood pressure monitoring in evaluation and treatment of essential hypertension. *Am J Hypertens*. 1994;7:464-468.
6. Tunis S, Kendall P, Londner M, Whyte J. *Medicare Coverage Policy — Decisions: Ambulatory Blood Pressure Monitoring (#CAG-00067N): Decision Memorandum*. Washington, DC: Health Care Financing Administration; October 17, 2001. http://www.hcfa.gov/coverage/8b3-ff2.htm. Accessed April 01, 2002.
7. Gaziano TA. Accurate hypertension diagnosis is key in efficient control [Editorial]. *Lancet*. 2011;278:1199-1200.

The angiotensin-receptor blocker candesartan for treatment of acute stroke (SCAST): a randomised, placebo-controlled, double-blind trial
Sandset EC, on behalf of the SCAST Study Group (Oslo Univ Hosp Ullevål, Norway; et al)
Lancet 377:741-750, 2011

Background.—Raised blood pressure is common in acute stroke, and is associated with an increased risk of poor outcomes. We aimed to examine whether careful blood-pressure lowering treatment with the angiotensin-receptor blocker candesartan is beneficial in patients with acute stroke and raised blood pressure.

Methods.—Participants in this randomised, placebo-controlled, double-blind trial were recruited from 146 centres in nine north European countries. Patients older than 18 years with acute stroke (ischaemic or haemorrhagic) and systolic blood pressure of 140 mm Hg or higher were included within 30 h of symptom onset. Patients were randomly allocated to candesartan or placebo (1:1) for 7 days, with doses increasing from 4 mg on day 1 to 16 mg on days 3 to 7. Randomisation was stratified by centre, with blocks of six packs of candesartan or placebo. Patients and investigators were masked to treatment allocation. There were two co-primary effect variables: the composite endpoint of vascular death, myocardial infarction, or stroke during the first 6 months; and functional outcome at 6 months, as measured by the modified Rankin Scale. Analyses were by intention to treat. The study is registered, number NCT00120003 (ClinicalTrials.gov), and ISRCTN13643354.

Findings.—2029 patients were randomly allocated to treatment groups (1017 candesartan, 1012 placebo), and data for status at 6 months were available for 2004 patients (99%; 1000 candesartan, 1004 placebo). During the 7-day treatment period, blood pressures were significantly lower in patients allocated candesartan than in those on placebo (mean 147/82 mm Hg [SD 23/14] in the candesartan group on day 7 vs 152/84 mm Hg [22/14] in the placebo group; p<0·0001). During 6 months' follow-up, the risk of the composite vascular endpoint did not differ between treatment groups (candesartan, 120 events, vs placebo, 111 events; adjusted hazard ratio 1·09, 95% CI 0·84−1·41; p=0·52). Analysis of functional outcome suggested a higher risk of poor outcome in the candesartan group (adjusted common odds ratio 1·17, 95% CI 1·00−1·38; p=0·048 [not significant at p≤0·025 level]). The observed effects were similar for all prespecified secondary endpoints (including death from any cause, vascular death, ischaemic stroke, haemorrhagic stroke, myocardial infarction, stroke progression, symptomatic hypotension, and renal failure) and outcomes (Scandinavian Stroke Scale score at 7 days and Barthel index at 6 months), and there was no evidence of a differential effect in any of the prespecified subgroups. During follow-up, nine (1%) patients on candesartan and five (<1%) on placebo had symptomatic hypotension, and renal failure was reported for 18 (2%) patients taking candesartan and 13 (1%) allocated placebo.

Interpretation.—There was no indication that careful blood-pressure lowering treatment with the angiotensin-receptor blocker candesartan is beneficial in patients with acute stroke and raised blood pressure. If anything, the evidence suggested a harmful effect.

▶ The role of blood pressure lowering during or immediately after a stroke (ischemic or hemorrhagic), specifically using angiotensin receptor blockers, is quite controversial. Current US guidelines recommend lowering blood pressure only if it is "extremely high" in the setting of an acute stroke,[1] and most American neurologists prefer to hold antihypertensive drug therapy until stroke rehabilitation is underway, for fear of "increasing the ischemic penumbra" and decreasing blood flow into "watershed areas of the brain." This traditional dogma is being challenged by clinical trials done outside the United States, but so far only one relatively small trial (using candesartan) has shown such a significant benefit of antihypertensive drugs on all cardiovascular events and mortality that it was stopped early, which reduced its already limited power to compare recurrent stroke rates.[2] Another epidemiologic study suggested that patients who suffered a stroke had better outcomes if they were taking antihypertensive drug therapy, especially ARBs, before the stroke.[3] The authors therefore designed and executed the Scandinavian Candesartan Acute Stroke Trial to test the hypothesis that careful lowering of blood pressure with candesartan, given within 30 hours (average, 18 hours) of the onset of stroke symptoms, would improve prognosis, as defined by the 2 coprimary endpoints of first cardiovascular event or functional status (using the modified Rankin scale), 6 months after randomization. By all criteria, this was a well-done study that basically showed no benefit of early antihypertensive treatment and a trend for both primary endpoints in the adverse direction, which was consistent across all prespecified subgroups. In addition, the authors performed, and report in this article, a meta-analysis that included the results of the 9 previous (and smaller) trials and their study, using death or dependency as the outcome variable. This showed only a tightening of the 95% confidence intervals, but no overall change in the point estimate, which was a nonsignificant 4% increase in risk associated with blood pressure—lowering treatment.

The authors and the editorialist for this publication[4] both discuss recent (eg, INTERACT[5] and COSSACS[6]) and ongoing trials that attempt to address variations of the research hypothesis, using, for example, only patients with acute hemorrhagic (INTERACT-2[7]) or ischemic (ENOS[8]) stroke. Until these larger trials are complete, however, SCAST will doubtless be the best current single trial (which was confirmed by the embedded meta-analysis) to support the contention that acute lowering of blood pressure in patients with stroke-in-evolution should not be routinely attempted.

W. J. Elliott, MD, PhD

References

1. Adams HP Jr, del Zoppo G, Alberts MJ, et al. Guidelines for the early management of adults with ischemic stroke: a guideline from the American Heart Association/American Stroke Association Stroke Council, Clinical Cardiology Council, Cardiovascular Radiology and Intervention Council, and the Atherosclerotic Peripheral Vascular Disease and Quality of Care Outcomes in Research Interdisciplinary Working Groups: the American Academy of Neurology affirms the value of this guideline as an educational tool for neurologists. *Stroke.* 2007;38:1655-1711.
2. Schrader J, Lüders S, Kulschewski A, et al. The ACCESS Study: evaluation of Acute Candesartan Cilexetil Therapy in Stroke Survivors. *Stroke.* 2003;34:1699-1703.
3. Fuentes B, Fernández-Domínguez J, Ortega-Casarrubios MA, et al. Treatment with angiotensin receptor blockers before stroke could exert a favourable effect in acute cerebral infarction. *J Hypertens.* 2010;28:575-581.
4. Hankey GJ. Lowering blood pressure in acute stroke: the SCAST trial. *Lancet.* 2011;377:696-698.
5. Anderson CS, Huang Y, Wang JG, et al; INTERACT Investigators. Intensive blood pressure reduction in acute cerebral hemorrhage trial (INTERACT): a randomized pilot trial. *Lancet Neurol.* 2008;7:391-399.
6. Robinson TG, Potter JF, Ford GA, et al; COSSACS Investigators. Effects of antihypertensive treatment after acute stroke in the Continue Or Stop post-Stroke Antihypertensives Collaborative Study (COSSACS): a prospective, randomised, open, blinded-endpoint trial. *Lancet Neurol.* 2010;9:767-775.
7. Delcourt C, Huang Y, Wang J, et al; INTERACT2 Investigators. The second (main) phase of an open, randomized, multicentre study to investigate the

effectiveness of an intensive blood pressure reduction in acute cerebral haemorrhage trial (INTERACT2). *Int J Stroke.* 2010;5:110-116.

8. The ENOS Trial Investigators. Glyceryl trinitrate vs. control, and continuing vs. stopping temporarily prior antihypertensive therapy, in acute stroke: rationale and design of the Efficacy of Nitric Oxide in Stroke (ENOS) trial (ISRCTN99414122). *Int J Stroke.* 2006;1:245-249.

Moderate dietary sodium restriction added to angiotensin converting enzyme inhibition compared with dual blockade in lowering proteinuria and blood pressure: randomised controlled trial

Slagman MCJ, for the HONEST (HOlland NEphrology STudy) Group (Univ Med Ctr Groningen, Netherlands; et al)
BMJ 343:d4366, 2011

Objective.—To compare the effects on proteinuria and blood pressure of addition of dietary sodium restriction or angiotensin receptor blockade at maximum dose, or their combination, in patients with non-diabetic nephropathy receiving background treatment with angiotensin converting enzyme (ACE) inhibition at maximum dose.

Design.—Multicentre crossover randomised controlled trial.

Setting.—Outpatient clinics in the Netherlands.

Participants.—52 patients with non-diabetic nephropathy.

Interventions.—All patients were treated during four 6 week periods, in random order, with angiotensin receptor blockade (valsartan 320 mg/day) or placebo, each combined with, consecutively, a low sodium diet (target 50 mmol Na$^+$/day) and a regular sodium diet (target 200 mmol Na$^+$/day), with a background of ACE inhibition (lisinopril 40 mg/day) during the entire study. The drug interventions were double blind; the dietary interventions were open label.

Main Outcome Measures.—The primary outcome measure was proteinuria; the secondary outcome measure was blood pressure.

Results.—Mean urinary sodium excretion, a measure of dietary sodium intake, was 106 (SE 5) mmol Na$^+$/day during a low sodium diet and 184 (6) mmol Na$^{(+)}$/day during a regular sodium diet (P<0.001). Geometric mean residual proteinuria was 1.68 (95% confidence interval 1.31 to 2.14) g/day during ACE inhibition plus a regular sodium diet. Addition of angiotensin receptor blockade to ACE inhibition reduced proteinuria to 1.44 (1.07 to 1.93) g/day (P=0.003), addition of a low sodium diet reduced it to 0.85 (0.66 to 1.10) g/day (P<0.001), and addition of angiotensin receptor blockade plus a low sodium diet reduced it to 0.67 (0.50 to 0.91) g/day (P<0.001). The reduction of proteinuria by the addition of a low sodium diet to ACE inhibition (51%, 95% confidence interval 43% to 58%) was significantly larger (P<0.001) than the reduction of proteinuria by the addition of angiotensin receptor blockade to ACE inhibition (21%, 8% to 32%) and was comparable (P=0.009, not significant after Bonferroni correction) to the reduction of proteinuria by the addition of both angiotensin receptor blockade and a low sodium diet to ACE inhibition (62%, 53% to 70%). Mean systolic blood pressure was 134 (3) mm Hg during ACE inhibition plus a regular sodium diet. Mean systolic blood pressure was not significantly altered by the addition of angiotensin receptor blockade (131 (3) mm Hg; P=0.12) but was reduced by the addition of a low sodium diet (123 (2) mm Hg; P<0.001) and angiotensin receptor blockade plus a low sodium diet (121 (3) mm Hg; P<0.001) to ACE inhibition. The reduction of systolic blood pressure by the addition of a low sodium diet (7% (SE 1%)) was significantly larger (P=0.003) than the reduction of systolic blood pressure by the addition of angiotensin receptor blockade (2% (1)) and was similar (P=0.14) to the reduction of systolic blood pressure by the addition of both angiotensin receptor blockade and low sodium diet (9% (1)), to ACE inhibition.

Conclusions.—Dietary sodium restriction to a level recommended in guidelines was more effective than dual blockade for reduction of proteinuria and blood pressure in non-diabetic nephropathy. The findings support the combined endeavours of patients and health professionals to reduce sodium intake.

Trial Registration.—Netherlands Trial Register NTR675.

▶ In patients with chronic kidney disease, nephrologists often use the degree of proteinuria as a surrogate endpoint because in several long-term studies, it correlated in direction and degree with both renoprotection (a composite of doubling of serum creatinine, end-stage renal disease, or death[1-4]) and prevention of cardiovascular events. In general, proteinuria can be reduced by lowering blood pressure, adding 1 or more inhibitors of the renin-angiotensin-aldosterone system, or reducing dietary sodium intake, but the relative contributions of each (especially when combined) are not well known. For many patients, long-term dietary sodium restriction is more difficult to sustain than taking more medications (either a very high dose of an angiotensin-converting enzyme [ACE] inhibitor or an angiotensin receptor blocker [ARB], the combination, or the addition of spironolactone). This trial was therefore organized to compare protein excretion rates and blood pressures during periods of high- and low-sodium intake with dual blockade of the renin-angiotensin system (using an ACE-inhibitor + ARB).

For ethical reasons, all patients received traditional lisinopril at 40 mg/d because their urinary protein excretion was in the 1.5 to 2.0 g/d range.[4] The various treatment regimens were given in random order for 6 weeks, without a wash-out phase in between. Dietitians provided advice to participants on 2 to 4 occasions, with the intent of achieving a 24-hour urinary sodium level of 50 (low sodium) or 200 mEq per day (high sodium); on average, participants achieved 106 and 184 mEq per day, respectively. In this "Latin square" design, each participant received each of the 4 regimens, so a paired *t* test was used to compare protein excretion rates and systolic and diastolic blood pressures, resulting in 6 comparisons requiring a Bonferroni adjustment of the acceptable *P* value to .05/(26 − 1), or .0083. The major conclusions of the trial were that the low-sodium diet was both more effective than, and additive to, the effects of full doses of an ARB in reducing both proteinuria and blood pressures, with remarkably few adverse effects (only 7 of 54 patients experienced symptomatic hypotension).

Some limitations are notable. The US Food and Drug Administration still does not recognize proteinuria or albumin/creatinine ratios as useful surrogate endpoints, even in patients with chronic kidney disease. Only 54 of the original 58 patients completed the study; 2 withdrew during the run-in period (ie, before randomization). Each intervention period lasted only 6 weeks, and all patients had nondiabetic nephropathy (a similar trial by the same investigators in subjects with diabetic nephropathy is ongoing and is likely to require many more subjects). Stable doses of diuretics were given to 13 of the 54 patients throughout the protocol, making it difficult to assess whether intensifying diuretic therapy might have had similar effects as reducing dietary sodium.

These data suggest that a low-sodium diet has substantial benefit in patients with proteinuric, nondiabetic chronic kidney disease; the challenge for most patients (both with and without renal disease) is how to achieve and maintain the recommended level of dietary sodium restriction. The fact that the effects of the low-sodium diet are larger than those of adding another drug may help convince some patients (who often wish to avoid taking more medication, especially with hyperkalemia as a known adverse effect) to adopt this lifestyle modification. Future studies are needed to see how well this strategy can be implemented in routine clinical practice. How applicable these data are to patients with lower degrees of urinary protein excretion is also controversial and probably will not be addressed in upcoming guidelines.

W. J. Elliott, MD, PhD

References

1. Lewis EJ, Hunsicker LG, Bain RP, Rohde RD. The effect of angiotensin-converting-enzyme inhibition on diabetic nephropathy. The Collaborative Study Group. *N Engl J Med*. 1993;323:1456-1462.
2. Lewis EJ, Hunsicker LG, Clarke WR, et al; Collaborative Study Group. Renoprotective effect of the angiotensin-receptor antagonist irbesartan in patients with nephropathy due to Type 2 diabetes. *N Engl J Med*. 2001;345:851-860.
3. Brenner BM, Cooper ME, de Zeeuw D, et al; RENAAL Study Investigators. Effects of losartan on renal and cardiovascular outcomes in patients with type 2 diabetes and nephropathy. *N Engl J Med*. 2001;345:861-869.
4. Jafar TH, Stark PC, Schmid CH, et al. Progression of chronic kidney disease: the role of blood pressure control, proteinuria, and angiotensin-converting enzyme inhibition: a patient-level meta-analysis. *Ann Intern Med*. 2003;139:244-252.

A double-blind, randomized study comparing the antihypertensive effect of eplerenone and spironolactone in patients with hypertension and evidence of primary aldosteronism
Parthasarathy HK, Ménard J, White WB, et al (Papworth Hosp, Cambridge, UK; Paris-Descartes Univ, Paris, France; Univ of Connecticut School of Medicine, Farmington; et al)
J Hypertens 29:980-990, 2011

Background.—Eplerenone is claimed to be a more selective blocker of the mineralocorticoid receptor than spironolactone being associated with fewer antiandrogenic side-effects. We compared the efficacy, safety and tolerability of eplerenone versus spironolactone in patients with hypertension associated with primary aldosteronism.

Methods.—The study was multicentre, randomized, double-blind, active-controlled, and parallel group design. Following a single-blind, placebo run-in period, patients were randomized 1 : 1 to a 16-week double-blind, treatment period of spironolactone (75−225 mg once daily) or eplerenone (100−300 mg once daily) using a titration-to-effect design. To be randomized, patients had to meet biochemical criteria for primary aldosteronism and have a seated DBP at least 90 mmHg and less than 120 mmHg and SBP less than 200 mmHg. The primary efficacy endpoint was the antihypertensive effect of eplerenone versus spironolactone to establish noninferiority of eplerenone in the mean change from baseline in seated DBP.

Results.—Changes from baseline in DBP were less on eplerenone ($-5.6 \pm$ 1.3 SE mmHg) than spironolactone (-12.5 ± 1.3 SE mmHg) [difference, -6.9 mmHg (-10.6, -3.3); $P<0.001$]. Although there were no significant differences between eplerenone and spironolactone in the overall incidence of adverse events, more patients randomized to spironolactone developed male gynaecomastia (21.2 versus 4.5%; $P=0.033$) and female mastodynia (21.1 versus 0.0%; $P=0.026$).

Conclusion.—The antihypertensive effect of spironolactone was significantly greater than that of eplerenone in hypertension associated with primary aldosteronism.

▶ Eplerenone is a more selective aldosterone receptor antagonist than spironolactone, with fewer adverse effects; spironolactone's side effects have been attributed to its antiandrogenic and progestin-like effects.[1] Despite the fact that eplerenone became generically available in the United States in 2008, it is still far more expensive than spironolactone ($3.07/50 mg pill vs $0.91/100 mg pill at drugstore.com on December 27, 2011), and many formularies do not include it. These drugs have an important role in severe heart failure[2,3] (and left ventricular dysfunction postmyocardial infarction),[4] hyperaldosteronism (and obstructive sleep apnea),[5,6] and resistant hypertension.[7] Many physicians believe that the 2 drugs are equipotent, because there is only 1 small study in 34 subjects that compared the 2 in a head-to-head fashion.

These authors therefore performed a multicenter, randomized trial comparing the 2 drugs, head-to-head, in patients with proven hyperaldosteronism. They titrated the doses of each agent (300 mg/d for eplerenone, 225 mg/d of spironolactone) to well beyond what the US Food and Drug Administration considers the maximum dose for each to allay concerns about a possible comparison at subtherapeutic doses. The study was designed as a "noninferiority trial," perhaps to obtain funding from the developer of eplerenone, which has since been acquired. This is one of the few trials that, despite its design as an "equivalence trial," was able to prove superiority of the conventional over the experimental agent. The authors' conclusion seems fair: spironolactone is a far more potent antihypertensive agent than eplerenone. However, the brief abstract does not include what may be a more important point: 80.3% of the subjects receiving spironolactone and 62.9% given eplerenone completed the study. Withdrawals for adverse events included 11.3% of those given spironolactone, compared with 10.0% given eplerenone; fully 20% of the eplerenone-treated group withdrew because of treatment failure (ie, inability to lower blood pressure in accord with the investigator's desires). As expected, fewer subjects experienced breast discomfort or tenderness with eplerenone, but comparison of most symptoms during treatment favored spironolactone.

It is perhaps fortunate that eplerenone was never promoted for hypertension, because these data indicate that it is much less effective than the far less expensive spironolactone. It is likely that managed care pharmacies can use this important article to enforce a "step-edit" for the more expensive drug and insist that it be given only to patients who develop breast complaints or other sexual adverse effects after a specific number of weeks of spironolactone.

W. J. Elliott, MD, PhD

References

1. Croom KF, Perry CM. Eplerenone: a review of its use in essential hypertension. *Am J Cardiovasc Drugs*. 2008;5:51-69.
2. Pitt B, Zannad F, Remme WJ, et al. The effect of spironolactone on morbidity and mortality in patients with severe heart failure. Randomized Aldactone Evaluation Study Investigators. *N Engl J Med*. 1999;341:709-717.
3. Zannad F, McMurray JJ, Krum H, et al; EMPHASIS-HF Study Group. Eplerenone in patients with systolic heart failure and mild symptoms. *N Engl J Med*. 2011; 364:11-21.
4. Pitt B, Remme W, Zannad F, et al; Eplerenone Post-Acute Myocardial Infarction Heart Failure Efficacy and Survival Study Investigators. Eplerenone, a selective aldosterone blocker, in patients with left ventricular dysfunction after myocardial infarction. *N Engl J Med*. 2003;348:1309-1321.
5. Funder JW, Carey RM, Fardella C, et al. Case detection, diagnosis, and treatment of patients with primary aldosteronism: an endocrine society clinical practice guideline. *J Clin Endocrinol Metab*. 2008;93:3266-3281.
6. Epstein LJ, Kristo D, Strollo PJ Jr, et al. Clinical guideline for the evaluation, management and long-term care of obstructive sleep apnea in adults. *J Clin Sleep Med*. 2009;5:263-276.
7. Calhoun DA, Jones D, Textor S, et al. Resistant hypertension: Diagnosis, evaluation, and treatment. A Scientific Statement from the American Heart Association Professional Education Committee of the Council for High Blood Pressure Research. *Hypertension*. 2008;51:1403-1419.

Is a systolic blood pressure target <140 mmHg indicated in all hypertensives? Subgroup analyses of findings from the randomized FEVER trial

Zhang Y, for the FEVER Study Group (FuWai Hosp and Cardiovascular Inst, Beijing, China; et al)
Eur Heart J 32:1500-1508, 2011

Aims.—Major guidelines recommend lowering systolic blood pressure (SBP) to <140 mmHg in all hypertensives, but evidence is missing whether this is beneficial in (i) uncomplicated hypertensives, (ii) grade 1 hypertensives, and (iii) elderly hypertensives. Providing this missing evidence is important to justify efforts and costs of aggressive therapy in all hypertensives.

Methods and Results.—Felodipine Event Reduction (FEVER) was a double-blind, randomized trial on 9711 Chinese hypertensives, in whom cardiovascular outcomes were significantly reduced by more intense therapy (low-dose hydrochlorothiazide and low-dose felodipine) achieving a mean of 138 mmHg SBP compared with less-intense therapy (low-dose hydro-chlorothiazide and placebo) achieving a mean of 142 mmHg. FEVER included older and younger patients, and patients with and without diabetes or cardiovascular disease. In the analyses here reported, Cox regression models assessed outcome differences between more and less-intense treatments in groups of patients with different baseline characteristics. Significant reductions in stroke were found in uncomplicated hypertensives (-39%, $P = 0.002$), in hypertensives with randomization SBP, 153 mmHg (-29%, $P = 0.03$), and in elderly hypertensives (-44%, $P < 0.001$), when their SBP was lowered by more intense treatment. Significant reductions (between -29 and -47%, $P = 0.02$ to <0.001) were also found in all cardiovascular events and all deaths. Achieving mean SBP values <140 mmHg by adding a small dose of a generic drug prevented 2.1 (uncomplicated hypertensives) and 5.2 (elderly) cardiovascular events every 100 patients treated for 3.3 years.

Conclusions.—These analyses provide strong support, missing so far, to guidelines recommending goal SBP <140 mmHg in uncomplicated hypertensives, individuals with moderately elevated BP and elderly hypertensives.

The FEVER trial has been registered on www.clinicaltrials.gov, n. NCT01136863.

▶ There is new, pervasive emphasis among guideline writers to require that all recommendations be very evidence based, using clinical trials or meta-analyses of clinical trials as the highest-ranking evidence.[1] As noted by these authors, clinical trial evidence for a systolic blood pressure less than 140 mm Hg is lacking, primarily because diastolic blood pressure was the major target of treatment until about the year 2000. The clinical trial evidence for a benefit of lower blood pressure targets for patients with diabetes,[2-4] chronic kidney disease,[5] or established heart disease[6] has not been statistically significant when rigorously evaluated recently. Many anticipate that the soon-to-be-released Eighth Report of the Joint National Committee on Prevention, Detection, Evaluation, and Treatment of High Blood Pressure will also follow recent hypertension guidelines from the United Kingdom[1] and rescind these lower blood pressure targets due to lack of evidence that they are effective in preventing cardiovascular or renal disease events.

The Felodipine EVEnt Reduction trial provided the data for this posthoc analysis that, by happy coincidence, compared outcomes in hypertensive Chinese patients whose blood pressures were not adequately controlled with a low dose of hydrochlorothiazide and who were then randomly assigned to continue the hydrochlorothiazide and add either low-dose felodipine or placebo. The mean on-treatment systolic blood pressure for the latter was 142 mm Hg, whereas that of the former was 138 mm Hg, allowing a comparison between groups above and below 140 mm Hg. These specific analyses were done to explore the outcome differences in 3 subgroups: (1) otherwise uncomplicated hypertensives, (2) hypertensive patients ≥65 years of age (elderly), and (3) "high-risk" hypertensive patients (eg, diabetics, previous cardiovascular disease events, or left ventricular hypertrophy).

The data suggest that outcomes are improved if the achieved systolic blood pressure is, on average, less than 140 mm Hg, compared with greater than 140 mm Hg. The authors recognize the many limitations of their data and conclusions, the most important of which is that the trial did not prespecify the target blood pressures (unlike the Hypertension Optimal Treatment study did for diastolic blood pressure,[7] for example). The analyses performed preserve randomization and are therefore less likely to be biased than similar analyses done with other clinical trials,[8] although it is probably tempting for the FEVER authors to perform a supplemental analysis that explores outcomes according to achieved systolic blood pressure, regardless of randomized treatment. It seems likely, however, that conclusions of such an analysis would not be much different than those seen here, which, in fact, may be the most direct evidence in favor of the less-than 140 mm Hg systolic blood pressure goal.

W. J. Elliott, MD, PhD

References

1. NICE clinical guideline 127: Hypertension: Clinical management of primary hypertension in adults. http://www.nice.org.uk/CG127. Accessed 24 Aug 2011.
2. Cushman WC, Evans GW, Byington RP, et al; on behalf of The Action to Control Cardiovascular Risk in Diabetes (ACCORD) Study Group. Effects of intensive blood-pressure control in type 2 diabetes mellitus. *N Engl J Med.* 2010;362: 1575-1585.
3. Turnbull F, Neal B, Algert C, et al; Blood Pressure Lowering Treatment Trialists' Collaboration. Effects of different blood pressure-lowering regimens on major cardiovascular events in individuals with and without diabetes mellitus: results of prospectively designed overviews of randomized trials. *Arch Intern Med.* 2005;165:1410-1419.
4. Elliott WJ. What should be the blood pressure target for diabetics patients? *Curr Opin Cardiol.* 2011;26:308-313.
5. Upadhyay A, Earley A, Haynes SM, Uhlig K. Systematic review: blood pressure target in chronic kidney disease and proteinuria as an effect modifier. *Ann Intern Med.* 2011;154:541-548.
6. Rosendorff C, Black HR, Cannon CP, et al. Treatment of hypertension in the prevention and management of ischemic heart disease: a scientific statement from the American Heart Association Council for High Blood Pressure Research and the Councils on Clinical Cardiology and Epidemiology and Prevention. *Circulation.* 2007;115:2761-2788.
7. Hansson L, Zanchetti A, Carruthers SG, et al. Effects of intensive blood-pressure lowering and low-dose aspirin in patients with hypertension: principal results of the Hypertension Optimal Treatment (HOT) randomised trial. HOT Study Group. *Lancet.* 1998;351:1755-1762.
8. Weber M, Julius S, Kjeldsen KE, et al. Blood pressure dependent and independent effects of antihypertensive treatment on clinical events in the VALUE trial. *Lancet.* 2004;363:2049-2051.

Effects of Manidipine and Delapril in Hypertensive Patients With Type 2 Diabetes Mellitus: The Delapril and Manidipine for Nephroprotection in Diabetes (DEMAND) Randomized Clinical Trial

Ruggenenti P, for the DEMAND Study Investigators (Mario Negri Inst for Pharmacological Res, Ranica, Bergamo, Italy; et al)
Hypertension 58:776-783, 2011

To assess whether angiotensin-converting enzyme inhibitors and third-generation dihydropyridine calcium channel blockers ameliorate diabetic complications, we compared glomerular filtration rate (GFR; primary outcome), cardiovascular events, retinopathy, and neuropathy in 380 hypertensive type 2 diabetics with albuminuria <200 mg/min included in a multicenter, double-blind, placebo-controlled trial (DEMAND [Delapril and Manidipine for Nephroprotection in Diabetes]) and randomized to 3-year treatment with manidipine/delapril combination (10/30 mg/d; n=126), delapril (30 mg/d; n=127), or placebo (n=127). GFR was centrally measured by iohexol plasma clearance. Median monthly GFR decline (interquartile range [IQR]) was 0.32 mL/min per 1.73 m^2 (IQR: 0.16−0.50 mL/min per 1.73 m^2) on combined therapy, 0.36 mL/min per 1.73 m^2 (IQR: 0.18−0.53 mL/min per 1.73 m^2) on delapril, and 0.30 mL/min per 1.73 m^2 (IQR: 0.12−0.50 mL/min per 1.73 m^2) on placebo ($P=0.87$ and $P=0.53$ versus combined therapy or delapril, respectively). Similar findings were observed when baseline GFR values were not considered for slope analyses. Albuminuria was stable in the 3 treatment groups. The hazard ratio (95% CI) for major cardiovascular events between combined therapy and placebo was 0.17 (0.04−0.78; $P=0.023$). Among 192 subjects without retinopathy at inclusion, the hazard ratio for developing retinopathy between combined therapy and placebo was 0.27 (0.07−0.99; $P=0.048$). Among 200 subjects with centralized neurological evaluation, the odds ratios for peripheral neuropathy at 3 years between combined therapy or delapril and placebo were 0.45 (0.24−0.87; $P=0.017$) and 0.52 (0.27−0.99; $P=0.048$), respectively. Glucose disposal rate decreased from 5.8 ± 2.4 to 5.3 ± 1.9 mg/kg per min on placebo ($P=0.03$) but did not change on combined or delapril therapy. Treatment was well tolerated. In hypertensive type 2 diabetic patients, combined manidipine and delapril therapy failed to slow GFR decline but safely ameliorated cardiovascular disease, retinopathy, and neuropathy and stabilized insulin sensitivity.

▶ This rather bold clinical trial was designed to test the effects on renal function of 2 therapies against placebo in hypertensive diabetics at very low risk for doubling serum creatinine, end-stage renal disease, or renal replacement therapy (a composite endpoint used previously for "renoprotection").[1-5] The recruited patients had a baseline glomerular filtration rate (GFR) of about 100 mL/min/ 1.73 m^2; an average age of 60 years; only 6 years of diabetes (which was extremely well controlled); and an average urinary albumin excretion of 5−7 µg/min (~80-95 mg/d). Data from these investigators and others suggested that such patients usually lose about 0.33 mL/min/1.73 m^2 of GFR per month (if blood pressure were to remain untreated)[6] but remain stable in those with well-controlled blood pressures. The authors chose active antihypertensive drug therapy that was predicted to maximize renal benefits. They and others have found that angiotensin-converting enzyme (ACE) inhibitors blunt the decline in renal function and many other adverse outcomes in diabetics. Manidipine, a "third-generation" dihydropyridine calcium antagonist that also blocks T-type calcium channels in postglomerular arterioles, and has reduced albuminuria in hypertensive type 2 diabetics, even when treated with angiotensin receptor blockers,[7] was expected to further improve prognosis in these patients.

Many would characterize the primary results of this trial as negative. Despite a great effort to control confounders and a very large number of secondary exploratory analyses, they found no significant difference across randomized groups in the loss of renal function, which was, in fact, almost exactly the predicted mean fall in untreated subjects (and 3–6 times the rate of normotensive, nondiabetic subjects). This must have been very disappointing to the investigators. They claim that the failure to detect a difference across treatments was not due to lack of statistical power and therefore is likely due to pathogenic factors that were not specifically treated in the trial, such as metabolic factors in diabetes, oxidative stress, or inflammation.

The authors claim that their secondary outcomes data on cardiovascular events, retinopathy, and glucose disposal rates do show advantages for the combined treatment versus placebo. It is notable, however, that their statistics were not adjusted for multiple comparisons, which would make their threshold P-values smaller than those that were reported. Their very carefully worded Statistical Methods section suggests that the favored comparison was between placebo and combination therapy, but they report performing "adjusted Cox proportional hazards analyses" for the composite cardiovascular outcome when there were only 2 versus 8 afflicted patients in the 2 compared groups. Nonetheless, the trends they observed are similar to those seen in treated type 1 diabetics (for retinopathy),[8] and in hypertensive diabetics and nondiabetics given an ACE-inhibitor plus dihydropyridine calcium antagonist (for cardiovascular events).[9,10] The editorialist for this article agrees with the authors that more research is needed to identify strategies that can blunt the decline in loss of renal function in early diabetes.[11]

W. J. Elliott, MD, PhD

References

1. Lewis EJ, Hunsicker LG, Bain RP, Rohde RD. The effect of angiotensin converting enzyme inhibition in diabetic nephropathy. The Collaborative Study Group. *N Engl J Med.* 1993;329:1456-1462.
2. Lewis EJ, Hunsicker LG, Clarke WR, et al; Collaborative Study Group. Renoprotective effect of the angiotensin-receptor antagonist irbesartan in patients with nephropathy due to type 2 diabetes. *N Engl J Med.* 2001;345:851-860.
3. Brenner BM, Cooper ME, de Zeeuw D, et al; RENAAL Study Investigators. Effects of losartan on renal and cardiovascular outcomes in patients with Type 2 diabetes and nephropathy. *N Engl J Med.* 2001;345:861-869.
4. Mann JF, Schmieder RE, McQueen M; ONTARGET Investigators. Renal outcomes with telmisartan, ramipril, or both, in people at high vascular risk

(the ONTARGET study): a multicentre, randomised, double-blind, controlled trial. *Lancet.* 2008;372:547-553.

5. Bakris GL, Sarafidis PA, Weir MR, et al; ACCOMPLISH Trial Investigators. Renal outcomes with different fixed-dose combination therapies in patients with hypertension at high risk for cardiovascular events (ACCOMPLISH): a pre-specified secondary analysis of a randomised controlled trial. *Lancet.* 2010;375: 1173-1181.

6. Lebovitz HE, Wiegmann TB, Cnaan A, et al. Renal protective effects of enalapril in hypertensive NIDDM: role of baseline albuminuria. *Kidney Int.* 1994;45: S150-S155.

7. Fogari R, Corradi L, Zoppi A, et al. Addition of manidipine improves the anti-proteinuric effect of candesartan in hypertensive patients with type II diabetes and microalbuminuria. *Am J Hypertens.* 2007;20:1092-1096.

8. Mauer M, Zinman B, Gardiner R, et al. Renal and retinal effects of enalapril and losartan in type 1 diabetes. *N Engl J Med.* 2009;361:40-51.

9. Jamerson K, Weber MA, Bakris GL, et al; ACCOMPLISH Trial Investigators. Benazepril plus amlodipine or hydrochlorothiazide for hypertension in high-risk patients. *N Engl J Med.* 2008;359:2417-2428.

10. Weber MA, Bakris GL, Jamerson K, et al; ACCOMPLISH Investigators. Cardio-vascular events during differing hypertension therapies in patients with diabetes. *J Am Coll Cardiol.* 2010;56:77-85.

11. Weir MR. Optimal treatment strategies for patients with hypertension and dia-betes: are effects on metabolism important [Editorial]? *Hypertension.* 2011;58: 758-759.

Aliskiren and the calcium channel blocker amlodipine combination as an initial treatment strategy for hypertension control (ACCELERATE): a randomised, parallel-group trial

Brown MJ, McInnes GT, Papst CC, et al (Univ of Cambridge, UK; British Hypertension Society, London, UK; Novartis Pharma AG, Basel, Switzerland)
Lancet 377:312-320, 2011

Background.—Short-term studies have suggested that the use of initial combination therapy for the control of blood pressure improves early effectiveness. We tested whether a combination of aliskiren and amlodi-pine is superior to each monotherapy in early control of blood pressure without excess of adverse events, and if initial control by monotherapy impairs subsequent control by combination therapy.

Methods.—We did a double-blind, randomised, parallel-group, superi-ority trial at 146 primary and secondary care sites in ten countries, with enrolment from Nov 28, 2008, to July 15, 2009. Patients eligible for enrol-ment had essential hypertension, were aged 18 years or older, and had systolic blood pressure between 150 and 180 mm Hg. Patients were ran-domly assigned (1:1:2) to treatment with 150 mg aliskiren plus placebo, 5 mg amlodipine plus placebo, or 150 mg aliskiren plus 5 mg amlodipine. Random assignment was through a central interactive voice response system and treatment allocation was masked from the patients. From 16–32 weeks, all patients received combination therapy with 300 mg aliskiren plus 10 mg amlodipine. Our primary endpoints, assessed on an intention-to-treat basis (ie, in patients who received the allocated treatment), were the adjusted mean reduction in systolic blood pressure from baseline over 8 to 24 weeks, and then the final reduction at 24 weeks. This trial is registered with ClinicalTrials.gov, number NCT00797862.

Findings.—318 patients were randomly assigned to aliskiren, 316 to amlodipine, and 620 to aliskiren plus amlodipine. 315 patients initially allocated to aliskiren, 315 allocated to amlodipine, and 617 allocated to aliskiren plus amlodipine were available for analysis. Patients given initial combination therapy had a 6·5 mm Hg (95% CI 5·3 to 7·7) greater reduction in mean systolic blood pressure than the monotherapy groups (p<0·0001). At 24 weeks, when all patients were on combination treatment, the difference was 1·4 mm Hg (95% CI −0·05 to 2·9; p=0·059). Adverse events caused withdrawal of 85 patients (14%) from the initial aliskiren plus amlodipine group, 45 (14%) from the aliskiren group, and 58 (18%) from the amlodipine group. Adverse events were peripheral oedema, hypotension, or orthostatic hypotension.

Interpretation.—We believe that routine initial reduction in blood pressure (>150 mm Hg) with a combination such as aliskiren plus amlodipine can be recommended.

▶ The role of initial combination drug therapy for hypertension is expanding. The Seventh Report of the Joint National Committee on Prevention, Detection, Evaluation and Treatment of High Blood Pressure recommended that "consideration be given to initiating therapy with a 2-drug regimen, either as a fixed-dose combination or separate prescriptions," if the initial blood pressure was greater than 20/10 mm Hg higher than the target blood pressure.[1] In the last 5 years, the US Food and Drug Administration has approved more 2-drug anti-hypertensive combinations for initial therapy than in the prior 30 years, particularly "if the probability of achieving blood pressure goals with monotherapy is small." Progress in approval of initial 2-drug therapies in the United Kingdom has apparently been slower, as only combinations of a diuretic and beta-blocker are marketed for initial therapy there.

The evidence base for this strategy has been strengthened, but not really proven, in post-hoc analyses from the Valsartan Antihypertensive Long-term Use Evaluation (VALUE)[2] and the Systolic Hypertension in Europe (Syst-Eur) Trials[3] and by a recent meta-analysis that suggests that even after initial randomized therapies are stopped at the end of a trial's planned follow-up, significant differences in cardiovascular endpoints persist.[4]

This trial was therefore undertaken to compare the blood pressure control rates and safety data in hypertensive people who were given either initial combination therapy or who could be given such therapy after monotherapy when one or the other option was insufficient. The study design was a traditional parallel-group randomized trial, but the same question was asked by Canadian investigators,[5] who found the same answer: initial combination therapy lowers blood pressure more quickly to target, and when the initial combination has fewer adverse effects than high-dose monotherapy, results show fewer discontinuations of therapy and higher quality-of-life and health care provider satisfaction scores (neither of which was studied in this trial).

Many unanswered questions remain about ACCELERATE and its implications. The significant differences in systolic and diastolic blood pressures across treatment groups 16 weeks after randomization (ie, after dose doubling) were not significant thereafter, suggesting that, in the end, each strategy controls blood pressure equally well after 24 weeks. This is important because the post-hoc data from VALUE used the 6-month blood pressure control to dichotomize "responders" and showed they had improved long-term outcomes.[2] There are no data to suggest that attaining blood pressure control at 16 weeks makes a difference with regard to adverse cardiovascular or renal outcomes. The addition of hydrochlorothiazide to any of the 3 regimens for the last 8 weeks of the trial seemed to have little, if any, benefit on blood pressure, consistent with a recent systematic review and meta-analysis regarding this diuretic.[6]

Other concerns result from the reported adverse effects observed during the trial. The addition of aliskiren to amlodipine appears to have a small and nonsignificant effect on peripheral edema (21.4%) compared with amlodipine alone (24.1%), contrary to the conclusion of a recent meta-analysis of the addition of an angiotensin-converting enzyme inhibitor or an angiotensin receptor blocker to a dihydropyridine calcium antagonist.[7] To be fair, there was a significant ($P = .04$) difference in discontinuations for pedal edema, but this was not corrected for multiple comparisons. Lastly, angioedema, cardiac failure, and hypertensive crises were observed during the trial, but details regarding drug therapy in the affected patients were not provided. Several correspondents have also expressed concern about the authors' opinion that "a combination such as aliskiren + amlodipine can be recommended."[8]

W. J. Elliott, MD, PhD

References

1. Chobanian AV, Bakris GL, Black HR, et al; Joint National Committee on Prevention, Detection, Evaluation, and Treatment of High Blood Pressure. National Heart, Lung, and Blood Institute; National High Blood Pressure Education Program Coordinating Committee. Seventh report of the Joint National Committee on Prevention, Detection, Evaluation, and Treatment of High Blood Pressure. *Hypertension.* 2003;42: 1206-1252.
2. Weber MA, Julius S, Kjeldsen SE, et al. Blood pressure dependent and independent effects of antihypertensive treatment on clinical events in the VALUE trial. *Lancet.* 2004;363:2049-2051.
3. Staessen JA, Thijisq L, Fagard R, et al. Effects of immediate versus delayed antihypertensive therapy on outcome in the Systolic Hypertension in Europe trial. *J Hypertens.* 2004;22:847-857.
4. Kostis WJ, Thijs L, Richart T, Kostis JB, Staessen JA. Persistence of mortality reduction after the end of randomized therapy in clinical trials of blood pressure-lowering medications. *Hypertension.* 2010;56:1060-1068.
5. Feldman RD, Zou GY, Vandervoort MK, Wong CJ, Nelson SA, Feagan BG. A simplified approach to the treatment of uncomplicated hypertension: a cluster randomized, controlled trial. *Hypertension.* 2009;53:646-653.
6. Messerli FH, Makani H, Benjo A, Romero J, Alviar C, Bangalore S. Antihypertensive efficacy of hydrochlorothiazide as evaluated by ambulatory blood pressure monitoring: a meta-analysis of randomized trials. *J Am Coll Cardiol.* 2011;57: 590-600.

7. Makani H, Bangalore S, Romero J, Wever-Pinzon O, Messerli FH. Effect of renin-angiotensin system blockade on calcium channel blocker-associated peripheral edema. *Am J Med.* 2011;124:128-135.
8. Chan SS-W, Rainer TH, Ruggenenti P, Remuzzi G. Initial combination therapy for treatment of hypertension [Letters]. *Lancet.* 2011;377:1490-1492.

Conventional versus automated measurement of blood pressure in primary care patients with systolic hypertension: randomised parallel design controlled trial

Myers MG, Godwin M, Dawes M, et al (Univ of Toronto, Ontario, Canada; Memorial Univ of Newfoundland, St John's, Canada; McGill Univ, Montreal, Quebec, Canada; et al)
BMJ 342:d286, 2011

Objective.—To compare the quality and accuracy of manual office blood pressure and automated office blood pressure using the awake ambulatory blood pressure as a gold standard.

Design.—Multi-site cluster randomised controlled trial.

Setting.—Primary care practices in five cities in eastern Canada.

Participants.—555 patients with systolic hypertension and no serious comorbidities under the care of 88 primary care physicians in 67 practices in the community.

Interventions.—Practices were randomly allocated to either ongoing use of manual office blood pressure (control group) or automated office blood pressure (intervention group) using the BpTRU device. The last routine manual office blood pressure (mm Hg) was obtained from each patient's medical record before enrolment. Office blood pressure readings were compared before and after enrolment in the intervention and control groups; all readings were also compared with the awake ambulatory blood pressure.

Main Outcome Measure.—Difference in systolic blood pressure between awake ambulatory blood pressure minus automated office blood pressure and awake ambulatory blood pressure minus manual office blood pressure.

Results.—Cluster randomisation allocated 31 practices (252 patients) to manual office blood pressure and 36 practices (303 patients) to automated office blood pressure measurement. The most recent routine manual office blood pressure (149.5 (SD 10.8)/81.4 (8.3)) was higher than automated office blood pressure (135.6 (17.3)/77.7 (10.9)) (P<0.001). In the control group, routine manual office blood pressure before enrolment (149.9 (10.7)/81.8 (8.5)) was reduced to 141.4 (14.6)/80.2 (9.5) after enrolment (P<0.001/P=0.01), but the reduction in the intervention group from manual office to automated office blood pressure was significantly greater (P<0.001/P=0.02). On the first study visit after enrolment, the estimated-mean difference for the intervention group between the awake ambulatory systolic/diastolic blood pressure and automated office blood pressure (−2.3 (95% confidence interval −0.31 to −4.3)/−3.3 (−2.7 to −4.4)) was less (P=0.006/P=0.26) than the difference in the control group between the awake ambulatory blood pressure and the manual office blood pressure (−6.5 (−4.3 to −8.6)/−4.3 (−2.9 to −5.8)). Systolic/diastolic automated office blood pressure showed a stronger (P<0.001) within group correlation (r=0.34/r=0.56) with awake ambulatory blood pressure after enrolment compared with manual office blood pressure versus awake ambulatory blood pressure before enrolment (r=0.10/r=0.40); the mean difference in r was 0.24 (0.12 to 0.36)/0.16 (0.07 to 0.25)). The between group correlation comparing diastolic automated office blood pressure and awake ambulatory blood pressure (r=0.56) was stronger (P<0.001) than that for manual office blood pressure versus awake ambulatory blood pressure (r=0.30); the mean difference in r was 0.26 (0.09 to 0.41). Digit preference with readings ending in zero was substantially reduced by use of automated office blood pressure.

Conclusion.—In compliant, otherwise healthy, primary care patients with systolic hypertension, introduction of automated office blood pressure measurement into routine primary care significantly reduced the white coat response compared with the ongoing use of manual office blood pressure measurement. The quality and accuracy of automated office blood pressure in relation to the awake ambulatory blood pressure was also significantly better when compared with manual office blood pressure.

Trial Registration.—Clinical trials NCT 00214053.

▶ Obtaining accurate office blood pressure measurements is challenging because few medical offices routinely take the appropriate steps (and 14 minutes per patient) to standardize the process, despite recently updated national guidelines regarding the procedure.[1] To identify the approximately 20% of patients with "white-coat hypertension" and another 10% to 15% with "masked hypertension," the recent British National Institute of Health and Clinical Excellence guidelines recommend that every person suspected of hypertension should undergo 24-hour ambulatory blood pressure monitoring[2] because it is cost-effective in the United Kingdom.[3] An alternative to this technically complex and potentially costly procedure would be simple protocols for office blood pressure measurements, which this investigative group has developed and validated for more than a decade. This report summarizes the results of the first phase of the Conventional versus Automated Measurement of Blood pressure in the Office (CAMBO) trial.

The authors' data suggest that a series of automated office blood pressures reduces the "white-coat response" and correlates better with awake ambulatory blood pressure monitoring readings than traditional, manual office readings. Although this does not necessarily prove that the automated readings better predict prognosis, the fact that automated office readings correlate better with 24-hour ambulatory readings (which most see as the best predictor of both target-organ damage and prognosis[4]) is strong evidence in their favor.

The authors point out several limitations of their study, including that it was conducted in reasonably adherent primary care patients with no major comorbidities with their hypertension. Because it was not designed to interfere much with the daily practice of medicine, they did not undertake extensive staff training in measuring blood pressure (using either the automated device or traditional methods). This accounts for some of the differences in results between this study and several others they have done before, which were meant to demonstrate the validity of the automated readings.[5] However, it seems likely that this "demonstration project" could easily be transitioned to other primary care practices with little increase in staff time, training, or effort. Other investigators have also reported that a series of automated blood pressure measurements, without the health care provider in the room, improved several measures of quality related to blood pressure measurements.[6,7]

W. J. Elliott, MD, PhD

References

1. Pickering TG, Hall JE, Appel LJ, et al; Subcommittee of Professional and Public Education of the American Heart Association Council on High Blood Pressure Research. Recommendations for blood pressure measurement in humans and experimental animals: Part 1: blood pressure measurement in humans: a statement for professionals from the Subcommittee of Professional and Public Education of the American Heart Association Council on High Blood Pressure Research. *Hypertension.* 2005;45: 142-161.
2. Williams B, Williams H, Northedge J, et al; for The Guideline Development Groups, National Collaborating Centres, and NICE Project Team. NICE Clinical Guideline 127: Hypertension: Clinical Management of Primary Hypertension in Adults. United Kingdom National Health Service: National Institute for Health and Clinical Excellence. http://www.nice.org.uk/CG127. Accessed August 24, 2011.
3. Lovibond K, Jowett S, Barton P, et al. Cost-effectiveness of options for the diagnosis of high blood pressure in primary care: a modelling study. *Lancet.* 2011; 378:1219-1230.
4. Hodgkinson J, Mant J, Martin U, et al. Relative effectiveness of clinic and home blood pressure monitoring compared with ambulatory blood pressure monitoring in diagnosis of hypertension: systematic review. *BMJ.* 2011;342:d3621.
5. Myers MG, Valdivieso M, Kiss A. Optimum frequency of office blood pressure measurement using an automated sphygmomanometer. *Blood Press Monit.* 2008; 13:333-338.
6. Godwin M, Birtwhistle R, Delva D, et al. Manual and automated office measurements in relation to awake ambulatory blood pressure monitoring. *Fam Pract.* 2011;28:110-117.
7. Eaton C, Rucker-Whitaker C, Liebson PR, Elliott WJ. Terminal digit preference in blood pressure measurements is reduced by automated sphygmomanometers in routine use [abstract]. *J Clin Hypertens (Greenwich).* 2008;10:A67-A68.

Home Blood Pressure Management and Improved Blood Pressure Control: Results From a Randomized Controlled Trial

Bosworth HB, Powers BJ, Olsen MK, et al (Durham Veterans Affairs Med Ctr, NC; et al)
Arch Intern Med 171:1173-1180, 2011

Background.—To determine which of 3 interventions was most effective in improving blood pressure (BP) control, we performed a 4-arm randomized trial with 18-month follow-up at the primary care clinics at a Veterans Affairs Medical Center.

Methods.—Eligible patients were randomized to either usual care or 1 of 3 telephone-based intervention groups: (1) nurse-administered behavioral management, (2) nurse- and physician-administered medication management, or (3) a combination of both. Of the 1551 eligible patients, 593 individuals were randomized; 48% were African American. The intervention telephone calls were triggered based on home BP values transmitted via telemonitoring devices. Behavioral management involved promotion of health behaviors. Medication management involved adjustment of medications by a study physician and nurse based on hypertension treatment guidelines.

Results.—The primary outcome was change in BP control measured at 6-month intervals over 18 months. Both the behavioral management and medication management alone showed significant improvements at 12 months—12.8% (95% confidence interval [CI], 1.6%–24.1%) and 12.5% (95% CI, 1.3%–23.6%), respectively—but not at 18 months. In subgroup analyses, among those with poor baseline BP control, systolic BP decreased in the combined intervention group by 14.8 mm Hg (95% CI, −21.8 to −7.8 mm Hg) at 12 months and 8.0 mm Hg (95% CI, −15.5 to −0.5 mm Hg) at 18 months, relative to usual care.

Conclusions.—Overall intervention effects were moderate, but among individuals with poor BP control at baseline, the effects were larger. This study indicates the importance of identifying individuals most likely to benefit from potentially resource intensive programs.

Trial Registration.—clinicaltrials.gov Identifier: NCT00237692.

▶ Some years ago, the US Department of Veterans Affairs (VA) funded a number of clinical trials, involving many different strategies, to improve blood pressure management and control in the world's largest managed care organization.[1] This article reports the results of the multifaceted intervention tested in Duke University–affiliated outpatient VA facilities. These investigators combined several different interventions that have shown short-term improvements in blood pressure control; all groups received a home blood pressure monitoring and a device that transmitted readings to a secure central computer, which was monitored by nurses for both hypertension and hypotension.[2] The group randomly assigned to behavioral modification received 11 modules pertaining to health beliefs related to hypertension, each of which lasted 12 to 14 minutes and were nurse led.[3] The group randomly assigned to medication management had their antihypertensive drug therapy changed in response to home blood pressures; this effort was also nurse led but physician controlled and documented.[4] The last randomized group received both behavioral modification and medication management.

The interventions were implemented for 18 months, and blood pressures were systematically measured in the office by an observer blinded to the randomized group at 6-month intervals. The major challenge to the interpretation of the results is the fact that, although the inclusion criteria prohibited enrollment of patients with controlled hypertension, fully 59% of the enrolled patients had, at randomization, controlled blood pressures, using the standardized research method for measuring blood pressures. This reduced the statistical power of the interventions to improve blood pressure control, particularly as the passage of time reduced the numbers of participating subjects. The authors also compared the costs of the different interventions (which averaged about $1100 per patient per year), but because the long-term blood pressure results were not significant, the economic analyses were not explored in detail.

These rather disappointing results are perhaps understandable because of the dilutional effect of the patients who were enrolled with "controlled blood pressures." These results are likely to dampen the enthusiasm of payors to implement such intensive interventions, as the primary endpoint of the study was not met at 18 months.

W. J. Elliott, MD, PhD

References

1. Green BB, Cook AJ, Ralston JD, et al. Effectiveness of home blood pressure monitoring, web communication, and pharmacist care on hypertension control: a randomized controlled trial. *JAMA.* 2008;299:2857-2867.
2. Walsh JM, McDonald KM, Shojania KG, et al. Quality improvement strategies for hypertension management: a systematic review. *Med Care.* 2006;44:646-657.
3. Clark CE, Smith LF, Taylor RS, Campbell JL. Nurse led interventions to improve control of blood pressure in people with hypertension: systematic review and meta-analysis. *BMJ.* 2010;341:c3995.
4. McManus RJ, Mant J, Bray EP, et al. Telemonitoring and self-management in the control of hypertension (TASMINH2): a randomised controlled trial. *Lancet.* 2010;376:163-172.

Culturally Appropriate Storytelling to Improve Blood Pressure: A Randomized Trial

Houston TK, Allison JJ, Sussman M, et al (Bedford Veterans Affairs Med Ctr, MA; Univ of Massachusetts Med School, Worcester; Cooper Green Mercy Hosp and Univ of Alabama at Birmingham, Alabama; et al)
Ann Intern Med 154:77-84, 2011

Background.—Storytelling is emerging as a powerful tool for health promotion in vulnerable populations. However, these interventions remain largely untested in rigorous studies.

Objective.—To test an interactive storytelling intervention involving DVDs.

Design.—Randomized, controlled trial in which comparison patients received an attention control DVD. Separate random assignments were performed for patients with controlled or uncontrolled hypertension. (ClinicalTrials.gov registration number: NCT00875225).

Setting.—An inner-city safety-net clinic in the southern United States.

Patients.—230 African Americans with hypertension.

Intervention.—3 DVDs that contained patient stories. Storytellers were drawn from the patient population.

Measurements.—The outcomes were differential change in blood pressure for patients in the intervention versus the comparison group at baseline, 3 months, and 6 to 9 months.

Results.—299 African American patients were randomly assigned between December 2007 and May 2008 and 76.9% were retained throughout the study. Most patients (71.4%) were women, and the mean age was 53.7 years. Baseline mean systolic and diastolic pressures were similar in both groups. Among patients with baseline uncontrolled hypertension, reduction favored the intervention group at 3 months for both systolic (11.21 mm Hg [95% CI, 2.51 to 19.9 mm Hg]; $P = 0.012$) and diastolic (6.43 mm Hg [CI, 1.49 to 11.45 mm Hg]; $P = 0.012$) blood pressures. Patients with baseline controlled hypertension did not significantly differ over time between study groups. Blood pressure subsequently increased for both groups, but between-group differences remained relatively constant.

Limitation.—This was a single-site study with 23% loss to follow-up and only 6 months of follow-up.

Conclusion.—The storytelling intervention produced substantial and significant improvements in blood pressure for patients with baseline uncontrolled hypertension.

▶ Engaging patients in, and increasing their motivation to continuously take, their treatment is often challenging, especially with a chronic, often asymptomatic condition like hypertension.[1] The burden of hypertension is especially large in African Americans, who (as a group) have hypertension more frequently than most other populations worldwide. Many interventions, including case managers, lay advocates, peer-group counselors, support groups, cognitive behavioral therapy, and others, have been tested, with little success in improving hypertension control rates. "Storytelling" (a type of interactive, narrative communication) by culturally appropriate individuals (who usually have faced the same or similar medical problem) has been posited to promote meaningful therapeutic choices, allow patients to identify with the storyteller, and imagine themselves as making similar, valid choices, including drug therapy, lifestyle modifications, and attending follow-up appointments.[2] This clinical trial was therefore designed to assess whether such a multistage intervention, specially produced and recorded by peer patients, and delivered via mailed digital video disks (DVDs) to the subjects' homes, would improve blood pressure control rates in an inner-city "safety-net" clinic serving African American hypertensive patients.

The rationale and design of the DVD program is fascinating and tells much about the expected behaviors of the patients. Apparently DVD players are currently more ubiquitous in the United States than CD-ROM players or Internet access, which prompted this method of delivery of the health education. The authors recruited 14 hypertensive patients who provided clear and persuasive video clips (1–3 minutes per topic) about their experience with hypertension and amassed 80 hours of footage, which were severely edited into a documentary-style DVD movie comprising 3 DVDs in 2 major sections. Unfortunately, there was no objective quality control or assessment of whether the mailed DVDs were watched by the participants. All participants in the intervention group said they had watched at least 1 video segment from each of the 3 DVDs. Sadly, there was no relationship between the minutes of DVD watched and change in blood pressure.

The clinical trial methodology was traditional, but the baseline blood pressures were about 133/76 mm Hg, and a full 58% of the patients were controlled at randomization. There was little effect on the blood pressures of patients who were controlled at randomization, but the changes in blood pressure over time (using a very sophisticated time-series modeling method) were significantly lower for those provided the DVDs than controls, by 11.2/6.4 mm Hg for the 3-month follow-up, but decreased to 6.4/4.2 mm Hg at 6 to 9 months of follow-up. Sadly, about 23% of the subjects did not follow up at 6 months. The editorialists point out several positive aspects of this study[3] but are suitably disappointed that the benefit on blood pressure was not longer lived. They concluded that "stories are unlikely to become a routine part of treatment" based on this trial, which is more conservative than the discussion in this article.

W. J. Elliott, MD, PhD

References

1. Miller NH, Hill M, Kottke T, Ockene IS. The multilevel compliance challenge: recommendations for a call to action. A statement for healthcare professionals. *Circulation.* 1997;95:1085-1090.
2. Slater MD, Rouner D. Entertainment—education and elaboration likelihood: understanding the processing of narrative persuasion. *Commun Theory.* 2002;12:173-191.
3. Myers KR, Green MJ. Storytelling: a novel intervention for hypertension. *Ann Intern Med.* 2011;154:129-130.

2 Pediatric Cardiovascular Disease

Tetralogy of Fallot

The evolving role of intraoperative balloon pulmonary valvuloplasty in valve-sparing repair of tetralogy of Fallot

Robinson JD, Rathod RH, Brown DW, et al (Children's Hosp, Boston, MA)
J Thorac Cardiovasc Surg 142:1367-1373, 2011

Objective.—The late morbidity of pulmonary regurgitation has intensified the interest in valve-sparing repair of tetralogy of Fallot. This study reviewed a single institution's experience with valve-sparing repair and investigated the role of intraoperative balloon valvuloplasty.

Methods.—A retrospective chart review identified 238 patients who underwent complete primary repair of tetralogy of Fallot at less than 180 days of age. Patients were divided into 4 groups on the basis of the type of right ventricular outflow tract repair: transannular patch (n = 111), commissurotomy or standard rigid dilation (n = 71), intraoperative balloon pulmonary valvuloplasty (n = 32), or no valvar intervention (n = 24).

Results.—Baseline demographic and anatomic factors differed among the 4 procedural groups with substantial overlap. Among 142 patients with pulmonary valve hypoplasia (z score, -2 to -4), 37% had valve-sparing repair. These patients had significant annular growth over time: z score increased 0.67 and 1.00 per year in the intraoperative balloon valvuloplasty ($P < .001$) and traditional valve-sparing ($P < .001$) groups, respectively. Rates of valve growth did not differ across groups, but z scores were 0.58 lower for the balloon valvuloplasty group across all time points ($P = .001$). Freedom from reintervention and surgery was shorter for the balloon valvuloplasty group than for the other groups ($P < .001$).

Conclusions.—Patients with tetralogy of Fallot and pulmonary valve hypoplasia who undergo valve-sparing repair with intraoperative balloon valvuloplasty have significant longitudinal annular growth, with normalization of annular size over time. Despite application in patients with more hypoplastic valves, balloon valvuloplasty resulted in similar valve growth and pulmonary regurgitation as traditional methods, but higher rates of reintervention. Although the precise role of this technique needs further refinement, it is likely to be most useful in patients with moderate pulmonary stenosis and moderate pulmonary valve dysplasia.

▶ This article details the use of balloon pulmonary valvuloplasty during infant surgery for tetralogy of Fallot with a valve-sparing approach. This approach was applied in 32 of 142 infants undergoing repair at approximately 3 months of age. It appeared to be useful as applied to the more hypoplastic valves. There was a higher rate of reintervention for right ventricular outflow tract (RVOT) obstruction than with rigid dilatation with a Hegar dilator. Surgical preference for pulmonary valve (PV)—sparing techniques increased over the time of this study (1997—2008) and the percentage of patients treated by catheter-based therapy alone for residual RVOT obstruction also increased. The authors note that intraoperative balloon pulmonary valvuloplasty may play an important role in achieving a more competent PV with little RVOT obstruction particularly in patients with a PV Z-score of −2.5 to −3.5.

T. P. Graham, Jr, MD

Late Repair of the Native Pulmonary Valve in Patients With Pulmonary Insufficiency After Surgery for Tetralogy of Fallot

Mainwaring RD, Pirolli T, Punn R, et al (Lucile Packard Children's Hosp at Stanford, CA)
Ann Thorac Surg 93:677-679, 2012

Pulmonary regurgitation developing late after tetralogy of Fallot repair is now recognized as a serious threat to the long-term welfare of these patients. This article summarizes our experience with 5 patients who underwent reoperations for treatment of severe pulmonary regurgitation after transannular patch repair of tetralogy of Fallot. In each case, the intraoperative findings revealed anatomy favorable for valve repair and enabled preservation of the native pulmonary valves.

▶ This is a great solution for a limited number of postoperative tetralogy patients who have a native bicuspid valve, preserved valve leaflets, growth of the native leaflets with retained mobility, and minimal gradient across the annulus. These are rare findings in postoperative patients but when present should present a golden opportunity for these patients.

T. P. Graham, Jr, MD

Long-term results of pulmonary artery rehabilitation in patients with pulmonary atresia, ventricular septal defect, pulmonary artery hypoplasia, and major aortopulmonary collaterals

Dragulescu A, Kammache I, Fouilloux V, et al (Hôpital de la Timone-Enfants, Marseille, France; Hôpital d'Enfants de la Timone, Pierre, Marseille, France; et al)

J Thorac Cardiovasc Surg 142:1374-1380, 2011

Objective.—The study objective was to report the long-term results of pulmonary artery rehabilitation in patients with pulmonary atresia, ventricular septal defect, hypoplastic pulmonary arteries, and major aortopulmonary collaterals.

Methods.—Since 1991, 20 patients with profound pulmonary artery hypoplasia (mean Nakata index 26 ± 14 mm^2/m^2) have undergone a medicosurgical strategy of native pulmonary artery rehabilitation to achieve complete repair with satisfactory hemodynamics (right ventricle to aortic pressure ratio < 0.8).

Results.—The first step, right ventricle to pulmonary artery connection, was performed at a median age of 4.1 (0.1−18.7) months with 1 operative death. After a median duration of 4.3 (1.1−26) months, the second step of interventional catheterizations followed (median, 2 (1−7)/patient), consisting of 36 pulmonary angioplasties, 11 stent implantations, and 20 collateral occlusions. Significant pulmonary artery growth was obtained in all cases with a Nakata index of 208 ± 85 mm^2/m^2 before surgical correction ($P < .001$). The third step of surgical repair was performed at a median age of 1.9 (0.6−10.7) years, with right ventricular outflow reconstruction and ventricular septal defect closure fenestrated in 3 cases. During a mean follow-up of 8.2 ± 4.5 years, pulmonary artery rehabilitation was pursued in most patients, with 47 pulmonary angioplasties, 15 stent implantations, and 11 collateral occlusions. Three patients with a poor hemodynamic result died. At last visit, the 16 survivors are in New York Heart Association class I (n = 12) or II (n = 4) with satisfactory hemodynamics in 13 cases.

Conclusions.—Pulmonary artery rehabilitation allows complete repair in the majority of patients with pulmonary atresia, ventricular septal defect, hypoplastic pulmonary arteries, and major aortopulmonary collaterals. However, long-term management often requires pursuit of the rehabilitation process.

▶ This is a positive report on some difficult patients; generally there are very good results with a medico-surgical approach to pulmonary artery rehabilitation of hypoplastic pulmonary arteries, including major aortopulmonary collateral arteries in patients with pulmonary atresia and ventricular septal defect. This is difficult surgery, and good long-term results require a skilled interventional catheter team to dilate and stent these pulmonary arteries multiple times in many instances. This approach continues to provide new hope to many infants.

T. P. Graham, Jr, MD

Pulmonary Atresia, Ventricular Septal Defect, and Major Aortopulmonary Collaterals: Neonatal Pulmonary Artery Rehabilitation Without Unifocalization

Liava'a M, Brizard CP, Konstantinov IE, et al (Univ of Melbourne and the Murdoch Children's Res Inst, Victoria, Australia; Adelaide Women's and Children's Hosp, Adelaide, South Australia, Australia)

Ann Thorac Surg 93:185-192, 2012

Background.—This study analyzed a protocol of neonatal rehabilitation of hypoplastic pulmonary arteries in the management of pulmonary atresia, ventricular septal defect (VSD), and major aortopulmonary collateral arteries (MAPCAs). Ideal management of patients with pulmonary atresia, VSD, and MAPCAs is the subject of controversy.

Methods.—From June 2003 to December 2008, 25 consecutive patients were diagnosed with pulmonary atresia, VSD, and MAPCAs, and 20 were entered into a neonatal shunting regimen. The median age at the first operation was 3.6 weeks (range, 0.7 to 17 weeks). All patients underwent an initial central or modified Blalock-Taussig shunt, or both. Further preparatory procedures included 26 pulmonary artery patch reconstructions, 19 right ventricle- to-pulmonary artery conduits, 4 MAPCA ligations, and 4 further shunts. No patient underwent translocation of the collateral arteries.

Results.—At the latest follow-up, 12 of 20 patients have had a complete repair at a median age of 18 months (range, 11 to 48 months), 6 are awaiting repair, and 2 are considered unlikely to be repaired. No patient was missing follow-up. Median pulmonary artery indices had grown from 14.51 to 118.7 in 17 patients. Postoperative angiograms were performed at a median of 8 months (range, 1.9 to 32.7 months) in 9 of 12 completely repaired patients. The median right/left ventricular pressure ratio was 0.64 (range, 0.54 to 0.91).

Conclusions.—Rehabilitation of hypoplastic native pulmonary arteries by a neonatal shunting regimen, without MAPCA translocation, for pulmonary atresia, VSD, and MAPCAs, provides encouraging results with excellent early survival.

▶ This is the alternative approach to unifocalization; no attempt is made to incorporate major aortopulmonary collateral arteries (MAPCAs) into the central pulmonary arterial tree. Indeed, no catheterization is done initially; computed tomography or CMR is used to try to identify the pulmonary artery (PA) anatomy followed by central shunting or modified Blalock-Taussig shunt to enlarge the central PAs. This is followed by right ventricle-to-PA conduits, PA patch reconstructions, further shunts when needed, and occasionally MAPCA ligations. They question whether their recent success may have been due to a favorable cluster of patients. Time will tell, but the results to date look good. Certainly, a debate on how to handle these infants between this approach and the early unifocalization groups would be ideal. The variable anatomy of these complex patients makes the comparison of methods difficult. There is a need to clarify the preoperative anatomy in each patient and look at results of such an approach: a long-term goal but a laudable one.

T. P. Graham, Jr, MD

Pulmonary valve replacement in chronic pulmonary regurgitation in adults with congenital heart disease: Impact of preoperative QRS-duration and NT-proBNP levels on postoperative right ventricular function
Westhoff-Bleck M, Girke S, Breymann T, et al (Hannover Med School, Germany; et al)
Int J Cardiol 151:303-306, 2011

Background.—Chronic severe pulmonary regurgitation (PR) causes progressive right ventricular (RV) dysfunction and heart failure. Parameters defining the optimal time point for surgery of chronic PR are lacking. The present study prospectively evaluated the impact of preoperative clinical parameters, cardiorespiratory function, QRS duration and NT-proBNP levels on postoperative RV function and volumes assessed by cardiac magnetic resonance imaging (CMR) in patients with chronic severe PR undergoing pulmonary valve replacement.

Methods and Results.—CMR was performed pre- and 6 months postoperatively in 27 patients (23.6 ± 2.9 years, 15 women) with severe PR. Postoperatively, RV endsystolic (RVESVI) and enddiastolic volume indices (RVEDVI) decreased significantly (RVESVI pre 78.2 ± 20.4 ml/m^2 BSA vs. RVESVI post 52.2 ± 16.8 ml/m^2 BSA, $p<0.001$; RVEDVI pre 150.7 ± 27.7 ml/m^2 BSA vs. RVEDVI post 105.7 ± 26.7 ml/m^2 BSA; $p<0.001$). With increasing preoperative QRS-duration, postoperative RVEF decreased significantly ($r=-0.57$; $p<0.005$). Preoperative QRS-duration smaller than the median (156 ms) predicted an improved RVEF compared to QRS-duration ≥156 ms (54.9% vs 46.8%, $p<0.05$). Multivariate analysis identified preoperative QRS duration as an independent predictor of postoperative RVEF ($p<0.005$). NT-proBNP levels correlated with changes in RVEDI ($r=0.58$ $p<0.005$) and RVESVI ($r=0.63$; $p<0.0001$). Multivariate analysis identified NT-proBNP levels prior to PVR as an independent predictor of volume changes ($p<0.05$).

Conclusion.—Valve replacement in severe pulmonary regurgitation causes significant reduction of RV volumes. Both preoperative NT-proBNP level elevation and QRS prolongation indicate patients with poorer outcome regarding RV function and volumes.

▶ This study shows that a preoperative QRS duration is a good predictor of improvement in right ventricular ejection fraction (RVEF) after PVR; in addition, preoperative higher levels of NT-proBNP were associated with a reduced capability for RV remodeling. These patients were characterized as being only mildly symptomatic preoperatively and did improve their exercise test postoperatively. What do we do with these data? One approach would be to monitor the QRS duration and the NT-proBNP in patients with significant pulmonary regurgitation before PVR as well as Trail Making Test results and RVEF to hopefully get a clearer consensus on when to intervene for PVR. This sounds like a long-range, expensive study, but these patients do need our help; there are a lot of them in clinics for adults with congenital heart disease with these issues to solve.

T. P. Graham, Jr, MD

Long term outcome of mechanical valve prosthesis in the pulmonary position
Dos L, Muñoz-Guijosa C, Mendez AB, et al (Hospital de la Santa Creu i Sant Pau, Barcelona, Spain)
Int J Cardiol 150:173-176, 2011

Objectives.—Assessment of the long term outcome of mechanical valve prosthesis at pulmonary position in a population of grown-up congenital heart disease patients from a tertiary referral center.

Methods.—From 1977 to 2007, 22 consecutive patients underwent a total of 25 pulmonary valve replacements with mechanical prosthesis. The most frequent underlying cardiac condition was tetralogy of Fallot ($n = 16, 64\%$) and the mean age at the time of pulmonary valve replacement was 32 ± 11 years (range 14–50 years).

Results.—The postoperative mortality rate was 4% ($n = 1$) with no late deaths documented after a mean follow-up of 7.6 ± 7.6 years (range 0.29–24 years). No major bleeding episodes occurred. Three patients presented with valve thrombosis in the setting of long term anticoagulation withdrawal and required valve re-replacement. Two of these patients, both with poor right ventricular function and overt clinical signs of right heart failure at the time of valve re-replacement, experienced further episodes of thrombosis despite correct anticoagulation. All episodes resolved with thrombolysis. After addition of antiplatelet treatment in one case and anticoagulation self-control, in the other, no further thrombosis has been documented.

Conclusions.—Mechanical valve prosthesis may be an alternative to tissue valve prosthesis in patients with congenital heart disease requiring pulmonary valve replacement. Optimal anticoagulation is crucial and additional antiplatelet treatment should be considered. Our data also suggest that patients with severe right ventricular dysfunction and congestive heart failure might be at particular risk for valve thrombosis.

▶ These authors present an alternative to valved conduits for pulmonary valve replacement (PVR) in older children and adults. The positive aspects of this approach include potential increased longevity of the prosthesis and good hemodynamic profile in the absence of thrombosis. Negative aspects include the need for anticoagulation, the risk of bleeding or thrombosis, and the inability to intervene with a percutaneous PVR.

T. P. Graham, Jr, MD

Transposition of the Great Arteries

Anatomic repair for congenitally corrected transposition of the great arteries: A single-institution 19-year experience

Murtuza B, Barron DJ, Stumper O, et al (Birmingham Children's Hosp, UK)
J Thorac Cardiovasc Surg 142:1348-1357, 2011

Objective(s).—Anatomic repair for congenitally corrected transposition of the great arteries (ccTGA) has been shown to improve patient survival. We sought to examine long-term outcomes in patients after anatomic repair with focus on results in high-risk patients, the fate of the neo-aortic valve, and occurrence of morphologically left ventricular dysfunction.

Methods.—We conducted a retrospective, single-institution study of patients undergoing anatomic repair for ccTGA. A total of 113 patients from 1991 to March 2011 were included. Double-switch (DS) repair was performed in 68 patients, with Rastelli-Senning (RS)—type repair in 45. Pulmonary artery banding for retraining was performed in 23 cases. Patients were followed up for survival status, morbidity, and reinterventions. A subgroup of 17 high-risk patients in severe heart failure, ventilated, and on inotropes before repair, were included.

Results.—Median age at repair was 3.2 years (range, 25 days to 40 years) and weight was 14.3 kg (3.2-61.4). There were 5 (of 68; 7.4%) early deaths in the DS group and 0 (of 45) in the RS group. Actuarial survivals in the DS group were 87.6%, 83.9%, 83.9% at 1, 5, and 10 years versus 91.6%, 91.6%, 77.3% in the RS group (log—rank: $P=.98$). Freedom from death, transplantation, or heart failure was significantly better in the RS group at 10 years ($P=.03$). There was no difference in reintervention at 10 years (DS, 50.3%; RS, 49.1%; $P=.44$). In the DS group, the Lecompte maneuver was associated with late reinterventions on the pulmonary arteries. Overall survival in the high-risk group was 70.6%. During follow-up, 14.2% patients had poor function of the morphologically left ventricle, all in the DS group, but this was not related to preoperative status or previous banding. The majority of patients after DS had mild aortic incompetence, which appeared well tolerated. Annuloplasty of the aortic root at time of DS reduced the risk of late aortic valve replacement.

Conclusions.—There is significant morbidity after anatomic repair of ccTGA, which is higher in the DS than the RS group. Nevertheless, the majority of patients are free of heart failure at 10 years, including high-risk patients in severe heart failure before repair. Aortic annuloplasty may reduce risk of late aortic insufficiency.

▶ This is an excellent contribution to the ongoing story of the anatomic repair of congenitally corrected transposition of the great arteries patients. There is a significant incidence of left ventricular (LV) dysfunction occurring after the double-switch (DS) operation, which is worrisome and not always predicted by preoperative factors. The Rastelli-Senning repair group did not show late LV dysfunction. These authors do not recommend preoperative autologous blood donation (PABD) in infants or young children who are asymptomatic and have no or very mild TR; progression to moderate TR would alter their approach to definitely consider PABD, which can only successfully be done in the early preadolescent years. AR can be an issue in the DS group, and these authors recommend aortic root annuloplasty to attempt to ameliorate this problem.

T. P. Graham, Jr, MD

Congenitally Corrected Transposition of the Great Arteries: Ventricular Function at the Time of Systemic Atrioventricular Valve Replacement Predicts Long-Term Ventricular Function

Mongeon F-P, Connolly HM, Dearani JA, et al (Mayo Clinic, Rochester, MN)
J Am Coll Cardiol 57:2008-2017, 2011

Objectives.—The objective was to evaluate the systemic ventricular ejection fraction (SVEF) at the time of systemic atrioventricular valve (SAVV) replacement as a predictor of SVEF ≥1 year after surgery in patients with congenitally corrected transposition of the great arteries (CCTGA).

Background.—Progressive SAVV regurgitation causes systemic ventricular failure in CCTGA patients, who are commonly referred late for intervention. Survival after surgery is poor when the pre-operative SVEF is <44%.

Methods.—We retrospectively reviewed 46 patients (pre-operative SVEF ≥40% in 27 patients and <40% in 19 patients) with 2 good-sized ventricles, a morphologically right systemic ventricle, and SAVV regurgitation requiring surgery. Median follow-up was not different in patients with a pre-operative SVEF ≥40% (8.8 years) or <40% (7.7 years, p = 0.36).

Results.—Pre-operative SVEF was the only independent predictor of ≥1-year post-operative SVEF (p < 0.0001). The late SVEF was preserved (defined as ≥40%) in 63% of patients who underwent surgery with an SVEF <40% compared with 10.5% of patients who underwent surgery with an SVEF <40%. Pre-operative variables associated with late mortality were an SVEF ≤40%, a subpulmonary ventricular systolic pressure ≥50 mm Hg, atrial fibrillation, and New York Heart Association functional class III to IV.

Conclusions.—Post-operative systemic ventricular function after SAVV replacement can be predicted from the pre-operative SVEF. For best results, operation should be considered at an earlier stage, before the SVEF falls below 40% and the subpulmonary ventricular systolic pressure rises above 50 mm Hg.

▶ These authors propose that congenitally corrected transposition of the great arteries in patients with moderate/severe tricuspid regurgitation have tricuspid valve replacement before the systemic ventricular ejection fraction (SVEF) falls below 40%. The data support this approach. The difficulty arises when the patient arrives with an SVEF considerably below 40% that does not improve with maximal medical therapy. The decision then is to proceed with transplant and band the pulmonary artery in an attempt to decrease the TR. The double switch with banding is rarely, if ever, possible in patients older than late child-hood. Hopefully there will be other methods to improve RV function in the future.

T. P. Graham, Jr, MD

Fontan Operation

A Multicenter, Randomized Trial Comparing Heparin/Warfarin and Acetylsalicylic Acid as Primary Thromboprophylaxis for 2 Years After the Fontan Procedure in Children

Monagle P, for the Fontan Anticoagulation Study Group (Univ of Melbourne, Victoria, Australia; et al)
J Am Coll Cardiol 58:645-651, 2011

Objectives.—The purpose of this study was to compare the safety and efficacy of acetylsalicylic acid (ASA) and warfarin for thromboprophylaxis after the Fontan procedure.

Background.—Fontan surgery is the definitive palliation for children with single-ventricle physiology. Thrombosis is an important complication; the optimal thromboprophylaxis strategy has not been determined.

Methods.—We performed a multicenter international randomized trial of primary prophylactic anticoagulation after Fontan surgery. Patients were randomized to receive for 2 years either ASA (5 mg/kg/day, no heparin phase) or warfarin (started within 24 h of heparin lead-in; target international normalized ratio: 2.0 to 3.0). Primary endpoint (intention to treat) was thrombosis, intracardiac or embolic (all events adjudicated). At 3 months and 2 years after the Fontan procedure, transthoracic and transesophageal echocardiograms were obtained as routine surveillance. Major bleeding and death were primary adverse outcomes.

Results.—A total of 111 eligible patients were randomized (57 to ASA, 54 to heparin/warfarin). Baseline characteristics for each group were similar. There were 2 deaths unrelated to thrombosis or bleeding. There were 13 thromboses in the heparin/warfarin group (3 clinical, 10 routine echo) and 12 thromboses in the ASA group (4 clinical, 8 routine echo). Overall freedom from thrombosis 2 years after Fontan surgery was 19%, despite thrombosis prophylaxis. Cumulative risk of thrombosis was persistent but varying and similar for both groups (p = 0.45). Major bleeding occurred in 1 patient in each group.

Conclusions.—There was no significant difference between ASA and heparin/warfarin as primary thromboprophylaxis in the first 2 years after Fontan surgery. The thrombosis rate was suboptimal for both regimens, suggesting alternative approaches should be considered. (International Multi Centre Randomized Clinical Trial Of Anticoagulation In Children Following Fontan Procedures; NCT00182104).

▶ This is the first and only multicenter, randomized controlled trial comparing acetylsalicylic acid with warfarin for primary prophylactic anticoagulation after Fontan surgery. There was excellent matching of pre- and postoperative patient diagnoses and characteristics. The study revealed no significant differences in thrombosis rate, which was not optimal for either arm of the study. Major complications of the treatment groups also did not differ. This study did show the enhanced ability to detect thrombosis by transesophageal echocardiography. There continues to be a need for optimal strategies for thrombosis prophylaxis in these patients.

T. P. Graham, Jr, MD

Cavopulmonary pathway modification in patients with heterotaxy and newly diagnosed or persistent pulmonary arteriovenous malformations after a modified Fontan operation
McElhinney DB, Marx GR, Marshall AC, et al (Harvard Med School, Boston, MA)
J Thorac Cardiovasc Surg 141:1362-1370, 2011

Objective.—Pulmonary arteriovenous malformations are an important but uncommon complication of cavopulmonary connection, particularly in patients with heterotaxy. Absence of hepatic venous effluent in pulmonary arterial blood seems to be a predisposing factor. Pulmonary arteriovenous malformations are most common after superior cavopulmonary anastomosis, but may develop, progress, or persist in 1 lung after Fontan completion if hepatic venous blood streams completely or primarily to the contralateral lung.

Methods.—Among 53 patients with heterotaxy and inferior vena cava interruption who underwent a modified Fontan procedure from 1985 to 2005, 8 had unilateral streaming of hepatic venous flow and clinically significant pulmonary arteriovenous malformations after hepatic venous inclusion and underwent reconfiguration of the cavopulmonary pathway. In all 8 patients, the hepatic vein-pulmonary artery pathway was contralateral to and offset from the pulmonary artery anastomosis of the single or dominant superior vena cava. Pathway reconfiguration included pulmonary arterial stenting (n = 2), revision of the superior vena cava-pulmonary artery connection (n = 1), construction of a branched hepatic vein-pulmonary artery conduit (n = 2), and surgical or transcatheter construction of a direct hepatic vein-azygous vein pathway (n = 5).

Results.—Hepatic vein-azygous vein connection led to improvement in 4 of 5 patients; other approaches typically did not lead to improvement.

Conclusions.—Resolution of hypoxemia after cavopulmonary pathway reconfiguration in patients with unilateral pulmonary arteriovenous malformations and hepatic venous flow-streaming after Fontan completion supports the importance of hepatic venous effluent in the pathogenesis of pulmonary arteriovenous malformations and the practice of cavopulmonary pathway revision in such patients. Completion or reconfiguration of the Fontan circulation with direct hepatic vein-azygous vein connection may provide the most reliable mixing and bilateral distribution of hepatic venous blood in this population of patients.

▶ This is an interesting article on attempts to modify pulmonary pathways because of persistent significant cyanosis late (range 3.6—10.1, median 8 years) after superior caval (Fontan) "completion" in 8 patients. In this setting, most patients have heterotaxy with hepatic venous flow not going to 1 lung, which then develops pulmonary arteriovenous malformations because of the lack of a putative hepatic factor that presumably can prevent this complication. Multiple approaches were used, but direct hepatic venous-azygous vein connections proved to be the most reliable method to treat this condition. This article is a must read for any physicians dealing with these complex patients.

T. P. Graham, Jr, MD

Center Variation in Patient Age and Weight at Fontan Operation and Impact on Postoperative Outcomes

Wallace MC, Jaggers J, Li JS, et al (Duke Univ Med Ctr, Durham, NC; Univ of Colorado School of Medicine, Denver; Cleveland Clinic, OH; et al)
Ann Thorac Surg 91:1445-1452, 2011

Background.—The impact of age and weight on outcomes after the Fontan operation is unclear. Previous analyses have suggested that lower weight-for-age z-score is an important predictor of poor outcome in patients undergoing bidirectional Glenn. We evaluated variation in age, weight, and weight-for-age z-score at Fontan across institutions, and the impact of these variables on postoperative morbidity and mortality.

Methods.—Patients in The Society of Thoracic Surgeons Congenital Heart Surgery Database undergoing the Fontan operation (2000 to 2009) were included. Center variation in age, weight, and weight-for-age z-score were described. Multivariable analysis was performed to evaluate the impact of age, weight, and weight-for-age z-score on in-hospital mortality, Fontan failure (combined in-hospital mortality and Fontan takedown/revision), postoperative length of stay, and complications, adjusting for other patient and center factors.

Results.—A total of 2,747 patients (68 centers) were included: 61% male; 45% right dominant lesions (38% left dominant, 17% undifferentiated). An extracardiac conduit Fontan (versus lateral tunnel) was performed in 63%; 65% were fenestrated. Median age, median weight at Fontan operation, and proportion with weight-for-age z-score less than -2 varied across centers and ranged from 1.7 to 4.8 years, 10.5 to 16.1 kg, and 0% to 30%, respectively. In multivariable analysis, age and weight were not significantly associated with outcome. Weight-for-age z-score less than -2 was associated with increased in-hospital mortality (odds ratio 2.73, 95% confidence interval: 1.09 to 6.86), Fontan failure (odds ratio 2.59, 95% confidence interval: 1.24 to 5.40), and longer length of stay (+1.2 days, 95% confidence interval: 0.1 to 2.4).

Conclusions.—Weight-for-age z-score less than −2 is associated with significant morbidity and mortality after the Fontan operation independent of other patient and center characteristics.

▶ The impact of weight and age on Fontan outcome has been debated for many years. This large multicenter study shows that it is weight for age that is the important variable. The potential good news is that this is a modifiable variable as shown by the Milwaukee group with a comprehensive feeding and monitoring plan despite comorbidities.[1]

T. P. Graham, Jr, MD

Reference

1. Fischbach P, Cole W, Mahle W, Rastagar D, Frias P. Outpatient evaluation of chest pain in children: utilization benchmarking. *Congenit Heart Dis.* 2010;5:512.

Clinical outcomes of prophylactic Damus-Kaye-Stansel anastomosis concomitant with bidirectional Glenn procedure

Shimada M, Hoashi T, Kagisaki K, et al (Natl Cerebral and Cardiovascular Ctr, Suita, Japan)

J Thorac Cardiovasc Surg 143:137-143, 2012

Objective.—We evaluated prophylactic Damus-Kaye-Stansel (DKS) anastomosis in association with the timing of a bidirectional Glenn (BDG) procedure as second-stage palliation aiming at Fontan completion to prevent late systemic ventricular outflow tract obstruction.

Methods.—Between 1996 and 2005, 25 patients (14 boys; median age, 12 months) underwent a BDG procedure concomitant with DKS anastomosis. All had a systemic ventricular outflow tract through an intraventricular communication or morphologically developed subaortic conus and had previously undergone pulmonary artery banding. Enlargement of intraventricular communication and/or resection of a subaortic conus were not performed before or during the operation.

Results.—Twenty-one (84%) patients subsequently underwent a Fontan operation, with a follow-up period of 6.8 ± 1.9 years (range, 4-11 years), with no mortalities after the Fontan operation. Cardiac catheterization showed that systemic ventricular end-diastolic volume was significantly decreased from 187% ± 74% of normal before BDG to 139% ± 35% after ($P = .038$) and to 73% ± 14% at 4.3 years after the Fontan operation ($P < .001$). However, the pressure gradient across the systemic ventricular outflow tract remained at 0.5 ± 0.8 mm Hg after DKS anastomosis and 0.6 ± 2.3 mm Hg at 4.6 years after the Fontan operation. None of the patients showed more than moderate aortic or neoaortic regurgitation, except 1 who progressed to pulmonary regurgitation after DKS anastomosis and required a reoperation for a systemic ventricular outflow tract. No anatomic properties affected late neoaortic valve function.

Conclusions.—Regardless of a significant reduction in systemic ventricular volume, DKS anastomosis concomitant with a BDG procedure shows promise for a nonobstructive systemic ventricular outflow tract after a Fontan operation.

▶ This aggressive approach to a potential obstructive systemic ouflow tract in patients with a Fontan procedure has worked well for this group. The risk of later obstruction to systemic outflow obstruction can be estimated in these patients with measurement of the ventricular septal defect (VSD) or bulboventricular foramen; these authors felt that this method was not sensitive enough to prevent narrowing of the systemic outflow between follow-up visits. Certainly this problem can occur rapidly with the decrease in ventricular volume known to occur with the bidirectional Glenn or the Fontan procedures resulting in ventricular hypertrophy and marked decrease in ventricular distensibility, which renders these patients very poor candidates for successful Fontan viability. This approach has much to recommend it but does carry a risk of development of significant semilunar valvular regurgitation. It seems appropriate to proceed with this approach if the measured VSD of bulboventricular foramen is even borderline small after pulmonary artery banding. Hopefully, other investigators have data or will acquire data using this approach to determine if such a plan is feasible to avoid Damus-Kaye-Stansel in certain patients with relatively widely patent outflow to the systemic circuit.

T. P. Graham Jr, MD

Early Results of the "Clamp and Sew" Fontan Procedure Without the Use of Circulatory Support

Shinkawa T, Anagnostopoulos PV, Johnson NC, et al (Univ of California, San Francisco)
Ann Thorac Surg 91:1453-1459, 2011

Background.—A modification of the Fontan operation was recently applied, which includes anastomoses of the extracardiac conduit to the right pulmonary artery and inferior vena cava using simple clamping with no additional circulatory support, venous shunting, pulmonary artery preparation, or prior maintenance of azygos vein patency. The objective of this study is to assess the outcomes of this novel off-pump "clamp and sew" Fontan procedure.

Methods.—This is a retrospective review of all patients having a Fontan procedure between January 2009 and October 2010 at a single institution.

Results.—Twelve patients had a Fontan procedure with the use of cardiopulmonary bypass (CPB group), and 12 had an off-pump Fontan procedure (off-pump group). Preoperative demographic and hemodynamic data were similar except for higher mean pulmonary artery pressure in the CPB group

(12.2 ± 1.6 mm Hg versus 9.9 ± 2.4 mm Hg; $p = 0.02$). No patients in the off-pump group required conversion to CPB. The mean inferior vena cava clamp time in the off-pump group patients was 10 ± 3 minutes. There were no early or midterm deaths. No patients exhibited postoperative hepatic or renal dysfunction. Postoperative maximal serum creatinine and aspartate transaminase were significantly lower in the off-pump group compared with the CPB group (0.59 ± 0.12 versus 0.77 ± 0.22 mg/dL; $p = 0.03$ and 35.5 ± 8.3 versus 53.1 ± 19.0 U/L; $p = 0.02$, respectively). At median follow-up of 13 months (range, 1 to 20 months), all but 1 patient in the CPB group are in New York Heart Association class I with unobstructed Fontan circulation.

Conclusions.—The clamp and sew technique for completion of an extra-cardiac conduit Fontan procedure appears safe and feasible for selected patients.

▶ This is a new concept for me, and the authors make a good case for continuing this technique for selected patients. It does require a rapid anastomosis of the inferior vena cava to the pulmonary artery conduit to avoid prolonged abdominal congestion and possible liver or other end-organ damage. Hopefully a large multi-institutional study can be put together to determine the benefits and/or risks of this technique.

T. P. Graham, Jr, MD

Impact of the Evolution of the Fontan Operation on Early and Late Mortality: A Single-Center Experience of 405 Patients Over 3 Decades

Ohuchi H, Kagisaki K, Miyazaki A, et al (Natl Cerebral and Cardiovascular Ctr, Osaka, Japan)
Ann Thorac Surg 92:1457-1467, 2011

Background.—Postoperative mortality has decreased in patients undergoing the Fontan operation, and the determinants of such mortality may also have changed significantly.

Methods.—We conducted a study intended to focus on clarifying the determinants of mortality in 405 consecutive patients who had undergone a Fontan operation (62 patients after an atriopulmonary connection, 105 after an intra-atrial rerouting, and 238 patients after an extracardiac rerouting) between 1979 and 2010.

Results.—The overall 1-year, 5-year, 10-year, and 15-year rates of survival were 87.1%, 84.6%, 83.4%, and 81.6%, respectively, and the type of procedure as well as heterotaxy syndrome, ventricular ejection fraction, and atrioventricular valve repair at the time of the Fontan operation were independent predictors of overall mortality ($p < 0.05$ for all). Heterotaxy syndrome and atrioventricular (AV) valve repair were independent predictors of early (less than 6 months postoperative) mortality and the type of procedure was an independent predictor of late (6 or more months postoperative) mortality ($p < 0.05$ to 0.01). In the era of intra-atrial rerouting, heterotaxy syndrome was the only independent predictor of total, early, and late mortality ($p < 0.05$ for all), whereas a low ejection fraction, AV valve repair, and repair of a total anomalous pulmonary vein connection, rather than heterotaxy syndrome, were independent predictors of total or early mortality or both ($p < 0.05$ for all) in the era of extracardiac rerouting.

Conclusions.—Even in the modern era of extracardiac rerouting in the Fontan operation, a low ventricular ejection fraction, AV valve dysfunction, or a total anomalous pulmonary vein connection remain significant risk factors for mortality in patients with a single-ventricle physiology.

▶ This comprehensive review of Fontan surgery over the past 31 years shows a remarkable improvement in outcome, as would be expected, but continued lower survival related to lower ejection fraction, atrioventricular valve repair, and total anomalous pulmonary vein connection. Future improvements in outcome may depend on preserving ventricular function, improving the methods of atrioventricular valve repair, and possibly resorting to transplant in certain patients.

T. P. Graham, Jr, MD

Comparison of risk factors and outcomes for pediatric patients listed for heart transplantation after bidirectional Glenn and after Fontan: An analysis from the Pediatric Heart Transplant Study

Kovach JR, Naftel DC, Pearce FB, et al (Med College of Wisconsin, Milwaukee; Univ of Alabama at Birmingham; et al)
J Heart Lung Transplant 31:133-139, 2012

Background.—Patients listed for transplant after the bidirectional Glenn (BDG) may have better outcomes than patients listed after Fontan. This study examined and compared outcomes after listing for BDG and Fontan patients.

Methods.—All patients listed for transplant after the BDG in the Pediatric Heart Transplant Study between January 1993 and December 2008 were evaluated. Comparisons were made with Fontan patients and with a matched cohort of congenital heart disease patients. Competing outcomes analysis and actuarial survival were evaluated for the study populations, including an examination of various risk factors.

Results.—Competing outcomes analysis for BDG and Fontan patients after listing were similar. There was no difference in actuarial survival after listing or transplant among the 3 cohorts. Mechanical ventilation, United Network of Organ Sharing status, and age were risk factors for death after listing in BDG and Fontan patients, but ventilation at the time of transplant was significant only for the Fontan patients. Mortality was increased in Fontan patients listed < 6 months after surgery compared with patients listed > 6 months after surgery, but no difference was observed in BDG patients. There was a trend toward improved survival after listing for both populations across 3 eras of the study, but this did not reach statistical significance.

Conclusion.—Outcomes after listing for BDG and Fontan patients are similar. Mechanical ventilation at the time of transplant remains a significant risk factor for death in the Fontan population, as does listing for transplant soon after the Fontan, suggesting that some patients may benefit from transplant instead of Fontan completion.

▶ This is an intriguing report. I hoped that it would give us more data on when to use transplant instead of Fontan completion in patients with complex heart disease. It does suggest that earlier listing for transplant may be a useful strategy in this difficult group of patients. The data do show a half-life of approximately 10 years for transplant recipients, which is similar to that found in pediatric patients with any diagnosis, a remarkable achievement by these transplant teams.

T. P. Graham, Jr, MD

Hypoplastic Left Heart Syndrome

A Comparison of the Modified Blalock-Taussig Shunt With the Right Ventricle-to-Pulmonary Artery Conduit
Fiore AC, Tobin C, Jureidini S, et al (St Louis Univ School of Medicine, MO)
Ann Thorac Surg 91:1479-1485, 2011

Background.—This study compared the modified Blalock-Taussig (MBT) shunt with the right ventricle-to-pulmonary artery (RVPA) conduit with respect to outcome and PA growth.

Methods.—PA growth was assessed in 19 MBT patients and in 15 RVPA patients before stage 2 palliation for hypoplastic left heart syndrome. The RVPA was done with a ringed Gore-Tex tube (W. L. Gore and Assoc, Flagstaff, AZ) at each anastomosis.

Results.—The two cohorts had similar pre-Glenn demographic and hemodynamic data. No patient required transcatheter or surgical intervention on the shunt or PAs after stage 1 palliation. The branch PA growth was better in RVPA (McGoon ratio: MBT, 1.5 ± 0.2 vs RVPA, 2.0 ± 0.6; $p < 0.003$) and was significantly more balanced (right-to-left PA area ratio: MBT, 1.5 ± 0.5 vs RVPA, 0.9 ± 0.6; $p = 0.002$). The Nakata index trended higher in RVPA (MBT, $242A \pm 90$ mm^2/m^2 vs RVPA, 267 ± 95 mm^2/m^2, $p = 0.2$). After stage 2 palliation, oxygen saturation trended higher in the RVPA ($81\% \pm 5\%$) vs MBT cohort ($77\% \pm 8\%$, $p < 0.08$).

Conclusions.—The Norwood operation using a RVPA nonvalved conduit is associated with improved branch PA growth.

▶ This relatively small study in terms of patient numbers is indicative of an improved pulmonary artery flow and ultimate size of the pulmonary proximal bed after surgery. This would certainly be advantageous in terms of pulmonary flow post-Fontan. Hopefully the incision will not result in right ventricular dysfunction later in life.

T. P. Graham, Jr, MD

Changes of Right Ventricular Function and Longitudinal Deformation in Children with Hypoplastic Left Heart Syndrome Before and After the Norwood Operation
Petko C, Uebing A, Furck A, et al (Univ Hosp of Schleswig-Holstein, Kiel, Germany)
J Am Soc Echocardiogr 24:1226-1232, 2011

Background.—The purpose of this study was to investigate changes in right ventricular (RV) function and deformation parameters before and at steady state after the Norwood operation in neonates with hypoplastic left heart syndrome. A further aim was to delineate factors that affected these changes.

Methods.—On echocardiograms before and 21 days (range, 10—35 days) after the Norwood operation, the two-dimensional speckle-tracking parameters global and regional peak systolic longitudinal strain and strain rate were retrospectively compared in 33 patients with hypoplastic left heart syndrome. In addition, RV functional assessment included RV fractional area change and tricuspid annular plane systolic excursion. The associations between postoperative echocardiographic findings and preoperative or postoperative complications, prenatal diagnosis, postoperative heart rate, oxygen saturation, and medication use as well as cardiopulmonary bypass and aortic cross-clamp times were tested.

Results.—Global strain ($-18.3 \pm 3.6\%$ vs $-16.8 \pm 3.8\%$, $P = .02$) and global strain rate (-1.6 ± 0.3 vs -1.2 ± 0.3 sec^{-1}, $P < .0001$) decreased significantly. Regional strain decreased significantly in the apical and mid lateral segments, while regional strain rate decreased significantly in all but the basal septal segments. Tricuspid annular plane systolic excursion of the lateral annulus decreased significantly, while RV fractional area change remained the same. No significant associations were found between postoperative RV function and potential impact factors.

Conclusions.—Two-dimensional global and regional longitudinal strain and strain rate as well as tricuspid annular plane systolic excursion were reduced in patients with hypoplastic left heart syndrome after the Norwood operation. None of the examined preoperative and postoperative patient or surgical factors was found to explain this decrease.

▶ These investigators have provided new data on right ventricular (RV) size and function after the first stage of surgery for hypoplastic left heart syndrome. As might be expected, global and regional functions are decreased and RV size increased despite no detectable change in TR. Hopefully, more longitudinal studies on these patients will help to clarify the significance of these changes and provide management changes to ameliorate these effects.

T. P. Graham, Jr, MD

Comprehensive evaluation of right ventricular function in children with different anatomical subtypes of hypoplastic left heart syndrome after Fontan surgery

Petko C, Möller P, Hoffmann U, et al (Univ Hosp of Schleswig-Holstein, Kiel, Germany)

Int J Cardiol 150:45-49, 2011

Background.—There is some evidence that hypoplastic left heart syndrome (HLHS) survivors with a larger left ventricular (LV) cavity may have poorer long-term outcome than those with mitral and aortic valve atresia (MA/AA) and negligible LV. A negative impact of the LV remnant on right ventricular (RV) function may contribute to this.

Methods.—We retrospectively evaluated RV function echocardiographically using 2D, Doppler and colour tissue Doppler techniques in 42 children with HLHS after Fontan surgery. Patients diagnosed with MA/AA at birth (group 1, $n=20$) were compared to all the remaining anatomical subgroups of HLHS (group 2, $n=22$).

Results.—The MA/AA group had a smaller diameter of the ascending aorta at birth ($p<0.0001$), smaller LV area ($p<0.0001$) and larger RV area at end-diastole ($p=0.004$) and end-systole ($p=0.01$) after Fontan. All parameters of RV function including the myocardial performance index, tricuspid annular plane systolic excursion, RV fractional area change and all regional colour Doppler derived myocardial velocities were not different between groups.

Conclusion.—In our cohort, RV function in HLHS after Fontan surgery was not different for the subgroup with MA/AA when compared to the remaining subgroups.

▶ These authors have brought comprehensive echo measurements of right ventricular (RV) function to the question regarding the possible disadvantage of having a relatively larger left ventricular (LV; "piggyback" ventricle) in patients with hypoplastic left heart syndrome. There were no differences in resting RV function by this methodology. These data do not provide information on the potential detrimental effect of the larger LV on RV function with increased afterload, heart rate, and volume loading.

T. P. Graham, Jr, MD

Regional Myocardial Dysfunction following Norwood with Right Ventricle to Pulmonary Artery Conduit in Patients with Hypoplastic Left Heart Syndrome

Menon SC, Minich LL, Casper TC, et al (Univ of Utah, Salt Lake City)
J Am Soc Echocardiogr 24:826-833, 2011

Background.—Improved early survival has led many centers to use the right ventricle—to—pulmonary artery (RVPA) conduit instead of the modified Blalock-Taussig shunt for Norwood palliation of hypoplastic left-heart syndrome. However, there is concern regarding the potential deleterious effects of the required right ventriculotomy for placement of the RVPA conduit on global and regional right ventricular (RV) function. The purpose of this study was to investigate global and regional RV wall motion abnormalities after Norwood palliation with RVPA conduit using Velocity Vector Imaging (VVI).

Methods.—Thirty consecutive patients with hypoplastic left-heart syndrome who underwent stage 2 palliation between January 2007 and December 2009 were identified from the surgical database. VVI was performed on two-dimensional echocardiographic images obtained before second-stage palliation. Peak systolic circumferential and radial velocity, strain, and strain rate were measured from parasternal short-axis and apical four-chamber views. RV ejection fraction was measured using the biplane modified Simpson's rule. Regional RV systolic deformations were compared between different RV segments. VVI measures were also compared with RV systolic function. In a subgroup ($n = 14$), VVI was repeated on follow-up after stage 2 palliation to evaluate changes in regional and global RV deformation.

Results.—A total of 30 patients (20 males) were studied. The median age at the time of interstage echocardiography was 12 weeks (range, 8—18 weeks). In the short axis, average peak systolic circumferential strain values for the anterior, posterior, septal, and RV free wall segments were 3.79 ± 2.52%, 11.4 ± 5.2%, 13.3 ± 6.5%, and 11.1 ± 5.0%, respectively. From the short-axis view, the anterior RV segment (ventriculotomy site) exhibited significantly reduced circumferential velocity, peak systolic strain, and strain rate ($P < .0001$). Mean global VVI measurements were correlated with RV ejection fraction. On follow-up after stage 2 palliation, the ventriculotomy region showed persistently reduced velocity, peak systolic strain, and strain rate compared with all other segments.

Conclusions.—In patients with hypoplastic left-heart syndrome after Norwood palliation with RVPA conduit, RV myocardial deformation was significantly reduced at the ventriculotomy site, which persisted after stage 2 palliation. VVI-derived measures demonstrating impairment of global systolic myocardial deformation were correlated with RV systolic function. Long-term multicenter studies to evaluate the effects of ventriculotomy scar on single systemic right ventricle are required.

▶ This report shows a decrease in right ventricle (RV) function associated with stage 1 palliation of hypoplastic left-heart syndrome patients with the use of an

RV conduit. This abnormality persisted after stage 2 palliation and was associated with specific wall motion abnormalities at the ventriculotomy site. Unfortunately, they did not have patients to compare who had palliation with a BT shunt nor data on possible arch obstruction, which could exacerbate regional and global myocardial function. Nevertheless, these data do suggest that further analysis of regional and global function of post–stage 1 palliation patients should be very helpful in furthering our ability to maximize the long-term outlook for these patients.

T. P. Graham, Jr, MD

New approach to interstage care for palliated high-risk patients with congenital heart disease

Dobrolet NC, Nieves JA, Welch EM, et al (Congenital Heart Inst at Miami Children's Hosp and Arnold Palmer Children's Hosp, Miami, FL)
J Thorac Cardiovasc Surg 142:855-860, 2011

Objective.—Home surveillance monitoring might identify patients at risk for interstage death after stage 1 palliation for hypoplastic left heart syndrome. We sought to identify the effect that a high-risk program might have on interstage mortality and identification of residual/recurrent lesions after neonatal palliative operations.

Methods.—Between January 2006 to January 2010, newborns after stage 1 palliation for hypoplastic left heart syndrome or shunt placement were invited to participate in our high-risk program. Patients enrolled in our high-risk program comprise the study group. Patients who had similar operations between January 2002 and December 2005 comprise the control group. Comparisons are made between the 2 groups with respect to interstage mortality and the frequency and timing of interstage admissions requiring medical, catheter, or surgical treatment.

Results.—Seventy-two patients met the criteria for our high-risk program. Fifty-nine (82%) of 72 patients were enrolled. Among 19 patients with hypoplastic left heart syndrome in our high-risk program, outpatient interstage mortality was zero. Outpatient interstage mortality for the 36 control subjects with hypoplastic left heart syndrome was 6%. Among 40 patients with shunts in the study group, there was 1 outpatient interstage death compared with 4 (6%) deaths in 68 subjects in the control group. Significant residual/recurrent lesions were identified with similar frequency between the 2 groups. However, after shunt operations, these lesions were detected and treated at significantly younger mean ages for patients followed in the high-risk program ($P < .005$).

Conclusions.—Initiation of a high-risk program might decrease interstage mortality after high-risk neonatal palliative operations. Such an approach might contribute to earlier detection of significant residual/recurrent lesions amenable to therapy.

▶ This type of intensive interstage care for high-risk patients included hypoplastic left heart syndrome, other univentricular heart palliation with a shunt, or dKS shunt. Comparisons with similar patients before the institution of the new approach were performed. Significant residual/recurrent lesions were detected in both groups, but were treated earlier in the high group. This type of interstage care will become the norm in programs that are dealing with these fragile infants and hopefully will improve long-term outcome.

T. P. Graham Jr, MD

Pulmonary Artery and Conduit Reintervention Rates After Norwood Using a Right Ventricle to Pulmonary Artery Conduit
Mery CM, LaPar DJ, Seckeler MD, et al (Univ of Virginia, Charlottesville; Levine Children's Hosp, Charlotte, NC)
Ann Thorac Surg 92:1483-1489, 2011

Background.—There is a high incidence of cardiovascular reintervention in patients undergoing a Norwood procedure (NP). The goal of this study was to analyze the rate of pulmonary artery (PA) and conduit stenosis using the right ventricle (RV)-to-PA modification of the NP.

Methods.—Patients who underwent a NP January 2005 to December 2009 were included. The procedure was performed with a ringed conduit sutured to a membrane to form a patch. The patch was sutured to the PA confluence, and the spatulated conduit was anastomosed to an appropriately sized right ventriculotomy. Rates of PA and conduit stenosis requiring reintervention were calculated based on cardiac catheterization data.

Results.—Thirty-three patients with hypoplastic left heart syndrome underwent a NP. Perioperative mortality was 6% (2 of 33). Twenty-eight patients (85%) had a Glenn procedure 5 ± 1 months later, and 12 patients (36%) had a Fontan procedure 34 ± 2 months after the Glenn. Pulmonary artery stenosis occurred in 11 patients (33%), and RV-PA conduit stenosis occurred only in 2 patients (6%). One-year and 3-year actuarial survival rates were 82% and 77%, respectively. Both branch PAs showed good and symmetric growth at cardiac catheterization before Glenn.

Conclusions.—The NP with RV-PA conduit using a ringed graft and a pulmonary patch is a technique associated with a low rate of PA and conduit stenosis, and good outcomes.

▶ These authors have done an excellent job using the right ventricle (RV)-to-pulmonary artery (PA) conduit for stage I Norwood procedure; avoiding the conduit stenosis that plagued some groups as they began using this technique. In addition, they have produced excellent right PA and left PA symmetrical growth with the modification of the surgical technique as shown in Fig 1 and with reintervention for PA stenosis when required. The Nakata indices were essentially normal at the time of the bidirectional Glenn procedure, which could be performed off pump in the majority of cases. The issue of possible

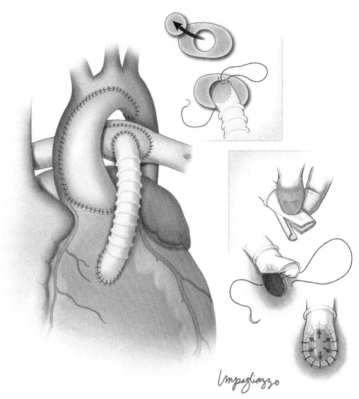

FIGURE 1.—Surgical technique for construction of the Norwood procedure with right ventricle to pulmonary artery conduit. (Reprinted from Mery CM, LaPar DJ, Seckeler MD, et al. Pulmonary Artery and Conduit Reintervention Rates After Norwood Using a Right Ventricle to Pulmonary Artery Conduit. *Ann Thorac Surg.* 2011;92:1483-1489. Copyright 2011, with permission from The Society of Thoracic Surgeons.)

RV dysfunction from the RV incision is still a potential problem for the future, but no evidence for this complication has been seen to date in this cohort.

T. P. Graham, Jr, MD

Pulmonary Atresia/Intact Ventricular Septum

Interstage attrition between bidirectional Glenn and Fontan palliation in children with hypoplastic left heart syndrome

Carlo WF, Carberry KE, Heinle JS, et al (Univ of Alabama at Birmingham; Texas Children's Hosp, Houston; et al)

J Thorac Cardiovasc Surg 142:511-516, 2011

Objective.—With improving operative mortality for staged palliation of hypoplastic left heart syndrome, interstage death accounts for an increasing proportion of hypoplastic left heart syndrome mortality. We investigated risk factors for death or cardiac transplantation during the interstage period between bidirectional Glenn and Fontan procedures in children with hypoplastic left heart syndrome.

Methods.—Patients with hypoplastic left heart syndrome who underwent bidirectional Glenn between August 1995 and June 2007 were screened. Standard risk patients, defined by having been discharged after both Norwood and bidirectional Glenn, were included for analysis. Patient demographic, echocardiographic, cardiac catheterization, and operative data were reviewed. Interstage attrition was defined as death or cardiac transplantation more than 30 days after bidirectional Glenn and before the Fontan procedure. Statistical analysis was carried out using the Student *t* test, Pearson chi-square correlation, and Cox proportional hazard modeling for multivariable analysis.

Results.—Ninety-two patients with hypoplastic left heart syndrome were alive at 30 days after bidirectional Glenn. Of these patients, 8 died and 3 underwent cardiac transplantation at a median of 391 days (range, 59—1175 days) after bidirectional Glenn, yielding an interstage attrition rate of 12%. Removing the 7 patients who are still awaiting Fontan (but all of whom are at least 3.5 years after bidirectional Glenn) adjusts the attrition rate to 13%. Interstage attrition did not correlate with hemodynamic data obtained at cardiac catheterization, aortic arch obstruction, or right ventricular dysfunction. Multivariable analysis demonstrated that the presence of moderate or severe tricuspid valve regurgitation (hazard ratio, 6.02; 95% confidence interval, 1.56—23.24; $P < .01$) and weight z score (hazard ratio, 0.38; 95% confidence interval, 0.16—0.88; $P = .02$) were independent preoperative risk factors for interstage attrition.

Conclusions.—Interstage attrition between bidirectional Glenn and Fontan procedures occurred in 12% of our study population. Moderate or greater tricuspid valve regurgitation and low weight z score at the time of bidirectional Glenn are important risk factors for interstage attrition between the bidirectional Glenn and Fontan procedures in children with hypoplastic left heart syndrome.

▶ Interstage attrition between stage I Norwood surgery for hypoplastic left heart syndrome and BDG has received far more attention than attrition between bidirectional Glenn (BDG) and Fontan as reported here. The potential for this later risk is not trivial as shown by this and other studies. The major risks appear to be moderate or severe TR and slow weight gain. One would think that poor right ventricular function would also be a risk, but it did not show up on the statistical analysis.

T. P. Graham, Jr, MD

Concomitant stenting of the patent ductus arteriosus and radiofrequency valvotomy in pulmonary atresia with intact ventricular septum and intermediate right ventricle: Early in-hospital and medium-term outcomes

Alwi M, Choo K-K, Radzi NAM, et al (Institut Jantung Negara (Natl Heart Inst), Kuala Lumpur, Malaysia)

J Thorac Cardiovasc Surg 141:1355-1361, 2011

Objectives.—Our objective was to determine the feasibility and early to medium-term outcome of stenting the patent ductus arteriosus at the time of radiofrequency valvotomy in the subgroup of patients with pulmonary atresia with intact ventricular septum and intermediate right ventricle.

Background.—Stenting of the patent ductus arteriosus and radiofrequency valvotomy have been proposed as the initial intervention for patients with intermediate right ventricle inasmuch as the sustainability for biventricular circulation or 1½-ventricle repair is unclear in the early period.

Methods.—Between January 2001 and April 2009, of 143 patients with pulmonary atresia and intact ventricular septum, 37 who had bipartite right ventricle underwent radiofrequency valvotomy and stenting of the patent ductus arteriosus as the initial procedure. The mean tricuspid valve z-score was -3.8 ± 2.2 and the mean tricuspid valve/mitral valve ratio was 0.62 ± 0.16.

Results.—Median age was 10 days (3—65 days) and median weight 3.1 kg (2.4—4.9 kg). There was no procedural mortality. Acute stent thrombosis developed in 1 patient and necessitated emergency systemic—pulmonary shunt. There were 2 early in-hospital deaths owing to low cardiac output syndrome. One late death occurred owing to right ventricular failure after the operation. Survival after the initial procedure was 94% at 6 months and 91% at 5 years. At a median follow-up of 4 years (6 months to 8 years), 17 (48%) attained biventricular circulation with or without other interventions and 9 (26%) achieved 1½-ventricle repair. The freedom from reintervention was 80%, 68%, 58%, and 40% at 1, 2, 3, and 4 years, respectively.

Conclusions.—Concomitant stenting of the patent ductus arteriosus at the time of radiofrequency valvotomy in patients with pulmonary atresia with intact ventricular septum and intermediate right ventricle is feasible and safe with encouraging medium-term outcome.

▶ This approach to pulmonary atresia with intact ventricular septum—that is, ductal stenting for only the severely diminutive right ventricle (RV), usually associated with coronary sinusoids and frequently associated with coronary obstruction (the single ventricle/Fontan pathway)—seems reasonable and "kinder-gentler." The infant with a tripartite RV can usually be treated with just radiofrequency-assisted valvotomy and balloon dilatation (RFV) and weaning off prostaglandine before discharge. This leaves the infant with a bipartite RV (22% of the infants in this study) who were treated with RFV plus patent ductus arteriosus stenting; 48% achieved a biventricular repair, and 26% achieved a 1.5 ventricular repair.

Hopefully these results or better can be achieved in future studies. The question of narrowing or closing an atrial defect to enhance RV inflow and possibly improve the chances for a 2-ventricle repair is for another study to determine.

T. P. Graham, Jr, MD

Surgical Therapy

Surgical Interventions for Atrioventricular Septal Defect Subtypes: The Pediatric Heart Network Experience
Kaza AK, for the Pediatric Heart Network Investigators (Univ of Utah, Salt Lake City; et al)
Ann Thorac Surg 92:1468-1475, 2011

Background.—The influence of atrioventricular septal defect (AVSD) subtype on outcomes after repair is poorly understood.

Methods.—Demographic, procedural, and outcome data were obtained 1 and 6 months after AVSD repair in an observational study conducted at 7 North American centers.

Results.—The 215 AVSD patients were subtyped as 60 partial, 27 transitional, 120 complete, and 8 with canal-type VSD. Preoperatively, transitional patients had the highest prevalence of moderate or severe left atrioventricular valve regurgitation (LAVVR, $p = 0.01$). At repair, complete AVSD and canal-type VSD patients, both with the highest prevalence of trisomy 21 ($p < 0.001$), were younger ($p < 0.001$), had lower weight-for-age z scores ($p = 0.005$), and had more associated cardiac defects ($p < 0.001$). Annuloplasty was similar among subtypes ($p = 0.91$), with longer duration of ventilation and hospitalization for complete AVSD ($p < 0.001$). Independent predictors of moderate or severe LAVVR at the 6-month follow-up were older log(age) at repair ($p = 0.02$) but not annuloplasty, subtype, or center ($p > 0.4$). Weight-for-age z scores improved in all subtypes at the 6-month follow-up, and improvement was similar among subtypes ($p = 0.17$).

Conclusions.—AVSD subtype was significantly associated with patient characteristics and clinical status before repair and influenced age at repair. Significant postoperative LAVVR is the most common sequela, with a similar prevalence across centers 6 months after the intervention. Annuloplasty failed to decrease the postoperative prevalence of moderate or severe LAVVR at 6 months. After accounting for age at repair, AVSD subtype was not associated with postoperative LAVVR severity or growth failure at 6 months. Further investigation is needed to determine if interventional strategies specific to AVSD subtype improve surgical outcomes.

▶ Surgery for atrioventricular septal defects (AVSDs) has certainly improved over the past 20 to 30 years, but postoperative left atrioventricular valve regurgitation (LAVVR) continues to plague these patients. It is important to perform a postrepair transesophageal echocardiogram in the operating room to be sure the surgeon has done all he or she can do to minimize the postoperative LAVVR. However, if the LAVVR is minimal at that point and suddenly becomes severe postoperatively, during reoperation one will usually find that a stitch has pulled out; resuturing it can lead to a dramatic sudden cure of the AVVR, and the patient will immediately be asymptomatic with no need for further medication and an excellent long-term result.

T. P. Graham, Jr, MD

Adolescents With d-Transposition of the Great Arteries Corrected With the Arterial Switch Procedure: Neuropsychological Assessment and Structural Brain Imaging

Bellinger DC, Wypij D, Rivkin MJ, et al (Children's Hosp Boston, MA; et al)
Circulation 124:1361-1369, 2011

Background.—We report neuropsychological and structural brain imaging assessments in children 16 years of age with d-transposition of the great arteries who underwent the arterial switch operation as infants. Children were randomly assigned to a vital organ support method, deep hypothermia with either total circulatory arrest or continuous low-flow cardiopulmonary bypass.

Methods and Results.—Of 159 eligible adolescents, 139 (87%) participated. Academic achievement, memory, executive functions, visual-spatial skills, attention, and social cognition were assessed. Few significant treatment group differences were found. The occurrence of seizures in the postoperative period was the medical variable most consistently related to worse outcomes. The scores of both treatment groups tended to be lower than those of the test normative populations, with substantial proportions scoring ≥ 1 SDs below the expected mean. Although the test scores of most adolescents in this trial cohort are in the average range, a substantial proportion have received remedial academic or behavioral services (65%). Magnetic resonance imaging abnormalities were more frequent in the d-transposition of the great arteries group (33%) than in a referent group (4%).

Conclusions.—Adolescents with d-transposition of the great arteries who have undergone the arterial switch operation are at increased neurodevelopmental risk. These data suggest that children with congenital heart disease may benefit from ongoing surveillance to identify emerging difficulties.

Clinical Trial Registration.—URL: http://www.clinicaltrials.gov. Unique identifier: NCT00000470.

▶ These data are both encouraging and sobering. Most adolescents post arterial switch do reasonably well from a neurodevelopmental standpoint, but there are certainly caveats to warrant continued follow-up. There does appear to be a neurodevelopmental price to pay for cardiac surgery at a young age; however, these changes are not all caused by the surgical technique used but by other factors such as whether seizures occurred in the postoperative period. There have continued to be changes in the operative suite, particularly related to this and other studies, which hopefully will continue to minimize any effect on long-term neurodevelopmental outcome of these amazing operations on the youngest cardiac patients.

T. P. Graham, Jr, MD

Anomalous Aortic Origin of a Coronary Artery: Medium-Term Results After Surgical Repair in 50 Patients
Mainwaring RD, Reddy VM, Reinhartz O, et al (Lucile Packard Children's Hosp/Stanford Univ, CA; Oakland Children's Hosp, CA; Children's Hosp of Central California, Madera; et al)
Ann Thorac Surg 92:691-697, 2011

Background.—Anomalous aortic origin of a coronary artery (AAOCA) is a rare congenital heart defect that has been associated with myocardial ischemia and sudden death. Controversies exist regarding the diagnosis, treatment, and long-term recommendations for patients with AAOCA. The purpose of this study is to evaluate the medium-term results of surgical repair for AAOCA.

Methods.—From January 1999 through August 2010, 50 patients underwent surgical repair of AAOCA. The median age at surgery was 14 years (range, 5 days to 47 years). Thirty-one patients had the right coronary originate from the left sinus of Valsalva, 17 had the left coronary originate from the right sinus, and 2 had an eccentric single coronary ostium. Twenty six of the 50 patients had symptoms of myocardial ischemia preoperatively, and 14 patients had associated congenital heart defects. Repair was accomplished by unroofing in 35, reimplantation in 6, and pulmonary artery translocation in 9.

Results.—There was no operative mortality. The median time of follow-up has been 5.7 years. Two patients were lost to follow-up, and 1 patient required heart transplantation 1 year after AAOCA repair. In the remaining 47 postoperative patients, all have remained free of cardiac symptoms and no one has experienced a sudden death event.

Conclusions.—The surgical treatment of AAOCA is safe and appears to be highly effective in eliminating ischemic symptoms. These medium-term results are encouraging and suggest that many patients may be able to resume normal activities.

▶ This report deals with the difficult decisions regarding the surgical treatment of patients who have this coronary anomaly and no symptoms of coronary ischemia. There is general agreement regarding surgery for patients with symptoms or with the left coronary arising from the right cusp. The anomalous right coronary arising from the left cusp is felt to be usually a benign lesion that can be followed up without treatment in the absence of signs or symptoms of myocardial ischemia. These authors indicate that these patients should also have surgery, particularly if there is evidence of an intramural course of the anomalous coronary. This issue needs more data, and there are plans for a multi-institutional registry to be developed.

T. P. Graham, Jr, MD

Follow-up and Outcome Studies

Best Practices in Managing Transition to Adulthood for Adolescents With Congenital Heart Disease: The Transition Process and Medical and Psychosocial Issues: A Scientific Statement From the American Heart Association

Sable C, on behalf of the American Heart Association Congenital Heart Defects Committee of the Council on Cardiovascular Disease in the Young, Council on Cardiovascular Nursing, Council on Clinical Cardiology, and Council on Peripheral Vascular Disease

Circulation 123:1454-1485, 2011

Background.—Children with complex childhood diseases are more likely to survive into adulthood than previously and can expect to live meaningful, productive lives. Ultimately it is necessary to transition them from their pediatric care providers to adult care practitioners. Often there are no structured programs to guide this transition, causing patients and their families as well as the healthcare delivery system emotional and financial stress. Many patients are simply lost to follow-up at this point. At least half of the adults with congenital heart disease (CHD) have complex disease and require specialized providers. Looking ahead, adolescent patients with CHD will require a well-planned, well-executed transition process to be able to successfully transfer to adult care providers. A formal transition program should prepare young adults for the transfer of care while providing uninterrupted care that is patient centered, age and developmentally appropriate, flexible, and comprehensive. The ultimate goal is to optimize the patient's quality of life (QOL), life expectancy, and future productivity. The American Heart Association (AHA) has offered recommendations for this transition process, which were presented in the context of topics pertaining to the care of adolescents and young adults with CHD.

Topics.—The topics explored included underlying concepts specific to transition care; timing for transitions; social and/or family dynamics; health supervision issues; anticipatory guidance with respect to genetic counseling, sexuality, pregnancy, and reproductive issues, exercise, education and career choices, end-of-life, mortality, and advance directives; and issues relevant to patients with developmental delay or disabilities. These were approached from the standpoint of the patient, the family, and the health care practitioner. Also offered was a description of the transition clinic and how it would facilitate the process of transferring care from pediatric to adult providers. The key elements relate to the pretransition phase, which involves preparation for transitioning and focuses on educating the patient and family about what is to come; the transition itself, which is only undertaken when the patient is developmentally mature and includes a standard core educational curriculum; and the transfer phase, which is ideally accomplished after the successful completion of a thoughtful transition process. It is recommended that there be a policy on timing, but that this policy be flexible to meet individual patient needs.

Recommendations.—AHA recommendations and levels of evidence for practice guidelines were provided as appropriate. These were also directed toward the adolescent, parents, or health care provider and offered specific actions to be taken.

Conclusions.—There is an urgent need for programs designed to facilitate the smooth transition of adolescent CHD patients to adult CHD care situations. It is hoped that transition programs will soon become the standard of care so that these patients can achieve their full potential under excellent medical supervision and live meaningful and productive lives.

▶ This very comprehensive statement regarding transition from pediatric cardiac centers to adult congenital heart disease centers contains information for all who are involved with these patients. I have not seen any center that has seamlessly, completely solved the multiple issues involved with this process. This treatise gives the optimal management all can strive for.

T. P. Graham, Jr, MD

Comprehensive Use of Cardiopulmonary Exercise Testing Identifies Adults With Congenital Heart Disease at Increased Mortality Risk in the Medium Term
Inuzuka R, Diller G-P, Borgia F, et al (Royal Brompton Hosp and Harefield NHS Foundation Trust, UK)
Circulation 125:250-259, 2012

Background.—Parameters of cardiopulmonary exercise testing were recently identified as strong predictors of mortality in adults with congenital heart disease. We hypothesized that combinations of cardiopulmonary exercise testing parameters may provide optimal prognostic information on midterm survival in this population.

Methods and Results.—A total of 1375 consecutive adult patients with congenital heart disease (age, 33 ± 13 years) underwent cardiopulmonary exercise testing at a single center over a period of 10 years. Peak oxygen consumption (peak $\dot{V}O_2$), ventilation per unit of carbon dioxide production ($\dot{V}E/\dot{V}CO_2$ slope), and heart rate reserve were measured. During a median follow-up of 5.8 years, 117 patients died. Peak $\dot{V}O_2$, heart rate reserve, and $\dot{V}E/\dot{V}CO_2$ slope were related to midterm survival in adult patients with congenital heart disease. Risk of death increased with lower peak $\dot{V}O_2$ and heart rate reserve. A higher $\dot{V}E/\dot{V}CO_2$ slope was also related to increased risk of death in noncyanotic patients, whereas the $\dot{V}E/\dot{V}CO_2$ slope was not predictive of mortality in cyanotic patients. The combination of peak $\dot{V}O_2$

and heart rate reserve provided the greatest predictive information after adjustment for clinical parameters such as negative chronotropic agents, age, and presence of cyanosis. However, the incremental value of these exercise parameters was reduced in patients with peak respiratory exchange ratio <1.0.

Conclusions.—Cardiopulmonary exercise testing provides strong prognostic information in adult patients with congenital heart disease. Prognostication should be approached differently, depending on the presence of cyanosis, use of rate-lowering medications, and achieved level of exercise. We provide 5-year survival prospects based on cardiopulmonary exercise testing parameters in this growing population.

▶ This very large dataset of cardiopulmonary exercise in adult congenital heart disease patients provides interesting information on outcome, specifically mortality over 5 years after cardiopulmonary exercise. How does one use these data to improve outcome? Possibly, one could do so by increasing follow-up, improving ventricular function, being aware of negative chronotropic agents, paying particular attention to possible arrhythmia symptoms, and involving electrophysiologists in the care of these patients.

T. P. Graham, Jr, MD

Geriatric Congenital Heart Disease: Burden of Disease and Predictors of Mortality
Afilalo J, Therrien J, Pilote L, et al (McGill Univ, Montreal, Quebec, Canada; McGill Univ Health Ctr, Montreal, Quebec, Canada)
J Am Coll Cardiol 58:1509-1515, 2011

Objectives.—The study sought to measure the prevalence, disease burden, and determinants of mortality in geriatric adults with congenital heart disease (ACHD).

Background.—The population of ACHD is increasing and aging. The geriatric ACHD population has yet to be characterized.

Methods.—Population-based cohort study using the Quebec Congenital Heart Disease Database of all patients with congenital heart disease coming into contact with the Quebec healthcare system between 1983 and 2005. Subjects with specific diagnoses of congenital heart disease and age 65 years at time of entry into the cohort were followed for up to 15 years. The primary outcome was all-cause mortality.

Results.—The geriatric ACHD cohort consisted of 3,239 patients. From 1990 to 2005, the prevalence of ACHD in older adults remained constant from 3.8 to 3.7 per 1,000 indexed to the general population (prevalence odds ratio: 0.98; 95% confidence interval [CI]: 0.93 to 1.03). The age-stratified population prevalence of ACHD was similar in older and younger adults. The most common types of congenital heart disease lesions in older adults were shunt lesions (60%), followed by valvular lesions (37%) and severe congenital heart lesions (3%). Type of ACHD and ACHD-related complications had a minor impact on mortality, which was predominantly driven by acquired comorbid conditions. The most powerful predictors of mortality in the Cox proportional hazards model were: dementia (hazard ratio [HR]: 3.24; 95% CI: 1.53 to 6.85), gastrointestinal bleed (HR: 2.79; 95% CI: 1.66 to 4.69), and chronic kidney disease (HR: 2.50; 95% CI: 1.72 to 3.65).

Conclusions.—The prevalence of geriatric ACHD is substantial, although severe lesions remain uncommon. ACHD patients that live long enough acquire general medical comorbidities, which are the pre-eminent determinants of their mortality.

▶ Treating geriatric patients with congenital heart disease (CHD) could be the new frontier for growth in the field, with a critical need for physicians specializing in the treatment of adults with CHD projected for the future. Certainly physicians choosing to care for adult CHD patients will have to become familiar with the many geriatric issues we senior citizens deal with.

T. P. Graham, Jr, MD

Coarctation, Interrupted Arch

Cardiovascular changes after transcatheter endovascular stenting of adult aortic coarctation

Babu-Narayan SV, Mohiaddin RH, Cannell TM, et al (Royal Brompton Hosp, London, UK)
Int J Cardiol 149:157-163, 2011

Background.—Longer term data on efficacy and clinical endpoints relating to transcatheter endovascular stenting in adults with aortic coarctation remains limited. We hypothesised that stenting would have effects on blood pressure, presence and extent of collaterals, left ventricular (LV) mass and vascular function.

Methods.—Eighteen patients mean age 31.6 ± 12.8 years were studied with clinical assessment and cardiovascular magnetic resonance before and after (10.2 ± 2.2 months) aortic coarctation endovascular stenting. Fredriksen coarctation index increased and using this index no patient had significant coarctation (index <0.25) after stenting.

Results.—Blood pressure decreased ($153 \pm 17/82 \pm 14$ *versus* $130 \pm 21/69 \pm 13$ mm Hg; $p<0.001$) unrelated to change in existing anti-hypertensive therapy. LV ejection fraction increased (70 ± 10 *versus* $74 \pm 8\%$; $p=0.01$) and LV mass index decreased (91 ± 24 *versus* 82 ± 20g/m^2; $p=0.003$). Collaterals appeared smaller and the degree of flow through collateral arteries decreased (40 ± 29 *versus* $-1 \pm 33\%$; $p<0.001$). Distensibility of the ascending aorta increased (4.0 ± 2.5 *versus* $5.6 \pm 3.5 \times 10^{-3}$ mm Hg^{-1}; $p=0.04$). Unexpectedly, right ventricular mass index decreased (35 ± 7 *versus* 30 ± 10g/m^2; $p=0.01$).

Conclusion.—All patients underwent successful relief of coarctation by endovascular stenting. Both cardiac and vascular beneficial outcomes were demonstrated. The reduction in LV mass suggests a potential for reduction in risk of adverse events and warrants further study.

▶ This comprehensive cardiovascular magnetic resonance (CMR) study indicates very good results of stenting coarctation in adults with marked improvements in blood pressure, left ventricular mass, left ventricular ejection fraction, aortic distensibility, right ventricular mass, and collateral flow. There were significant complications, including 2 small aneurysms and a transient loss of normal vision. This study shows the excellent data obtained by CMR in both pre- and posttreatment of coarctation patients. A pressing need in this area is for a long-term prospective study of both catheter-treated and surgically treated patients using these or similar CMR studies.

T. P. Graham, Jr, MD

Comparison of Risk of Hypertensive Complications of Pregnancy Among Women With Versus Without Coarctation of the Aorta
Krieger EV, Landzberg MJ, Economy KE, et al (Children's Hosp Boston, MA; Brigham and Women's Hosp, Boston, MA; et al)
Am J Cardiol 107:1529-1534, 2011

Hypertension is a common consequence of coarctation of the aorta. The frequency of hypertensive complications of pregnancy in women with coarctation in the general population is undefined. In this study, we used the 1998 to 2007 Nationwide Inpatient Sample, a nationally representative data set, to identify patients admitted to an acute care hospital for delivery. The frequency of hypertensive complications of pregnancy was compared between women with and without coarctation. Secondary outcomes, including length of stay, hospital charges, Caesarean delivery, and adverse maternal outcomes, were also assessed. There were an estimated 697 deliveries among women with coarctation, compared to 42,601,409 deliveries by women without coarctation. The frequency of hypertensive complications of pregnancy was 24.1 ± 3.3% for women with coarctation compared to 8.0 ± 0.1% for women without coarctation (multivariate odds ratio [OR] 3.6, 95% confidence interval [CI] 2.5 to 5.2). Preexisting hypertension complicating pregnancy (10.2 ± 2.5% vs 1.0% ± 0.02%, multivariate OR 10.8, 95% CI 5.9 to 19.8) and pregnancy-induced hypertension (13.9 ± 3.0% vs 7.0% ± 0.1%, multivariate OR 2.1, 95% CI 1.3 to 3.3) were more common in women with coarctation. Women with coarctation were more likely to deliver by Caesarean section (41.6 ± 3.3% vs 26.4% ± 0.2%, multivariate OR 2.0, 95% CI 1.4 to 2.8), have adverse cardiovascular outcomes (4.8 ± 2.2% vs 0.3 ± 0.01%, multivariate OR 16.7, 95% CI 6.7 to 41.5), have longer hospital stays, and incur higher hospital charges (both p values <0.0001) than women without coarctation.

In conclusion, women with coarctation are more likely to have hypertensive complications of pregnancy, deliver by Caesarean section, have adverse cardiovascular outcomes, have longer hospitalizations, and incur higher hospital charges than women without coarctation.

▶ This article documents the presence of an increased risk of hypertensive problems and cesarean delivery in women with coarctation. Many women have had coarctation surgical repair or percutaneous treatment; these all need follow-up in a center for adults with congenital heart disease and planned obstetric care in collaboration with such a center.

T. P. Graham, Jr, MD

Miscellaneous

Alternative approach for selected severe pulmonary hypertension of congenital heart defect without initial correction — Palliative surgical treatment
Lin M-T, Chen Y-S, Huang S-C, et al (Natl Taiwan Univ Hosp, Taipei)
Int J Cardiol 151:313-317, 2011

Objectives.—Uncorrected congenital heart defects (CHD) with severe pulmonary hypertension (sPH, systolic pulmonary artery >70% of systolic pressure) are usually considered inoperable. We are curious to know if some selected patients might benefit from palliative operation for those sPH with uncorrected CHD.

Methods.—Adults or adolescents with sPH associated with ventricular septal defect (VSD) with/without great artery anomalies were selected for pulmonary artery banding (PAB) to reduce sPH. The target pulmonary pressure was less than half of the systolic blood pressure after arch or great arteries reconstruction. Repeated catheterization was performed to evaluate the feasibility of defect closure.

Results.—Consecutively, 8 patients (age 26 ± 9 years) received PAB as a palliative procedure in the past 8 years without mortality. The pre-PAB systolic pulmonary pressure was 119 ± 9 mmHg. Additional PAB had been applied in 4 of them. All patients showed significant improvement in function class (III to I or II). The mean post-PAB pulmonary pressure decreased significantly (77.5 ± 9.2 mmHg to 42.0 ± 9.0 mmHg) and 6-minute walk test was also found to have great improvement (270 ± 86 m to 414 ± 49 m), but the saturation at rest did not show a difference. Three of them received corrective surgery to close defects over 3-5 years.

Conclusion.—For some selected adult sPH with uncorrected CHD, PAB can work as a palliative procedure to improve their functional class and even provide a chance of total repair.

▶ These authors have tackled a very difficult, but very important problem. Are some patients, previously felt to be inoperable, candidates for palliative pulmonary artery banding and possibly for later repair? The results are quite good in the small number of patients reported to date. The selection of patients was of interest; no patient had a systemic 02 saturation < 87%. The authors wanted to give the patients pulmonary vasodilators after banding, but were not able to do so because of cost. These studies hopefully can be extended to a larger series and criteria developed to select patients for this procedure.

T. P. Graham, Jr, MD

Cardiac resynchronization therapy in paediatric and congenital heart disease patients
van der Hulst AE, Delgado V, Blom NA, et al (Leiden Univ Med Ctr, The Netherlands)
Eur Heart J 32:2236-2246, 2011

The number of patients with congenital heart disease (CHD) has significantly increased over the last decades. The CHD population has a high prevalence of heart failure during late follow-up and this is a major cause of mortality. Cardiac resynchronization therapy (CRT) may be a promising therapy to improve the clinical outcome of CHD and paediatric patients with heart failure. However, the CHD and paediatric population is a highly heterogeneous group with different anatomical substrates that may influence the effects of CRT. Echocardiography is the mainstay imaging modality to evaluate CHD and paediatric patients with heart failure and novel echocardiographic tools permit a comprehensive assessment of cardiac dyssynchrony that may help selecting candidates for CRT. This article reviews the role of CRT in the CHD and paediatric population with heart failure. The current inclusion criteria for CRT as well as the outcomes of different anatomical subgroups are evaluated. Finally, echocardiographic assessment of mechanical dyssynchrony in the CHD and paediatric population and its role in predicting response to CRT is comprehensively discussed.

▶ This is an excellent review of the relatively small number of studies in cardiac resynchronization therapy in congenital heart disease. The studies to date do show promise for improving ventricular function of the left, right, and single ventricle in these patients, but criteria for use and objective methods for evaluating the response remain issues to resolve. This is another area in which a longer term study with a larger patient base is a clear need.

T. P. Graham, Jr, MD

Left Ventricular Function After Left Ventriculotomy for Surgical Treatment of Multiple Muscular Ventricular Septal Defects

Shin HJ, Jhang WK, Park J-J, et al (Konkuk Univ Med Ctr, Seoul, Republic of Korea; Unive of Ulsan College of Medicine, Seoul, Republic of Korea)
Ann Thorac Surg 92:1490-1493, 2011

Background.—Optimal management of muscular ventricular septal defects (MVSD) is still not determined in the current era. Moreover, long-term left ventricular function after closure of MVSD is not well known. Thus, we investigated surgical outcomes including long-term left ventricular function after closure of MVSD through left ventriculotomy.

Methods.—We conducted a retrospective review of medical records of 20 children who underwent MVSD closure between March 1993 and August 2010. There were 10 boys (50%) and 10 girls (50%). Patient age ranged from 1.6 to 103.4 months (median, 26.4 months), and body weight from 2.8 to 31.5 kg (median, 11.9 kg). Electrocardiogram results were normal sinus rhythm in all except 1 patient with congenital complete atrioventricular block. There were 16 patients who previously had palliative pulmonary artery banding procedures before closure of MVSD. There were 13 patients (65%) with Swiss-cheese type VSD.

Results.—There was 1 hospital death of a patient with congenital complete atrioventricular block with pacemaker malfunction (5%). There was 1 late death of a patient with del 22q with adenoviral pneumonia. There was no reoperation. Median follow-up duration was 85.9 months (range, 4.7 to 166.7). The location of MVSD was apical portion in 10 patients (50%) and midtrabecular portion in 9 patients (45%). There were 6 Dacron patch closures and 13 direct closures of MVSD through left ventriculotomy. There was no complete atrioventricular block. Last follow-up echocardiographic data showed normal ejection fraction with 65.2% ± 8.2% after closure of MVSDs. There was no leakage in 8 patients; 11 patients had insignificant leakage, which disappeared spontaneously in 4 patients 17.9 months (median value) after operation.

Conclusions.—Our acceptable long-term results of left ventricular function after left ventriculotomy proved that this technique might be a viable option in the management of MVSD.

▶ This article is potential good news for many patients who had a previous left ventriculotomy for ventricular septal defect closure. I thought that most of these patients would have significant left ventricular (LV) dyskinesia and be at risk for dysfunction and possible arrhythmia in the future. Apparently, these surgeons were able to repair these defects with relatively small patches and preserve normal LV function. Hopefully, long-term data can be obtained from these and similar patients repaired by surgery and compare them with patients with hybrid or percutaneous closure.

T. P. Graham, Jr, MD

Coronary Artery Disease in Adult Congenital Heart Disease: Outcome After Coronary Artery Bypass Grafting

Stulak JM, Dearani JA, Burkhart HM, et al (Mayo Clinic and Foundation, Rochester, MN)
Ann Thorac Surg 93:116-123, 2012

Background.—Atherosclerotic coronary artery disease may be seen during repair of adult congenital heart disease (ACHD). There are few data outlining outcomes of concomitant coronary artery bypass grafting (CABG) in these patients.

Methods.—Between February 1972 and August 2009, 122 patients (77 men) underwent concomitant CABG at the time of ACHD repair; median age was 64 years (range 40 to 85 years). Thirty patients (25%) had preoperative angina, 7 patients (6%) had previous myocardial infarction (MI), and 6 patients (5%) had previous percutaneous intervention. Most common primary cardiac diagnoses included secundum atrial septal defect (ASD) in 73 patients (60%), Ebstein's anomaly in 14 patients (11%), and partial anomalous pulmonary venous connection in 8 patients (7%).

Results.—Operations included ASD repair in 78 patients (64%), tricuspid/pulmonary valve procedures in 23 patients (19%), and ventricular septal defect repair in 10 patients (8%). One bypass graft procedure was performed in 69 patients (57%), 2 bypass graft procedures were performed in 32 patients (26%), 3 bypass graft procedures were performed in 14 patients (11%), 4 bypass graft procedures were performed in 5 patients (4%), and 5 bypass graft procedures were performed in 2 patients (2%). There were 4 early deaths (3.3%). During a median follow-up of 6 years (maximum follow-up, 32 years), actuarial survival was 76% at 5 years and 56% at 10 years. In patients with left anterior descending (LAD) artery disease, survival was higher when a left internal mammary graft (LIMA) was used (5 years, 86% versus 66%; 10 years, 66% versus 36%; $p < 0.05$).

Conclusions.—Concomitant CABG may be required at the time of correction of ACHD. Survival is higher when a LIMA graft is used, and late functional outcome is good, with a low incidence of late angina and need for reintervention.

▶ This is an interesting study of a problem that is certain to occur with greater frequency as the adult congenital heart disease (ACHD) population grows and ages. The bottom line is that surgery for coronary artery disease (CAD) performed with excellent outcome at the time of cardiac surgery for atrial septal defect (ASD), ventricular septal defect (VSD), Ebstein disease, or pulmonary valvotomy as well as for other less-common conditions. In addition, the left internal mammary graft (LIMA) operation outperformed other grafts, and late survival for women with ASD repair was inferior to ASD repair alone. The possible explanation for this finding is that female patients may have more advanced disease because of the perception that women have less CAD than men and have a decreased referral rate for testing for this problem. These authors suggest that all ACHD patients ≥40 years have coronary arteriograms prior to ACHD surgery. In addition, workup for ACHD surgery at a younger age should include consideration for coronary arteriograms and patients who have risk factors for early-onset CAD.

T. P. Graham, Jr, MD

Evaluation of image quality and radiation dose at prospective ECG-triggered axial 256-slice multi-detector CT in infants with congenital heart disease
Huang M-P, Liang C-H, Zhao Z-J, et al (Guangdong General Hosp, Guangzhou, People's Republic of China; et al)
Pediatr Radiol 41:858-866, 2011

Background.—There are a limited number of reports on the technical and clinical feasibility of prospective electrocardiogram (ECG)-gated multi-detector computed tomography (MDCT) in infants with congenital heart disease (CHD).

Objective.—To evaluate image quality and radiation dose at weight-based low-dose prospectively gated 256-slice MDCT angiography in infants with CHD.

Materials and Methods.—From November 2009 to February 2010, 64 consecutive infants with CHD referred for pre-operative or post-operative CT were included. All were scanned on a 256-slice MDCT system utilizing a low-dose protocol (80 kVp and 60−120 mAs depending on weight: 60 mAs for ≤3 kg, 80 mAs for 3.1−6 kg, 100 mAs for 6.1−10 kg, 120 mAs for 10.1−15 kg).

Results.—No serious adverse events were recorded. A total of 174 cardiac deformities, confirmed by surgery or heart catheterization, were studied. The sensitivity of MDCT for cardiac deformities was 97.1%; specificity, 99.4%; accuracy, 95.9%. The mean heart rate during scan was 136.7 ± 14.9/min (range, 91−160) with a corresponding heart rate variability of 2.8 ± 2.2/min (range, 0−8). Mean scan length was 115.3 ± 11.7 mm (range, 93.6−143.3). Mean volume CT dose index, mean dose-length product and effective dose were 2.1 ± 0.4 mGy (range, 1.5−2.8), 24.7 ± 5.9 mGy·cm (range, 14.7−35.8) and 1.6 ± 0.3 mSv (range, 1.1−2.5), respectively. Diagnostic-quality images were achieved in all cases. Satisfactory diagnostic quality for visualization of all/proximal/distal coronary artery segments was achieved in 88.4/98.8/80.0% of the scans.

Conclusion.—Low-dose prospectively gated axial 256-slice CT angiography is a valuable tool in the routine clinical evaluation of infants with CHD, providing a comprehensive three-dimensional evaluation of the cardiac anatomy, including the coronary arteries.

▶ I am always impressed by the high-quality images produced by CT scans of the heart and great vessels. I am also concerned about radiation dosages, which are of concern to all who deal with patients with congenital heart disease who will undoubtedly need multiple imaging studies during their lifetime. These authors show some exquisitely detailed images. It is hoped that further studies will result in even additional decreases in radiation dose.

T. P. Graham, Jr, MD

Left Ventricular Function in Adult Patients With Atrial Septal Defect: Implication for Development of Heart Failure After Transcatheter Closure
Masutani S, Senzaki H (Saitama Med Univ, Japan)
J Card Fail 17:957-963, 2011

Despite advances in device closure for atrial septal defect (ASD), post-closure heart failure observed in adult patients remains a clinical problem. Although right heart volume overload is the fundamental pathophysiology in ASD, the post-closure heart failure characterized by acute pulmonary congestion is likely because of age-related left ventricular diastolic dysfunction, which is manifested by acute volume loading with ASD closure. Aging also appears to play important roles in the pathophysiology of heart failure through several mechanisms other than diastolic dysfunction, including ventricular systolic and vascular stiffening and increased incidence of comorbidities that significantly affect cardiovascular function. Recent studies suggested that accurate assessment of preclosure diastolic function, such as test ASD occlusion, may help identify high-risk patients for post-closure heart failure. Anti—heart failure therapy before device closure or the use of fenestrated device appears to be effective in preventing post-closure heart failure in the high-risk patients. However, the long-term outcome of such patients remains to be elucidated. Future studies are warranted to construct an algorithm to identify and treat patients at high risk for heart failure after device closure of ASD.

▶ This interesting review of congestive heart failure (CHF) in adults after percutaneous atrial septal defect (ASD) closure provides a clear picture of the important physiologic mechanisms in this process. It is known that the left ventricle (LV) is smaller than normal in patients with a large atrial left to right shunt (approximately 75% to 85% of normal); in younger patients, the inherent stiffness of the LV is usually not increased, and LV diastolic pressure does not increase to high levels under these conditions. The data in older adults indicate that LV diastolic dysfunction is the cause of postclosure CHF. Current management of this problem includes ASD test occlusion to determine the increase in LV end-diastole and left atrial pressure (LAP) associated with this maneuver (defined as an increase in mean LAP > 10 mm Hg). If such an increase is seen, pretreatment with furosemide, dopamine, and milrinone has proven effective. This is an important problem to be aware of and provides more evidence for closure of ASDs in childhood.

T. P. Graham, Jr, MD

Costs of Prenatal Detection of Congenital Heart Disease

Jegatheeswaran A, Oliveira C, Batsos C, et al (Univ of Toronto, Ontario, Canada; et al)
Am J Cardiol 108:1808-1814, 2011

Little information is available about the transportation costs incurred from the missed prenatal diagnosis of congenital heart disease (CHD). The objectives of the present study were to analyze the costs of emergency transportation related to the postnatal diagnosis of major CHD and to perform a cost/benefit analysis of additional training for ultrasound technicians to study the implications of improved prenatal detection rates. The 1-year costs incurred for emergency transportation of pre- and postnatally diagnosed infants with CHD in Northern California and North Western Nevada were calculated and compared. The prenatal detection rate in our cohort (n = 147) was 30.6%. Infants postnatally diagnosed were 16.5 times more likely (p <0.001) to require emergency transport. The associated emergency transportation costs were US$542,143 in total for all patients with CHD. The mean cost per patient was $389.00 versus $5,143.51 for prenatally and postnatally diagnosed infants, respectively (p <0.001). Assuming an improvement in detection rates after 1-day training for ultrasound technicians, the investment in training cost can be recouped in 1 year if the detection rate increased by 2.4% to 33%. Savings of $6,543,476 would occur within 5 years if the detection rate increased to 50%. In conclusion, CHD diagnosed postnatally results in greater costs related to emergency transportation of ill infants. Improving the prenatal detection rates through improved ultrasound technician training could result in considerable cost savings.

▶ This thoughtful study about the costs and benefits of prenatal diagnosis of congenital heart disease is a useful paradigm to explore in many situations. There is definitely going to be a decrease in reimbursement for medical care in this country and undoubtedly worldwide. Hopefully, this type of research can prove meaningful in the long run for reducing costs as well as improving outcome.

T. P. Graham, Jr, MD

Generalised muscle weakness in young adults with congenital heart disease

Greutmann M, Le TL, Tobler D, et al (Univ of Toronto, Ontario, Canada; Toronto General Hosp, Ontario, Canada)
Heart 97:1164-1168, 2011

Background.—In patients with heart failure from acquired cardiomyopathy, respiratory and skeletal muscle weakness is common and is an independent predictor for adverse events. Despite a different underlying pathology, many young adults with congenital heart disease (CHD) develop a syndrome comparable to heart failure from acquired cardiomyopathy and may be at risk for a similar skeletal muscle weakness.

Objectives.—To assess respiratory and skeletal muscle strength in adults with complex CHD.

Methods.—Respiratory and skeletal muscle function was assessed in 51 adults; 41 with complex CHD (16 tetralogy of Fallot, 11 univentricular anatomy with Fontan operation and 14 with subaortic right ventricles) and 10 controls. Maximal inspiratory (MIPs) and expiratory (MEPs) pressures, handgrip strength, lung volumes and aerobic capacity (peak VO_2) were measured.

Results.—In patients with CHD (age 34 ± 13 years), average% predicted MIPs, MEPs and handgrip strength were lower than in controls ($77 \pm 27\%$ vs $106 \pm 28\%$, $85 \pm 32\%$ vs $116 \pm 41\%$ and $72 \pm 15\%$ vs $93 \pm 14\%$, respectively, $p \leq 0.01$). There was no significant difference in muscle weakness between CHD subgroups. In 39% of patients with CHD, the handgrip strength, and in 22%, respiratory muscle strength was <70% predicted. These patients had a significantly lower peak VO_2 ($50 \pm 12\%$ vs $64 \pm 14\%$ predicted, $p=0.008$).

Conclusion.—Respiratory and skeletal muscle weakness is common in young adults with complex CHD and similar to that found in older adults with advanced heart failure from acquired heart disease.

▶ This study indicates a significant number of adults with congenital heart disease have muscle weakness that can affect both respiratory and skeletal muscles. The next step seems to be to try to enhance muscle strength by exercise, which hopefully would significantly improve patient lifestyle and potentially long-term outcome.

T. P. Graham, Jr, MD

Erosion of an Amplatzer Septal Occluder Device Into the Aortic Root
Kamouh A, Osman MN, Rosenthal N, et al (Univ Hosps Case Med Ctr, Cleveland, OH)
Ann Thorac Surg 91:1608-1610, 2011

Atrial septal defects can be closed surgically or percutaneously. We report a patient who underwent percutaneous closure of an atrial septal defect with an Amplatzer septal occluder device (AGA Medical Corp, Golden Valley, MN). The patient presented 4 months later with congestive heart failure secondary to an erosion of the Amplatzer septal occluder into the aortic root. The device was removed surgically, and the fistula was repaired. Amplatzer septal occluder indications, selection criteria, and complications are discussed.

▶ This is just a reminder that there is no free lunch. Percutaneous atrial septal defect closure has increased almost exponentially over the past several years.

These procedures are usually noneventful in experienced hands, but the physician performing them must be aware of when to back off and send the patient to surgery. These danger signs have been documented and include an atrial rim less than 5 mm, excessive mobility of the device, excessive oversizing of the device (> 1.5 times the size of the atrial septal defect), splaying of the atrial disks across the aortic root, and extreme movement of the device deployed before release.

T. P. Graham, Jr, MD

A genetic contribution to risk for postoperative junctional ectopic tachycardia in children undergoing surgery for congenital heart disease
Borgman KY, Smith AH, Owen JP, et al (Vanderbilt Univ School of Medicine, Nashville, TN)
Heart Rhythm 8:1900-1904, 2011

Background.—Junctional ectopic tachycardia (JET) is a common arrhythmia complicating pediatric cardiac surgery, with many identifiable clinical risk factors but no genetic risk factors to date.

Objective.—To test the hypothesis that the angiotensin-converting enzyme insertion/deletion (ACE I/D) polymorphism associates with postoperative JET.

Methods.—DNA samples were collected from children undergoing the Norwood procedure; arterial switch operation; and repairs of Tetralogy of Fallot, balanced atrioventricular septal defect, and ventricular septal defect at a single center. The incidence of postoperative JET was associated with previously identified clinical risk factors and ACE I/D genotype.

Results.—Of the 174 children who underwent the above-mentioned surgeries, 21% developed JET. Postoperative JET developed in 31% of children with the D/D genotype but only in 16% of those with the I/I genotype or the I/D genotype ($P = .02$). Clinical predictors of JET were selected a priori and included age, inotrope score, cardiopulmonary bypass time, and cross-clamp time. Multivariable logistic regression identified a significant correlation between the D/D genotype and postoperative JET independent of these predictors (odds ratio = 2.4; 95% confidence interval, 1.04−5.34; $P = .04$). A gene−dose effect was apparent in the homogeneous subset of subjects with atrioventricular septal defect (58% JET in D/D subjects, 12% JET in I/D subjects, and 0% JET in I/I subjects; $P < .01$).

Conclusion.—The common ACE deletion polymorphism is associated with a greater than 2-fold increase in the odds of developing JET in children undergoing surgical repair of atrioventricular septal defect, Tetralogy of Fallot, ventricular septal defect or the Norwood and arterial switch procedures. These findings may support the potential role of the renin−angiotensin−aldosterone system in the etiology of JET.

▶ This study emphasizes the new possibility for genetic-based prescription in the management of patients with congenital heart disease. This study suggests that prescription with a beta-blocker or angiotensin converting enzyme inhibitors might decease the occurrence of junctional ectopic tachycardia in patients with the D/D genotype.

T. P. Graham, Jr, MD

Cardiovascular Screening with Electrocardiography and Echocardiography in Collegiate Athletes

Magalski A, McCoy M, Zabel M, et al (Saint Luke's Mid America Heart and Vascular Inst, Kansas City, MO; Lawrence Memorial Hosp, KS; et al)
Am J Med 124:511-518, 2011

Background.—Current guidelines for preparticipation screening of competitive athletes in the US include a comprehensive history and physical examination. The objective of this study was to determine the incremental value of electrocardiography and echocardiography added to a screening program consisting of history and physical examination in college athletes.

Methods.—Competitive collegiate athletes at a single university underwent prospective collection of medical history, physical examination, 12-lead electrocardiography, and 2-dimensional echocardiography. Electrocardiograms (ECGs) were classified as normal, mildly abnormal, or distinctly abnormal according to previously published criteria. Eligibility for competition was determined using criteria from the 36th Bethesda Conference on Eligibility Recommendations for Competitive Athletes with Cardiovascular Abnormalities.

Results.—In 964 consecutive athletes, ECGs were classified as abnormal in 334 (35%), of which 95 (10%) were distinctly abnormal. Distinct ECG abnormalities were more common in men than women (15% vs 6%, *P*<.001) as well as black compared with white athletes (18% vs 8%, *P*<.001). Echocardiographic and electrocardiographic findings initially resulted in exclusion of 9 athletes from competition, including 1 for long QT syndrome and 1 for aortic root dilatation; 7 athletes with Wolff-Parkinson-White patterns were ultimately cleared for participation. (Four received further evaluation and treatment, and 3 were determined to not need treatment.) After multivariable adjustment, black race was a statistically significant predictor of distinctly abnormal ECGs (relative risk 1.82, 95% confidence interval, 1.22-2.73; *P*=.01).

Conclusions.—Distinctly abnormal ECGs were found in 10% of athletes and were most common in black men. Noninvasive screening using both electrocardiography and echocardiography resulted in identification of 9 athletes with important cardiovascular conditions, 2 of whom were excluded from competition. These findings offer a framework for performing preparticipation screening for competitive collegiate athletes.

▶ This study indicates that the addition of an electrocardiogram (ECG) to history and physical exam is useful to identify athletes with cardiovascular abnormalities that require further evaluation and possible treatment before participation in competitive sports. Interestingly, there were no athletes found with hypertrophic cardiomyopathy. The majority of abnormalities were Wolff-Parkinson-White, which resulted in 4 of 7 receiving further evaluation and treatment, and 3 of 7 were determined not to require treatment. Ultimately, 2 athletes were excluded from competition. These data suggest that ECG screening can be useful in this screening process.

T. P. Graham, Jr, MD

3 Cardiac Surgery

Coronary Artery Disease

2011 ACCF/AHA guideline for coronary artery bypass graft surgery: Executive summary: A report of the American College of Cardiology Foundation/American Heart Association Task Force on Practice Guidelines
Hillis LD, Smith PK, Anderson JL, et al
J Thorac Cardiovasc Surg 143:4-34, 2012

Background.—Guidelines were developed by the American College of Cardiology Foundation/American Heart Association Task Force on Practice Guidelines regarding the use of coronary artery bypass graft (CABG) surgery. These were designed to provide for the safe, appropriate, and efficacious performance of CABG. Included were procedural areas, coronary artery disease (CAD) revascularization, perioperative management, CABG-associated morbidity and mortality, and treatment of special patient subsets.

Procedural Issues.—Anesthetic management is directed at early postoperative extubation and accelerated recovery for patients at low to medium risk who are having uncomplicated CABG. Volatile anesthetic-based regimens are useful, but high thoracic epidural anesthesia/analgesia is not well supported. Cyclooxygenase-2 inhibitors are not recommended for pain relief postoperatively.

The left internal mammary artery is preferred for bypass of the left anterior descending artery when required. Other options for bypass grafting include the right internal mammary artery and a second internal mammary artery to graft the left circumflex or right coronary artery. Complete arterial revascularization may help in patients age 60 years or younger with few or no comorbidities. With critical stenosis, a right coronary artery or radial artery graft may be needed.

When acute, persistent, and life-threatening hemodynamic disturbances do not respond to treatment and when valvular surgery is done concomitantly, intraoperative transesophageal echocardiography is indicated. This helps to monitor hemodynamic status, ventricular function, regional wall motion, and valvular function. To reduce the risk of perioperative myocardial ischemia and infarction, the determinants of coronary arterial perfusion should optimized. However, prophylactic pharmacologic therapies or controlled reperfusion strategies as well as postconditioning strategies have uncertain value. Mechanical preconditioning may reduce the risk of myocardial ischemia and infarction in patients having off-pump CABG. Remote ischemic preconditioning strategies (peripheral extremity occlusion/reperfusion) may attenuate the adverse effects of myocardial reperfusion injury. Specific recommendations vary with clinical status.

CAD Revascularization.—Revascularization is done in patients with CAD to relieve symptoms and improve survival. A Heart Team approach is recommended for patients with unprotected left main or complex CAD. Patients with significant left main coronary artery stenosis should undergo CABG. Selected stable patients with significant unprotected left main CAD and anatomic and clinical characteristics predicting a significantly higher risk of adverse surgical outcomes and those who have unstable acute ST-elevation myocardial infarction (UA/STEMI) can be managed by percutaneous coronary intervention (PCI). Either CABG or PCI is useful in patients with one or more significant coronary artery stenoses amenable to revascularization and unacceptable angina unresponsive to guideline-directed medical therapy (GDMT). Certain conditions are best approached using hybrid coronary revascularization procedures.

Perioperative Management.—Preoperative antiplatelet therapy with aspirin is used for all CABG patients. Patients having elective CABG must discontinue clopidogrel and ticagrelor at least 5 days preoperatively and prasugrel at least 7 days preoperatively. In urgent CABG, clopidogrel and ticagrelor should be suspended for at least 24 hours before surgery. Short-acting intravenous glycoprotein inhibitors should be discontinued at least 2 to 4 hours preoperatively. Aspirin is initiated within 6 hours of surgery and continued indefinitely. Clopidogrel can be given to patients intolerant of or allergic to aspirin.

All patients having CABG should receive statin therapy unless contraindicated. The statin dose should reduce low-density lipoprotein (LDL) cholesterol to less than 100 mg/dL and lower LDL cholesterol by at least 30%. Very high-risk patients should receive statins to lower LDL cholesterol to less than 70 mg/dL. For urgent or emergency CABG in patients not taking statins, high-dose statin therapy is initiated immediately.

Intravenous insulin is administered continuously to achieve and maintain an early postoperative blood glucose concentration of 180 mg/dL or less. Women undergoing CABG should not be receiving postmenopausal hormone therapy. Beta blockers are given to all patients (unless contraindicated) for at least 24 hours before CABG and continued postoperatively. Similar guidelines apply to angiotensin-converting enzyme inhibitors and angiotensin-receptor blockers.

All smokers should be given in-hospital counseling and offered smoking cessation therapy during their stay. Patients with depression should also receive cognitive behavioral therapy or collaborative care. In addition, all eligible patients should undergo cardiac rehabilitation after CABG. Perioperatively patients have central nervous system monitoring, electrocardiographic monitoring, and pulmonary artery catheter placement.

CABG-Associated Morbidity and Mortality.—Epiaortic ultrasound imaging allows assessment of the presence, location, and severity of plaque in the ascending aorta, reducing the incidence of atheroembolic complications. Patients with clinically significant carotid artery disease should be managed via a multidisciplinary team approach. Possible approaches include carotid artery duplex scanning and carotid revascularization in conjunction with CABG.

All patients should receive prophylactic antibiotics preoperatively, usually a first- or second-generation cephalosporin for patients without methicillin-resistant *Staphylococcus aureus* colonization and vancomycin alone or with other antibiotics to cover patients with proved or suspected methicillin-resistant *S aureus* colonization. Leukocyte-filtered blood is recommended for all transfusions.

Patients with preexisting renal dysfunction may benefit from off-pump CABG. Perioperative hematocrit is maintained over 19% and mean arterial pressure over 60 mm Hg. Surgery may be delayed after coronary angiography to assess the effect of contrast material on the kidney.

Patients at high risk for myocardial dysfunction perioperatively can be managed by inserting an intra-aortic balloon. Biomarkers of myonecrosis are monitored for the first 24 hours after CABG. Blood conservation measures are advised.

Special Patients.—Some patients need special handling. Included are those with anomalous coronary arteries, chronic obstructive pulmonary disease and/or respiratory insufficiency, end-stage renal disease who are undergoing dialysis, concomitant valvular disease, and previous cardiac surgery.

Conclusions.—The practice guidelines are designed to help healthcare providers make clinical decisions by providing generally acceptable approaches to the diagnosis, management, and prevention of specific diseases or conditions. The practices described meet the needs of most patients in most situations. Ultimately, however, the care of a specific patient will be determined by the health care provider and patient considering all the circumstances present.

▶ This latest report from American College of Cardiology (ACC) and American Heart Association (AHA) task force on clinical guidelines for management of coronary artery disease (CAD) includes strong participation from Society of Thoracic (STS) and American Association for Thoracic Surgery (AATS). Of note, the Society of Cardiovascular Anesthesiologists also participated in the task force. These comprehensive guidelines cover a broad range of issues related to CAD, from preoperative assessment, intraoperative management, options of management, to postoperative care, as well as measurement of outcomes. This document is a must read for those participating in the treatment of patients with coronary disease. One key area of focus is the emphasis on development of the "heart team approach" to revascularization decisions. The task force recognizes the current assessment, management, and treatment of CAD predominantly by cardiology is suboptimal and encourages increased collaboration between cardiology and cardiac surgery. The development of these heart teams will likely improve quality of care for cardiac patients. Another noteworthy contribution of this report is its stance that hybrid revascularization is reasonable if there are poor targets for coronary artery bypass graft, lack of suitable grafts, or unfavorable left anterior descending artery for percutaneous coronary intervention. These guidelines are the product of an effort by a large task force after thorough review of the literature, current methodology, and techniques. As such, they form the cornerstone for effective medical practice.

S. R. Neravetla, MD

V. H. Thourani, MD

Coronary-Artery Bypass Surgery in Patients with Left Ventricular Dysfunction

Velazquez EJ, for the STICH Investigators (Duke Univ Med Ctr, Durham, NC; et al)

N Engl J Med 364:1607-1616, 2011

Background.—The role of coronary-artery bypass grafting (CABG) in the treatment of patients with coronary artery disease and heart failure has not been clearly established.

Methods.—Between July 2002 and May 2007, a total of 1212 patients with an ejection fraction of 35% or less and coronary artery disease amenable to CABG were randomly assigned to medical therapy alone (602 patients) or medical therapy plus CABG (610 patients). The primary outcome was the rate of death from any cause. Major secondary outcomes included the rates of death from cardiovascular causes and of death from any cause or hospitalization for cardiovascular causes.

Results.—The primary outcome occurred in 244 patients (41%) in the medical-therapy group and 218 (36%) in the CABG group (hazard ratio with CABG, 0.86; 95% confidence interval [CI], 0.72 to 1.04; P=0.12). A total of 201 patients (33%) in the medicaltherapy group and 168 (28%) in the CABG group died from an adjudicated cardiovascular cause (hazard ratio with CABG, 0.81; 95% CI, 0.66 to 1.00; P=0.05). Death from any cause or hospitalization for cardiovascular causes occurred in 411 patients (68%) in the medical-therapy group and 351 (58%) in the CABG group (hazard ratio with CABG, 0.74; 95% CI, 0.64 to 0.85; P<0.001). By the end of the followup period (median, 56 months), 100 patients in the medical-therapy group (17%) underwent CABG, and 555 patients in the CABG group (91%) underwent CABG.

Conclusions.—In this randomized trial, there was no significant difference between medical therapy alone and medical therapy plus CABG with respect to the primary end point of death from any cause. Patients assigned to CABG, as compared with those assigned to medical therapy alone, had lower rates of death from cardiovascular causes and of death from any cause or hospitalization for cardiovascular causes. (Funded by the National Heart, Lung, and Blood Institute and Abbott Laboratories; STICH ClinicalTrials.gov number, NCT00023595.)

▶ The role of coronary artery bypass grafting (CABG) in patients with coronary artery disease and heart failure remains unclear. This particular portion of the

Surgical Treatment for Ischemic Heart Failure (STICH) trial reports the results of the medical therapy plus CABG versus medical therapy alone in patients with left ventricular systolic dysfunction. This was an international multicenter, randomized study across 127 clinical sites. Because of enrollment difficulty, the study design was modified by increasing follow-up time to allow smaller enrollment. Overall, 1212 patients were enrolled in this arm of the study. Six hundred ten patients were assigned to CABG and 602 patients were assigned to medical therapy alone. One hundred patients (17%) of the medical therapy group underwent CABG before the end of the follow-up. Although not statistically significant, overall mortality in the medical therapy group was 41% and 36% in the CABG group. With as-treated analysis, the hazard ratio of the CABG arm was 0.70 ($P < .001$). Patients in the medical therapy alone arm did have statistically significant higher rates of cardiovascular deaths and death from any cause or hospitalization for cardiovascular cause. It is not surprising to note that early deaths were higher in the surgical arm. After the first 2 years, however, survival in the surgical arm improved, and the question arises whether the surgical therapy group would have had statistically significant all-cause mortality reduction if the study had continued longer. This was a large study that attempted to elucidate a complex disease. Other reports from the STICH trial expound further on the algorithm for coronary artery disease and heart failure, including defining the impact of myocardial viability on treatment outcomes. Further studies will need to be performed to more definitely define the role of CABG in patients with heart failure. However, long-term follow-up will have to be a critical component of this study, because these data appear to show an increasing trend in benefit of CABG with time.

S. R. Neravetla, MD

V. H. Thourani, MD

Long-Term Outcomes of Endoscopic Vein Harvesting After Coronary Artery Bypass Grafting

Dacey LJ, for the Northern New England Cardiovascular Disease Study Group (Dartmouth-Hitchcock Med Ctr, Hanover, NH; et al)
Circulation 123:147-153, 2011

Background.—Use of endoscopic saphenous vein harvesting has developed into a routine surgical approach at many cardiothoracic surgical centers. The association between this technique and long-term morbidity and mortality has recently been called into question. The present report describes the use of open versus endoscopic vein harvesting and risk of mortality and repeat revascularization in northern New England during a time period (2001 to 2004) in which both techniques were being performed.

Methods and Results.—From 2001 to 2004, 8542 patients underwent isolated coronary artery bypass grafting procedures, 52.5% with endoscopic vein harvesting. Surgical discretion dictated the vein harvest approach. The main outcomes were death and repeat revascularization (percutaneous coronary intervention or coronary artery bypass grafting) within 4 years of the index admission. The use of endoscopic vein harvesting increased from 34% in 2001 to 75% in 2004. In general, patients undergoing endoscopic vein harvesting had greater disease burden. Endoscopic vein harvesting was associated with an increased adjusted risk of bleeding requiring a return to the operating room (2.4 versus 1.7; $P=0.03$) but a decreased risk of leg wound infections (0.2 versus 1.1; $P<0.001$). Use of endoscopic vein harvesting was associated with a significant reduction in long-term mortality (adjusted hazard ratio, 0.74; 95% confidence interval, 0.60 to 0.92) but a nonsignificant increased risk of repeat revascularization (adjusted hazard ratio, 1.29; 95% confidence interval, 0.96 to 1.74). Similar results were obtained in propensity-stratified analysis.

Conclusions.—During 2001 to 2004 in northern New England, the use of endoscopic vein harvesting was not associated with harm. There was a nonsignificant increase in repeat revascularization, and survival was not decreased.

▶ The traditional open harvesting of the saphenous vein (OVH) for a conduit for coronary artery bypass grafting (CABG) has long been considered the standard. Over the last decade, vast improvements in optics and endoscopic tools from a variety of surgical fields have helped in the development and wide adoption of endoscopic saphenous vein harvesting (EVH). Over the last 2 years, the usage of EVH has been criticized for leading to decreased saphenous vein patency. The inferiority of EVH was reported by Lopes and colleagues[1] in an ad-hoc analysis of a randomized study evaluating OVH versus EVH in those undergoing CABG. Graft failure rates were significantly higher in the EVH group 12 to 18 months after surgery. At 3 years, the composite endpoint of death, myocardial infarction, or repeat revascularization was 20.2% for EVH versus 17.4% for OVH ($P < .001$). This study was conducted in the early days of EVH and, since that time, the devices have been modified at least 5 times. Furthermore, it is possible that evolution of EVH devices, operator experience, and administration of anticoagulation before harvesting the veins undoubtedly would yield different results if the same study were repeated today.

Dr Dacey, on behalf of the Northern New England Cardiovascular Disease Study Group, has reported on 8542 patients from 2001 to 2004 who underwent isolated CABG procedures. In this propensity-stratified analysis, 4480 patients underwent EVH and 4062 underwent OVH. To date, this is the largest patient cohort evaluating the use of EVH versus OVH. The authors noted that during this period, the adoption of EVH increased from 34% of the patients in 2001 to 75% in 2004. Despite the EVH patients having greater disease burden, they concluded that EVH was not associated with harm, as measured by significant diminished long-term survival or repeat revascularization. The key advantage of decreased leg wound infections with endoscopic vein harvesting and the decrease in the morbidity associated with OVH was clearly demonstrated in this study. This is an important study in that it evaluates a more modern perspective and the nuisances that are common in the harvesting of vein conduits. Further studies are underway to evaluate and refine the specific techniques of EVH, and prospective, randomized double-blind trials comparing the

2 techniques are warranted; long-term graft patency continues to be a concern. However, patient demand and satisfaction with minimally invasive procedures will continue to drive further improvements in endoscopic vein harvesting techniques and likely make it the gold standard.

A. R. Khan, MD

V. H. Thourani, MD

Reference

1. Lopes RD, Hafley GE, Allen KB, et al. Endoscopic versus open vein-graft harvesting in coronary-artery bypass surgery. *N Engl J Med.* 2009;361:235-244.

Quality of Life after PCI with Drug-Eluting Stents or Coronary-Artery Bypass Surgery
Cohen DJ, for the Synergy between PCI with Taxus and Cardiac Surgery (SYNTAX) Investigators (Univ of Missouri—Kansas City; et al)
N Engl J Med 364:1016-1026, 2011

Background.—Previous studies have shown that among patients undergoing multivessel revascularization, coronary-artery bypass grafting (CABG), as compared with percutaneous coronary intervention (PCI) either by means of balloon angioplasty or with the use of bare-metal stents, results in greater relief from angina and improved quality of life. The effect of PCI with the use of drug-eluting stents on these outcomes is unknown.

Methods.—In a large, randomized trial, we assigned 1800 patients with three-vessel or left main coronary artery disease to undergo either CABG (897 patients) or PCI with paclitaxeleluting stents (903 patients). Health-related quality of life was assessed at baseline and at 1, 6, and 12 months with the use of the Seattle Angina Questionnaire (SAQ) and the Medical Outcomes Study 36-Item Short-Form Health Survey (SF-36). The primary end point was the score on the angina-frequency subscale of the SAQ (on which scores range from 0 to 100, with higher scores indicating better health status).

Results.—The scores on each of the SAQ and SF-36 subscales were significantly higher at 6 and 12 months than at baseline in both groups. The score on the angina-frequency subscale of the SAQ increased to a greater extent with CABG than with PCI at both 6 and 12 months (P = 0.04 and P = 0.03, respectively), but the between-group differences were small (mean treatment effect of 1.7 points at both time points). The proportion of patients who were free from angina was similar in the two groups at 1 month and 6 months and was higher in the CABG group than in the PCI group at 12 months (76.3% vs. 71.6%, P = 0.05). Scores on all the other SAQ and SF-36 subscales were either higher in the PCI group (mainly at 1 month) or were similar in the two groups throughout the follow-up period.

Conclusions.—Among patients with three-vessel or left main coronary artery disease, there was greater relief from angina after CABG than after

PCI at 6 and 12 months, although the extent of the benefit was small. (Funded by Boston Scientific; ClinicalTrials.gov number, NCT00114972.)

▶ The most well-known and largest contemporary trial comparing percutaneous coronary intervention (PCI) and coronary artery bypass grafting (CABG) is the Synergy between PCI with Taxus and Cardiac Surgery (SYNTAX Trial) study. This is the large, randomized trial in which the outcomes of PCI with the use of the paclitaxel-eluting stents were compared with those of CABG among patients with 3-vessel or left main coronary artery disease. In the original publication, it was reported that although the rate of the composite primary endpoint (death, myocardial infarction, stroke, or repeat revascularization) was lower with CABG than with PCI at 1 year, the composite endpoint of death, myocardial infarction, or stroke was not different between groups. An important adjunct to the clinical outcomes of morbidity and mortality include the prospectively collected quality-of-life (QOL) substudy within the SYNTAX trial.

In this large, randomized trial (CABG group, n = 897 and PCI group, n = 903), the Seattle Angina Questionnaire (SAQ) and the Medical Outcomes Study 36-Item Short-Form Health Survey (SF-36) were administered at baseline and 1, 6, and 12 months. It is comforting that in both groups, SAQ and SF-36 subscales were significantly higher at 6 and 12 months when compared with baseline. As expected, the SAQ physical limitation and SF-36 physical functioning was improved in the PCI group at 1 month compared with CABG. However, at 6 and 12 months, these differences abated with no significant difference between groups. In terms of the primary QOL endpoint, the extent of improvement was slightly but significantly greater with CABG than with PCI at 6 and 12 months. Interestingly, in those patients with daily or weekly angina, CABG was associated with greater relief from angina than with PCI at 6 and 12 months, whereas there was no difference between groups in those with less-frequent angina.

This very informative and interesting study allows an objective analysis of QOL measures in a contemporary era for the treatment of coronary artery disease. This should allow practicing physicians to relate to the patient a more realistic expectation and discussion for not only morbidity and mortality but also quality of life following the management of their disease process.

S. R. Neravetla, MD
V. H. Thourani, MD

Randomized Comparison of Percutaneous Coronary Intervention With Sirolimus-Eluting Stents Versus Coronary Artery Bypass Grafting in Unprotected Left Main Stem Stenosis
Boudriot E, Thiele H, Walther T, et al (Univ of Leipzig—Heart Ctr, Germany; et al)
J Am Coll Cardiol 57:538-545, 2011

Objectives.—The purpose of this randomized study was to compare sirolimus-eluting stenting with coronary artery bypass grafting (CABG) for patients with unprotected left main (ULM) coronary artery disease.

Background.—CABG is considered the standard of care for treatment of ULM. Improvements in percutaneous coronary intervention (PCI) with use of drug-eluting stents might lead to similar results. The effectiveness of drug-eluting stenting versus surgery has not been established in a randomized trial.

Methods.—In this prospective, multicenter, randomized trial, 201 patients with ULM disease were randomly assigned to undergo sirolimus-eluting stenting (n = 100) or CABG using predominantly arterial grafts (n = 101). The primary clinical end point was noninferiority in freedom from major adverse cardiac events, such as cardiac death, myocardial infarction, and the need for target vessel revascularization within 12 months.

Results.—The combined primary end point was reached in 13.9% of patients after surgery, as opposed to 19.0% after PCI (p = 0.19 for noninferiority). The combined rates for death and myocardial infarction were comparable (surgery, 7.9% vs. stenting, 5.0%; noninferiority p < 0.001), but stenting was inferior to surgery for repeat revascularization (5.9% vs. 14.0%; noninferiority p = 0.35). Perioperative complications including 2 strokes were higher after surgery (4% vs. 30%; p < 0.001). Freedom from angina was similar between groups (p = 0.33).

Conclusions.—In patients with ULM stenosis, PCI with sirolimus-eluting stents is inferior to CABG at 12-month follow-up with respect to freedom from major adverse cardiac events, which is mainly influenced by repeated revascularization, whereas for hard end points, PCI results are favorable. A longer follow-up is warranted. (Percutaneous Coronary Intervention [PCI] With Drug-Eluting Stents [DES] Versus Coronary Artery Bypass Graft [CABG] for Patients With Significant Left Main Stenosis; NCT00176397.)

▶ The unprotected left main stem stenosis (ULM) is well documented to have a worse outcome than any other form of coronary artery disease. The gold standard for the treatment of ULM is considered to be coronary artery bypass grafting (CABG). With the significant advancements in percutaneous coronary procedures (PCIs) and improvements in stent technology, PCI is increasingly being adopted for the treatment of ULM even in the presence of the increased risk with this type of stenosis. This prospective, randomized study attempted to compare PCI with sirolimus drug-eluting stent versus CABG in the setting of ULM. This was a noninferiority trial; therefore, the study endpoint was freedom from any major adverse cardiac events, such as myocardial infarction, cardiac death, or need for revascularization. An important point about this study was the stringent exclusion criteria for patients, which included distal left main disease, total occlusions, left dominant coronary anatomy, renal failure, recent myocardial infarction (< 48 h), and congestive heart failure. With such stringent exclusion criteria, this trial only enrolled the elective patient incidentally found to have proximal left main disease, a rare scenario in most community centers. Strokes were observed in patients during this study but did not affect the study results or statistical analysis. DES was shown to be inferior to CABG because of the increased rate of revascularizations. Limitations of this study included the short time interval (12-month follow-up) of the analysis, a smaller sample size (201 patients), and the fact that all aspects of major adverse cardiac and cerebrovascular events were not used as endpoints. This study posed a good starting point for future trials with larger multicenter enrollment; larger study samples and longer time of follow-up, such as the ongoing SYNTAX trial, are warranted. Patients with ULM remain a challenging subgroup for cardiologists and surgeons alike, but currently, CABG remains the standard-of-care in this patient population. Only consultation with a cardiac surgeon leading to high-risk operability should lead to elective ULM PCI.

A. R. Khan, MD
V. H. Thourani, MD

Valve Disease

Elevated parathyroid hormone predicts mortality in dialysis patients undergoing valve surgery
Yan H, Sharma J, Weber CJ, et al (Emory Univ School of Medicine, Atlanta, GA)
Surgery 150:1095-1101, 2011

Background.—Dialysis patients requiring valve surgery have high morbidity and mortality rates. Although elevated serum parathyroid hormone (PTH) levels are associated with increased mortality in dialysis patients, this correlation has not been investigated in patients undergoing cardiac valve operations. This study assesses the impact of PTH levels on mortality in dialysis patients undergoing valve operations.

Methods.—A retrospective analysis of 109 dialysis patients undergoing valve operation with preoperative PTH levels between 1996 and 2007 at a US academic center was performed. Cox regression analyses were done using PTH as a binary variable. The patients were followed from the date of the operative procedure until death or loss to follow-up.

Results.—Higher mortality risk was seen once preoperative PTH exceeded 200 pg/mL (hazard ratio [HR], 3.43; $P = .003$). Mean survival was improved in the PTH < 200 pg/mL group when compared with the PTH ≥ 200 pg/mL group (86.7 vs 40.3 months, respectively). Other independent predictors of mortality included serum phosphate (HR, 1.20; $P = .017$), calcium–phosphate product (HR, 1.02; $P = .038$), and history of myocardial infarction (HR, 2.12; $P = .015$).

Conclusion.—Preoperative PTH level ≥ 200 pg/mL is predictive of increased mortality after valve surgery among dialysis patients. Hyperparathyroidism should be investigated further as a possible modifiable risk factor for postoperative mortality in this high-risk patient cohort.

▶ More than 300 000 people in the United States are currently undergoing therapy for stage 5 chronic kidney disease with most receiving hemodialysis. Over time, the majority of these patients develop secondary hyperparathyroidism (SHPT) and its associated abnormalities in mineral metabolism. The resultant altered levels of serum calcium, phosphorus, and parathyroid hormone (PTH) have been associated with increased bone disease, vascular calcification, and mortality. The negative impact of PTH on survival has been previously demonstrated in the general dialysis population, but this study is unique in that it investigates this association in dialysis patients after valve replacement surgery. Although dialysis patients generally have poor survival compared with nondialysis patients after valve surgery, they are not a homogeneous group, and this article suggests that their survival can be stratified based on preoperative PTH. The authors note higher mortality risk was seen once preoperative PTH rose above 200 pg/mL, which is within the National Kidney Foundation's Kidney Disease Outcomes Quality Initiative target range of 150 to 300 pg/mL. Although previous correlation between elevated PTH and increased mortality has been well studied, the previous studies have primarily found mortality to increase once PTH exceeded 300 pg/mL instead of 200 pg/mL. The plot of the PTH residuals revealed that although mortality continued to increase with higher PTH, the relationship was not linear. The greatest mortality risk increase occurred in the 300 to 700 pg/mL range, and the rate at which risk increased became attenuated above that range. Consequently, further elevation in PTH resulted in more modest rises in mortality risk. This is possibly due to the smaller number of patients in the higher PTH groups after they were separated into 4 groups.

Although no previous study has investigated the association between PTH and postoperative mortality in dialysis patients undergoing valve surgery, these novel results are consistent with other studies investigating the general dialysis population. In summary, the authors conclude that severe secondary hyperparathyroidism is a strong predictor of mortality in dialysis patients after cardiac valve surgery. Although these patients have high mortality as a group, they can be stratified based on their preoperative PTH levels. Therefore, present severe secondary hyperparathyroidism as a possible modifiable risk factor in this patient population may be feasible.

A. R. Khan, MD

V. H. Thourani, MD

Percutaneous Repair or Surgery for Mitral Regurgitation

Feldman T, for the EVEREST II Investigators (NorthShore Univ Health System, Evanston, IL; et al)
N Engl J Med 364:1395-1406, 2011

Background.—Mitral-valve repair can be accomplished with an investigational procedure that involves the percutaneous implantation of a clip that grasps and approximates the edges of the mitral leaflets at the origin of the regurgitant jet.

Methods.—We randomly assigned 279 patients with moderately severe or severe (grade 3+ or 4+) mitral regurgitation in a 2:1 ratio to undergo either percutaneous repair or conventional surgery for repair or replacement of the mitral valve. The primary composite end point for efficacy was freedom from death, from surgery for mitral-valve dysfunction, and from grade 3+ or 4+ mitral regurgitation at 12 months. The primary safety end point was a composite of major adverse events within 30 days.

Results.—At 12 months, the rates of the primary end point for efficacy were 55% in the percutaneous-repair group and 73% in the surgery group (P = 0.007). The respective rates of the components of the primary end point were as follows: death, 6% in each group; surgery for mitral-valve dysfunction, 20% versus 2%; and grade 3+ or 4+ mitral regurgitation, 21% versus 20%. Major adverse events occurred in 15% of patients in the percutaneous-repair group and 48% of patients in the surgery group at 30 days (P<0.001). At 12 months, both groups had improved left ventricular size, New York Heart Association functional class, and quality-of-life measures, as compared with baseline.

Conclusions.—Although percutaneous repair was less effective at reducing mitral regurgitation than conventional surgery, the procedure was associated with superior safety and similar improvements in clinical outcomes. (Funded by Abbott Vascular; EVEREST II ClinicalTrials.gov number, NCT00209274.)

▶ If untreated, severe mitral regurgitation (MR) can lead to heart failure symptoms and reduced survival. The goal should be to intervene to eliminate MR at the onset of symptoms or before any irreversible changes in cardiac function occur. Currently, our choices for intervention are surgical mitral valve repair or replacement, with repair preferred whenever possible because it has a low operative mortality rate (about 2%), restores normal valve function, and provides excellent long-term outcomes. Over the last 5 years, the treatment of severe MR has evolved such that in some patients, a third option is a viable alternative: the percutaneous treatment modality.

Feldman and colleagues report the results of a randomized, prospective trial of a percutaneously inserted mitral valve clip for the treatment of severe regurgitation (EVEREST II: Endovascular Valve Edge-to-Edge Repair Study). The idea that MR may be treated with a nonsurgical approach is exciting, particularly if the new procedure effectively reduces MR severity with a low morbidity and mortality. However, as is optimal for new less invasive technology, outcomes should at least be noninferior to the tried and tested surgical valve repair in terms of safety, valve function, durability, and long-term outcomes. The mitral valve clip that was evaluated in this study fulfills some of these criteria. As compared with mitral valve surgery, the mitral clip was associated with a lower rate of complications at 30 days. However, it is disappointing that by 1 year after the procedure, 20% of patients in the percutaneous treatment group required surgery for mitral valve dysfunction compared with 2% of patients in the surgical group who required repeat surgery. It is of particular concern that substantial residual regurgitation (grade 2 + or more) was present in 46% of patients in the percutaneous treatment group compared with 17% in the surgical group at 12 months. However, it is important to note that the trial was reported with the use of an intention-to-treat analysis, so patients who were assigned to surgery but did not undergo surgery (15 of 95 patients) were considered to have the same degree of mitral regurgitation at 1 and 2 years as at baseline; this group accounted for most of the patients with residual mitral regurgitation and reflected the reality that some patients do not undergo surgery. Among the 80 patients assigned to and treated with surgery, 3% had grade 3+ or 4+ mitral regurgitation at 1-year follow-up. This modest reduction in regurgitant severity might be associated with favorable short-term and midterm outcomes, but surgical series suggest that residual mitral regurgitation predicts adverse long-term clinical outcomes. Another confounding issue remains the heterogeneity of the MR patient cohort. In this study, both patients with primary leaflet disease and those with functional regurgitation were evaluated.

Similar to the treatment of aortic stenosis in high-risk patients using transcatheter aortic valve replacement, it is incumbent for the heart valve team consisting of echocardiographers, interventional cardiologists, and cardiac surgeons to make appropriate decisions regarding the choices of watchful waiting, medical therapy, percutaneous intervention, or surgical valve repair or replacement.

S. R. Neravetla, MD

V. H. Thourani, MD

Valve Configuration Determines Long-Term Results After Repair of the Bicuspid Aortic Valve

Aicher D, Kunihara T, Abou Issa O, et al (Univ Hosp of Saarland, Homburg, Germany)

Circulation 123:178-185, 2011

Background.—Reconstruction of the regurgitant bicuspid aortic valve has been performed for >10 years, but there is limited information on long-term results. We analyzed our results to determine the predictors of suboptimal outcome.

Methods and Results.—Between November 1995 and December 2008, 316 patients (age, 49 ± 14 years; male, 268) underwent reconstruction of a regurgitant bicuspid aortic valve. Intraoperative assessment included extent of fusion, root dimensions, circumferential orientation of the 2 normal commissures (>160°, ≤160°), and effective height after repair. Cusp pathology was treated by central plication (n=277), triangular resection (n=138), or pericardial patch (n=94). Root dilatation was treated by subcommissural plication (n=100), root remodeling (n=122), or valve reimplantation (n=2). All patients were followed up echocardiographically (cumulative follow-up, 1253 years; mean, 4 ± 3.1 years). Clinical and morphological parameters were analyzed for correlation with 10-year freedom from reoperation with the Cox proportional hazards model. Hospital mortality was 0.63%; survival was 92% at 10 years. Freedom from reoperation at 5 and 10 years was 88% and 81%; freedom from valve replacement, 95% and 84%. By univariable analysis, statistically significant predictors of reoperation were age (hazard ratio [HR]=0.97), aortoventricular diameter (HR=1.24), effective height (HR=0.76), commissural orientation (HR=0.95), use of a pericardial patch (HR=7.63), no root replacement (HR=3.80), subcommissural plication (HR=2.07), and preoperative aortic regurgitation grade 3 or greater.

By multivariable analysis, statistically significant predictors for reoperation were age (HR=0.96), aortoventricular diameter (HR=1.30), effective height (HR=0.74), commissural orientation (HR=0.96), and use of a pericardial patch (HR=5.16).

Conclusions.—Reconstruction of bicuspid aortic valve can be performed reproducibly with good early results. Recurrence and progression of regurgitation, however, may occur, depending primarily on anatomic features of the valve.

▶ In the last 15 years, reconstruction of the aortic valve has become an increasingly attractive alternative to replacement in those patients with a bicuspid aortic valve (BAV) anatomy. This represents the most common congenital cardiovascular malformation, with relevant aortic stenosis at a mean age of approximately 60 years or relevant regurgitation at a mean age of approximately 30 years of age. Aortic dilatation may be associated with bicuspid valve anatomy in 50% to 60% of individuals. Although reconstruction of the BAV was proposed as early as 1992, repair failures have stymied the generalization of this technique within the surgical community. Furthermore, very little data regarding mid- to long-term results have been published in a large cohort of patients.

The current analysis is from unarguably one of the largest sites in the world performing bicuspid aortic valve repair. This analysis on 316 patients from 1995 to 2008 confirms previous data showing a low incidence of valve-related complications after reconstruction of the regurgitant BAV from a highly experience single institution. A detailed pre- and intraoperative echocardiographic and computed tomography analysis was performed to assess extent of fusion, root dimensions, circumferential orientation of the 2 normal commissures, and effective height after repair. There were very low hospital mortality and excellent 92% survival at 10 years. At 5 years, the freedom from reoperation (88%) or valve replacement (95%) at 5 years is acceptable. Aortic stenosis was infrequent up to 14 years after surgery. Repair failure is the most frequent complication, and it is influenced by such anatomic characteristics of the valves as commissural orientation or prerepair root dimensions. Repair works well with excellent durability in certain anatomic situations but should be avoided, at least with current reconstructive techniques, in others. A strong influence of anatomic characteristics on long-term durability of repair was found, with commissural orientation and degree of annular dilatation as the 2 most important predictors. The findings of this study highlight that bicuspid anatomy is not constant but rather includes a wide spectrum of anatomic variations. Therefore, specific strategies still have to be developed and proven for the subtypes of bicuspid valves that will most likely lead to further generalization of this technique.

S. R. Neravetla, MD

V. H. Thourani, MD

Transplantation/Ventricular Assist Devices

Continuous Flow Left Ventricular Assist Device Outcomes in Commercial Use Compared With the Prior Clinical Trial

John R, Naka Y, Smedira NG, et al (Univ of Minnesota, Minneapolis; Columbia Presbyterian Hosp, NY; Cleveland Clinic, OH; et al)
Ann Thorac Surg 92:1406-1413, 2011

Background.—A multicenter clinical trial conducted from 2005 to 2008 of a continuous flow left ventricular assist device (LVAD) resulted in Food and Drug Administration approval for bridge to transplantation. The purpose of this analysis was to determine changes in posttrial outcomes in widespread commercial use since the clinical trial.

Methods.—We compared outcomes of 486 patients who received a continuous flow LVAD as a bridge to transplantation at 36 centers during the clinical trial (March 2005 to April 2008) with outcomes of 1,496 posttrial patients who received a continuous flow LVAD at 83 centers (April 2008 to September 2010 as reported to the Interagency Registry for Mechanically Assisted Circulatory Support).

Results.—Baseline data were comparable between groups. Cumulative follow-up was 511 and 1,082 patient-years for trial and posttrial patients, respectively, and average support duration was 12.6 ± 14.0 and 8.7 ± 7.1 months. Kaplan-Meier survival improved at 1 year from 76% (trial) to 85% (posttrial). The percentage of patients undergoing transplantation in the first year decreased from 48% in the trial period to 39% in the posttrial period. Quality of life metrics improved by 3 months in both groups.

Conclusions.—The survival rate of a large group of continuous flow LVAD patients in a real-world setting after Food and Drug Administration market approval for bridge to transplantation has improved since the clinical trial. These data show that excellent outcomes have been maintained with dissemination of new LVAD technology from a clinical trial phase to more broad based use in the period after market approval.

▶ The promising data from the trial conducted on continuous flow left ventricular assist device (LVAD) led to its commercial approval. Since approval, it has been implanted in approximately 1500 patients. The initial trial showed increased survival in the bridge to transplant (BTT) patients with continuous-flow LVAD. This study examined the results of the large number of implants since commercial approval to assess its impact in the real world. The posttrial patients had a lower mortality rate (4.5%) and increased 1-year survival rate (85% compared with 76%). Although most of the patients in this group were very ill, they actually required less inotropic or intra-aortic balloon pump support than patients in the trial period. The patients in the posttrial period had better results despite having a decreased rate of transplant (22% posttrial vs 32% trial period). These results show that as experience with continuous flow LVADs has increased, the patients in the "real world" have actually done better despite the expansion of use into smaller, less-experienced centers. This was an impressive large study that confirmed the utility of continuous-flow LVADs in the BTT patient population.

S. R. Neravetla, MD
V. H. Thourani, MD

Inhaled nitric oxide after left ventricular assist device implantation: A prospective, randomized, double-blind, multicenter, placebo-controlled trial

Potapov E, Meyer D, Swaminathan M, et al (Deutsches Herzzentrum Berlin, Germany; Univ of Texas Southwestern/St Paul Med Ctr, Dallas; Duke Univ Med Ctr, Durham, NC; et al)
J Heart Lung Transplant 30:870-878, 2011

Background.—Used frequently for right ventricular dysfunction (RVD), the clinical benefit of inhaled nitric oxide (iNO) is still unclear. We conducted a randomized, double-blind, controlled trial to determine the effect of iNO on post-operative outcomes in the setting of left ventricular assist device (LVAD) placement.

Methods.—Included were 150 patients undergoing LVAD placement with pulmonary vascular resistance ≥ 200 dyne/sec/cm^{-5}. Patients received iNO (40 ppm) or placebo (an equivalent concentration of nitrogen) until 48 hours after separation from cardiopulmonary bypass, extubation, or upon meeting study-defined RVD. For ethical reasons, crossover to open-label iNO was allowed during the 48-hour treatment period if RVD criteria were met.

Results.—RVD criteria were met by 7 of 73 patients (9.6%; 95% confidence interval, 2.8–16.3) in the iNO group compared with 12 of 77 (15.6%; 95% confidence interval, 7.5–23.7) who received placebo ($p = 0.330$). Time on mechanical ventilation decreased in the iNO group (median days, 2.0 vs 3.0; $p = 0.077$), and fewer patients in the iNO group required an RVAD (5.6% vs 10%; $p = 0.468$); however, these trends did not meet statistical boundaries of significance. Hospital stay, intensive care unit stay, and 28-day mortality rates were similar between groups, as were adverse events. Thirty-five patients crossed over to open-label iNO (iNO, $n = 15$; placebo, $n = 20$). Eighteen patients (iNO, $n = 9$; placebo, $n = 9$) crossed over before RVD criteria were met.

Conclusions.—Use of iNO at 40 ppm in the perioperative phase of LVAD implantation did not achieve significance for the primary end point of reduction in RVD. Similarly, secondary end points of time on mechanical ventilation, hospital or intensive care unit stay, and the need for RVAD support after LVAD placement were not significantly improved.

▶ Right heart failure is a difficult complication after left ventricular assist device (LVAD) placement in patients with end-stage cardiac failure. Inhaled nitric oxide (iNO) has been used anecdotally based on small studies both for prophylaxis and treatment of right heart failure, but it is a very expensive intervention.

This randomized, multicenter trial examined the effectiveness of iNO in preventing right heart failure after LVAD. The study did find a decrease (but not statistically significant) duration of mechanical ventilation in the iNO arm, but it did not translate to decrease in intensive care unit or hospital length of stay. Most importantly, there was no difference in survival at 1 month or need for right ventricular assist device within 1 month. One inevitable drawback of the article is the high crossover rate from placebo to open label (20 of 77). Patients crossed over because of physician decision, and 11 patients met right heart failure criteria and therefore switched from study drug to open label. However, the iNO arm also had a high crossover rate (15 of 73). These crossovers were included in the intention-to-treat analysis. Despite these limitations, the authors of this study should be commended for undertaking such a timely and relevant protocol. While this study is not definitive due to its inherent limitations, it raises questions regarding the prevalent use of empiric use of iNO. This treatment warrants further investigation, which may lead to decreased use of a costly intervention.

S. R. Neravetla, MD

V. H. Thourani, MD

Outcomes and Quality Assessment

Changing outcomes in patients bridged to heart transplantation with continuous- versus pulsatile-flow ventricular assist devices: An analysis of the registry of the International Society for Heart and Lung Transplantation

Nativi JN, Drakos SG, Kucheryavaya AY, et al (Univ of Utah, Salt Lake City; International Society for Heart and Lung Transplantation, Addison, TX; et al)
J Heart Lung Transplant 30:854-861, 2011

Background.—Patients bridged to heart transplantation with left ventricular assist devices (LVADs) have been reported to have higher post-transplant mortality compared with those without LVADs. Our aim was to determine the impact of the type of LVAD and implant era on post-transplant survival.

Methods.—In this study we included 8,557 patients from the registry of the International Society for Heart and Lung Transplantation. We examined post-transplant outcomes in 1,100 patients bridged to transplant with pulsatile-flow LVADs between January 2000 and June 2004 (first era), 880 patients bridged with pulsatile-flow LVADs between July 2004 and May 2008 (second era), and 417 patients bridged with continuous-flow LVADs in the second era. Patients who required intravenous inotropes but not LVAD support ($n = 2,728$) and patients who did not require either LVAD or inotropes ($n = 3,432$) served as controls.

Results.—Post-transplant survival of patients bridged with pulsatile LVADs improved significantly between the first and the second era ($p = 0.03$). In the second era, there was no significant difference in post-transplant survival of patients bridged with pulsatile- vs continuous-flow LVADs ($p = 0.26$), and survival rates in the 2 groups were not statistically different from that of the non-LVAD group. Graft rejection was similar in patients bridged with LVADs compared to those without LVADs.

Conclusions.—In the most recent era, the use of either pulsatile- or continuous-flow LVADs did not result in increased post-transplant mortality. This finding is important as the proportion of patients with LVADs at the time of transplant has been rising.

▶ The advent of continuous flow, nonpulsatile flow, left ventricular assist devices (LVADs) has led to a paradigm shift in the management of end-stage heart failure. The efficacy of newer, more efficient nonpulsatile LVAD as a bridge to transplant (BTT) is assessed in this article by analyzing the outcome data from registry of the International Society of Heart and Lung Transplant (ISHLT). This article addresses the concern for negative outcomes from the current trend toward using nonpulsatile LVAD. In the ISHLT database, 880 patients received pulsatile LVADs at the same time period that 417 patients received nonpulsatile LVADs as a bridge to transplant. A number of different devices were used at multiple transplant centers around the world, although Heartmate II was used most commonly. The demographic data, preoperative status, and overall post-transplant outcomes were also compared with patients who did not receive any LVAD before transplant. It is encouraging to find that the overall outcomes for all heart transplant patients who were bridged with LVAD have significantly improved. In the recent group of patients with the pulsatile LVAD, about 68% were not hospitalized before being placed on LVAD compared with only 37% before 2004. This likely reflects better understanding and management of patients before and after heart transplant. Of note, this data analysis shows the use of pulsatile or nonpulsatile LVAD as a bridge to heart transplant had equally good outcomes across multiple institutions worldwide. This is in contrast to prior data from 2000 to 2004, which showed an increased risk of mortality after transplant following BTT. BTT patients did have a higher rate of renal failure compared with non-LVAD transplant patients. One interesting finding was an increase level in allosensitization in pulsatile versus continuous-flow LVAD patients, although this was not associated with increase in rejection. Although allosensitization is thought to impact long-term survival, it is unclear based on this study if this is a clinically significant difference. This large registry review shows promising results for BTT, which would encourage more widespread use of LVAD, especially the newer-generation continuous flow LVADs.

S. R. Neravetla, MD

V. H. Thourani, MD

Mitral valve repair in heart failure: Five-year follow-up from the mitral valve replacement stratum of the Acorn randomized trial
Acker MA, Jessup M, Bolling SF, et al (Univ of Pennsylvania, Philadelphia; Univ of Michigan, Ann Arbor; et al)
J Thorac Cardiovasc Surg 142:569-574, 2011

Objective.—The study objective was to evaluate the long-term (5-year) safety and efficacy of mitral valve surgery with and without the CorCap cardiac support device (Acorn Cardiovascular, St Paul, Minn) in patients with dilated cardiomyopathy and New York Heart Association class II–IV heart failure.

Background.—The Acorn trial provided a unique opportunity to assess the long-term safety and efficacy of mitral valve surgery because clinical visits and echocardiograms (read by a core laboratory) were completed for 5 years of follow-up. Further, this study provided follow-up data on the long-term effect of the CorCap cardiac support device as an adjunct to mitral valve surgery.

Methods.—From the original Acorn trial (n = 300 patients), 193 patients were enrolled in the mitral valve repair/replacement stratum. A total of 102 were randomized to mitral valve surgery alone (control group) and 91 were randomized to mitral valve surgery with implantation of the CorCap cardiac support device (treatment group). Patients were followed up for 5 years.

Results.—As previously reported, 30-day operative mortality was only 1.6%. At 5 years, the total mortality was 30% with an average annual mortality rate of approximately 6% per year. The effects of mitral valve surgery led to a progressive decrease in left ventricular end-diastolic and end-systolic volumes, which were highly significant at all time points. At the end of 5 years, there was an average reduction in left ventricular end-diastolic volume of 75 mL, which represents a 28% reduction from baseline. During 5 years of follow-up, 29 patients had recurrent mitral regurgitation and 5 patients underwent repeat mitral valve surgery. The addition of the CorCap device led to greater decreases in left ventricular end-diastolic volume (average difference of 16.5 mL; $P = .05$), indicating that the CorCap device had an additive effect to the mitral valve operation.

Conclusions.—This study demonstrates long-term improvement in left ventricular structure and function after mitral valve surgery for up to 5 years. These data provide evidence supporting mitral valve repair in combination with the Acorn CorCap device for patients with nonischemic heart failure with severe left ventricular dysfunction who have been medically optimized yet remain symptomatic with significant mitral regurgitation.

▶ Heart failure and dilated cardiomyopathy secondary to mitral regurgitation (MR) is associated with a poor prognosis secondary to chronic volume overload leading to ventricular remodeling from conical to spherical shape progressively. This study examined the role of mitral valve (MV) surgery and the CorCap device and its role in improving ventricular structure and, ultimately, ventricular function. Patients were randomly assigned to MV surgery alone versus MV surgery plus CorCap device if they had a clinically significant MR and an indication for MV repair. The CorCap cardiac support device is a fabric mesh device that is implanted around the heart to theoretically decrease left ventricular (LV) wall stress. Eighty-four percent of patients underwent MV repair with ring, and approximately 16% underwent MV replacement. Both arms had progressive improvement in LV wall remodeling leading to decreased LV end diastolic volume (LVEDV) that continued to improve. This study shows that MV surgery not only improves LV remodeling but also decreases LVEDV. In addition to the significant improvement with MV surgery alone, CorCap further improves remodeling. The improvement in the sphericity index, a measure of remodeling, is further improved in the CorCap group compared with the MV surgery—alone group. Because the CorCap device adds further improvement with minimal increase in operating time, it should be considered as an adjunct in the treatment of cardiomyopathy. These results support the use of the CorCap device for patients with nonischemic heart failure secondary to severe LV dysfunction who have been medically optimized with improvement. With the advent of newer noninvasive techniques for the treatment of MR and heart failure, this device may add to the physician's armamentarium for treatment of concomitant MR and left ventricular dysfunction.

V. H. Thourani, MD

S. R. Neravetla, MD

Miscellaneous

Bypass Versus Drug-Eluting Stents at Three Years in SYNTAX Patients With Diabetes Mellitus or Metabolic Syndrome

Mack MJ, Banning AP, Serruys PW, et al (Heart Hosp Baylor Plano, Dallas, TX; John Radcliffe Hosp, Oxford, UK; Erasmus Univ Med Ctr Rotterdam, The Netherlands; et al)

Ann Thorac Surg 92:2140-2146, 2011

Background.—Diabetes mellitus increases adverse outcomes after coronary revascularization; however, the impact of metabolic syndrome is unclear. We examined the impact of diabetes and metabolic syndrome on coronary artery bypass graft surgery (CABG) and stenting outcomes to determine the optimal revascularization option for the treatment of complex coronary artery disease.

Methods.—Patients (n = 1,800) with left main or three-vessel disease or both were randomly allocated to treatment with a TAXUS Express^2 paclitaxel-eluting stent (PES) or CABG, and were included in predefined nondiabetic (n = 1,348) or diabetic subgroups (n = 452); 258 patients with diabetes also had metabolic syndrome.

Results.—Among diabetic patients, the 3-year major adverse cardiac and cerebrovascular event (MACCE) rate (22.9% CABG, 37.0% PES; $p =$ 0.002) and revascularization rate (12.9% CABG, 28.0% PES; $p < 0.001$) were higher after PES treatment. Diabetes increased MACCE rates among PES-treated patients, but had little impact on results after CABG. Compared with CABG, PES treatment yielded comparable MACCE in diabetic patients (30.5% versus 29.8%, $p = 0.98$) and nondiabetic patients (20.2% versus 20.3%, $p = 0.99$) with low Synergy Between Percutaneous Coronary Intervention With Taxus and Cardiac Surgery (SYNTAX) study scores of 22 or less. For patients with SYNTAX Scores of 33 or greater, MACCE rates were lower with CABG (18.5% versus 45.9%, $p < 0.001$ diabetic; 19.8% versus 30.0%, $p = 0.01$ nondiabetic). Metabolic syndrome did not significantly predict MACCE or repeat revascularization.

Conclusions.—These exploratory analyses suggest that among diabetic patients with complex left main or three-vessel disease, or both, 3-year MACCE is higher after PES compared with CABG. Although PES is a potential treatment option in patients with less complex lesions, CABG should be the revascularization option of choice for patients with more complex anatomic disease, especially with concurrent diabetes. Metabolic syndrome had little impact on 3-year outcomes.

▶ The World Health Organization definition of metabolic syndrome is the presence of diabetes and any 2 of the following: hypertension, central obesity (body mass index > 30 kg/m^2), dyslipidemia, or microalbuminuria. The impact of diabetes mellitus as a significant risk factor for cardiovascular disease and its deleterious effects following both coronary artery bypass grafting (CABG) and percutaneous coronary interventions (PCI) have been well documented and studied. However, the effects of metabolic syndrome in relation to coronary artery disease are still not fully understood. This interval analysis (3 years) of subgroups of the SYNTAX trial patients evaluates the outcomes of CABG versus paclitaxel drug-eluting stent (PES) in patients with or without diabetes and patients with metabolic syndrome. The goal of this study and the SYNTAX trial is to guide in the optimal strategy, CABG versus PES, for patients with cardiovascular disease in a prospective, randomized fashion. According to the results, diabetic patients had worse major adverse cardiac and cerebrovascular events (MACCE) and repeat revascularization rates following PES. In patients with less complex coronary artery disease, both with or without diabetes, PCI is a potential treatment option. However, CABG was shown to be the treatment of choice for patients with complex coronary disease and in patients with diabetes. This analysis failed to show a significant effect of metabolic syndrome in this set of patients in relation to MACCE or repeat revascularization. A limitation of this study was that it was a post-hoc analysis of patients with metabolic syndrome in the SYNTAX trial. Future studies need to be focused on the evaluation of metabolic syndrome and cardiovascular disease, specifically. The 5-year results and eventual completion of the SYNTAX trial will greatly help in the guidance of the best treatment options of patients with cardiovascular disease.

A. R. Khan, MD

V. H. Thourani, MD

Cardiac stem cells in patients with ischaemic cardiomyopathy (SCIPIO): initial results of a randomised phase 1 trial
Bolli R, Chugh AR, D'Amario D, et al (Univ of Louisville, KY; et al)
Lancet 378:1847-1857, 2011

Background.—c-kit-positive, lineage-negative cardiac stem cells (CSCs) improve post-infarction left ventricular (LV) dysfunction when administered to animals. We under took a phase 1 trial (Stem Cell Infusion in

Patients with Ischemic cardiOmyopathy [SCIPIO]) of autologous CSCs for the treatment of heart failure resulting from ischaemic heart disease.

Methods.—In stage A of the SCIPIO trial, patients with post-infarction LV dysfunction (ejection fraction [EF] ≤40%) before coronary artery bypass grafting were consecutively enrolled in the treatment and control groups. In stage B, patients were randomly assigned to the treatment or control group in a 2:3 ratio by use of a computer-generated block randomisation scheme. 1 million autologous CSCs were administered by intracoronary infusion at a mean of 113 days (SE 4) after surgery; controls were not given any treatment. Although the study was open label, the echocardiographic analyses were masked to group assignment. The primary endpoint was short-term safety of CSCs and the secondary endpoint was efficacy. A per-protocol analysis was used. This study is registered with ClinicalTrials.gov, number NCT00474461.

Findings.—This study is still in progress. 16 patients were assigned to the treatment group and seven to the control group; no CSC-related adverse effects were reported. In 14 CSC-treated patients who were analysed, LVEF increased from 30·3% (SE 1·9) before CSC infusion to 38·5% (2·8) at 4 months after infusion (p=0·001). By contrast, in seven control patients, during the corresponding time interval, LVEF did not change (30·1% [2·4] at 4 months after CABG *vs* 30·2% [2·5] at 8 months after CABG). Importantly, the salubrious effects of CSCs were even more pronounced at 1 year in eight patients (eg, LVEF increased by 12·3 ejection fraction units [2·1] *vs* baseline, p=0·0007). In the seven treated patients in whom cardiac MRI could be done, infarct size decreased from 32·6 g (6·3) by 7·8 g (1·7; 24%) at 4 months (p=0·004) and 9·8 g (3·5; 30%) at 1 year (p=0·04).

Interpretation.—These initial results in patients are very encouraging. They suggest that intracoronary infusion of autologous CSCs is effective in improving LV systolic function and reducing infarct size in patients with heart failure after myocardial infarction, and warrant further, larger, phase 2 studies.

▶ Heart failure is responsible for more morbidity and mortality compared with acute myocardial infarction (MI). Stem cell use for the treatment of heart failure is an area of great interest. This is one of the first adult human cardiac stem cell clinical trials using stem cells that normally reside in the adult heart. It is worthwhile to note that the investigators sought to treat chronic ischemic cardiomyopathy rather than acute MI. This phase 1 trial is ongoing, and some patients have been followed up for 1 year after stem cell infusion. The intervention was performed around 4 months after coronary artery bypass grafting (CABG) with the rationale that any LV function improvement due to CABG would have been seen by 4 months. Of surgical significance is the fact that intracoronary infusion does not require a thoracotomy like other methods of delivery. From a phase 1 safety standpoint, the results are promising, as adverse events and complications were minimal. Although this trial is not meant to assess efficacy, an increase in ejection fraction by 8.2 units 4 months after CABG—although higher than other trials—does not seem clinically significant. Further studies regarding the efficacy of stem cells are underway, and those results will need to be noted to determine the role of stem cells in the management of heart failure.

S. R. Neravetla, MD

V. H. Thourani, MD

Effect of Everolimus Introduction on Cardiac Allograft Vasculopathy—Results of a Randomized, Multicenter Trial

Arora S, Ueland T, Wennerblom B, et al (Oslo Univ Hosp, Norway; Sahlgrenska Univ Hosp, Gothenburg, Sweden; et al)

Transplantation 92:235-243, 2011

Background.—Everolimus reduces the progression of cardiac allograft vasculopathy (CAV) in de novo heart transplant (HTx) recipients, but the influence on established CAV is unknown.

Methods.—In this Nordic Certican Trial in Heart and lung Transplantation substudy, 111 maintenance HTx recipients (time post-HTx 5.8 ± 4.3 years) randomized to everolimus+reduced calcineurin inhibitor (CNI) or standard CNI had matching (intravascular ultrasound) examinations at baseline and 12 months allowing accurate assessment of CAV progression.

Results.—No significant difference in CAV progression was evident between the treatment groups ($P=0.30$). When considering patients receiving concomitant azathioprine (AZA) therapy (n=39), CAV progression was attenuated with everolimus versus standard CNI (Δmaximal intimal thickness 0.00 ± 0.04 and 0.04 ± 0.04 mm, Δpercent atheroma volume $0.2\% \pm 3.0\%$ and $2.6\% \pm 2.5\%$, and Δtotal atheroma volume 0.25 ± 14.1 and 19.8 ± 20.4 mm^3, respectively [$P<0.05$]). When considering patients receiving mycophenolate mofetil (MMF), accelerated CAV progression occurred with everolimus versus standard CNI (Δmaximal intimal thickness 0.06 ± 0.12 vs. 0.02 ± 0.06 mm and Δpercent atheroma volume $4.0\% \pm 6.3\%$ vs. $1.4\% \pm 3.1\%$, respectively; $P<0.05$). The levels of C-reactive protein and vascular cell adhesion molecule-1 declined significantly with AZA+everolimus, where as MMF+everolimus patients demonstrated a significant increase in levels of C-reactive protein, vascular cell adhesion molecule-1, and von Wille brand factor.

Conclusions.—Conversion to everolimus and reduced CNI does not influence CAV progression among maintenance HTx recipients. However, background immunosuppressive therapy is important as AZA+everolimus patients demonstrated attenuated CAV progression and a decline in inflammatory markers, whereas the opposite pattern was seen with everolimus+MMF. The different effect of everolimus when combined with AZA versus MMF could potentially reflect hitherto unknown interactions.

▶ Cardiac allograft vasculopathy (CAV) is the most common cause of death after heart transplant. Although proliferation signal inhibitors such as everolimus have been found to slow CAV progression in de novo heart transplants, its effectiveness in CAV prevention among maintenance heart transplant patients has not been demonstrated. This study found no difference in CAV progression between study arms. However, further analysis found reduced rate of CAV progression in everolimus with azathioprine (AZA) versus calcineurin inhibitor (CNI) plus AZA, whereas everolimus plus mycophenolate mofetil (MMF) was associated with increased rate of CAV compared with CNI plus MMF. Because both AZA and MMF are purine synthesis inhibitors, the reason for this paradoxical response remains unclear, and further studies are warranted. MMF has previously been found to be associated with lower rates of acute rejection and improved survival. Thus, the timing and interaction between everolimus and MMF should be further elucidated. These results indicate that everolimus should be started early for CAV prophylaxis and that late introduction of everolimus may lead to an undesired effect, especially when adding to MMF. Further study with patients also randomly assigned to AZA or MMF as background immunosuppresion is necessary to further examine this relationship.

V. H. Thourani, MD

S. R. Neravetla, MD

Transcatheter versus Surgical Aortic-Valve Replacement in High-Risk Patients
Smith CR, for the PARTNER Trial Investigators (Columbia Univ Med Ctr—New York Presbyterian Hosp; et al)
N Engl J Med 364:2187-2198, 2011

Background.—The use of transcatheter aortic-valve replacement has been shown to reduce mortality among high-risk patients with aortic stenosis who are not candidates for surgical replacement. However, the two procedures have not been compared in a randomized trial involving high-risk patients who are still candidates for surgical replacement.

Methods.—At 25 centers, we randomly assigned 699 high-risk patients with severe aortic stenosis to undergo either transcatheter aortic-valve replacement with a balloon-expandable bovine pericardial valve (either a transfemoral or a transapical approach) or surgical replacement. The primary end point was death from any cause at 1 year. The primary hypothesis was that transcatheter replacement is not inferior to surgical replacement.

Results.—The rates of death from any cause were 3.4% in the transcatheter group and 6.5% in the surgical group at 30 days (P = 0.07) and 24.2% and 26.8%, respectively, at 1 year (P = 0.44), a reduction of 2.6 percentage points in the transcatheter group (upper limit of the 95% confidence interval, 3.0 percentage points; predefined margin, 7.5 percentage points; P = 0.001 for noninferiority). The rates of major stroke were 3.8% in the transcatheter group and 2.1% in the surgical group at 30 days (P = 0.20) and 5.1% and 2.4%, respectively, at 1 year (P = 0.07). At 30 days, major vascular complications were significantly more frequent with transcatheter replacement (11.0% vs. 3.2%, P<0.001); adverse events that were more frequent after surgical replacement included major bleeding (9.3% vs. 19.5%, P<0.001) and new-onset atrial fibrillation (8.6% vs. 16.0%, P = 0.006). More patients undergoing transcatheter replacement had an improvement in symptoms at 30 days, but by 1 year, there was not a significant between-group difference.

Conclusions.—In high-risk patients with severe aortic stenosis, transcatheter and surgical procedures for aortic-valve replacement were associated with similar rates of survival at 1 year, although there were important differences in periprocedural risks.

▶ The treatment of aortic stenosis in patients considered at high risk for traditional surgical aortic valve replacement (AVR) has had a remarkable transformation over the last couple of years. As one of the high-volume early adopters of this technology at Emory University, I have seen firsthand the impact associated with this technology. In this article by Smith et al, a review of the results of these data from the randomized Placement of Aortic Transcatheter Valves (PARTNER) trial is presented. The PARTNER trial tested the hypothesis that transcatheter aortic valve replacement (TAVR, with transfemoral or transapical techniques) would be noninferior to surgical replacement in the 1-year survival of patients with severe aortic-valve stenosis and high operative risk. The high-risk nature was determined by the Predicted Risk of Mortality of the Society of Thoracic Surgeons database. Overall, perioperative rates of death were low for these patients. In the intention-to-treat population, 30-day mortality rate was 3.4% in the TAVR group and 6.5% in the surgical group (*P* = .07), and the 1-year overall mortality rate was 24.2% versus 26.8%, confirming noninferiority. However, TAVR did come at the price of increased serious vascular complications and increased hazards of embolic stroke and paravalvular leakage. It is feasible that the technical problems and imperfect seating of the SAPIEN valve may be eliminated with increased operator experience. Furthermore, newer, more flexible, and smaller delivery systems (XT device) should increase the number of patients who are eligible for transfemoral insertion and may decrease vascular injury. With regard to increased risk of stroke, it is plausible that embolic protection devices or other refinements in techniques, including anticoagulation and atrial fibrillation management, should decrease this complication.

Continued surveillance of patients in this study will be critically important to determine the durability of the prosthesis, to assess the risk of late thromboembolic events, and to monitor the effects of the paravalvular leaks. Database and registry, as proposed by the Society of Thoracic Surgeons and the American College of Cardiology Foundation, are a start in the right direction.

V. H. Thourani, MD

S. R. Neravetla, MD

4 Coronary Heart Disease

Acute ST-Segment Elevation Myocardial Infarction

30-Year Trends in Heart Failure in Patients Hospitalized With Acute Myocardial Infarction

McManus DD, Chinali M, Saczynski JS, et al (Univ of Massachusetts Med School, Worcester; et al)
Am J Cardiol 107:353-359, 2011

Despite significant advances in its treatment, acute myocardial infarction (AMI) remains an important cause of heart failure (HF). Contemporary data remain lacking, however, describing long-term trends in incidence rates, demographic and clinical profiles, and outcomes of patients who develop HF as a complication of AMI. Our study sample consisted of 11,061 residents of the Worcester (Massachusetts) metropolitan area hospitalized with AMI at all greater Worcester hospitals in 15 annual study periods from 1975 to 2005. Overall, 32.4% of patients (n = 3,582) with AMI developed new-onset HF during their acute hospitalization. Patients who developed HF were generally older, more likely to have pre-existing cardiovascular disease, and were less likely to receive cardiac medications or undergo revascularization procedures during their hospitalization than patients who did not develop HF (p <0.001). Incidence rates of HF remained relatively stable from 1975 to 1991 at 26% but decreased thereafter. Decreases were also noted in hospital and 30-day death rates in patients with acute HF (p <0.001). However, patients who developed new-onset HF remained at significantly higher risk for dying during their hospitalization (21.6%) than patients who did not develop this complication (8.3%, p <0.001). Our large community-based study of patients hospitalized with AMI demonstrates that incidence rates of and mortality attributable to HF have decreased over the previous 3 decades. In conclusion, HF remains a common and frequently fatal complication of AMI to which increased surveillance and treatment efforts should be directed (Fig 1).

▶ It has been suggested that one of the unwanted benefits of reducing the acute mortality of myocardial infarction in the reperfusion era would be an

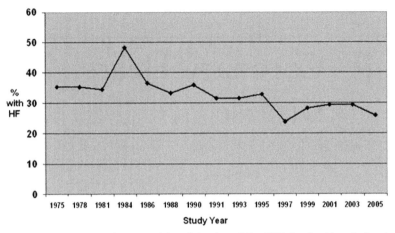

FIGURE 1.—Percentages of patients with heart failure from 1975 to 2005. (Reprinted from the American Journal of Cardiology, McManus DD, Chinali M, Saczynski JS, et al. 30-year trends in heart failure in patients hospitalized with acute myocardial infarction. *Am J Cardiol*. 2011;107:353-359. Copyright 2011, with permission from Elsevier.)

increase in late deaths caused by heart failure. The postulate is that patients with severe left ventricular function who previously would have died in the hospital now survive only to develop heart failure at a later date.

This analysis from the long-running Worcester (Massachusetts) Heart Attack Study provides more encouraging information. Although the incidence of heart failure during the initial hospitalization for myocardial infarction was high (32%), after being relatively stable between 1975 and 1991 the incidence decreased thereafter and was 25.8% in 2005. An age- and gender-adjusted model documented a quite striking reduction in the odds of developing heart failure and in comparison with 1975, the adjusted odds ratio of developing heart failure was 0.47 (0.37–0.60). What is also encouraging is that the mortality after developing heart failure has also declined over the last 3 decades, although it is still approximately 2.5 or greater than among patients without heart failure, and this is consistent with other studies.[1] Not surprisingly, the incidence of heart failure after revascularization procedures was significantly lower. This study, however, only answers the question in part because mortality is based on the initial hospitalization.

Nonetheless, a prior study from the Mayo Clinic using the Olmsted County database also reported an encouraging trend with a decline of 28% in incident heart failure after myocardial infarction between 1994 and 1979.[2] This study had a mean follow-up of approximately 7.5 years and also demonstrated a favorable impact of reperfusion therapy. These data also suggest that improved survival after myocardial infarction is unlikely to be a major contributor to the current epidemic of heart failure.

B. J. Gersh, MB, ChB, DPhil, FRCP

References

1. Hellermann JP, Jacobsen SJ, Gersh BJ, Rodeheffer RJ, Reeder GS, Roger VL. Heart failure after myocardial infarction: a review. *Am J Med.* 2002;113:324-330.
2. Hellermann JP, Goraya TY, Jacobsen SJ, et al. Incidence of heart failure after myocardial infarction: is it changing over time? *Am J Epidemiol.* 2003;157: 1101-1107.

Acute coronary syndrome and cocaine use: 8-year prevalence and inhospital outcomes
Carrillo X, Curós A, Muga R, et al (Hospital Universitari Germans Trias i Pujol, Badalona, Spain)
Eur Heart J 32:1244-1250, 2011

Aims.—The use of cocaine as a recreational drug has increased in recent years. The aims of this study were to analyse the prevalence and inhospital evolution of acute coronary syndrome (ACS) associated with cocaine consumption (ACS-ACC).

Methods and Results.—Prospective analysis of ACS patients admitted to a coronary care unit from January 2001 to December 2008. During the study period, 2752 patients were admitted for ACS, and among these 479 were ≤50 years of age. Fifty-six (11.7%) patients had a medical history of cocaine use with an increase in prevalence from 6.8% in 2001 to 21.7% in 2008 ($P = 0.035$). Among patients younger than 30 years of age, 25% admitted to being users compared with 5.5% of those aged 45−50 years ($P = 0.007$). Similarly, the prevalence of positive urine tests for cocaine was four times higher in the younger patients (18.2 vs. 4.1%, $P = 0.035$). Acute coronary syndrome associated with cocaine consumption patients ($n = 24$; those who had a positive urine test for cocaine or who admitted to being users upon admission) had larger myocardial infarcts as indicated by troponin I levels (52.9 vs. 23.4 ng/mL, $P < 0.001$), lower the left ventricular ejection fraction (44.5 vs. 52.2%, $P = 0.049$), and increased inhospital mortality (8.3 vs. 0.8%, $P = 0.030$).

Conclusions.—The association between cocaine use and ACS has increased significantly over the past few years. Young adults with ACS-ACC that require admission to the coronary care unit have greater myocardial damage and more frequent complications (Figs 1 and 2).

▶ This is an unusual study confined to patients younger than 50 years with acute coronary syndromes from the University Hospital in Barcelona. The authors analyze the prevalence of cocaine use in patients admitted with acute coronary syndromes and the impact of this on the natural history. Cocaine is said to cause more cardiovascular complications than any other illegal drug, including arterial hypertension, aortic dissection, arrhythmias, acute pulmonary edema, coronary vasospasm, cardiomyopathy, and sudden cardiac death.[1] An association between cocaine and acute coronary syndromes was first documented in the early 1980s and then in a large series in the 1990s.[2]

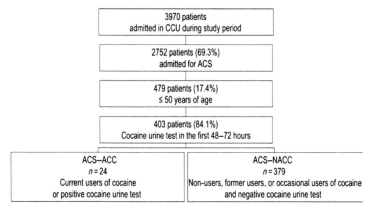

FIGURE 1.—Patients admitted to the coronary care unit between 1 January 2001 and 31 December 2008. ACS-ACC, acute coronary syndrome associated with cocaine consumption; ACS-NACC, acute coronary syndrome not associated with cocaine consumption. (Reprinted from Carrillo X, Curós A, Muga R, et al, Acute coronary syndrome and cocaine use: 8-year prevalence and inhospital outcomes. *Eur Heart J*. 2011;32:1244-1250, by permission of The European Society of Cardiology.)

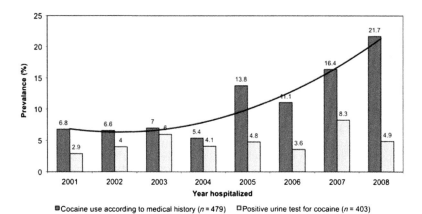

FIGURE 2.—Annual prevalence of cocaine use according to patient history and urine test for cocaine. (Reprinted from Carrillo X, Curós A, Muga R, et al, Acute coronary syndrome and cocaine use: 8-year prevalence and inhospital outcomes. *Eur Heart J*. 2011;32:1244-1250, by permission of The European Society of Cardiology.)

Among patients younger than 50 years 11.7% had a medical history of cocaine use. As expected, the prevalence of a history of cocaine use increased steadily between 2001 and 2008 from 6.8% to an alarming 21.7%. What is also notable but not surprising is the young age of the patients, and in patients under the age of 45 years, cocaine use ranged from 17.3% (age 40–44 years) to 25% in those younger than 30 years. Mortality and infarct size were greater in cocaine users, and left ventricular ejection fraction was lower. Moreover, the impact on mortality was huge (8.3% in cocaine users vs 0.8% among nonusers). The marked adverse prognosis is particularly disturbing given the young age of the patients. Interestingly, acute coronary syndromes occurred among both acute and chronic cocaine users, and the prevalence of 2- and 3-vessel disease was significantly higher among cocaine users.

The explanation for these adverse outcomes are multifactorial and might reflect a lack of prior beta blocker use, adrenergic hyperactivity secondary to cocaine leading to increased myocardial oxygen demands, and perhaps concomitant vasospasm or vasoconstriction. In addition, cocaine users had more Q-wave myocardial infarctions and a greater proportion of multivessel disease. These data certainly reinforce the need for a physician to take a specific medical history with regard to cocaine use and to use urine testing, particularly in younger patients with acute coronary syndromes. I suspect that these data also reinforce the need for beta blockers, and although there is no evidence to support this, there are data to suggest a hyperadronergic state in cocaine users, which might interfere with them.

B. J. Gersh, MB, ChB, DPhil, FRCP

References

1. Lange RA, Hillis LD. Cardiovascular complications of cocaine use. *New Engl J Med*. 2001;345:351-358.
2. Mittleman MA, Mintzer D, Maclure M, Tofler GH, Sherwood JB, Muller JE. Triggering of myocardial infarction by cocaine. *Circulation*. 1999;99:2737-2741.

Association Between Adoption of Evidence-Based Treatment and Survival for Patients With ST-Elevation Myocardial Infarction

Jernberg T, for SWEDEHEART/RIKS-HIA (Karolinska Univ Hosp, Stockholm, Sweden; et al)
JAMA 305:1677-1684, 2011

Context.—Only limited information is available on the speed of implementation of new evidence-based and guideline-recommended treatments and its association with survival in real life health care of patients with ST-elevation myocardial infarction (STEMI).

Objective.—To describe the adoption of new treatments and the related chances of short- and long-term survival in consecutive patients with STEMI in a single country over a 12-year period.

Design, Setting, and Participants.—The Register of Information and Knowledge about Swedish Heart Intensive Care Admission (RIKS-HIA) records baseline characteristics, treatments, and outcome of consecutive patients with acute coronary syndrome admitted to almost all hospitals in Sweden. This study includes 61 238 patients with a first-time diagnosis of STEMI between 1996 and 2007.

Main Outcome Measures.—Estimated and crude proportions of patients treated with different medications and invasive procedures and mortality over time.

Results.—Of evidence based-treatments, reperfusion increased from 66% (95%, confidence interval [CI], 52%-79%) to 79% (95% CI, 69%-89%; $P < .001$), primary percutaneous coronary intervention from 12% (95%

CI, 11%-14%) to 61% (95% CI, 45%-77%; $P < .001$), and revascularization from 10% (96% CI, 6%-14%) to 84% (95% CI, 73%-95%; $P < .001$). The use of aspirin, clopidogrel, β-blockers, statins, and angiotensin-converting enzyme (ACE) inhibitors all increased: clopidogrel from 0% to 82% (95% CI, 69%-95%; $P < .001$), statins from 23% (95% CI, 12%-33%) to 83% (95% CI, 75%-91%; $P < .001$), and ACE inhibitor or angiotensin II receptor blockers from 39% (95% CI, 26%-52%) to 69% (95% CI, 58%-70%; $P < .001$). The estimated in-hospital, 30-day and 1-year mortality decreased from 12.5% (95% CI, 4.3%-20.6%) to 7.2% (95% CI, 1.7%-12.6%; $P < .001$); from 15.0% (95% CI, 6.2%-23.7%) to 8.6% (95% CI, 2.7%-14.5%; $P < .001$); and from 21.0% (95% CI, 11.0%-30.9%) to 13.3% (95% CI, 6.0%-20.4%; $P < .001$), respectively. After adjustment, there was still a consistent trend with lower standardized mortality over the years. The 12-year survival analyses showed that the decrease of mortality was sustained over time.

Conclusion.—In a Swedish registry of patients with STEMI, between 1996 and 2007, there was an increase in the prevalence of evidence-based treatments. During this same time, there was a decrease in 30-day and 1-year mortality that was sustained during long-term follow-up.

▶ The results of this national registry from Sweden, which includes all 72 hospitals that provide care for patients with acute cardiac diseases, are indeed gratifying. This analysis was confined to the 61 238 patients with ST-elevation myocardial infarction (STEMI), and the strength of the study is the inclusion of every STEMI patient in the whole of Sweden for 10 years and the fact that most patients were included for an additional 2 years. This virtually eliminates selection bias; follow-up was also complete.

Over the last 12 years there has been a steady increase in the use of evidence-based pharmacologic therapies, an increase in the proportion of patients receiving reperfusion therapy, and a marked switch from fibrinolysis to primary percutaneous coronary intervention. At the same time, there has been a marked reduction in both early and late mortality, and it would appear that this trend is continuing. This appears to be a great example of translating the results of clinical trials into evidence-based clinical practice.

Notably, however, there was a wide variation between hospitals as to how quickly new therapies based on guidelines and evidence were implemented into the clinical protocols, and in many centers the adoption of these treatments was slow and gradual. This is one area amenable to a quality improvement initiative that apparently is already an ongoing process in Sweden.

An accompanying editorial does point out that data do not definitively confirm a cause-and-effect relationship between new therapies and the decline in mortality.[1] Nonetheless, the results certainly suggest a strong association and at a minimum confirm that guideline-based treatment works. What is also encouraging is to see the efficacy outcomes of clinical trials reflected in clinical practice.

B. J. Gersh, MB, ChB, DPhil, FRCP

Reference

1. Mukherjee D. Implementation of evidence-based therapies for myocardial infarction and survival. *JAMA*. 2011;305:1710-1711.

Association of Door-In to Door-Out Time With Reperfusion Delays and Outcomes Among Patients Transferred for Primary Percutaneous Coronary Intervention

Wang TY, Nallamothu BK, Krumholz HM, et al (Duke Univ Med Ctr, Durham, NC; Univ of Michigan Med School, Ann Arbor; Yale Univ School of Medicine and Yale—New Haven Hosp Ctr for Outcomes Res and Evaluation, CT; et al)
JAMA 305:2540-2547, 2011

Context.—Patients with ST-elevation myocardial infarction (STEMI) requiring interhospital transfer for primary percutaneous coronary intervention (PCI) often have prolonged overall door-to-balloon (DTB) times from first hospital presentation to second hospital PCI. Door-in to door-out (DIDO) time, defined as the duration of time from arrival to discharge at the first or STEMI referral hospital, is a new clinical performance measure, and a DIDO time of 30 minutes or less is recommended to expedite reperfusion care.

Objective.—To characterize time to reperfusion and patient outcomes associated with a DIDO time of 30 minutes or less.

Design, Setting, and Patients.—Retrospective cohort of 14 821 patients with STEMI transferred to 298 STEMI receiving centers for primary PCI in the ACTION Registry—Get With the Guidelines between January 2007 and March 2010.

Main Outcome Measures.—Factors associated with a DIDO time greater than 30 minutes, overall DTB times, and risk-adjusted in-hospital mortality.

Results.—Median DIDO time was 68 minutes (interquartile range, 43-120 minutes), and only 1627 patients (11%) had DIDO times of 30 minutes or less. Significant factors associated with a DIDO time greater than 30 minutes included older age, female sex, off-hours presentation, and non—emergency medical services transport to the first hospital. Patients with a DIDO time of 30 minutes or less were significantly more likely to have an overall DTB time of 90 minutes or less compared with patients with DIDO times greater than 30 minutes (60% [95% confidence interval {CI}, 57%-62%] vs 13% [95% CI, 12%-13%]; $P < .001$). Among patients with DIDO times greater than 30 minutes, only 0.6% (95% CI, 0.5%-0.8%) had an absolute contraindication to fibrinolysis. Observed in-hospital mortality was significantly higher among patients with DIDO times greater than 30 minutes vs patients with DIDO times of 30 minutes or less (5.9% [95% CI, 5.5%-6.3%] vs 2.7% [95% CI, 1.9%-3.5%]; $P < .001$; adjusted odds ratio for in-hospital mortality, 1.56 [95% CI, 1.15-2.12]).

Conclusion.—A DIDO time of 30 minutes or less was observed in only a small proportion of patients transferred for primary PCI but was associated with shorter reperfusion delays and lower in-hospital mortality.

▶ It is generally accepted that primary percutaneous coronary intervention (PPCI) is the optimal method of reperfusion therapy, but 75% of US hospitals do not have acute PCI capability and, as such, need to transfer patients to a PCI center when logistically feasible. The processes involved in transfer are a potential Achilles heel, and several studies have documented substantial delays both in patients receiving lytics and in those transferred directly for PPCI.[1] Moreover, these delays have been associated with worse outcomes, although it is unclear whether this is directly a time-related phenomenon or a reflection of the overall standard of care.

The door-in to door-out (DIDO) measure is increasingly being recognized as an important metric that places the burden of responsibility on both the transferring and receiving hospitals. This large study makes several important points. First, only 11% of patients had DIDO times of 30 minutes or less, and factors associated with longer times were older age, female sex, off-hours presentation, and nonemergency medical services transportation to the first hospital. Moreover, a DIDO time of less than 30 minutes was associated with an overall door-to-balloon time of 90 minutes or less (the guideline recommendation for PPCI without preceding lytics). In addition, there was a statistically significant reduction in risk-adjusted in-hospital mortality in patients with a DIDO of 30 minutes or less versus greater than 30 minutes (2.7% vs 5.9% $P > .001$).

These data suggest that DIDO is important as a metric for assessing the quality of reperfusion therapy, and the data really do also show that there is ample room for improvement. We have done well in shortening door-to-balloon times, but the major advances in the delivery of reperfusion therapy will come from steps taken outside the PCI-capable hospital.

B. J. Gersh, MB, ChB, DPhil, FRCP

Reference

1. McMullan JT, Hinckley W, Bentley J, et al. Reperfusion is delayed beyond guideline recommendations in patients requiring interhospital helicopter transfer for treatment of ST-segment elevation myocardial infarction. *Ann Emerg Med.* 2011;57:213-220.

Association of Mortality With Years of Education in Patients With ST-Segment Elevation Myocardial Infarction Treated With Fibrinolysis
Mehta RH, O'Shea JC, Stebbins AL, et al (Duke Clinical Res Inst and Duke Univ Med Ctr, Durham, NC; Bon Secours Hosp, Cork, Ireland; et al)
J Am Coll Cardiol 57:138-146, 2011

Objectives.—The purpose of this study was to examine the association between lower socioeconomic status (SES), as ascertained by years of education, and outcomes in patients with acute ST-segment elevation myocardial infarction (STEMI).

Background.—Previous studies have shown an inverse relationship between SES and coronary heart disease and mortality. Whether a similar association between SES and mortality exists in STEMI patients is unknown.

Methods.—We evaluated 11,326 patients with STEMI in the GUSTO-III (Global Use of Strategies to Open Occluded Coronary Arteries) trial study from countries that enrolled >500 patients. We evaluated clinical outcomes (adjusted using multivariate regression analysis) according to the number of years of education completed.

Results.—One-year mortality was inversely related to years of education and was 5-fold higher in patients with <8 years compared with those with >16 years of education (17.5% vs. 3.5%, p < 0.0001). The strength of the relationship between education and mortality varied among different countries. Nonetheless, years of education remained an independent correlate of mortality at day 7 (hazard ratio per year of increase in education: 0.86; 95% confidence interval: 0.83 to 0.88) and also between day 8 and 1 year (hazard ratio per year of increase in education: 0.96; 95% confidence interval: 0.94 to 0.98), even after adjustment for baseline characteristics and country of enrollment.

Conclusions.—When the number of years of education was used as a measure of SES, there was an inverse relationship such that significantly higher short-term and 1-year mortality existed beyond that accounted for by baseline clinical variables and country of enrollment. Future studies should account for and investigate the mechanisms underlying this link between SES and cardiovascular disease outcomes (Fig 2).

▶ This analysis from a large randomized, controlled trial of reperfusion therapy quite dramatically illustrates the impact of the socioeconomic gradient on outcomes in patients with cardiovascular disease. Impact of socioeconomic status is reflected in differences in coronary heart disease mortality between wealthier and underdeveloped countries[1] in addition to studies linking social class to the risk of myocardial infarction in single countries or regions.[2]

In this study, years of education are used as a good surrogate of socioeconomic status in approximately 11 000 patients with ST-elevation myocardial infarction. The results are quite emphatic and demonstrate a strong inverse association between mortality and years of education, and this is actually 5-fold greater in patients with less than 8 years of education compared with those with 16 years or more of education. The strength of the association varied among countries, but years of education nonetheless remained independently predictive of both early mortality at day 7 and 1-year mortality.

The explanations are multifactorial and are probably in part related to a greater proportion of risk factors and other adverse demographic variables in patients with a low level of education. Nonetheless, the independent predictive power of years of education is somewhat surprising but consistent with other studies performed 20 to 30 years ago.[3]

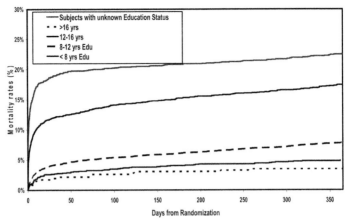

FIGURE 2.—Relationship of Years of Education With 1-Year Mortality. Note the significantly early hazard in those with education <8 years as well as in those with information on years of education missing. (Reprinted from the Journal of the American College of Cardiology, Mehta RH, O'Shea JC, Stebbins AL, et al. Association of mortality with years of education in patients with ST-segment elevation myocardial infarction treated with fibrinolysis. *J Am Coll Cardiol*. 2011;57:138-146. Copyright 2011, with permission from the American College of Cardiology.)

Other potential explanations are discussed by the authors, including longer times to treatment, lower subsequent revascularization rates, and other variables that were not collected in this study including life stresses, social isolation, lack of insurance, difficulty in entering rehabilitation programs, and affordability of medications. All of these could be playing a role.

Either way, this is an important and fertile area for research focusing on the behavioral, social, psychological, and biological mediators that link socioeconomic status with cardiovascular disease and its outcomes.

B. J. Gersh, MB, ChB, DPhil, FRCP

References

1. Gersh BJ, Sliwa K, Mayosi BM, Yusuf S. Novel therapeutic concepts: the epidemic of cardiovascular disease in the developing world: global implications. *Eur Heart J*. 2010;31:642-648.
2. Wilhelmsen L, Rosengren A. Are there socio-economic differences in survival after acute myocardial infarction? *Eur Heart J*. 1996;17:1619-1623.
3. Ruberman W, Weinblatt E, Goldberg JD, Chaudhary BS. Psychosocial influences on mortality after myocardial infarction. *N Engl J Med*. 1984;311:552-559.

Composition of Coronary Thrombus in Acute Myocardial Infarction

Silvain J, Collet J-P, Nagaswami C, et al (Université Paris 6, France; Univ of Pennsylvania School of Medicine, Philadelphia)

J Am Coll Cardiol 57:1359-1367, 2011

Objectives.—We sought to analyze the composition of coronary thrombus in vivo in ST-segment elevation myocardial infarction (STEMI) patients.

Background.—The dynamic process of intracoronary thrombus formation in STEMI patients is poorly understood.

Methods.—Intracoronary thrombi (n = 45) were obtained by thromboaspiration in 288 consecutive STEMI patients presenting for primary percutaneous intervention, and analyzed using high-definition pictures taken with a scanning electron microscope. Plasma biomarkers (TnI, CRPus, IL-6, PAI-1, sCD40 ligand, and TNF-α) and plasma fibrin clot viscoelastic properties were measured simultaneously on peripheral blood.

Results.—Thrombi were mainly composed of fibrin (55.9 ± 18%) with platelets (16.8 ± 18%), erythrocytes (11.5 ± 9%), cholesterol crystals (5.2 ± 8.4%), and leukocytes (1.3 ± 2.0%). The median ischemic time was 175 min (interquartile range: 140 to 297). Ischemic time impacted thrombi composition, resulting in a positive correlation with intracoronary thrombus fibrin content, r = 0.38, p = 0.01, and a negative correlation with platelet content, r = −0.34, p = 0.02. Thus, fibrin content increased with ischemic time, ranging from 48.4 ± 21% (<3 h) up to 66.9 ± 9% (>6 h) (p = 0.02), whereas platelet content decreased from 24.9 ± 23% (<3 h) to 9.1 ± 6% (>6 h) (p = 0.07). Soluble CD40 ligand was positively correlated to platelet content in the thrombus (r = 0.40, p = 0.02) and negatively correlated with fibrin content (r = −0.36; p = 0.04). Multivariate analysis indicated that ischemic time was the only predictor of thrombus composition, with a 2-fold increase of fibrin content per ischemic hour (adjusted odds ratio: 2.00 [95% confidence interval: 1.03 to 3.7]; p = 0.01).

Conclusions.—In acute STEMI, platelet and fibrin contents of the occlusive thrombus are highly dependent on ischemia time, which may have a direct impact on the efficacy of drugs or devices used for coronary reperfusion (Figs 5 and 6).

▶ This rather elegant study has taken advantage of the benefits of thromboaspiration and scanning electron microscopy to assess the dynamic process of thrombus formation in ST-segment elevation myocardial infarction in addition to the determinants of thrombus architecture, for example, the impact of coronary anatomy and reperfusion, ischemic time, patient characteristics, and biomarkers.

Fibrin accounted for about 60% of thrombus composition and other blood elements, including cholesterol crystals, approximately 40%. The greater the ischemic time the greater the amount of fibrin and the less the platelet content. Soluble CD40 ligand was correlated with platelet thrombus and negatively with fibrin content, but troponins only correlated with ischemic time. On multivariate analysis, ischemic time was the only independent determinant of thrombus composition.

This unique study shows the evolution of the thrombotic process and the constituents of thrombus (all of which are potential therapeutic targets) over time. Initially, thrombi are platelet rich, but this is rapidly stabilized by fibrin fibers with a decreasing proportion of platelets over time.[1] This has a clinical correlate as suggested by a study that found that thrombus composition was an independent predictor of mortality.[2] The data would also explain the declining success rates of fibrinolysis over time since early on the clot has a small and accessible amount of thrombin, and fibrinolysis has not yet been overcome by the intensive

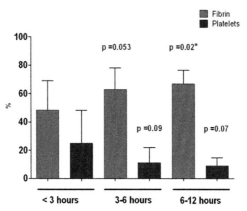

FIGURE 5.—Impact of Time on Thrombus Composition. The p values are given for comparison with the group <3 h as a reference with multiple Student *t* test. *p < 0.05. Multiple comparisons were done with the Dunnett's test, resulting in a p = 0.044 for fibrin and nonsignificant for platelet content. (Reprinted from the Journal of the American College of Cardiology, Silvain J, Collet J-P, Nagaswami C, et al. Composition of coronary thrombus in acute myocardial infarction. *J Am Coll Cardiol.* 2011;57:1359-1367. Copyright 2011, with permission from the American College of Cardiology.)

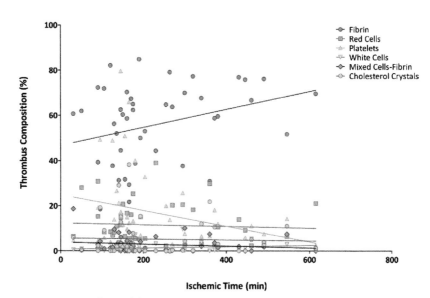

FIGURE 6.—Evolution of the Percentage Thrombus Composition for Each Component. The components in percentages (y-axis) are shown relative to ischemic times in minutes (x-axis). **Lines** represent linear regression for correlation with ischemic time. (Reprinted from the Journal of the American College of Cardiology, Silvain J, Collet J-P, Nagaswami C, et al. Composition of coronary thrombus in acute myocardial infarction. *J Am Coll Cardiol.* 2011;57:1359-1367. Copyright 2011, with permission from the American College of Cardiology.)

fibrin formation that occurs with stabilization and FXIII cross linking. These data also support other studies that show that the major benefit of GBIIb/IIIa inhibition is early in the course of the disease.[3] Limitations discussed by the authors include a surprisingly small number of erythrocytes with no change over time (this is perhaps outside the window of the study), the lack of collection of distal atherothrombotic debris, and damage to samples during aspiration.

Nonetheless, the study is valuable and an interesting addition to the literature.

B. J. Gersh, MB, ChB, DPhil, FRCP

References

1. Shand RA, Butler KD, Davies JA, Menys VC, Wallis RB. The kinetics of platelet and fibrin deposition on to damaged rabbit carotid arteries in vivo: involvement of platelets in the initial deposition of fibrin. *Thromb Res.* 1987;45:505-515.
2. Kramer MC, van der Wal AC, Koch KT, et al. Presence of older thrombus is an independent predictor of long-term mortality in patients with ST-elevation myocardial infarction treated with thrombus aspiration during primary percutaneous coronary intervention. *Circulation.* 2008;118:1810-1816.
3. Montalescot G, Antoniucci D, Kastrati A, et al. Abciximab in primary coronary stenting of ST-elevation myocardial infarction: a European meta-analysis on individual patients' data with long-term follow-up. *Eur Heart J.* 2007;28:443-449.

Causes of Delay and Associated Mortality in Patients Transferred With ST-Segment—Elevation Myocardial Infarction

Miedema MD, Newell MC, Duval S, et al (Minneapolis Heart Inst Foundation at Abbott Northwestern Hosp, MN)
Circulation 124:1636-1644, 2011

Background.—Regional ST-segment—elevation myocardial infarction systems are being developed to improve timely access to primary percutaneous coronary intervention (PCI). System delays may diminish the mortality benefit achieved with primary PCI in ST-segment—elevation myocardial infarction patients, but the specific reasons for and clinical impact of delays in patients transferred for PCI are unknown.

Methods and Results.—This was a prospective, observational study of 2034 patients transferred for primary PCI at a single center as part of a regional ST-segment—elevation myocardial infarction system from March 2003 to December 2009. Despite long-distance transfers, 30.4% of patients (n=613) were treated in ≤90 minutes and 65.7% (n=1324) were treated in ≤120 minutes. Delays occurred most frequently at the referral hospital (64.0%, n=1298), followed by the PCI center (15.7%, n=317) and transport (12.6%, n=255). For the referral hospital, the most common reasons for delay were awaiting transport (26.4%, n=535) and emergency department delays (14.3%, n=289). Diagnostic dilemmas (median, 95.5 minutes; 25th and 75th percentiles, 72—127 minutes) and nondiagnostic initial ECGs (81 minutes; 64—110.5 minutes) led to delays of the greatest magnitude. Delays caused by cardiac arrest and/or cardiogenic shock had the highest in-hospital mortality (30.6%), in contrast with nondiagnostic initial ECGs, which, despite long treatment delays, did not affect mortality (0%). Significant variation in both the magnitude and clinical impact of delays also occurred during the transport and PCI center segments.

Conclusions.—Treatment delays occur even in efficient systems for ST-segment–elevation myocardial infarction care. The clinical impact of specific delays in interhospital transfer for PCI varies according to the cause of the delay.

▶ The major advances in reperfusion therapy are going to be made outside the referral hospital setting. The emphasis has swung away from the specific nature of reperfusion therapy to the efficacy of its delivery, and the key to this is the establishment of regional systems or networks.[1] In this respect, one size does not fit all, and networks need to be adaptable and flexible in regard to local factors, including resources, ambulance systems, distances, climate, and the numbers and characteristics of hospitals in the area.

This prospective observational study from the state of Minnesota draws attention to the causes of delay and their effects on mortality. Approximately two-thirds of the delays occurred at the referral hospital and not the percutaneous coronary intervention (PCI) center. The most common reasons for delays at the referral hospital were awaiting transport and delays in the emergency department and other areas, and what is important is that these are all areas that are amenable to improvement. There were also significant variations in the magnitude and clinical impact of delays occurring during transport and at the PCI center. At the latter, the greatest delay was due to a diagnostic dilemma with little impact on mortality, whereas delays incurred by cardiogenic shock had the highest mortality.

This very nicely done study demonstrates opportunities for improvement in an already efficient system. Ongoing auditing and continuous quality improvement are essential components of a successful network.

B. J. Gersh, MB, ChB, DPhil, FRCP

Reference

1. Jollis JG, Roettig ML, Aluko AO, et al; Reperfusion of Acute Myocardial Infarction in North Carolina Emergency Departments (RACE) Investigators. Implementation of a statewide system for coronary reperfusion for ST-segment elevation myocardial infarction. *JAMA.* 2007;298:2371-2380.

Effect of upstream clopidogrel treatment in patients with ST-segment elevation myocardial infarction undergoing primary percutaneous coronary intervention

Koul S, Smith JG, Scherstén F, et al (Lund Univ, Sweden; et al)
Eur Heart J 32:2989-2997, 2011

Aims.—Immediate treatment with a loading dose of clopidogrel at diagnosis of ST-segment elevation myocardial infarction (STEMI) is recommended by ESC/AHA/ACC guidelines in patients eligible for primary percutaneous coronary intervention (PCI). However, the evidence for this practice is scarce.

Methods and Results.—All patients who underwent PCI for STEMI in Sweden between 2003 and 2008 were identified from the national Swedish Coronary Angiography and Angioplasty Registry (SCAAR). Patients with concomitant warfarin treatment and patients not having received aspirin upstream were excluded, leaving 13 847 patients for the analysis. Groups were compared for death and myocardial infarction (MI) during 1-year of follow-up using Cox regression models with adjustment for differences

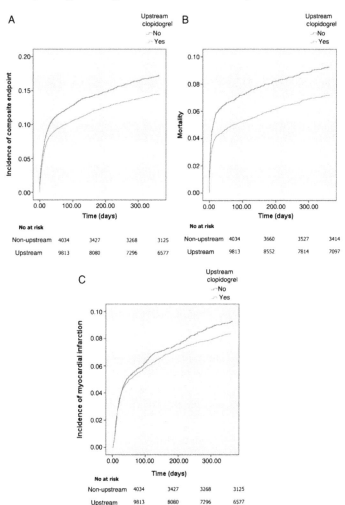

FIGURE 1.—Propensity score-adjusted incidence of (A) composite endpoint of death/myocardial infarction (B) mortality, and (C) myocardial infarction at 1 year. (Reprinted from Koul S, Smith JG, Scherstén F, et al. Effect of upstream clopidogrel treatment in patients with ST-segment elevation myocardial infarction undergoing primary percutaneous coronary intervention. *Eur Heart J.* 2011;32:2989-2997, by permission of The European Society of Cardiology.)

in baseline characteristics by propensity score methods. The combined primary endpoint of death or MI during 1-year follow-up occurred in 1325 of 9813 patients with upstream clopidogrel and in 364 out of 4034 patients without upstream treatment. After propensity score adjustment, a significant relative risk reduction (HR 0.82, 95% CI 0.73−0.93) in death/MI at 1-year was observed. The secondary endpoint of total 1-year death was significantly reduced (HR 0.76, 95% CI: 0.64−0.90), while the incidence of 1-year MI did not show any significant reduction (HR 0.90, 95% CI 0.77−1.06). Similar results were observed in multivariate analysis on top of propensity scoring and in sensitivity analyses excluding patients without clopidogrel and aspirin at discharge.

Conclusion.—This large observational study suggests that upstream clopidogrel treatment prior to arrival at the catheterization lab is associated with a reduction in the combined risk of death or MI as well as death alone in patients with STEMI treated with primary PCI (Fig 1).

▶ The role of clopidogrel in the management of acute coronary syndromes has been firmly established by the CURE trial of patients with non−ST-segment elevation myocardial infarction (STEMI) and in the COMMIT trial of patients with STEMI treated with fibrinolysis or primary PCI.[1] Current European Society of Cardiology guidelines recommend an immediate loading dose of clopidogrel at the time of diagnosis of STEMI but with a level of evidence C (consensus of expert opinion and/or small studies, retrospective studies).[2]

This large registry study from Sweden provides additional supportive evidence in favor of upstream clopidogrel in patients with STEMI. At 30 days and 1 year, multivariate analyses found a reduction in death and myocardial infarction. All observational studies have their limitations despite statistical methods of adjustment, and the loading dose of clopidogrel versus whether 300 or 600 mg is not known. Nonetheless, these data support a policy of administering clopidogrel as soon as possible after diagnosis. Of interest is the lack of effect on myocardial infarction in adjusted analyses, and it is possible that any effect on late myocardial infarction was diluted by the fact that all patients were discharged on similar doses of antiplatelet agents. In general, this and other studies show a trend toward a reduction in myocardial infarction with pretreatment clopidogrel, but achieving statistical significance has been difficult.

B. J. Gersh, MB, ChB, DPhil, FRCP

References

1. Sabatine MS, Cannon CP, Gibson CM, et al. Addition of clopidogrel to aspirin and fibrinolytic therapy for myocardial infarction with ST-segment elevation. *N Engl J Med.* 2005;352:1179-1189.
2. Van de Werf F, Bax J, Betriu A, et al; ESC Committee for Practice Guidelines (CPG). Management of acute myocardial infarction in patients presenting with persistent ST-segment elevation: the Task Force on the management of ST-Segment elevation acute myocardial infarction of the European Society of Cardiology. *Eur Heart J.* 2008;29:2909-2945.

Heparin plus a glycoprotein IIb/IIIa inhibitor versus bivalirudin monotherapy and paclitaxel-eluting stents versus bare-metal stents in acute myocardial infarction (HORIZONS-AMI): final 3-year results from a multicentre, randomised controlled trial
Stone GW, on behalf of the HORIZONS-AMI Trial Investigators (Columbia Univ Med Ctr and The Cardiovascular Res Foundation, NY; et al)
Lancet 377:2193-2204, 2011

Background.—Primary results of the HORIZONS-AMI trial have been previously reported. In this final report, we aimed to assess 3-year outcomes.

Method.—HORIZONS-AMI was a prospective, open-label, randomised trial undertaken at 123 institutions in 11 countries. Patients aged 18 years or older were eligible for enrolment if they had ST-segment elevation myocardial infarction (STEMI), presented within 12 h after onset of symptoms, and were undergoing primary percutaneous coronary intervention. By use of a computerised interactive voice response system, we randomly allocated patients 1:1 to receive bivalirudin or heparin plus a glycoprotein IIb/IIIa inhibitor (GPI; pharmacological randomisation; stratified by previous and expected drug use and study site) and, if eligible, randomly allocated 3:1 to receive a paclitaxel-eluting stent or a bare metal stent (stent randomisation; stratified by pharmacological group assignment, diabetes mellitus status, lesion length, and study site). We produced Kaplan-Meier estimates of major adverse cardiovascular events at 3 years by intention to treat. This study is registered with ClinicalTrials.gov, number NCT00433966.

Findings.—Compared with 1802 patients allocated to receive heparin plus a GPI, 1800 patients allocated to bivalirudin monotherapy had lower rates of all-cause mortality (5·9% *vs* 7·7%, difference −1·9% [−3·5 to −0·2], HR 0·75 [0·58−0·97]; $p = 0·03$), cardiac mortality (2·9% vs 5·1%, −2·2% [−3·5 to −0·9], 0·56 [0·40−0·80]; $p = 0·001$), reinfarction (6·2% *vs* 8·2%, −1·9% [−3·7 to −0·2], 0·76 [0·59−0·99]; $p = 0·04$), and major bleeding not related to bypass graft surgery (6·9% *vs* 10·5%, −3·6% [−5·5 to −1·7], 0·64 [0·51−0·80]; $p = 0·0001$) at 3 years, with no significant differences in ischaemia-driven target vessel revascularisation, stent thrombosis, or composite adverse events. Compared with 749 patients who received a bare-metal stent, 2257 patients who received a paclitaxel-eluting stent had lower rates of ischaemia-driven target lesion revascularisation (9·4% *vs* 15·1%, −5·7% [−8·6 to −2·7], 0·60 [0·48−0·76]; $p < 0·0001$) after 3 years, with no significant differences in the rates of death, reinfarction, stroke or stent thrombosis. Stent thrombosis was high (≥4·5%) in both groups.

Interpretation.—The effectiveness and safety of bivalirudin monotherapy and paclitaxel-eluting stenting are sustained at 3 years for patients with STEMI undergoing primary percutaneous coronary intervention.

▶ This is the 3-year follow-up of a large multicenter trial of patients with ST-segment elevation myocardial infarction (STEMI) randomly assigned to bare-metal versus drug-eluting stents and also to bivalirudin or the combination of heparin plus a glycoprotein IIb/IIIa inhibitor.

There are 2 interesting aspects of this trial. First, the trial essentially puts to rest previously expressed concerns about late outcomes with drug-eluting stents versus bare-metal stents.[1] Late stent thrombosis did not differ between the 2 groups but was quite high at 4% to 5%. The reduction in the need for ischemia-driven target revascularization was 5.7% less with paclitaxel-eluting stents, a finding that one would expect. Nonetheless, among patients not undergoing routine angiographic follow-up, the rates of revascularization were quite low in both groups, and this is perhaps a manifestation of the fact that stenotic lesions are supplying infracted myocardium and as such not causing symptoms. From a clinical perspective, however, these data are reassuring and support the use of bare-metal stents in patients undergoing primary percutaneous coronary intervention (PCI) in the presence of discrete, short lesions, and good distal vessels, particularly when one does not have the crucial information about compliance, ability to take long-term antiplatelet agents, and knowledge about the presence of comorbidities that might require noncardiac surgery. On the other hand, the relatively high rate of late stent thrombosis in both groups opens the window for additional improved antiplatelet medications.

Bivalirudin has in other studies been associated with less bleeding, and bleeding has been identified as a powerful independent predictor of subsequent mortality in patients with acute coronary syndromes and after PCI.[2] The mechanisms underlying this association are multifactorial and certainly complex.[3] To what extent the lower early and late mortality with bivalirudin in this trial is due to a reduction in major bleeding is uncertain. Moreover, the reduction in late mortality and reinfarction after the 30-day period is also difficult to explain since the half-life of the drug and duration of its administration is short lived. The limitations of the HORIZONS trial[4] have been previously discussed, but this is a landmark study that establishes the safety of drug-eluting stents in acute STEMI and raises intriguing questions in regard to the association between bivalirudin and a reduction in mortality.

B. J. Gersh, MB, ChB, DPhil, FRCP

References

1. Kaltoft A, Kelbaek H, Thuesen L, et al. Long-term outcome after drug-eluting versus bare-metal stent implantation in patients with ST-segment elevation myocardial infarction: 3-year follow-up of the randomized DEDICATION (Drug Elution and Distal Protection in Acute Myocardial Infarction) Trial. *J Am Coll Cardiol.* 2010;56:641-645.
2. Rao SV, Jollis JG, Harrington RA, et al. Relationship of blood transfusion in clinical outcomes in patients with acute coronary syndromes. *JAMA.* 2004;292:1555-1562.
3. Pocock SJ, Mehran R, Clayton TC, et al. Prognostic modeling of individual patient risk and mortality impact of ischemic and hemorrhagic complications: assessment from the Acute Catheterization and Urgent Intervention Triage Strategy trial. *Circulation.* 2010;121:43-51.
4. Stone GW, Witzenbichler B, Guagliumi G, et al. Bivalirudin during primary PCI in acute myocardial infarction. *N Engl J Med.* 2008;358:2218-2230.

Primary angioplasty vs. fibrinolysis in very old patients with acute myocardial infarction: TRIANA (TRatamiento del Infarto Agudo de miocardio eN Ancianos) randomized trial and pooled analysis with previous studies
Bueno H, on behalf of the TRIANA Investigators (Hospital General Universitario Gregorio Marañón, Madrid, Spain; et al)
Eur Heart J 32:51-60, 2011

Aims.—To compare primary percutaneous coronary intervention (pPCI) and fibrinolysis in very old patients with ST-segment elevation myocardial infarction (STEMI), in whom head-to-head comparisons between both strategies are scarce.
Methods and Results.—Patients ≥75 years old with STEMI <6 h were randomized to pPCI or fibrinolysis. The primary endpoint was a composite of all-cause mortality, re-infarction, or disabling stroke at 30 days. The trial was prematurely stopped due to slow recruitment after enroling 266 patients (134 allocated to pPCI and 132 to fibrinolysis). Both groups were well balanced in baseline characteristics. Mean age was 81 years. The primary endpoint was reached in 25 patients in the pPCI group (18.9%) and 34 (25.4%) in the fibrinolysis arm [odds ratio (OR), 0.69; 95% confidence interval (CI) 0.38−1.23; $P = 0.21$]. Similarly, non-significant reductions were found in death (13.6 vs. 17.2%, $P = 0.43$), re-infarction (5.3 vs. 8.2%, $P = 0.35$), or disabling stroke (0.8 vs. 3.0%, $P = 0.18$). Recurrent ischaemia was less common in pPCI-treated patients (0.8 vs. 9.7%, $P < 0.001$). No differences were found in major bleeds. A pooled analysis with the two previous reperfusion trials performed in older patients showed an advantage of pPCI over fibrinolysis in reducing death, re-infarction, or stroke at 30 days (OR, 0.64; 95% CI 0.45−0.91).
Conclusion.—Primary PCI seems to be the best reperfusion therapy for STEMI even for the oldest patients. Early contemporary fibrinolytic therapy may be a safe alternative to pPCI in the elderly when this is not available. Clinicaltrials.gov # NCT00257309 (Fig 4).

▶ It is generally and appropriately accepted, based on good evidence, that primary percutaneous coronary intervention (pPCI) is the preferred method of reperfusion therapy compared with thrombolysis. What has not been established is the amount of delay that is acceptable in regard to transferring a patient for pPCI versus prompt thrombolysis, and this is in part dependent on the duration of ischemia before therapy. Nonetheless, there is a paucity of data in patients of advanced age, the fastest growing population group in our society. Only 2 other small randomized controlled trials have compared pPCI versus thrombolysis.[1,2]

This trial from Spain (TRIANA) confined to patients aged 75 years and older encountered the same problems as the 2 other trials—namely, a difficulty in recruitment and that the trial was prematurely terminated on this account after enrolling 266 patients. Nonetheless, the results of this trial in addition to a meta-analysis including the other 2 trials does provide additional evidence that pPCI remains the preferred form of therapy in this age group (mean 81 years). This is not surprising given bleeding hazard in the elderly after

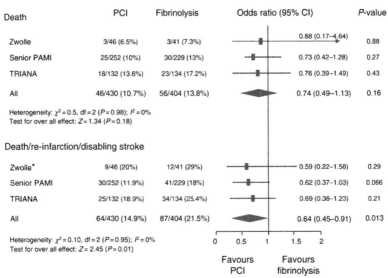

FIGURE 4.—Odd-ratios for mortality and the combined endpoint in the three randomized trials comparing primary percutaneous coronary intervention and fibrinolysis performed in very old patients with ST-segment elevation myocardial infarction. PCI, percutaneous coronary intervention. (Reprinted from Bueno H, on behalf of the TRIANA Investigators. Primary angioplasty vs. fibrinolysis in very old patients with acute myocardial infarction: TRIANA (TRatamiento del Infarto Agudo de miocardio eN Ancianos) randomized trial and pooled analysis with previous studies. *Eur Heart J.* 2011;32:51-60, by permission of The European Society of Cardiology.)

fibrinolytic therapy, especially among patients who are female, of low body mass, hypertensive, and with comorbidities. We should remember, however, that these characteristics also predict a higher risk of bleeding after pPCI.

The meta-analysis demonstrates a positive but nonsignificant trend in regard to death and a statistically significant benefit in regard to death, recurrent myocardial infarction, and disabling stroke. We probably will never get the definitive trial, and although it may be desirable from an evidence-based stand-point practically, it is extremely unlikely to happen.

Nonetheless, it appears that our preconceived perception that pPCI would be the best form of reperfusion therapy in patients of advanced age seems to be correct, and this conforms to current practice. In the event that pPCI is unavailable or delays in transfer are successive, we should still remember, however, that the prior trials of fibrinolytic therapy demonstrated a greater benefit in absolute terms over lytic therapy in the elderly.[3] The risk of bleeding is undoubtedly increased, but risk of no reperfusion therapy is much greater.

B. J. Gersh, MB, ChB, DPhil, FRCP

References

1. de Boer MJ, Ottervanger JP, van't Hof AW, et al; Zwolle Myocardial Infarction Study Group. Reperfusion therapy in elderly patients with acute myocardial infarction: a randomized comparison of primary angioplasty and thrombolytic therapy. *J Am Coll Cardiol.* 2002;39:1723-1728.

2. Senior PAMI. Primary PCI not better than lytic therapy in elderly patients. http://www.theheart.org/article/581549.do. Accessed May 14, 2010.
3. White HD. Thrombolytic therapy in the elderly. *Lancet.* 2000;356:2028-2030.

Randomized Comparison of Pre-Hospital—Initiated Facilitated Percutaneous Coronary Intervention Versus Primary Percutaneous Coronary Intervention in Acute Myocardial Infarction Very Early After Symptom Onset: The LIPSIA-STEMI Trial (Leipzig Immediate Prehospital Facilitated Angioplasty in ST-Segment Myocardial Infarction)

Thiele H, for the LIPSIA-STEMI Trial Group (Univ of Leipzig—Heart Ctr, Germany; et al)
JACC Cardiovasc Interv 4:605-614, 2011

Objectives.—This multicenter trial sought to assess the merits of facilitated percutaneous coronary intervention (PCI) versus primary PCI in an ST-segment elevation myocardial infarction (STEMI) network with long transfer distances in patients presenting early after symptom onset.

Background.—Facilitated PCI with fibrinolysis might be beneficial in specific high-risk STEMI situations to prevent myocardial necrosis expansion.

Methods.—Patients with STEMI (<3 h after symptom onset) were randomized to either pre-hospital—initiated facilitated PCI using tenecteplase (Group A; n = 81) or primary PCI (Group B; n = 81) plus optimal antithrombotic comedication. The primary endpoint was infarct size assessed by delayed-enhancement magnetic resonance imaging. Secondary endpoints were microvascular obstruction and myocardial salvage, early ST-segment resolution, and a composite of death, repeated myocardial infarctions, and congestive heart failure within 30 days.

Results.—The median time from symptom onset to randomization was 64 min (interquartile range [IQR]: 42 to 103 min) in Group A versus 55 min in Group B (IQR: 27 to 91 min; p = 0.26). Despite better pre-interventional TIMI (Thrombolysis In Myocardial Infarction) flow in Group A (71% vs. 35% TIMI flow grade 2 or 3; p < 0.001), the infarct size tended to be worse in Group A versus Group B (17.9% of left ventricle [IQR: 8.4% to 35.0%] vs. 13.7% [IQR: 7.5% to 24.0%]; p = 0.10). There was also a strong trend toward more early and late microvascular obstruction, (p = 0.06 and 0.09) and no difference in ST-segment resolution (p = 0.26). The combined clinical endpoint showed a trend toward higher event rates in Group A (19.8% vs. 13.6%; p = 0.13, relative risk: 0.52, 95% confidence interval: 0.23 to 1.18).

Conclusions.—In STEMI patients presenting early after symptom onset with relatively long transfer times, a fibrinolytic-based facilitated PCI approach with optimal antiplatelet comedication does not offer a benefit over primary PCI with respect to infarct size and tissue perfusion.

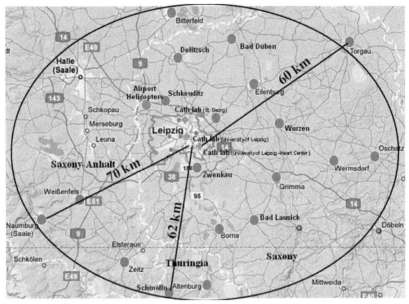

FIGURE 1.—The LIPSIA-STEMI network. Locations of the 24 mobile intensive care units (most of them with affiliated hospitals) are displayed with red dots, location of helicopters with green dot, and the 3 catheterization laboratories with blue crosses. LIPSIA-STEMI = Leipzig Immediate Prehospital Facilitated Angioplasty in ST-Segment Myocardial Infarction. For interpretation of the references to color in this figure legend, the reader is referred to web version of this article. (Reprinted from JAAC, Cardiovascular Interventions, Thiele H, for the LIPSIA-STEMI Trial Group. Randomized comparison of pre-hospital–initiated facilitated percutaneous coronary intervention versus primary percutaneous coronary intervention in acute myocardial infarction very early after symptom onset: the LIPSIA-STEMI Trial (Leipzig Immediate Prehospital Facilitated Angioplasty in ST-Segment Myocardial Infarction). *JACC Cardiovasc Interv.* 2011;4:605-614. Copyright 2011, with permission of Elsevier.)

([LIPSIA-STEMI] The Leipzig Immediate Prehospital Facilitated Angioplasty in ST-Segment Myocardial Infarction; NCT00359918) (Fig 1, Table 2).

▶ Facilitated percutaneous coronary intervention (PCI) is a logical concept in that fibrinolytics are given to restore patency during lengthy transfers from an outside hospital to a catheterization laboratory for primary PCI. Nonetheless, 2 large trials, namely ASSENT 4 and FINESSE, demonstrated no benefit on outcomes, and in ASSENT 4 the trend was in the wrong direction for facilitated PCI. Currently, the guidelines place facilitated PCI as a class 3 indication. There have been several proffered explanations for the negative results of what is intuitively an appealing strategy. These include design flaws in ASSENT 4, the possibility that very early routine PCI within 3 hours of receiving lytics may increase the risk of PCI-related complications, and the fact that fibrinolytic drugs may result in increased platelet aggregation.[1,2]

The current trial from Leipzig in Germany is well designed, and yet again the trend is in the wrong direction with increased infarct size and increased microvascular obstruction in the facilitated PCI group in addition to a trend toward more unfavorable events. Patients in this trial presented far earlier than those in the United States. It is interesting that in patients receiving prehospital lytic therapy,

TABLE 2.—MRI Results

Variable	Pre-Hospital Facilitated PCI (n = 69)	Primary PCI (n = 70)	p Value
LV ejection fraction, %	57.4 (49.7–66.9)	60.3 (51.5–67.0)	0.72
LV end-diastolic volume, ml	125.1 (100.9–153.9)	115.4 (104.2–140.0)	0.31
LV end-systolic volume, ml	55.5 (33.8–72.3)	47.3 (35.4–63.8)	0.47
Area at risk	33.1 (24.4–48.7)	32.2 (19.9–41.1)	0.34
Infarct size, % LV	17.9 (8.4–35.0)	13.7 (7.5–24.0)	0.10
Early MO, % LV	3.4 (1.0–7.9)	1.9 (0.0–5.9)	0.06
Late MO, % LV	1.3 (0.5–6.1)	0.9 (0.0–3.9)	0.09
Myocardial salvage, % LV	13.5 (5.1–23.7)	15.3 (9.1–21.6)	0.35
Myocardial salvage index	42.9 (27.0–66.9)	48.9 (33.7–68.5)	0.11

Values are median (interquartile range).
LV = left ventricle; MO = microvascular obstruction; PCI = percutaneous coronary intervention.

times to PCI were slightly longer because of the time spent in initiating lytic therapy prior to transfer. It is not clear why the lytic drugs themselves could not be started in the ambulance during the process of transfer as opposed to the administration of a lytic in a mobile intensive care unit followed by transfer. Another feature of this trial is that the delays to primary PCI were much shorter than expected, and in this situation the benefits of facilitation are likely to be far less than in patients in whom distances and transfer times are much longer. Nonetheless, any benefit would still likely be noted in patients who present early after symptom onset as in this German trial. In the 2 previous large trials, the time from symptom onset to randomization was long, and by then the patients are on the flat part of the curve with little benefit from earlier reperfusion.[3] In this study, patients presented early, but transfer delays were short, and the estimated time to reperfusion with TNK was probably no shorter than with primary PCI.

Currently, the guidelines recommend the pharmaco-invasive strategy in which fibrinolytic therapy is given at non-PCI hospitals, particularly those in rural communities in which the distances to a PCI center are substantial. Fibrinolytic therapy is followed by transfer for routine angiography at 3 to 24 hours unless rescue PCI is required. Obviously, if primary PCI can be performed within 90 minutes of presentation, there is no need for fibrinolytic drugs. Conceivably, there is a place for facilitated PCI in some patients who present early but are faced with lengthy transfer delays, but I suspect that the pharmaco-invasive strategy will prevail over the long term.[4]

B. J. Gersh, MB, ChB, DPhil, FRCP

References

1. Gersh BJ, Stone GW, White HD, Holmes DR Jr. Pharmacological facilitation of primary percutaneous coronary intervention for acute myocardial infarction: is the slope of the curve the shape of the future? *JAMA*. 2005;293:979-986.
2. Stone GW, Gersh BJ. Facilitated angioplasty: paradise lost. *Lancet*. 2006;367: 543-546.
3. Gersh BJ, Stone GW. Pharmacological facilitation of coronary intervention in ST-segment elevation myocardial infarction: time is of the essence. *JACC Cardiovasc Interv*. 2010;3:1292-1294.
4. Brodie BR. Facilitated percutaneous coronary intervention still searching for the right patients. *JACC Cardiovasc Interv*. 2011;4:615-617.

Sex Differences in Patient-Reported Symptoms Associated With Myocardial Infarction (from the Population-Based MONICA/KORA Myocardial Infarction Registry)

Kirchberger I, Heier M, Kuch B, et al (Central Hosp of Augsburg, Germany)
Am J Cardiol 107:1585-1589, 2011

Many studies have examined gender-related differences in symptoms of acute myocardial infarction (AMI). However, findings have been inconsistent, largely because of different study populations and different methods of symptom assessment and data analysis. This study was based on 568 women and 1,710 men 25 to 74 years old hospitalized with a first-ever AMI from January 2001 through December 2006 recruited from a population-based AMI registry. Occurrence of 13 AMI symptoms was recorded using standardized patient interview. After controlling for age, migration status, body mass index, smoking, some co-morbidities including diabetes, and type and location of AMI through logistic regression modeling, women were significantly more likely to complain of pain in the left shoulder/arm/hand (odds ratio [OR] 1.36, 95% confidence interval [CI] 1.10 to 1.69), pain in the throat/jaw (OR 1.78, 95% CI 1.43 to 2.21), pain in the upper abdomen (OR 1.39, 95% CI 1.02 to 1.91), pain between the shoulder blades (OR 2.22, 95% CI 1.78 to 2.77), vomiting (OR 2.23, 95% CI 1.67 to 2.97), nausea (OR 1.94, 95% CI 1.56 to 2.39), dyspnea (OR 1.45, 95% CI 1.17 to 1.78), fear of death (OR 2.17, 95% CI 1.73 to 2.72), and dizziness (OR 1.49, 95% CI 1.16 to 1.91) than men. Furthermore, women were more likely to report >4 symptoms (OR 2.14, 95% CI 1.72 to 2.66). No significant gender differences were found in chest pain, feelings of pressure or tightness, diaphoresis, pain in the right

TABLE 2.—Frequency of Symptoms

	Women (n = 568)	Men (n = 1,710)	Total (n = 2,278)
Number of symptoms, mean ± SD*	5.33 ± 2.38	4.37 ± 2.13	4.61 ± 2.23
Chest pain or feelings of pressure or tightness	531 (93.5%)	1,609 (94.2%)	2,140 (94.0%)
Only chest symptoms	15 (2.6%)	86 (5.0%)	101 (4.4%)
Pain left shoulder/arm/hand*	344 (60.7%)	941 (55.0%)	1,285 (56.4%)
Pain right shoulder/arm/hand	188 (33.1%)	517 (30.2%)	705 (31.0%)
Pain throat/jaw‡	226 (39.9%)	472 (27.6%)	698 (30.7%)
Pain upper abdomen*	76 (13.4%)	173 (10.1%)	249 (10.9%)
Pain between shoulder blades‡	227 (40.0%)	383 (22.4%)	610 (26.8%)
Vomiting‡	114 (20.1%)	183 (10.7%)	297 (13.0%)
Nausea‡	269 (47.4%)	549 (32.1%)	818 (35.9%)
Dyspnea‡	320 (56.3%)	787 (46.0%)	1,107 (48.6%)
Diaphoresis	335 (59.0%)	1,048 (61.3%)	1,383 (60.7%)
Fear of death‡	218 (38.4%)	402 (23.5%)	620 (27.2%)
Dizziness†	140 (24.7%)	332 (19.4%)	472 (20.7%)
Syncope	38 (6.7%)	83 (4.9%)	121 (5.3%)

*p <0.05.
†p <0.01.
‡p <0.001.

shoulder/arm/hand, and syncope. In conclusion, women and men did not differ regarding the chief AMI symptoms of chest pain or feelings of tightness or pressure and diaphoresis. However, women were more likely to have additional symptoms (Table 2).

▶ The data for this study were collected as part of the World Health Organization Monitoring Trends and Determinants in Cardiovascular Disease (MONICA) project, a population-based registry implemented in 1984. Subsequently, the registry was incorporated into the Cooperative Health Research Registry in the region of Augsburg, Germany.[1]

This study was based on 568 women and 1710 men aged 25 to 74 years from 2001 to 2006 with a diagnosis of an incident myocardial infarction. The most common reported symptoms were chest pain or feelings of pressure or tightness for both women (93.5%) and men (94.2%). After controlling for age, migration status, body mass index, smoking, and comorbidities including diabetes, and type and location of myocardial infarction, women were significantly more likely to complain of pain in the left shoulder, arm, or hand; pain in the throat or jaw, upper abdomen or between the shoulder blades; nausea, vomiting, and dyspnea; and fear of death. It would appear, therefore, that there are no gender differences in regard to the major symptoms of chest pain/pressure or diaphoresis, but women are much more likely to complain of additional symptoms, and the odds ratio for 4 or more symptoms was more than doubled in women.

A limitation of the study includes a lack of information on patients who were too ill to be interviewed or who died within 24 hours. In addition, the delay in interviews (on average 6 days after admission) may have introduced an element of recall bias. Furthermore, the age cutoff of 74 years is another limitation because it is well documented that the older the patient, the greater the frequency of atypical symptoms. What we also need to bear in mind is that clinically unrecognized myocardial infarction or "silent" myocardial infarction remains disturbingly common among the elderly and in the cardiovascular health study of individuals aged 65 years or older, 22.3% of myocardial infarctions were clinically unrecognized.[2]

B. J. Gersh, MB, ChB, DPhil, FRCP

References

1. Kuch B, von Scheidt W, Kling B, Heier M, Hoermann A, Meisinger C. Characteristics and outcome of patients with acute myocardial infarction according to presenting electrocardiogram (from the MONICA/KORA Augsburg Myocardial Infarction—Registry). *Am J Cardiol.* 2007;100:1056-1060.
2. Scheifer SE, Gersh BJ, Yanez ND 3rd, Ades PA, Burke GL, Manolio TA. Prevalence, predisposing factors, and prognosis of clinically unrecognized myocardial infarction in the elderly. *J Am Coll Cardiol.* 2000;35:119-126.

The Occluded Artery Trial (OAT) Viability Ancillary Study (OAT-NUC): Influence of infarct zone viability on left ventricular remodeling after percutaneous coronary intervention versus optimal medical therapy alone

Udelson JE, Pearte CA, Kimmelstiel CD, et al (Tufts Med Ctr, Boston, MA; New York Univ School of Medicine; et al)
Am Heart J 161:611-621, 2011

Background.—The Occluded Artery Trial (OAT) showed no difference in outcomes between percutaneous coronary intervention (PCI) versus optimal medical therapy (MED) in patients with persistent total occlusion of the infarct-related artery 3 to 28 days post–myocardial infarction. Whether PCI may benefit a subset of patients with preservation of infarct zone (IZ) viability is unknown.

Methods and Results.—The OAT nuclear ancillary study hypothesized that (1) IZ viability influences left ventricular (LV) remodeling and that (2) PCI as compared with MED attenuates adverse remodeling in post–myocardial infarction patients with preserved viability. Enrolled were 124 OAT patients who underwent resting nitroglycerin-enhanced technetium-99m sestamibi single-photon emission computed tomography (SPECT) before OAT randomization, with repeat imaging at 1 year. All images were quantitatively analyzed for infarct size, IZ viability, LV volumes, and function in a core laboratory. At baseline, mean infarct size was 26% ± 18 of the LV, mean IZ viability was 43% ± 8 of peak uptake, and most patients (70%) had at least moderately retained IZ viability. There were no significant differences in 1-year end-diastolic or end-systolic volume change between those with severely reduced versus moderately retained IZ viability, or when compared by treatment assignment PCI versus MED. In multivariable models, increasing baseline viability independently predicted improvement in ejection fraction ($P = .005$). There was no interaction between IZ viability and treatment assignment for any measure of LV remodeling.

Conclusions.—In the contemporary era of MED, PCI of the infarct-related artery compared with MED alone does not impact LV remodeling irrespective of IZ viability (Fig 4).

▶ Despite evidence from many sources suggesting that the open-artery concept was alive and well, the Open-Artery Trial (OAT) quite emphatically demonstrated no benefit to opening a totally occluded infarct-related artery 3 to 28 days post–myocardial infarction in stable patients.[1] Prior studies also suggested that preservation of myocardial viability within the infarct zone would attenuate left ventricular remodeling postinfarction and that this benefit could be potentiated by revascularization.[2] The aims of the OAT Nuclear Viability Ancillary Study were to look at the impact of viability on remodeling and to assess the effects of revascularization versus medical therapy on ventricular remodeling in patients with and without preserved viability. It should be emphasized that all patients had occluded coronary arteries at the time of the baseline angiography and were stable.

The study was completely neutral but limited by its small size—only 124 patients. There were no differences over 1 year in changes in volumes between

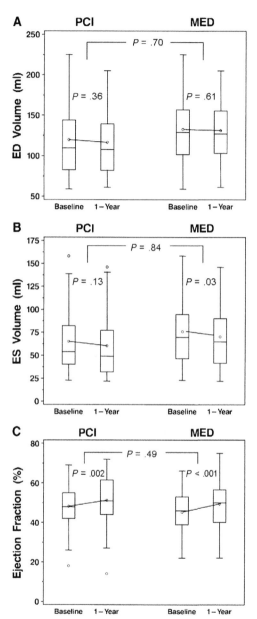

FIGURE 4.—One-year changes in end-diastolic (ED) and end-systolic (ES) volumes and EF, in patients who were randomized to the OAT PCI strategy compared with those randomized to MED. There were no significant between-group changes in any of the parameters. (Reprinted from the American Heart Journal, Udelson JE, Pearte CA, Kimmelstiel CD, et al. The Occluded Artery Trial (OAT) Viability Ancillary Study (OAT-NUC): influence of infarct zone viability on left ventricular remodeling after percutaneous coronary intervention versus optimal medical therapy alone. *Am Heart J*. 2011;161:611-621. Copyright 2011, with permission from Elsevier.)

those with severely reduced versus moderately reduced viability in the infarct zone or when compared by percutaneous coronary intervention (PCI) versus medical therapy. This is not what one would logically predict because viability is associated in most of our minds with reversibility.[3] A previous, even smaller study using cardiac magnetic resonance imaging demonstrated that PCI was associated with a statistically significant improvement in remodeling.[4] The OAT substudy in a more contemporary era used optimal medical therapies to prevent remodeling, and this may have limited the potential benefit of other nonpharmacologic modalities. Another potential explanation for the neutral findings is the relatively well-preserved baseline systolic function in these patients, because other studies have demonstrated the greatest benefit to be in those with the poorest baseline left ventricular function. A third possibility is the lack of ongoing severe ischemia in these patients, which also may have limited the benefit of revascularization.

Although these data suggest that there is no need to look for viability in otherwise stable patients in the contemporary era of comprehensive postinfarction medical therapy, I suspect that there is a good deal more that we need to learn about viability and its potential to limit revascularization, particularly in regard to the questions raised by the recently published and reviewed STICH trial.[5]

B. J. Gersh, MB, ChB, DPhil, FRCP

References

1. Hochman JS, Lamas GA, Buller CE, et al. Coronary intervention for persistent occlusion after myocardial infarction. *N Engl J Med.* 2006;355:2395-2407.
2. Sabia PJ, Powers ER, Ragosta M, Sarembock IJ, Burwell LR, Kaul S. An association between collateral blood flow and myocardial viability in patients with recent myocardial infarction. *N Engl J Med.* 1992;327:1825-1831.
3. Chareonthaitawee P, Gersh BJ, Araoz PA, Gibbons RJ. Revascularization in severe left ventricular dysfunction: the role of viability testing. *J Am Coll Cardiol.* 2005; 46:564-574.
4. Bellenger NG, Yousef Z, Rajappan K, Marber MS, Pennell DJ. Infarct zone viability influences ventricular remodelling after late recanalisation of an occluded infarct related artery. *Heart.* 2005;91:478-483.
5. Bonow RO, Maurer G, Lee KL, et al. Myocardial viability and survival in ischemic left ventricular dysfunction. *N Engl J Med.* 2011;364:1617-1625.

Ticagrelor Compared With Clopidogrel by Geographic Region in the Platelet Inhibition and Patient Outcomes (PLATO) Trial
Mahaffey KW, on behalf of the PLATO Investigators (Duke Clinical Res Inst, Durham, NC; et al)
Circulation 124:544-554, 2011

Background.—In the Platelet Inhibition and Patient Outcomes (PLATO) trial, a prespecified subgroup analysis showed a significant interaction between treatment and region ($P=0.045$), with less effect of ticagrelor in North America than in the rest of the world.

Methods and Results.—Reasons for the interaction were explored independently by 2 statistical groups. Systematic errors in trial conduct were investigated. Statistical approaches evaluated the likelihood of play of chance. Cox regression analyses were performed to quantify how much of the regional interaction could be explained by patient characteristics and concomitant treatments, including aspirin maintenance therapy. Landmark Cox regressions at 8 time points evaluated the association of selected factors, including aspirin dose, with outcomes by treatment. Systematic errors in trial conduct were ruled out. Given the large number of subgroup analyses performed and that a result numerically favoring clopidogrel in at least 1 of the 4 prespecified regions could occur with 32% probability, chance alone cannot be ruled out. More patients in the United States (53.6%) than in the rest of the world (1.7%) took a median aspirin dose ≥300 mg/d. Of 37 baseline and postrandomization factors explored, only aspirin dose explained a substantial fraction of the regional interaction. In adjusted analyses, both Cox regression with median maintenance dose and landmark techniques showed that, in patients taking low-dose maintenance aspirin, ticagrelor was associated with better outcomes compared with clopidogrel, with statistical superiority in the rest of the world and similar outcomes in the US cohort.

Conclusions.—The regional interaction could arise from chance alone. Results of 2 independently performed analyses identified an underlying statistical interaction with aspirin maintenance dose as a possible explanation for the regional difference. The lowest risk of cardiovascular death, myocardial infarction, or stroke with ticagrelor compared with clopidogrel is associated with a low maintenance dose of concomitant aspirin.

Clinical Trial Registration.—URL: http://www.clinicaltrials.gov. Unique identifier: NCT00391872.

▶ In the Platelet-Inhibition and Patient Outcomes (PLATO) trial of ticagrelor versus clopidogrel, ticagrelor was superior with regard to the composite endpoint of cardiovascular death, myocardial infarction, and stroke.[1] Preplanned exploratory analyses examined treatment effects in relation to 31 baseline variables, and to everyone's consternation, there was a nonsignificant trend toward worse outcomes with ticagrelor in North America versus the rest of the world, and the interaction term incorporating region was nominally significant. These findings certainly had an impact on the US Food and Drug Administration review process.

Several explanations for this were proffered, including the possibility that these regional differences were caused by the play of chance, and, given the large number of subset analyses, this can certainly not be ruled out. Additional analyses found no differences in trial conduct between the United States and the rest of the world, although drug adherence was less in the United States. Additional adjusted analyses, including landmark analyses, demonstrated that in patients taking lower-dose maintenance aspirin, ticagrelor was associated with better outcomes compared with clopidogrel. The greater use of higher-dose aspirin in the United States could explain these regional differences. Only a randomized, controlled trial would clarify this issue, but ticagrelor is now approved, and the current guidelines already recommend low-dose maintenance aspirin.

B. J. Gersh, MB, ChB, DPhil, FRCP

Reference

1. Wallentin L, Becker RC, Budaj A, et al; PLATO Investigators. Ticagrelor versus clopidogrel in patients with acute coronary syndromes. *N Engl J Med.* 2009; 361:1045-1057.

Chronic Coronary Artery Disease

Functional SYNTAX Score for Risk Assessment in Multivessel Coronary Artery Disease

Nam C-W, Mangiacapra F, Entjes R, et al (Stanford Univ Med Ctr, CA; Cardiovascular Ctr Aalst, Belgium; Catharina Hosp, Eindhoven, the Netherlands)
J Am Coll Cardiol 58:1211-1218, 2011

Objectives.—This study was aimed at investigating whether a fractional flow reserve (FFR)-guided SYNTAX score (SS), termed "functional SYNTAX score" (FSS), would predict clinical outcome better than the classic SS in patients with multivessel coronary artery disease (CAD) undergoing percutaneous coronary intervention (PCI).

Background.—The SS is a purely anatomic score based on the coronary angiogram and predicts outcome after PCI in patients with multivessel CAD. FFR-guided PCI improves outcomes by adding functional information to the anatomic information obtained from the angiogram.

Methods.—The SS was prospectively collected in 497 patients enrolled in the FAME (Fractional Flow Reserve versus Angiography for Multivessel Evaluation) study. FSS was determined by only counting ischemia-producing lesions (FFR $\leq$0.80). The ability of each score to predict major adverse cardiac events (MACE) at 1 year was compared.

Results.—The 497 patients were divided into tertiles of risk based on the SS. After determining the FSS for each patient, 32% moved to a lower-risk group as follows. MACE occurred in 9.0%, 11.3%, and 26.7% of patients in the low-, medium-, and high-FSS groups, respectively (p < 0.001). Only FSS and procedure time were independent predictors of 1-year MACE. FSS demonstrated a better predictive accuracy for MACE compared with SS (Harrell's C of FSS, 0.677 vs. SS, 0.630, p = 0.02; integrated discrimination improvement of 1.94%, p < 0.001).

Conclusions.—Recalculating SS by only incorporating ischemia-producing lesions as determined by FFR decreases the number of higher-risk patients and better discriminates risk for adverse events in patients with multivessel CAD undergoing PCI (Fig 2).

▶ The SYNTAX trial is a landmark study comparing percutaneous coronary intervention (PCI) with drug-eluting stents versus coronary bypass surgery in patients with triple vessel and left main coronary artery disease.[1] Overall at

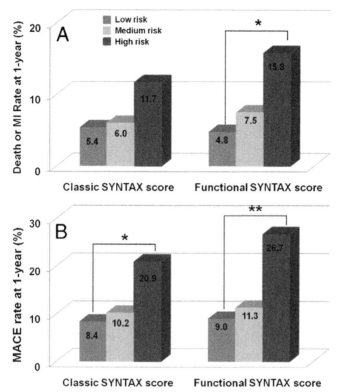

FIGURE 2.—Outcomes According to the SS. The rates of death or myocardial infarction (MI) (**A**), and the rates of major adverse cardiac events (MACE), as composite of death, MI, or any repeat revascularization including repeat percutaneous coronary intervention and coronary artery bypass graft (**B**) according to the tertiles of SS and FSS. The rate of death or MI as a critical hard endpoint was significantly different in the FSS groups unlike the SS groups. The rate of MACE was accordingly increased for the highest-risk group; this trend was attenuated in the FSS groups compared with the classic SS groups. *p < 0.01, **p < 0.001. Abbreviations as in Figure 1. (Reprinted from the Journal of the American College of Cardiology, Nam C-W, Mangiacapra F, Entjes R, et al. Functional SYNTAX score for risk assessment in multivessel coronary artery disease. *J Am Coll Cardiol.* 2011;58:1211-1218. Copyright 2011, with permission from the American College of Cardiology.)

1 year, rates of death and myocardial infarction were similar between the 2 groups with a higher rate of stroke after bypass surgery and a much higher rate of repeat revascularization after PCI. Perceptions of the results of this trial have been heavily influenced by the manner in which the components of the composite endpoints are perceived.

The SYNTAX score is an anatomic scoring system based on the extent of disease and lesion complexity on the angiogram.[2] It has been extremely helpful in identifying subgroups of patients with more complex disease who clearly benefit from bypass surgery and a lower-risk tertile in which PCI appears equally effective.

This study takes things a step further by integrating the anatomic score with an estimate of hemodynamic or functional severity based on measurements of fractional flow reserve as demonstrated in the FAME trial.[3] Measurement of fractional flow reserve resulted in 32% of patients being reclassified to a lower-risk group, and only the fractional flow reserve—guided SYNTAX score, which identifies ischemia producing lesions in addition to procedure times, were independent predictors of major adverse cardiac events at 1 year. It needs to be emphasized, however, that the population in this study who were part of the FAME trial was highly selected in that these were a much lower-risk subgroup than in the SYNTAX trial (corresponding to the lowest-risk tercile).

The trend is clear cut: identification of lesion severity by a visual estimate based on coronary angiography is being superseded by measurements of hemodynamic significance as performed in this study and by plaque characterization using intravascular ultrasound and other evolving technologies.

B. J. Gersh, MB, ChB, DPhil, FRCP

References

1. Serruys PW, Morice MC, Kappetein AP, et al. Percutaneous coronary intervention versus coronary-artery bypass grafting for severe coronary artery disease. *N Engl J Med.* 2009;360:961-972.
2. Serruys PW, Onuma Y, Garg S, et al. Assessment of the SYNTAX score in the Syntax study. *EuroIntervention.* 2009;5:50-56.
3. Pijls NH, Fearon WF, Tonino PA, et al. Fractional flow reserve versus angiography for guiding percutaneous coronary intervention in patients with multivessel coronary artery disease: 2-year follow-up of the FAME (Fractional Flow Reserve Versus Angiography for Multivessel Evaluation) study. *J Am Coll Cardiol.* 2010; 56:177-184.

Intra-aortic Balloon Counterpulsation and Infarct Size in Patients With Acute Anterior Myocardial Infarction Without Shock: The CRISP AMI Randomized Trial

Patel MR, Smalling RW, Thiele H, et al (Duke Univ Med Ctr, Durham, NC; Univ of Texas, Houston; Univ of Leipzig Heart Ctr, Germany; et al)
JAMA 306:1329-1337, 2011

Context.—Intra-aortic balloon counterpulsation (IABC) is an adjunct to revascularization in patients with cardiogenic shock and reduces infarct size when placed prior to reperfusion in animal models.

Objective.—To determine if routine IABC placement prior to reperfusion in patients with anterior ST-segment elevation myocardial infarction (STEMI) without shock reduces myocardial infarct size.

Design, Setting, and Patients.—An open, multicenter, randomized controlled trial, the Counterpulsation to Reduce Infarct Size Pre-PCI Acute Myocardial Infarction (CRISP AMI) included 337 patients with acute anterior STEMI but without cardiogenic shock at 30 sites in 9 countries from June 2009 through February 2011.

Intervention.—Initiation of IABC before primary percutaneous coronary intervention (PCI) and continuation for at least 12 hours (IABC plus PCI) vs primary PCI alone.

Main Outcome Measures.—Infarct size expressed as a percentage of left ventricular (LV) mass and measured by cardiac magnetic resonance imaging performed 3 to 5 days after PCI. Secondary end points included all-cause death at 6 months and vascular complications and major bleeding at 30 days. Multiple imputations were performed for missing infarct size data.

Results.—The median time from first contact to first coronary device was 77 minutes (interquartile range, 53 to 114 minutes) for the IABC plus PCI group vs 68 minutes (interquartile range, 40 to 100 minutes) for the PCI alone group (*P*=.04). The mean infarct size was not significantly different between the patients in the IABC plus PCI group and in the PCI alone group (42.1% [95% CI, 38.7% to 45.6%] vs 37.5% [95% CI, 34.3% to 40.8%], respectively; difference of 4.6% [95% CI, −0.2% to 9.4%], *P*=.06; imputed difference of 4.5% [95% CI, −0.3% to 9.3%], *P*=.07) and in patients with proximal left anterior descending Thrombolysis in Myocardial Infarction flow scores of 0 or 1 (46.7% [95% CI, 42.8% to 50.6%] vs 42.3% [95% CI, 38.6% to 45.9%], respectively; difference of 4.4% [95% CI, −1.0% to 9.7%], *P*=.11; imputed difference of 4.8% [95% CI, −0.6% to 10.1%], *P*=.08). At 30 days, there were no significant differences between the IABC plus PCI group and the PCI alone group for major vascular complications (n=7 [4.3%; 95% CI, 1.8% to 8.8%] vs n=2 [1.1%; 95% CI, 0.1% to 4.0%], respectively; *P*=.09) and major bleeding or transfusions (n=5 [3.1%; 95% CI, 1.0% to 7.1%] vs n=3 [1.7%; 95% CI, 0.4% to 4.9%]; *P*=.49). By 6 months, 3 patients (1.9%; 95% CI, 0.6% to 5.7%) in the IABC plus PCI group and 9 patients (5.2%; 95% CI, 2.7% to 9.7%) in the PCI alone group had died (*P*=.12).

Conclusion.—Among patients with acute anterior STEMI without shock, IABC plus primary PCI compared with PCI alone did not result in reduced infarct size.

Trial Registration.—clinicaltrials.gov Identifier: NCT00833612.

▶ This is a well-conducted trial demonstrating that among patients without cardiogenic shock, intra-aortic balloon counterpulsation (IABC) plus primary percutaneous coronary intervention (PCI) offered no benefits over primary PCI alone. In fact, in regard to infarct size, the trend was in the other direction, and there were no differences in clinical events other than a nonsignificant trend toward more vascular complications in the IABC group.

IABC is widely used in cardiogenic shock but also to provide circulatory support in high-risk PCI procedures, such as hemodynamic instability, post–myocardial infarction refractory angina, unprotected left main coronary artery disease, and severe left ventricular dysfunction. Several mechanisms may explain the lack of benefit in this group of stable patients without cardiogenic shock.[1] It is possible that the increase in diastolic perfusion pressure does not result in an increase in coronary blood flow, and even if coronary blood flow was increased, this could have the adverse consequence of improving contractility and increasing myocardial oxygen demands due to an increased stretch of myocardial fibers.[2] Another possibility is that the duration of symptoms before unloading is such that it is already too late to make a difference in terms of salvage. It is unlikely that the additional 10-minute delay to primary PCI incurred by balloon placement could have had a significant effect.

It appears, however, that in patients without shock, primary PCI with thrombectomy does pretty well, and it is difficult to improve on it. In patients with cardiogenic shock or hemodynamic instability, there will be no randomized trials, but clinical experience would suggest that the intra-aortic balloon does undoubtedly improve systemic hemodynamics. It is likely that the major advances in the management of ST-segment elevation myocardial infarction in the coming years will not be in the catheterization laboratory but in the community, with the emphasis of increasing the speed and utilization of reperfusion therapy to all who are eligible.

B. J. Gersh, MB, ChB, DPhil, FRCP

References

1. Ndrepepa G, Kastrati A. Need for critical reappraisal of intra-aortic balloon counterpulsation. *JAMA*. 2011;306:1376-1377.
2. Gregg DE. Effect of coronary perfusion pressure or coronary flow on oxygen usage of the myocardium. *Circ Res*. 1963;13:497-500.

Intramyocardial, Autologous CD34+ Cell Therapy for Refractory Angina
Losordo DW, the ACT34-CMI Investigators (Northwestern Univ, Chicago, IL; et al)
Circ Res 109:428-436, 2011

Rationale.—A growing number of patients with coronary disease have refractory angina. Preclinical and early-phase clinical data suggest that intramyocardial injection of autologous CD34+ cells can improve myocardial perfusion and function.

Objective.—Evaluate the safety and bioactivity of intramyocardial injections of autologous CD34+ cells in patients with refractory angina who have exhausted all other treatment options.

Methods and Results.—In this prospective, double-blind, randomized, phase II study (ClinicalTrials.gov identifier: NCT00300053), 167 patients with refractory angina received 1 of 2 doses (1×10^5 or 5×10^5 cells/kg) of mobilized autologous CD34+ cells or an equal volume of diluent (placebo). Treatment was distributed into 10 sites of ischemic, viable myocardium with a NOGA mapping injection catheter. The primary outcome measure was weekly angina frequency 6 months after treatment. Weekly angina frequency was significantly lower in the low-dose group than in placebo-treated patients at both 6 months (6.8 ± 1.1 versus 10.9 ± 1.2, $P=0.020$) and 12 months (6.3 ± 1.2 versus 11.0 ± 1.2, $P=0.035$); measurements in the high-dose group were also lower, but not significantly. Similarly, improvement in exercise tolerance was significantly greater in low-dose patients than in placebo-treated patients (6 months: 139 ± 151 versus 69 ± 122 seconds, $P=0.014$; 12 months: 140 ± 171 versus 58 ± 146 seconds, $P=0.017$) and

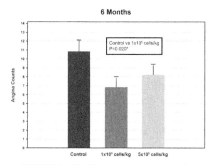
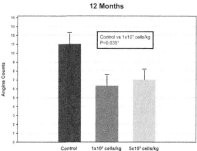

FIGURE 2.—Weekly angina incidence at 6 and 12 months. Least squares means and standard errors. *Probability values from pairwise comparisons of ratios from Poisson regression (log of baseline used as covariate). (Reprinted from Losordo DW, the ACT34-CMI Investigators. Intramyocardial, autologous CD34+ cell therapy for refractory angina. *Circ Res.* 2011;109:428-436. © American Heart Association, Inc.)

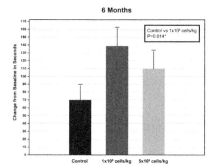
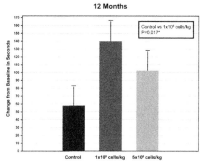

FIGURE 3.—Change in exercise time at 6 months and 12 months. Means and standard errors. *Probability values from analysis of covariance with repeated measures (baseline value used as covariate). (Reprinted from Losordo DW, the ACT34-CMI Investigators. Intramyocardial, autologous CD34+ cell therapy for refractory angina. *Circ Res.* 2011;109:428-436. © American Heart Association, Inc.)

greater, but not significantly, in the high-dose group. During cell mobilization and collection, 4.6% of patients had cardiac enzyme elevations consistent with non-ST segment elevation myocardial infarction. Mortality at 12 months was 5.4% in the placebo-treatment group with no deaths among cell-treated patients.

Conclusions.—Patients with refractory angina who received intramyocardial injections of autologous CD34+ cells (10^5 cells/kg) experienced significant improvements in angina frequency and exercise tolerance. The cell-mobilization and -collection procedures were associated with cardiac enzyme elevations, which will be addressed in future studies (Figs 2 and 3).

▶ This double-blind, randomized trial of autologous CD34＋ cells mobilized with granulocyte colony-stimulating factor in patients with refractory angina is extremely encouraging in that there appears to be a significant improvement in symptom status and exercise duration. Moreover, the trial was double blinded. In the current era, in which late mortality from symptomatic coronary disease has declined because of revascularization, improved medical therapy, and aggressive secondary prevention, we are now faced with an expanding population of "revascularization survivors" who are severely limited by refractory angina. Current estimates are that more than 850 000 people in the United States fall into this category.[1] The therapeutic options are limited but include enhanced external counterpulsation, spinal cord stimulation, transcutaneous nerve stimulation, and, until randomized trials demonstrated that it was ineffective, transcutaneous laser myocardial revascularization. New antianginal drugs have been slow to reach the market.

This trial is based on the fact that human CD34+ hematopoietic stem cells have also been shown to have endothelial lineage potential in vitro and in vivo. Furthermore, preclinical studies have suggested that the administration of these cells may improve perfusion and ischemia, perhaps by the stimulation of neovascularization in ischemic tissue and, in particular, the microvasculature.[2] This trial not only provides data on safety and efficacy but also demonstrates that the techniques of mobilizing, collecting, purifying, and delivering the cells via an intramyocardial approach is feasible at a large number of centers and is exemplified by those who took part in the trial.

What is a little puzzling about the data is the apparent decline in efficacy in the higher dose subgroup, but as pointed out by the authors, there is an extensive body of literature suggesting that the response to biological manipulation of angiogenesis may be biphasic.[3] The next step is a larger phase 3 clinical trial, but the data from this trial are certainly very encouraging.

B. J. Gersh, MB, ChB, DPhil, FRCP

References

1. Mannheimer C, Camici P, Chester MR, et al. The problem of chronic refractory angina: report from the esc joint study group on the treatment of refractory angina. *Eur Heart J.* 2002;23:355-370.
2. Kawamoto A, Iwasaki H, Kusano K, et al. CD34-positive cells exhibit increased potency and safety for therapeutic neovascularization after myocardial infarction compared with total mononuclear cells. *Circulation.* 2006;114:2163-2169.
3. Folkman J. Angiogenesis. *Annu Rev Med.* 2006;57:1-18.

Coronary Bypass Surgery and Percutaneous Coronary Intervention

Appropriateness of Percutaneous Coronary Intervention

Chan PS, Patel MR, Klein LW, et al (Saint Luke's Mid America Heart and Vascular Inst, Kansas City, MO; Duke Clinical Res Inst, Durham, NC; Advocate Illinois Masonic Med Ctr, Chicago; et al)
JAMA 306:53-61, 2011

Context.—Despite the widespread use of percutaneous coronary intervention (PCI), the appropriateness of these procedures in contemporary practice is unknown.

Objective.—To assess the appropriateness of PCI in the United States.

Design, Setting, and Patients.—Multicenter, prospective study of patients within the National Cardiovascular Data Registry undergoing PCI between July 1, 2009, and September 30, 2010, at 1091 US hospitals. The appropriateness of PCI was adjudicated using the appropriate use criteria for coronary revascularization. Results were stratified by whether the procedure was performed for an acute (ST-segment elevation myocardial infarction, non—ST-segment elevation myocardial infarction, or unstable angina with high-risk features) or nonacute indication.

Main Outcome Measures.—Proportion of acute and nonacute PCIs classified as appropriate, uncertain, or inappropriate; extent of hospital-level variation in inappropriate procedures.

Results.—Of 500 154 PCIs, 355 417 (71.1%) were for acute indications (ST-segment elevation myocardial infarction, 103 245 [20.6%]; non—ST-segment elevation myocardial infarction, 105 708 [21.1%]; high-risk unstable angina, 146 464 [29.3%]), and 144 737 (28.9%) for nonacute indications. For acute indications, 350 469 PCIs (98.6%) were classified as appropriate, 1055 (0.3%) as uncertain, and 3893 (1.1%) as inappropriate. For nonacute indications, 72 911 PCIs (50.4%) were classified as appropriate, 54 988 (38.0%) as uncertain, and 16 838 (11.6%) as inappropriate. The majority of inappropriate PCIs for nonacute indications were performed in patients with no angina (53.8%), low-risk ischemia on noninvasive stress testing (71.6%), or suboptimal (≤ 1 medication) antianginal therapy (95.8%). Furthermore, although variation in the proportion of inappropriate PCI across hospitals was minimal for acute procedures, there was substantial hospital variation for nonacute procedures (median hospital rate for inappropriate PCI, 10.8%; interquartile range, 6.0%-16.7%).

Conclusions.—In this large contemporary US cohort, nearly all acute PCIs were classified as appropriate. For nonacute indications, however, 12% were classified as inappropriate, with substantial variation across hospitals.

▶ The societal cost of percutaneous coronary intervention (PCI) in the United States is substantial; approximately 600 000 are performed annually at a cost exceeding 12 billion dollars per year.[1] Although there is abundant evidence supporting the benefits of PCI in acute coronary syndromes and in the relief of symptoms in chronic stable angina, several trials have failed to document any benefit from PCI over medical therapy in angiographically selected patients with mild to moderate chronic stable angina.[2] The appropriate use of PCI and other invasive and noninvasive therapeutic and imaging procedures is a major priority, but until recently a lack of a national standard for defining appropriate use has been a hindrance for prior studies aimed at defining appropriate patient selection criteria. Recently, a combined effort of 6 professional organizations determined appropriateness criteria for coronary revascularization,[3] and use of a large national registry of patients undergoing PCI has provided an ideal opportunity to evaluate the appropriateness of PCI in contemporary practice throughout the United States.

The results are somewhat mixed. As expected, nearly all PCIs performed acutely for patients with acute coronary syndromes were classified as appropriate. For nonacute indications, however, only 50.4% were classified as appropriate, 38% as uncertain, and 12% as inappropriate. Moreover, most inappropriate PCIs were in patients with no angina, low-risk ischemia on stress testing, or in patients on suboptimal antianginal therapy. There was, in addition, quite marked variability across hospitals and a trend suggesting lower volumes were associated with a greater rate of inappropriate procedures. These data do not address inappropriate underuse of the procedure, but the major issue confronting us is probably overuse.

The message is quite clear. The onus of responsibility for the appropriate performance of procedures rests upon us as cardiologists. If we do not exercise this judiciously, the decision will be taken out of our hands and driven by payers and not physicians.[4] This remains a critically important issue that must be addressed.

B. J. Gersh, MB, ChB, DPhil, FRCP

References

1. Mahoney EM, Wang K, Arnold SV, et al. Cost-effectiveness of prasugrel versus clopidogrel in patients with acute coronary syndromes and planned percutaneous coronary intervention: results from the trial to assess improvement in therapeutic outcomes by optimizing platelet inhibition with prasugrel-Thrombolysis in Myocardial Infarction TRITON-TIMI 38. *Circulation.* 2010;121:71-79.
2. Boden WE, O'Rourke RA, Teo KK, et al; COURAGE Trial Research Group. Optimal medical therapy with or without PCI for stable coronary disease. *N Engl J Med.* 2007;356:1503-1516.
3. Patel MR, Dehmer GJ, Hirshfeld JW, Smith PK, Spertus JA; American College of Cardiology Foundation Appropriateness Criteria Task Force; Society for Cardiovascular Angiography and Interventions; Society of Thoracic Surgeons; American Association for Thoracic Surgery; American Heart Association, and the American Society of Nuclear Cardiology Endorsed by the American Society of Echocardiography; Heart Failure Society of America; Society of Cardiovascular Computed Tomography. ACCF/SCAI/STS/AATS/AHA/ASNC 2009 Appropriateness Criteria for Coronary Revascularization: a report by the American College of Cardiology Foundation Appropriateness Criteria Task Force, Society for Cardiovascular Angiography and Interventions, Society of Thoracic Surgeons, American Association for Thoracic Surgery, American Heart Association, and the American Society of Nuclear Cardiology Endorsed by the American Society of Echocardiography, the Heart Failure Society of America, and the Society of Cardiovascular Computed Tomography. *J Am Coll Cardiol.* 2009;53:530-553.
4. Holmes DR Jr, Gersh BJ, Whitlow P, King SB 3rd, Dove JT. Percutaneous coronary intervention for chronic stable angina: a reassessment. *JACC Cardiovasc Interv.* 2008;1:34-43.

Aspirin Plus Clopidogrel Versus Aspirin Alone After Coronary Artery Bypass Grafting: The Clopidogrel After Surgery for Coronary Artery Disease (CASCADE) Trial

Kulik A, Le May MR, Voisine P, et al (Boca Raton Regional Hosp, FL; Univ of Ottawa Heart Inst, Ontario, Canada; Hôpital Laval, Quebec, Canada; et al)
Circulation 122:2680-2687, 2010

Background.—Clopidogrel inhibits intimal hyperplasia in animal studies and therefore may reduce saphenous vein graft (SVG) intimal hyperplasia after coronary artery bypass grafting. The Clopidogrel After Surgery for Coronary Artery DiseasE (CASCADE) study was undertaken to evaluate whether the addition of clopidogrel to aspirin inhibits SVG disease after coronary artery bypass grafting, as assessed at 1 year by intravascular ultrasound.

Methods and Results.—In this double-blind phase II trial, 113 patients undergoing coronary artery bypass grafting with SVGs were randomized to receive aspirin 162 mg plus clopidogrel 75 mg daily or aspirin 162 mg plus placebo daily for 1 year. The primary outcome was SVG intimal hyperplasia (mean intimal area) as determined by intravascular ultrasound at 1 year. Secondary outcomes were graft patency, major adverse cardiovascular events, and major bleeding. One-year intravascular ultrasound and coronary angiography were performed in 92 patients (81.4%). At 1 year, SVG intimal area did not differ significantly between the 2 groups (4.1 ± 2.0 versus 4.5 ± 2.1 mm^2, aspirinclopidogrel versus aspirin-placebo, $P = 0.44$). Overall 1-year graft patency was 95.2% in the aspirin-clopidogrel group compared with 95.5% in the aspirin-placebo group ($P = 0.90$), and SVG patency was 94.3% in the aspirin-clopidogrel group versus 93.2% in the aspirin-placebo group ($P = 0.69$). Freedom from major adverse cardiovascular events at 1 year was 92.9 ± 3.4% in the aspirin-clopidogrel group and 91.1 ± 3.8% in the aspirin-placebo group ($P = 0.76$). The incidence of major bleeding at 1 year was similar for the 2 groups (1.8% versus 0%, aspirin-clopidogrel versus aspirin-placebo, $P = 0.50$).

TABLE 3.—Primary and Secondary Outcomes Evaluated at the 1-Year IVUS and Coronary Angiogram

	Aspirin-Clopidogrel	Aspirin-Placebo	P
IVUS	n=46	n=44	
Mean intimal area, mm^2	4.1±2.0	4.5±2.1	0.44
Coronary angiography, %	n=46	n=46	
Any graft occlusion	4.8	4.5	0.90
Vein graft occlusion	5.7	6.8	0.69
Internal thoracic artery occlusion	3.4	0	0.50
Vein graft stenosis	2.8	2.9	1.00
Patients with vein graft occlusion	13.0	13.0	1.00

IVUS indicates intravascular ultrasound.

Conclusions.—Compared with aspirin monotherapy, the combination of aspirin plus clopidogrel did not significantly reduce the process of SVG intimal hyperplasia 1 year after coronary artery bypass grafting (Table 3).

▶ The Achilles heel of coronary bypass surgery (CABG) is the process of progressive saphenous vein graft (SVG) disease in addition to early occlusion. In some series, up to 20% of SVG occluded within the first year,[1] and by 10 years after surgery, approximately 60% are patent and about half of the patent grafts are severely diseased.[2]

The process of SVG disease is complex, including thrombosis, hyperplasia, and atherosclerosis, and there is evidence that platelet activity plays a key role in the progressive thickening of the vessel wall that characterizes intimal hyperplasia. As such, the process of intimal hyperplasia, which is in part platelet-mediated and which is linked to SVG stenosis, atherosclerosis, and occlusion, is an attractive target for pharmacologic intervention.

Unfortunately, this small double-blind Phase II trial of 1133 patients comparing aspirin and clopidogrel to aspirin alone had no effect on SVG intimal hyperplasia as determined by echocardiographic ultrasound (primary endpoint) nor on secondary outcomes including cardiovascular events and SVG patency, although the trial was not powered to detect differences in the latter. Whether the clopidogrel would have an effect on SVG patency or atherosclerosis cannot be answered by this trial. Nonetheless, it would appear that the benefit of aspirin and clopidogrel noted in patients with acute coronary syndromes and undergoing PCI do not translate into the CABG population.[3] This is in contrast to a trend noted in nonrandomized studies, but the lack of benefit is similar to that noted in one other randomized controlled trial.[4]

This trial may be underpowered to conclusively evaluate an effect of clopidogrel, and there was a trend in regard to SVG intimal hyperplasia, but it was not significant. It will be interesting to see the effects of newer agents such as prasugrel and ticagrelor, and this trial provides a useful template for the design of future intravascular ultrasound-based studies.

B. J. Gersh, MB, ChB, DPhil, FRCP

References

1. Alexander JH, Hafley G, Harrington RA, et al; PREVENT IV Investigators. Efficacy and safety of edifoligide, an E2F transcription factor decoy, for prevention of vein graft failure following coronary artery bypass graft surgery: PREVENT IV: a randomized controlled trial. *JAMA.* 2005;294:2446-2454.
2. Fitzgibbon GM, Kafka HP, Leach AJ, Keon WJ, Hooper GD, Burton JR. Coronary bypass graft fate and patient outcome: angiographic follow-up of 5,065 grafts related to survival and reoperation in 1,388 patients during 25 years. *J Am Coll Cardiol.* 1996;28:616-626.
3. Yusuf S, Zhao F, Mehta SR, Chrolavicious S, Tognoni G, Fox KK. Effects on clopidogrel in addition to aspirin in patient with acute coronary syndromes without ST-segment elevation. *N Engl J Med.* 2001;345:494-502.
4. Gao C, Ren C, Li D, Li L. Clopidogrel and aspirin versus clopidogrel alone on graft patency after coronary artery bypass grafting. *Ann Thorac Surg.* 2009;88:59-62.

Comparison of coronary bypass surgery with drug-eluting stenting for the treatment of left main and/or three-vessel disease: 3-year follow-up of the SYNTAX trial

Kappetein AP, Feldman TE, Mack MJ, et al (Erasmus Med Centre, Rotterdam, The Netherlands; NorthShore Univ Health System, Evanston, IL; Baylor Healthcare System, Dallas, TX; et al)
Eur Heart J 32:2125-2134, 2011

Aims.—Long-term randomized comparisons of percutaneous coronary intervention (PCI) to coronary artery bypass grafting (CABG) in left main coronary (LM) disease and/or three-vessel disease (3VD) patients have been limited. This analysis compares 3-year outcomes in LM and/or 3VD patients treated with CABG or PCI with TAXUS Express stents.

Methods and Results.—SYNTAX is an 85-centre randomized clinical trial ($n = 1800$). Prospectively screened, consecutive LM and/or 3VD patients were randomized if amenable to equivalent revascularization using either technique; if not, they were entered into a registry. Patients in the randomized cohort will continue to be followed for 5 years. At 3 years, major adverse cardiac and cerebrovascular events [MACCE: death, stroke, myocardial infarction (MI), and repeat revascularization; CABG 20.2% vs. PCI 28.0%, $P < 0.001$], repeat revascularization (10.7

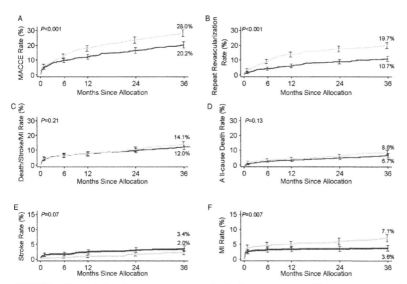

FIGURE 2.—Rates of clinical outcomes among randomized treatment groups. Time-to-event curves in patients treated with coronary artery bypass grafting (blue line) or percutaneous coronary intervention (yellow line) for the composite of major adverse cardiac and cerebrovascular events (*A*), repeat revascularization (*B*), death/stroke/myocardial infarction (*C*), all-cause death (*D*), stroke (*E*), and myocardial infarction (*F*) to 3 years. *P*-values from log-rank test. For interpretation of the references to color in this figure legend, the reader is referred to web version of this article. (Reprinted from Kappetein AP, Feldman TE, Mack MJ, et al. Comparison of coronary bypass surgery with drug-eluting stenting for the treatment of left main and/or three-vessel disease: 3-year follow-up of the SYNTAX trial. *Eur Heart J.* 2011;32:2125-2134, by permission of The European Society of Cardiology.)

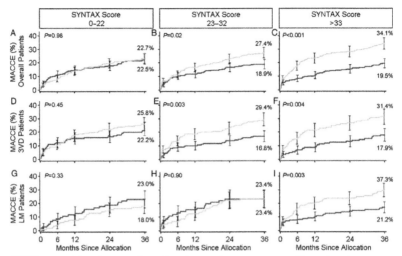

FIGURE 5.—Major adverse cardiac and cerebrovascular event rates according to the subset, treatment group, and SYNTAX score category. Time-to-event curves in the coronary artery bypass grafting (blue line) or percutaneous coronary intervention (yellow line) overall cohorts to 3 years according to the low (0–22, A), intermediate (23–32, B), or high (≥33, C) SYNTAX scores. (D–F) Major adverse cardiac and cerebrovascular events in three-vessel disease patients with low, intermediate, or high SYNTAX scores, respectively. (G–I) Major adverse cardiac and cerebrovascular events in patients with left main disease with low, intermediate, or high SYNTAX scores. P-value from log-rank test. For interpretation of the references to color in this figure legend, the reader is referred to web version of this article. (Reprinted from Kappetein AP, Feldman TE, MacK MJ, et al. Comparison of coronary bypass surgery with drug-eluting stenting for the treatment of left main and/or three-vessel disease: 3-year follow-up of the SYNTAX trial. *Eur Heart J.* 2011;32:2125-2134, by permission of The European Society of Cardiology.)

vs. 19.7%, $P < 0.001$), and MI (3.6 vs. 7.1%, $P = 0.002$) were elevated in the PCI arm. Rates of the composite safety endpoint (death/stroke/MI 12.0 vs. 14.1%, $P = 0.21$) and stroke alone (3.4 vs. 2.0%, $P = 0.07$) were not significantly different between treatment groups. Major adverse cardiac and cerebrovascular event rates were not significantly different between arms in the LM subgroup (22.3 vs. 26.8%, $P = 0.20$) but were higher with PCI in the 3VD subgroup (18.8 vs. 28.8%, $P < 0.001$).

Conclusions.—At 3 years, MACCE was significantly higher in PCI-compared with CABG-treated patients. In patients with less complex disease (low SYNTAX scores for 3VD or low/intermediate terciles for LM patients), PCI is an acceptable revascularization, although longer follow-up is needed to evaluate these two revascularization strategies (Figs 2 and 5).

▶ The SYNTAX trial is the most contemporary and largest randomized trial comparing coronary bypass surgery with drug-eluting stenting. It is confined to high-risk patients with 3-vessel disease and left main coronary artery disease. The initial results at 1 year demonstrated no difference in mortality between the 2 procedures, but the risk of stroke was higher in patients undergoing coronary artery bypass grafting (CABG), and the rate of myocardial infarction was higher in the percutaneous coronary intervention (PCI) group. The major difference between the 2 groups, however, was a much higher rate of repeat revascularization among stented patients—a finding that was not surprising. In terms of the primary composite endpoint of the trial, PCI failed to show a non-inferiority, but this was driven by the higher rate of repeat revascularization.[1] Not surprisingly, perceptions of the trial results vary substantially between surgeons and interventional cardiologists, which is a problem often introduced by the use of a composite endpoint as the primary endpoint.

The long-term results of this trial have been eagerly awaited, and patients will be followed for 5 years in total. The high number of stents implanted and the length of the stented segment of the vessel have raised questions about the long-term outcome in stented patients, and as such these 3-year data are important.

In regard to death, there remains no difference at 3 years, but the stroke rate remains slightly higher after CABG, although not quite statistically significant, but the difference in nonfatal myocardial infarction has increased and is significantly higher after stenting. The higher rate of repeat revascularization after PCI persists, and the gap is widening. However, among the triple-vessel disease patients, mortality and the combined endpoint of death, stroke, and myocardial infarction were increased in the PCI group.

Some of the most interesting data relate to the SYNTAX score, which is an index of lesion complexity and the severity and extent of disease. What we see is that in patients in the lowest tercile of the SYNTAX score, PCI is an acceptable form of revascularization, bearing in mind that these are patients with 3-vessel and left main coronary artery disease. On the other hand, among the highest tercile, CABG is clearly superior, and in the intermediate tercile of SYNTAX score, therapy with CABG is superior to stenting in those with triple vessel disease, but the 2 therapies were equivalent for left main coronary disease. In regard to left main disease, we need to await the results of larger ongoing trials of drug-eluting stents and coronary bypass surgery. In regard to SYNTAX, the 5-year data will be equally interesting.

B. J. Gersh, MB, ChB, DPhil, FRCP

Reference

1. Serruys PW, Morice MC, Kappetein AP, et al. Percutaneous coronary intervention versus coronary-artery bypass grafting for severe coronary artery disease. *N Engl J Med*. 2009;360:961-972.

Effect of Timing of Chronic Preoperative Aspirin Discontinuation on Morbidity and Mortality in Coronary Artery Bypass Surgery

Jacob M, Smedira N, Blackstone E, et al (Cleveland Clinic, OH)
Circulation 123:577-583, 2011

Background.—Aspirin (ASA) has been shown to reduce postoperative coronary artery bypass grafting (CABG) mortality and ischemic events; however, the timing of chronic ASA discontinuation before surgery is controversial because of concern about postoperative bleeding. We evaluated the effect of the timing of ASA discontinuation before CABG on major adverse cardiovascular outcomes and postoperative bleeding using the Cleveland Clinic Cardiovascular Information Registry database.

Methods and Results.—At the Cleveland Clinic between January 1, 2002, and January 31, 2008, 4143 patients undergoing CABG were taking preoperative chronic ASA. Of these, 2298 discontinued ASA 6 or more days before surgery (early discontinuation), and 1845 took ASA within 5 days of the surgery (late use). Because of substantial differences between these 2 groups, propensity score analysis, and matching based on 31 variables were used for fair comparison of outcomes. This resulted in 1519 well-matched pairs of patients (73%). There was no significant difference between those with early discontinuation and late ASA use with regard to the composite outcome of in-hospital mortality, myocardial infarction, and stroke (1.7% versus 1.8%, $P=0.80$). Late use was associated with more intraoperative transfusions (23% versus 20%, $P=0.03$) and postoperative transfusions (30% versus 26%, $P=0.009$) but a similar number of reoperations for bleeding (3.4% versus 2.4% $P=0.10$).

Conclusions.—Among patients undergoing isolated CABG, late discontinuation of ASA resulted in no difference in postoperative cardiovascular outcomes; however, there was an increased transfusion requirement. Thus, we recommend weighing the risks and benefits of late ASA use in these patients (Fig).

▶ I had not realized that the discontinuation of aspirin before coronary artery bypass surgery (CABG) was still an issue. Prior retrospective studies have suggested that the use of aspirin in the preoperative period reduces perioperative

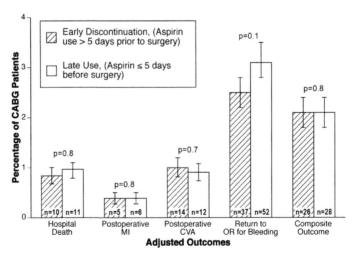

FIGURE.—Adjusted analysis of ASA discontinuation and post-CABG outcomes. Outcomes shown with 68% confidence intervals. CVA indicates cerebrovascular accident; OR, operating room. Composite outcome includes in-hospital death, postoperative MI, and postoperative CVA. (Reprinted Jacob M, Smedira N, Blackstone E, et al. Effect of timing of chronic preoperative aspirin discontinuation on morbidity and mortality in coronary artery bypass surgery. *Circulation.* 2011;123:577-583. © American Heart Association, Inc.)

mortality,[1] and there is general agreement that its use in the postoperative period is helpful.[2] It is interesting, however, to note that the American College of Cardiology/American Heart Association guidelines on CABG state that in stable patients, aspirin should be discontinued 10 or more days before surgery,[3] whereas the Society of Thoracic Surgeons 2005 guidelines give a Class IIa recommendation for aspirin to be discontinued 3 to 5 days before elective.[4]

This retrospective study from the large Cleveland Clinic database compared outcomes in patients in whom aspirin was discontinued 6 or more days before surgery and patients who took aspirin within 5 days of surgery. After propensity matching, there was no difference between the 2 groups in clinical outcomes, but late use was associated with more transfusions both intraoperatively and postoperatively. Nonetheless, there was no difference in rates of reoperation bleeding.

One cannot disagree with the authors' conclusions that the risks and benefits of continuing aspirin preoperatively need to be individualized. Nonetheless, I also agree with the majority who routinely continue aspirin prior to CABG unless there are contraindications. Trials suggesting that preoperative aspirin is associated with increased bleeding complications and offers no additional benefit in early vein graft patency took place more than 20 years ago. I think there is currently increasing concern that the discontinuation of aspirin, especially in patients with prior percutaneous coronary intervention, is linked to increased myocardial infarction, stroke, and death.[5] A limitation of this study as recognized by the authors is that the analysis is confined to patients who underwent surgery, and thus patients who had surgery planned but did not undergo operation because of an interim perioperative illness were excluded. I wonder how many patients who discontinued aspirin were in that group? Whether clopidogrel or prasugrel should be discontinued preoperatively is a different but related issue, and there is widespread agreement that these drugs should be discontinued if possible at least 5 to 7 days preoperatively.

B. J. Gersh, MB, ChB, DPhil, FRCP

References

1. Bybee KA, Powell BD, Valeti U, et al. Preoperative aspirin therapy is associated with improved postoperative outcomes in patients undergoing coronary artery bypass grafting. *Circulation*. 2005;112:I286-I292.
2. Dacey LJ, Munoz JJ, Johnson ER, et al. Effect of preoperative aspirin use on mortality in coronary artery bypass grafting patients. *Ann Thorac Surg*. 2000; 70:1986-1990.
3. Eagle KA, Guyton RA, Davidoff R, et al; American College of Cardiology/ American Heart Association Task Force on Practice Guidelines Committee to Update the 1999 Guidelines for Coronary Artery Bypass Graft Surgery, American Society for Thoracic Surgery, Society of Thoracic Surgeons. ACC/AHA 2004 guideline update for coronary artery bypass graft surgery: summary article. A report of the American College of Cardiology/American Heart Association Task Force on Practice Guidelines (Committee to Update the 1999 Guidelines for Coronary Artery Bypass Graft Surgery). *J Am Coll Cardiol*. 2004;44:e213-e310.
4. Ferraris VA, Ferraris SP, Moliterno DJ, et al; Society of Thoracic Surgerons. The Society of Thoracic Surgeons practice guideline series: aspirin and other antiplatelet agents during operative coronary revascularization (executive summary). *Ann Thorac Surg*. 2005;79:1454-1461.

5. Sethi GK, Copeland JG, Goldman S, Moritz T, Zadina K, Henderson WG. Implications of preoperative administration of aspirin in patients undergoing coronary artery bypass grafting. Department of Veterans Affairs Cooperative Study on Antiplatelet Therapy. *J Am Coll Cardiol.* 1990;15:15-20.

Effects of Optimal Medical Treatment With or Without Coronary Revascularization on Angina and Subsequent Revascularizations in Patients With Type 2 Diabetes Mellitus and Stable Ischemic Heart Disease

Dagenais GR, the Bypass Angioplasty Revascularization Investigation 2 Diabetes (BARI 2D) Study Group (Institut Universitaire de Cardiologie et de Pneumologie de Québec, Canada; et al)
Circulation 123:1492-1500, 2011

Background.—In the Bypass Angioplasty Revascularization Investigation 2 Diabetes (BARI 2D) trial, an initial strategy of coronary revascularization and optimal medical treatment (REV) compared with an initial optimal medical treatment with the option of subsequent revascularization (MED) did not reduce all-cause mortality or the composite of cardiovascular death, myocardial infarction, and stroke in patients with type 2 diabetes mellitus and stable ischemic heart disease. In the same population, we tested whether the REV strategy was superior to the MED strategy in preventing worsening and new angina and subsequent coronary revascularizations.

Methods and Results.—Among the 2364 men and women (mean age, 62.4 years) with type 2 diabetes mellitus, documented coronary artery disease, and myocardial ischemia, 1191 were randomized to the MED and 1173 to the REV strategy preselected in the percutaneous coronary intervention (796) and coronary artery bypass graft (377) strata. Compared with the MED strategy, the REV strategy at the 3-year follow-up had a lower rate of worsening angina (8% versus 13%; $P<0.001$), new angina (37% versus 51%; $P=0.001$), and subsequent coronary revascularizations (18% versus 33%; $P<0.001$) and a higher rate of angina-free status (66% versus 58%; $P=0.003$). The coronary artery bypass graft stratum patients were at higher risk than those in the percutaneous coronary intervention stratum, and had the greatest benefits from REV.

Conclusions.—In these patients, the REV strategy reduced the occurrence of worsening angina, new angina, and subsequent coronary revascularizations more than the MED strategy. The symptomatic benefits were observed particularly for high-risk patients.

Clinical Trial Registration.—URL: http://www.ClinicalTrials.gov. Unique identifier: NCT00006305 (Figs 1 and 3).

▶ The Bypass Angioplasty Revascularization Investigation 2 Diabetes (BARI 2D) trial in patients with type 2 diabetes stable coronary disease (defined by Canadian Cardiovascular Society [CCS] Class 1 and 2 and 18% without documented angina) did not show any benefit in terms of survival and myocardial

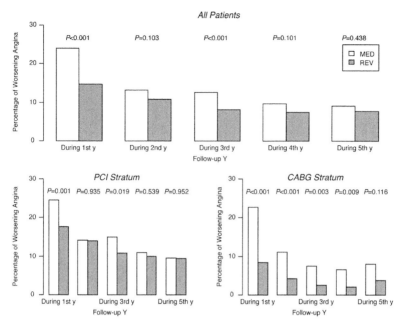

FIGURE 1.—Annual occurrence of worsening angina in optimal medical treatment with the option of subsequent revascularization (MED) and coronary revascularization and optimal medical treatment (REV) stratum. There was a significant decrease of worsening angina with REV compared with MED at 1 and 3 years in all patients and in the percutaneous coronary intervention (PCI) stratum patients. In the coronary artery bypass graft (CABG) stratum patients, the significant decrease with REV was observed during the first four years of follow-up. (Reprinted from Dagenais GR, the Bypass Angioplasty Revascularization Investigation 2 Diabetes (BARI 2D) Study Group. Effects of optimal medical treatment with or without coronary revascularization on angina and subsequent revascularizations in patients with type 2 diabetes mellitus and stable ischemic heart disease. *Circulation.* 2011;123:1492-1500. © American Heart Association, Inc.)

infarction between a strategy or optimal medical therapy with the option of subsequent revascularization versus the strategy of initial revascularization and optimal medical therapy.[1] Among patients with more severe disease, however, there was a benefit compared with medical therapy in regard to death and myocardial infarction in the stratum who underwent coronary artery bypass graft (CABG) but not in the percutaneous coronary intervention (PCI) group.[2]

Nonetheless, one of the main goals of therapy is to improve symptoms in quality of life. As pointed out in an accompanying editorial, we are limited, however, in our means of assessing clinically relevant differences in anginal severity, despite the use of the CCS classification and the Seattle anginal questionnaire.[3]

This is an important substudy from BARI 2D demonstrating a reduction in worsening angina, new-onset angina, and the need for revascularization at 3 years. This is more pronounced in the higher risk patients who had CABG. Notably, the initial differences declined over time and similar findings (ie, diminished effect size over time between therapies) were also noted in the

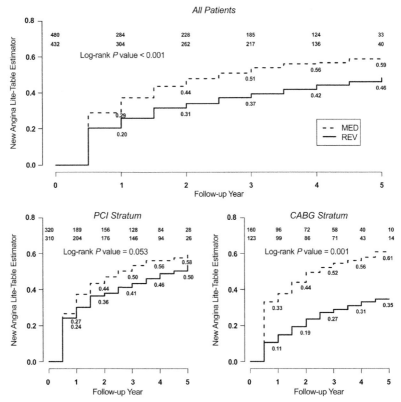

FIGURE 3.—Cumulative new angina rates for the 930 patients without angina at entry. For all patients and the coronary artery bypass graft (CABG) stratum patients, there were significantly lower rates of new angina throughout the follow-up in the entire and CABG stratum population randomized to coronary revascularization and optimal medical treatment (REV) compared with those randomized to the optimal medical treatment with the option of subsequent revascularization (MED) strategy. The lower rate in the percutaneous coronary intervention (PCI) stratum with the REV compared with MED strategy did not meet statistical significance. (Reprinted from Dagenais GR, the Bypass Angioplasty Revascularization Investigation 2 Diabetes (BARI 2D) Study Group. Effects of optimal medical treatment with or without coronary revascularization on angina and subsequent revascularizations in patients with type 2 diabetes mellitus and stable ischemic heart disease. *Circulation.* 2011;123:1492-1500. © American Heart Association, Inc.)

COURAGE trial. To some extent, this is because of crossover as patients who fail medical therapy had the option of subsequent revascularization, and in this respect, the trials are simply a mirror of clinical practice. Other contributing factors include efficacy of medications used to treat angina; self-imposed activity restriction, which may limit symptom severity; and the observation that angina in diabetics may wane over time, possibly as a result of ischemic preconditioning or the development of necrosis in areas of prior ischemia.

Taken in the context of the main trial results, these data support an initial strategy of medical therapy for patients with mild to moderate stable coronary artery disease (CCS Class 1–2) with the option of revascularization if this fails. The price to be paid for waiting is not an increased rate of death or myocardial infarction. Furthermore, there is no need for the trial of medical therapy to be drawn out: the drugs either work and are tolerated or they do not and are not; the decision in regard to revascularization can usually be made in a month or two. In patients with severe angina CCS Class 3—4 among whom medical therapy has probably already failed, I personally think that an additional trial of medical therapy is probably not required unless the patient is a bad surgical risk or anatomically unsuitable for PCI.

B. J. Gersh, MB, ChB, DPhil, FRCP

References

1. BARI 2D Study Group, Frye RL, August P, Brooks MM, et al. A randomized trial of therapies for type 2 diabetes and coronary artery disease. *N Engl J Med*. 2009; 360:2503-2515.
2. Chaitman BR, Hardison RM, Adler D, et al; Bypass Angioplasty Revascularization Investigation 2 Diabetes (BARI 2D) Study Group. The Bypass Angioplasty Revascularization Investigation 2 Diabetes randomized trial of different treatment strategies in type 2 diabetes mellitus with stable ischemic heart disease: impact of treatment strategy on cardiac mortality and myocardial infarction. *Circulation*. 2009;120:2529-2540.
3. Marso SP. Revascularization trumps medicine for patients with type 2 diabetes mellitus and chronic angina (or does it?). *Circulation*. 2011;123:1489-1491.

Impact of Angiographic Complete Revascularization After Drug-Eluting Stent Implantation or Coronary Artery Bypass Graft Surgery for Multivessel Coronary Artery Disease

Kim Y-H, Park D-W, Lee J-Y, et al (Univ of Ulsan College of Medicine, Seoul, South Korea)
Circulation 123:2373-2381, 2011

Background.—This study sought to evaluate the clinical impact of angiographic complete revascularization (CR) after drug-eluting stent implantation or coronary artery bypass graft surgery for multivessel coronary disease.

Methods and Results.—A total of 1914 consecutive patients with multivessel coronary disease undergoing drug-eluting stent implantation (1400 patients) or coronary artery bypass graft surgery (514 patients) were enrolled. Angiographic CR was defined as revascularization in all diseased segments according to the Synergy Between PCI With Taxus and Cardiac Surgery classification. The outcomes of patients undergoing CR were compared with those undergoing incomplete revascularization (IR) after adjustments with the inverse-probability-of-treatment weighting method. Angiographic CR was performed in 917 patients (47.9%) including 573 percutaneous coronary intervention (40.9%) and 344 coronary artery bypass graft (66.9%) patients. CR patients were younger and had more extensive coronary disease than IR patients. Over 5 years, CR patients had comparable incidences of death (8.9% versus 8.9%; adjusted hazard ratio, 1.04; 95% confidence interval, 0.76 to 1.43; $P=0.81$), the composite of death, myocardial infarction, and stroke (12.1% versus 11.9%; adjusted hazard ratio, 1.04; 95% confidence interval, 0.79 to 1.36; $P=0.80$), and the composite of death, myocardial infarction, stroke, and repeat revascularization (22.4% versus 24.9%; adjusted hazard ratio, 0.91; 95% confidence interval, 0.75 to 1.10; $P=0.32$) compared with IR patients. However, 368 patients (19.2%) with multivessel IR had a greater tendency toward higher risk of death, myocardial infarction, stroke, or repeat revascularization (30.3% versus 22.1%; adjusted hazard ratio, 1.27; 95% confidence interval, 0.97 to 1.66; $P=0.079$) than those without multivessel IR.

Conclusions.—Angiographic CR with drug-eluting stent implantation or coronary artery bypass grafting did not improve long-term clinical outcomes in patients with multivessel disease. This finding supports the strategy of ischemia-guided revascularization.

▶ The perceived advantages of complete revascularization are intuitively logical and have been the impetus for cardiac surgeons and interventionalists to perform complete revascularization (CR) when feasible. Nonetheless, the issue is not that clear cut, and the picture with regard to the advantages and disadvantages of CR versus incomplete revascularization (IR) are painted in shades of gray.

First, a major limiting factor is the lack of uniform definitions of completeness, and these are based on anatomy, the physiologic significance of lesion severity, and the presence of myocardial jeopardy in the area supplied by a stenotic vessel. Although many studies of both percutaneous coronary intervention and coronary bypass surgery have purported to demonstrate a benefit from CR, there are others in which the differences and survival are either not present or minimal, and the major impact has been on recurrent symptoms. Moreover, patients with IR are different compared with those with CR. Patients with IR are often "sicker" on the basis of age, comorbidities including diabetes and chronic renal failure, and the diffuseness of coronary artery disease. Multivariate analyses tend to adjust for baseline differences but cannot eliminate the effect of bypass because of confounders.

This study from Korea supports a prior surgical series suggesting that there is a spectrum of incompleteness.[1] Providing the left anterior descending territory is revascularized, it is not always necessary to revascularize all other diseased vessels. On the other hand, this study shows the potential hazard of leaving multiple vessels incompletely revascularized. Reasonable incomplete revascularization may be clinically indicated in certain situations guided by anatomic, functional, and physiologic parameters that define smaller areas of residual myocardium at risk.[2]

B. J. Gersh, MB, ChB, DPhil, FRCP

References

1. Rastan AJ, Walther T, Falk V, et al. Does reasonable incomplete surgical revascularization affect early or long-term survival in patients with multivessel coronary artery disease receiving left internal mammary artery bypass to left anterior descending artery? *Circulation.* 2009;120:S70-S77.
2. Dauerman HL. Reasonable incomplete revascularization. *Circulation.* 2011;123:2337-2340.

Long-Term Comparison of Drug-Eluting Stents and Coronary Artery Bypass Grafting for Multivessel Coronary Revascularization: 5-Year Outcomes From the Asan Medical Center-Multivessel Revascularization Registry
Park D-W, Kim Y-H, Song H-G, et al (Univ of Ulsan College of Medicine, Seoul, Korea)
J Am Coll Cardiol 57:128-137, 2011

Objectives.—We performed the long-term (5-year) follow-up of a large cohort of patients who underwent drug-eluting stent (DES) or coronary artery bypass graft (CABG) surgery for multivessel revascularization.

Background.—Limited information is available on very long-term outcomes after multivessel DES treatment relative to CABG.

Methods.—We evaluated 3,042 patients with multivessel disease who received DES (n = 1,547) or underwent CABG (n = 1,495) between January 2003 and December 2005, and for whom complete follow-up data were available for a median 5.6 years (interquartile range: 4.6 to 6.3 years). We compared adverse outcomes (death; a composite outcome of death, myocardial infarction, or stroke; and repeat revascularization).

Results.—After adjustment for differences in baseline risk factors, 5-year risk of death (hazard ratio [HR]: 1.00; 95% confidence interval [CI]: 0.76 to 1.32, p = 0.99) and the combined risk of death, myocardial infarction, or stroke (HR: 0.97; 95% CI: 0.76 to 1.24, p = 0.81) were similar between the DES group and the CABG group. However, the rates of revascularization were significantly higher in the DES group (HR: 2.93; 95% CI: 2.20 to 3.90, p < 0.001). Similar results were obtained in comparisons of DES with CABG for high-risk clinical and anatomic subgroups with diabetes mellitus, abnormal ventricular function, age 65 years or more, and 3-vessel and left main disease. However, mortality benefit with DES implantation relative to CABG was noted in patients with 2-vessel disease (HR: 0.57; 95% CI: 0.36 to 0.92, p = 0.02).

Conclusions.—or patients with multivessel disease, DES treatment, compared with CABG, showed similar rates of mortality and of the composite safety outcomes, but higher rates of revascularization up to 5 years (Fig 1).

▶ The strengths of this study are that it is a large registry with a 5-year follow-up, but its weakness is that it is just that—it is a registry, with all its limitations and advantages. Registries introduce selection bias but are of much greater relevance to the population at large.[1] On the other hand, a randomized trial is subject to entry bias because the inclusion criteria mandate clinical equipoise for both forms of therapy.[2] This is why the randomized trials are limited to a specific and minority proportion of all patients undergoing revascularization in a particular institution.

Nonetheless, with regard to registry studies, although multivariate models adjust for differences in baseline variables and confounders they simply cannot eliminate those differences. An interesting example of this with regard to patients who did or did not adhere to statin therapy was provided recently from a large database in British Columbia.[3]

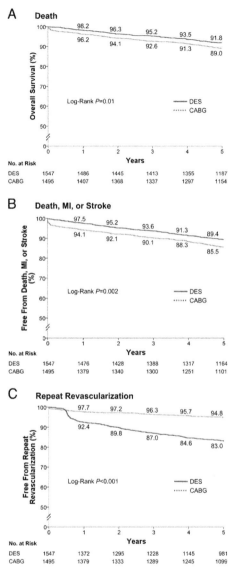

FIGURE 1.—Kaplan-Meier Curves of 5-Year Outcomes for Overall Patients Who Received DES or CABG. (**A**) Overall survival. (**B**) Freedom from death, myocardial infarction (MI), or stroke. (**C**) Repeat revascularization. CABG = coronary artery bypass graft surgery (**red line**); DES = drug-eluting stent(s) (**blue line**). For interpretation of the references to color in this figure legend, the reader is referred to web version of this article. (Reprinted from the Journal of the American College of Cardiology, Park D-W, Kim Y-H, Song H-G, et al. Long-term comparison of drug-eluting stents and coronary artery bypass grafting for multivessel coronary revascularization: 5-year outcomes from the Asan Medical Center-Multivessel Revascularization Registry. *J Am Coll Cardiol.* 2011;57:128-137. Copyright 2011, with permission from the American College of Cardiology.)

The 5-year data from this large single-center registry in Korea shows similar rates of mortality and composite safety outcomes with drug-eluting stents and coronary bypass surgery but higher rates of repeat revascularization after drug-eluting stents. These data are similar to those from the SYNTAX trial with a shorter length of follow-up, although recent data with patients stratified by the SYNTAX score are helpful by identifying high-risk patients who clearly benefit from bypass surgery and are a lower-risk minority who appear to do equally well with percutaneous coronary intervention versus coronary artery bypass graft. What remains to be seen is whether in certain subsets of patients, and particularly those at higher risk, whether the benefits of bypass surgery in terms of repeat revascularization may translate into mortality and safety benefits as well.[4,5]

B. J. Gersh, MB, ChB, DPhil, FRCP

References

1. Gersh BJ, Frye RL. Methods of coronary revascularization—things may not be as they seem. *N Engl J Med.* 2005;352:2235-2237.
2. Brown ML, Gersh BJ, Holmes DR, Bailey KR, Sundt TM 3rd. From randomized trials to registry studies: translating data into clinical information. *Nat Clin Pract Cardiovasc Med.* 2008;5:613-620.
3. Dormuth CR, Patrick AR, Shrank WH, et al. Statin adherence and risk of accidents: a cautionary tale. *Circulation.* 2009;119:2051-2057.
4. Banning AP, Westaby S, Morice MC. Diabetic and nondiabetic patients with left main and/or 3-vessel coronary artery disease: comparison of outcomes with cardiac surgery and paclitaxel-eluting stents. *J Am Coll Cardiol.* 2010;55:1067-1075.
5. Gulati R, Rihal CS, Gersh BJ. The SYNTAX trial: a perspective. *Circ Cardiovasc Interv.* 2009;2:463-467.

Radial Artery Grafts vs Saphenous Vein Grafts in Coronary Artery Bypass Surgery: A Randomized Trial

Goldman S, Sethi GK, Holman W, et al (Southern Arizona VA Health Care System, Tucson; Veterans Affairs Med Ctr, Birmingham, AL; et al)
JAMA 305:167-174, 2011

Context.—Arterial grafts are thought to be better conduits than saphenous vein grafts for coronary artery bypass grafting (CABG) based on experience with using the left internal mammary artery to bypass the left anterior descending coronary artery. The efficacy of the radial artery graft is less clear.

Objective.—To compare 1-year angiographic patency of radial artery grafts vs saphenous vein grafts in patients undergoing elective CABG.

Design, Setting, and Participants.—Multicenter, randomized controlled trial conducted from February 2003 to February 2009 at 11 Veterans Affairs medical centers among 757 participants (99% men) undergoing first-time elective CABG.

Interventions.—The left internal mammary artery was used to preferentially graft the left anterior descending coronary artery whenever possible;

the best remaining recipient vessel was randomized to radial artery vs saphenous vein graft.

Main Outcome Measures.—The primary end point was angiographic graft patency at 1 year after CABG. Secondary end points included angiographic graft patency at 1 week after CABG, myocardial infarction, stroke, repeat revascularization, and death.

Results.—Analysis included 733 patients (366 in the radial artery group, 367 in the saphenous vein group). There was no significant difference in study graft patency at 1 year after CABG (radial artery, 238/266; 89%; 95% confidence interval [CI], 86%-93%; saphenous vein, 239/269; 89%; 95% CI, 85%-93%; adjusted OR, 0.99; 95% CI, 0.56-1.74; $P=.98$). There were no significant differences in the secondary end points.

Conclusion.—Among Veterans Affairs patients undergoing first-time elective CABG, the use of a radial artery graft compared with saphenous vein graft did not result in greater 1-year patency.

Trial Registration.—clinicaltrials.gov Identifier: NCT00054847.

▶ This randomized trial is one of several studies from the Veterans Administration (VA) Cooperative Studies Program aimed at evaluating long-term graft patency after coronary bypass surgery (CABG). This particular trial compared radial artery grafts to saphenous vein grafts (SVG) in patients undergoing elective first-time CABG, among whom the left internal mammary artery (IMA) was used preferentially to bypass the left anterior descending coronary artery if possible, and this was the case in 86% of patients. At 1 year, there was no difference in angiographic graft patency or in clinical endpoints.

It is generally assumed that arterial conduits have superior patency rates compared with SVG, but there is a lack of data on radial artery grafts as opposed to the unequivocal evidence in regard to the IMA. A prior Canadian study demonstrated higher patency rates with radial versus SVG (92% vs 86%),[1] but in this trial, the patency of SVG was higher at 89%. Other studies have demonstrated excellent long-term patency rates with radial grafts.[2] Other potential differences between the 2 studies include the use of only 1 study graft per patient with the surgeon choosing the best recipient vessel, whereas in the Canadian study, each patient had both study grafts. Theoretically, the approach used in this VA trial should have resulted in the best chance for patency for each graft and an opportunity to define the patient characteristics that predict graft patency.

The radial artery can develop arteriosclerosis and calcification, especially in diabetics, in addition to propensity for increased vasoreactivity and coronary spasm, particularly if the underlying stenosis of the vessel being bypassed is less severe. In this trial, among diabetics, patency appeared higher with saphenous vein grafts. Another finding is the lower patency rate with endoscopic harvesting of SVG.

This study certainly suggests no advantage from using radial artery grafts as opposed to SVG, although one wonders what the 5- or 10-year data would look like. It appears, however, that the VA Cooperative Studies Program has funded a 5-year angiographic follow-up study. Another issue is the comparison of single versus bilateral internal mammary artery grafting. At 1 year in the Arterial Revascularization Trial, outcomes were similar but with a small increase in the need for sternal reconstruction after bilateral IMA grafting.[3] Ten-year data from this trial could provide answers to important clinical questions, but it will take many years before we have the final results of this study, and one concern is that too many patients will be lost to follow-up.[4]

B. J. Gersh, MB, ChB, DPhil, FRCP

References

1. Desai ND, Cohen EA, Naylor CD, Fremes SE; Radial Artery Patency Study Investigators. A randomized comparison of radial-artery and saphenous-vein coronary bypass grafts. *N Engl J Med.* 2004;351:2302-2309.
2. Tatoulis J, Buxton BF, Fuller JA, et al. Long-term patency of 1108 radial arterial-coronary angiograms over 10 years. *Ann Thorac Surg.* 2009;88:23-29.
3. Taggart DP, Altman DG, Gray AM, et al; ART Investigators. Randomized trial to compare bilateral vs. single internal mammary coronary artery bypass grafting: 1-year results of the Arterial Revascularisation Trial (ART). *Eur Heart J.* 2010; 31:2470-2481.
4. Kappetein AP. Bilateral mammary artery vs. single mammary artery grafting: promising early results: but will the match finish with enough players? *Eur Heart J.* 2010;31:2444-2446.

Radial versus femoral access for coronary angiography and intervention in patients with acute coronary syndromes (RIVAL): a randomised, parallel group, multicentre trial

Jolly SS, for the RIVAL trial group (McMaster Univ and the Population Health Res Inst, Hamilton, Ontario, Canada; et al)

Lancet 377:1409-1420, 2011

Background.—Small trials have suggested that radial access for percutaneous coronary intervention (PCI) reduces vascular complications and bleeding compared with femoral access. We aimed to assess whether radial access was superior to femoral access in patients with acute coronary syndromes (ACS) who were undergoing coronary angiography with possible intervention.

Methods.—The RadIal Vs femorAL access for coronary intervention (RIVAL) trial was a randomised, parallel group, multicentre trial. Patients with ACS were randomly assigned (1:1) by a 24 h computerised central automated voice response system to radial or femoral artery access. The primary outcome was a composite of death, myocardial infarction, stroke, or non-coronary artery bypass graft (non-CABG)-related major bleeding at 30 days. Key secondary outcomes were death, myocardial infarction, or stroke; and non-CABG-related major bleeding at 30 days. A masked central committee adjudicated the primary outcome, components of the primary outcome, and stent thrombosis. All other outcomes were as reported by the investigators. Patients and investigators were not masked to treatment allocation. Analyses were by intention to treat. This trial is registered with ClinicalTrials.gov, NCT01014273.

Findings.—Between June 6, 2006, and Nov 3, 2010, 7021 patients were enrolled from 158 hospitals in 32 countries. 3507 patients were randomly assigned to radial access and 3514 to femoral access. The primary outcome occurred in 128 (3·7%) of 3507 patients in the radial access group compared with 139 (4·0%) of 3514 in the femoral access group (hazard ratio [HR] 0·92, 95% CI 0·72−1·17; p=0·50). Of the six prespecified subgroups, there was a significant interaction for the primary outcome with benefit for radial access in highest tertile volume radial centres (HR 0·49, 95% CI 0·28−0·87; p=0·015) and in patients with ST-segment elevation myocardial infarction (0·60, 0·38−0·94; p=0·026). The rate of death, myocardial infarction, or stroke at 30 days was 112 (3·2%) of 3507 patients in the radial group compared with 114 (3·2%) of 3514 in the femoral group (HR 0·98, 95% CI 0·76−1·28; p=0·90). The rate of non-CABG-related major bleeding at 30 days was 24 (0·7%) of 3507 patients in the radial group compared with 33 (0·9%) of 3514 patients in the femoral group (HR 0·73, 95% CI 0·43−1·23; p=0·23). At 30 days, 42 of 3507 patients in the radial group had large haematoma compared with 106 of 3514 in the femoral group (HR 0·40, 95% CI 0·28−0·57; p<0·0001). Pseudoaneurysm needing closure occurred in seven of 3507 patients in the radial group compared with 23 of 3514 in the femoral group (HR 0·30, 95% CI 0·13−0·71; p=0·006).

Interpretation.—Radial and femoral approaches are both safe and effective for PCI. However, the lower rate of local vascular complications may be a reason to use the radial approach (Fig 2).

▶ In patients with acute coronary syndrome undergoing percutaneous coronary intervention (PCI), bleeding is not only a common complication, but it is an independent predictor of mortality, although confounding variables associated with bleeding, for example, age and renal dysfunction, are also contributory factors to adverse outcomes.[1] A substantial portion of bleeding occurs at vascular access sites, and observational studies and a meta-analysis have suggested a lower rate of bleeding with radial versus femoral access, a weak reduction in the incidence of death, myocardial infarction, or stroke, but a lower rate of angiographic PCI success.[2]

This large multinational trial of 7021 patients found that both procedures were safe and that the primary outcome of death, myocardial infarction, stroke, or non−coronary artery bypass graft−related bleeding was no different in the 2 groups at 30 days. However, radial access was significantly associated with fewer vascular complications but with similar PCI success rates and was also more commonly preferred among patients requiring an additional procedure. What is not at all clear to me is why the radial access appeared superior in terms of the primary endpoint in patients with ST-elevation myocardial infarction; it could be because there is a higher rate of bleeding in STEMI patients and because many are younger, and with less vascular disease, the procedure is easy to perform.

Clearly, there is a learning curve to the radial procedure, and the results are better in those centers that perform a higher number of radial procedures, but the converse was not seen in centers that performed a higher number of procedures by the femoral route. The data suggest that expertise in volume may be

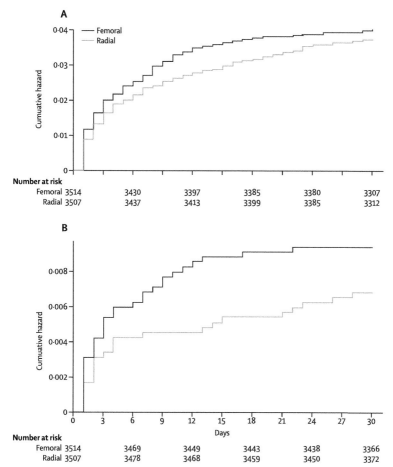

FIGURE 2.—Kaplan-Meier event curves for the primary outcome and a key secondary outcome. (A) Composite primary outcome of death, myocardial infarction, stroke, or non-coronary artery bypass graft related major bleeding. (B) Secondary outcome of non-coronary artery bypass graft related major bleeding. (Reprinted from The Lancet, Jolly SS, for the RIVAL trial group. Radial versus femoral access for coronary angiography and intervention in patients with acute coronary syndromes (RIVAL): a randomised, parallel group, multicentre trial. *Lancet.* 2011;377:1409-1420. © 2011, with permission from Elsevier.)

linked to outcomes in the case of the radial procedure, although other data would suggest that overall outcomes are related in any event to overall procedural volume.

B. J. Gersh, MB, ChB, DPhil, FRCP

References

1. Mehran R, Pocock SJ, Stone GW, et al. Associations of major bleeding and myocardial infarction with the incidence and timing of mortality in patients presenting with non-ST-elevation acute coronary syndromes: a risk model from the ACUITY trial. *Eur Heart J.* 2009;30:1457-1466.

2. Jolly SS, Amlani S, Hamon M, Yusuf S, Mehta SR. Radial versus femoral access for coronary angiography or intervention and the impact on major bleeding and ischemic events: a systematic review and meta-analysis of randomized trials. *Am Heart J.* 2009;157:132-140.

Recent Changes in Practice of Elective Percutaneous Coronary Intervention for Stable Angina

Ahmed B, on behalf of the Northern New England Cardiovascular Disease Study (Univ of New Mexico, Albuquerque; et al)
Circ Cardiovasc Qual Outcomes 4:300-305, 2011

Background.—The COURAGE (Clinical Outcomes Utilizing Revascularization and Aggressive Drug Evaluation) trial was designed to compare optimal medical therapy alone versus optimal medical therapy and percutaneous coronary intervention (PCI) for treatment of patients with stable coronary artery disease and showed equal efficacy for optimal medical therapy with or without PCI. The impact of results from the COURAGE trial on clinical practice is unknown.

Methods and Results.—We analyzed 26 388 consecutive patients from the Northern New England Cardiovascular Disease PCI Registry who underwent PCI between January 2006 and June 2009. We identified a COURAGE-like patient group as patients who were undergoing (1) an elective procedure; (2) for an indication of stable angina; and (3) on the day of admission (ie, the date of admission was the same as the procedure date). All other PCI patients were placed in an "other indications" cohort. We compared temporal trends in overall volume in PCI for stable angina and for other indications, comparing quarterly time periods before and after release of COURAGE in March 2007. Over the study period, there was a statistically significant decrease in total PCI volume from 2064 in Quarter 1 2006 (before COURAGE) to 1708 in Quarter 3 2007 (after COURAGE) ($P<0.01$). These trends were sustained through June 2009, with an approximate 16% peak relative reduction in all PCI compared with before COURAGE. As a percentage of all PCI, stable angina reached a high of 20.9% before COURAGE and began to decrease immediately after publication of COURAGE in Quarter 2 2007 to 16.1% ($P<0.01$). Among patients undergoing PCI for stable angina, there was a significant 26% peak decrease in post-COURAGE PCI volumes compared with pre-COURAGE Quarter 1 2006 (P trend, 0.01), which was maintained through the end of the study period.

Conclusions.—Publication of results from the COURAGE trial was temporally associated with a significant and sustained decline in the use of PCI to treat patients with stable angina. The long-term impact of this change in practice on patient outcomes remains to be determined (Fig 2).

▶ This is a rather encouraging article in that it suggests that in regard to coronary revascularization for chronic stable angina, we are adopting evidence-based

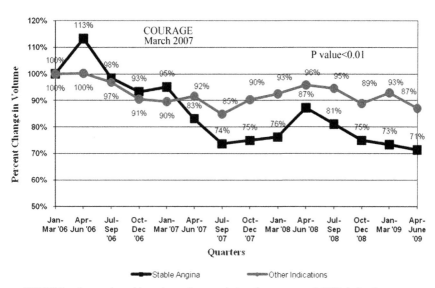

FIGURE 2.—Among the stable angina patient population, there was a peak 25% decline in percutaneous coronary intervention (PCI) for stable angina after COURAGE (Clinical Outcomes Utilizing Revascularization and Aggressive Drug Evaluation) relative to pre-COUARGE Quarter 1 2006. This change was maintained through June 2009. NNE indicates Northern New England Cardiovascular Disease Study Group. (Reprinted from Ahmed B, on behalf of the Northern New England Cardiovascular Disease Study. Recent changes in practice of elective percutaneous coronary intervention for stable angina. *Circ Cardiovasc Qual Outcomes.* 2011;4:300-305. © American Heart Association, Inc.)

therapies based on randomized clinical trials. This is an important issue because it is estimated that more than 16 million people in the United States have chronic stable angina.[1] Moreover, the current guidelines strongly recommend that in patients with mild to moderate chronic stable angina, initial therapy should be a trial of optimal medical treatment with revascularization as a subsequent option.

The COURAGE and BARI 2D trials strongly support the approach suggested by the guidelines.[2] Nonetheless, both trials also ignited a storm of controversy because they did not support a role for routine revascularization, contrary to the expectations in many. One caveat is that all of the patients in these trials were randomized after coronary angiography and as such are highly selected, but in the planning stage is an important clinical trial that will focus on randomization at the time of stress testing. This study from the Northern New England Cardiovascular Registry (NNECVR) suggests that we are behaving responsibly by demonstrating a temporarily associated, significant, and sustained decline in the use of percutaneous coronary intervention to treat patients with chronic stable angina. This is just as well because if we as cardiologists do not follow our own guidelines, particularly in the face of good evidence, then the decision to perform revascularization could be taken out of our hands. In this era of increasing evidence-based care, it is physicians who need to take the lead and not payors and administrators.[3]

B. J. Gersh, MB, ChB, DPhil, FRCP

References

1. Lloyd-Jones D, Adams RJ, Brown TM, et al; American Heart Association Statistics Committee and Stroke Statistics Subcommittee. Heart disease and stroke statistics—2010 update: a report from the American Heart Association. *Circulation.* 2010;121:e46-e215.
2. Boden WE, O'Rourke RA, Teo KK, et al. Optimal medical therapy with or without PCI for stable coronary disease. *N Engl J Med.* 2007;356:1503-1516.
3. Holmes DR Jr, Gersh BJ, Whitlow P, King SB 3rd, Dove JT. Percutaneous coronary intervention for chronic stable angina: a reassessment. *JACC Cardiovasc Interv.* 2008;1:34-43.

Secondary Prevention After Coronary Artery Bypass Graft Surgery: Findings of a National Randomized Controlled Trial and Sustained Society-Led Incorporation Into Practice

Williams JB, for the Society of Thoracic Surgeons and the National Cardiac Database (Duke Univ School of Medicine, Durham, NC; et al)
Circulation 123:39-45, 2011

Background.—Despite evidence supporting the use of aspirin, β-blockers, angiotensin-converting enzyme inhibitors, and lipid-lowering therapies in eligible patients, adoption of these secondary prevention measures after coronary artery bypass grafting has been inconsistent. We sought to rigorously test on a national scale whether low-intensity continuous quality improvement interventions can be used to speed secondary prevention adherence after coronary artery bypass grafting.

Methods and Results.—A total of 458 hospitals participating in the Society of Thoracic Surgeons National Cardiac Database and treating 361 328 patients undergoing isolated coronary artery bypass grafting were randomized to either a control or an intervention group. The intervention group received continuous quality improvement materials designed to influence the prescription of the secondary prevention medications at discharge. The primary outcome measure was discharge prescription rates of the targeted secondary prevention medications at intervention versus control sites, assessed by measuring preintervention and postintervention site differences. Prerandomization treatment patterns and baseline data were similar in the control (n = 234) and treatment (n = 224) groups. Individual medication use and composite adherence increased over 24 months in both groups, with a markedly more rapid rate of adherence uptake among the intervention hospitals and a statistically significant therapy hazard ratio in the intervention versus control group for all 4 secondary prevention medications.

Conclusions.—Provider-led, low-intensity continuous quality improvement efforts can improve the adoption of care processes into national practice within the context of a medical specialty society infrastructure. The findings of the present trial have led to the incorporation of study

TABLE 2.—Improvement in Secondary Prevention Medication Adherence Scores

	Control Mean Change (n=234), %	Intervention Mean Change (n=224), %	P
Discharge medications			
ASA	2.9	4.2	0.255
β-blockers	9.7	12.2	0.032
ACEIs	6.4	13.1	<0.001
Lipid lowering	13.1	15.7	0.017
All vs not all	12.1	16.7	0.001

P values refer to between-group changes.

outcome metrics into a medical society rating system for ongoing quality improvement (Table 2).

▶ This important article addresses the role of secondary prevention and continuous quality improvement (CQI). There is no doubt about the benefits of secondary prevention in patients who have undergone coronary bypass surgery, and the guidelines are quite clear about this, but the evidence suggests that the adoption of these measures has lagged behind implementation after percutaneous coronary intervention.[1]

This study using the Society of Thoracic Surgeons database was designed as a cluster randomized trial in which sites were randomized to control or an intervention; the latter was defined by the receipt of CQI materials designed to influence the discharge prescription rates of the targeted secondary prevention medications. It is of interest that the use of adherence to medications over 24 months improved in both groups, but there was a much more rapid rate of adherence uptake among intervention hospitals, and in this respect the intervention is judged to be successful.

The concepts of CQI in its current form emerged in the early 1980s.[2] At its core is the importance of process management and feedback in any system, whether industry or medical, designed to measure and manage quality.

The hospital environment, particularly after an invasive procedure or an acute event is the ideal environment for patient and health care provider education and is the ideal setting for the implementation of protocols designed to initiate secondary prevention before and after discharge. An unanswered question in regard to this study, however, is the long-term adherence rates after completion of the trial. Moreover, as pointed out in the accompanying editorial, adherence to discharge medications provides only part of the picture, although we do have good evidence that these drugs are effective.[3]

The message from this study is quite clear in that provider-led low-intensity continuous quality improvement efforts can certainly improve the adoption of clinical care processes in international practice. Such protocols need to be in place after bypass surgery, percutaneous coronary intervention, and in other cardiovascular care settings in addition to their value in patients hospitalized with other conditions. After all, cardiovascular disease remains the leading cause of mortality worldwide.

B. J. Gersh, MB, ChB, DPhil, FRCP

References

1. Hiratzka LF, Eagle KA, Liang L, Fonarow GC, LaBresh KA, Peterson ED; Get With the Guidelines Steering Committee. Atherosclerosis secondary prevention performance measures after coronary bypass graft surgery compared with percutaneous catheter intervention and nonintervention patients in the Get With the Guidelines database. *Circulation.* 2007;116:I207-I212.
2. Deming WE. *Out of the Crisis.* Boston, MA: Massachusetts Institute of Technology; 1986.
3. Gardner TJ. Can we take continuous quality improvement to the next level? *Circulation.* 2011;123:8-9.

Trends in Coronary Revascularization in the United States From 2001 to 2009: Recent Declines in Percutaneous Coronary Intervention Volumes

Riley RF, Don CW, Powell W, et al (Univ of Washington, Seattle)
Circ Cardiovasc Qual Outcomes 4:193-197, 2011

Background.—There is speculation that the volume of percutaneous coronary interventions (PCIs) has been decreasing over the past several years. Published studies of PCI volume have evaluated regional or hospital trends, but few have captured national data. This study describes the use of coronary angiography and revascularization methods in Medicare patients from 2001 to 2009.

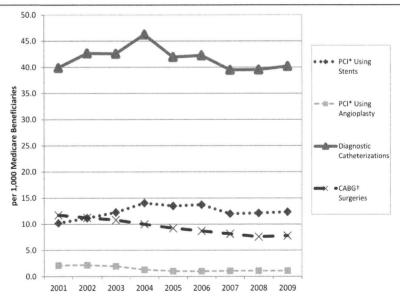

FIGURE 1.—Trends in total coronary procedures per 1000 Medicare beneficiaries from 2001 to 2009. (Reprinted from Riley RF, Don CW, Powell W, et al. Trends in coronary revascularization in the United States from 2001 to 2009: recent declines in percutaneous coronary intervention volumes. *Circ Cardiovasc Qual Outcomes.* 2011;4:193-197. © American Heart Association, Inc.)

Methods and Results.—This retrospective study used data from the Centers for Medicare & Medicaid Services from 2001 to 2009. The annual number of coronary angiograms, PCI, intravascular ultrasound, fractional flow reserve, and coronary artery bypass graft (CABG) surgery procedures were determined from billing data and adjusted for the number of Medicare recipients. From 2001 to 2009, the average year-to-year increase for PCI was 1.3% per 1000 beneficiaries, whereas the mean annual decrease for CABG surgery was 5%. However, the increase in PCI volume occurred primarily from 2001 to 2004, as there was a mean annual rate of decline of

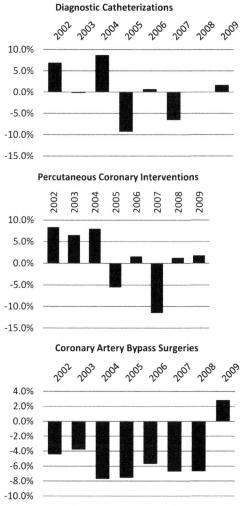

FIGURE 2.—Year-to-year percent change in coronary procedures per 1000 Medicare beneficiaries. (Reprinted from Riley RF, Don CW, Powell W, et al. Trends in coronary revascularization in the United States from 2001 to 2009: recent declines in percutaneous coronary intervention volumes. *Circ Cardiovasc Qual Outcomes.* 2011;4:193-197. © American Heart Association, Inc.)

2.5% from 2004 to 2009; similar trends were seen with diagnostic angiography. The use of intravascular ultrasound and fractional flow reserve steadily increased over time.

Conclusions.—This study confirms recent speculation that PCI volume has begun to decrease. Although rates of CABG have waned for several decades, all forms of coronary revascularization have been declining since 2004 (Figs 1 and 2).

▶ This retrospective study, using a massive billing database from the Centers for Medicaid and Medicare Services, demonstrates that the days of coronary artery bypass graft (CABG) and percutaneous coronary intervention (PCI) as a growth industry are probably over. Declines in the usage rates of CABG were demonstrated more than a decade ago both in the United States and Europe and are likely the direct result of the expansion of PCI.[1] More recently, the perception is that the volume of PCI procedures has also declined and the causes are likely multifactorial, including advances in medical therapy and in particular primary and secondary prevention; the use of drug-eluting stents, resulting in a dramatic reduction in restenosis; and hopefully some impact from the results of the COURAGE and BARI 2D trials.[2]

This study quite emphatically reinforces prior perceptions and reports and demonstrates the persistent decline in CABG utilization rates; with regard to PCI, after a peak in 2004, there has been a substantial decline, accompanied also by a decline in the use of diagnostic catheterization. The slight increases in the usage rates of PCI or CABG in 2009 is of uncertain significance, but regardless the numbers remain below their levels in prior years.

What is encouraging is the increase in the use of intravascular ultrasound and fractional flow reserve (FFR) studies, which suggest that the message that PCI needs to be directive toward physiologically and hemodynamically significant as opposed to visual assessment of stenoses is getting the attention it deserves.[3] Limitations to this study include the use of billing codes, which are subject to error, and the lack of clinical data in regard to the indications for the procedure and whether urgent or emergent.

Have these trends stabilized as would appear to be the case in 2009? It is too early to tell.

B. J. Gersh, MB, ChB, DPhil, FRCP

References

1. Gerber Y, Rihal CS, Sundt TM 3rd, et al. Coronary revascularization in the community. A population-based study, 1990 to 2004. *J Am Coll Cardiol.* 2007; 50:1223-1229.
2. Boden WE, O'Rourke RA, Teo KK, et al. Optimal medical therapy with or without PCI for stable coronary disease. *N Engl J Med.* 2007;356:1503-1516.
3. Pijls NH, Fearon WF, Tonino PA, et al; FAME Study Investigators. Fractional flow reserve versus angiography for guiding percutaneous coronary intervention in patients with multivessel coronary artery disease: 2-year follow-up of the FAME (Fractional Flow Reserve Versus Angiography for Multivessel Evaluation) study. *J Am Coll Cardiol.* 2010;56:177-184.

Epidemiology

Adolescent BMI Trajectory and Risk of Diabetes versus Coronary Disease

Tirosh A, Shai I, Afek A, et al (Boston Univ Med Ctr, MA; Ben-Gurion Univ of the Negev, Beer-Sheva, Israel; Chaim Sheba Med Ctr, Tel-Hashomer, Israel; et al)
N Engl J Med 364:1315-1325, 2011

Background.—The association of body-mass index (BMI) from adolescence to adulthood with obesity-related diseases in young adults has not been completely delineated.

Methods.—We conducted a prospective study in which we followed 37,674 apparently healthy young men for incident angiography-proven coronary heart disease and diabetes through the Staff Periodic Examination Center of the Israeli Army Medical Corps. The height and weight of participants were measured at regular intervals, with the first measurements taken when they were 17 years of age.

Results.—During approximately 650,000 person-years of follow-up (mean follow-up, 17.4 years), we documented 1173 incident cases of type 2 diabetes and 327 of coronary heart disease. In multivariate models adjusted for age, family history, blood pressure, lifestyle factors, and biomarkers in blood, elevated adolescent BMI (the weight in kilograms divided by the square of the height in meters; mean range for the first through last deciles, 17.3 to 27.6) was a significant predictor of both diabetes (hazard ratio for the highest vs. the lowest decile, 2.76; 95% confidence interval [CI], 2.11 to 3.58) and angiography-proven coronary heart disease (hazard ratio, 5.43; 95% CI, 2.77 to 10.62). Further adjustment for BMI at adulthood completely ablated the association of adolescent BMI with diabetes (hazard ratio, 1.01; 95% CI, 0.75 to 1.37) but not the association with coronary heart disease (hazard ratio, 6.85; 95% CI, 3.30 to 14.21). After adjustment of the BMI values as continuous variables in multivariate models, only elevated BMI in adulthood was significantly associated with diabetes ($\beta = 1.115$, $P = 0.003$; $P = 0.89$ for interaction). In contrast, elevated BMI in both adolescence ($\beta = 1.355$, $P = 0.004$) and adulthood ($\beta = 1.207$, $P = 0.03$) were independently associated with angiography-proven coronary heart disease ($P = 0.048$ for interaction).

Conclusions.—An elevated BMI in adolescence — one that is well within the range currently considered to be normal — constitutes a substantial risk factor for obesity-related disorders in midlife. Although the risk of diabetes is mainly associated with increased BMI close to the time of diagnosis, the risk of coronary heart disease is associated with an elevated BMI both in adolescence and in adulthood, supporting the hypothesis that the processes causing incident coronary heart disease, particularly atherosclerosis, are more gradual than those resulting in incident diabetes. (Funded by the

Chaim Sheba Medical Center and the Israel Defense Forces Medical Corps.) (Fig 2).

▶ This is a somewhat unique prospective longitudinal follow-up study from Israel. These data are extremely relevant from the standpoint of concern that the continued decline in cardiovascular mortality in the United States is starting to level off and, in fact, may be increasing in some young subgroups.[1] A key question is whether there will be a phase 5 of the epidemiologic transition as a consequence of the global epidemic of diabetes and obesity.[2]

It is well established that obesity in adulthood is a risk factor for both type 2 diabetes and coronary heart disease. What has been less clear is the role of obesity starting earlier in life, in particular, the interaction with other pathophysiologic mechanisms of obesity-related diseases and, if so, whether this occurs in a range of BMI that might be considered normal. This study comprises 37 000 apparently healthy young men who have 17.4 years of mean follow-up with initial measurements made at the age of 17 years. The results are sobering to say the least. An elevated BMI in adolescence (range, 17.3 in the bottom decile to 27.6 in the top decile—may therefore be in the normal range) was a significant predictor of both diabetes and angiographically documented coronary artery disease. Further adjusted analyses found that BMI in adulthood abolishes the statistical significance of adolescent BMI with regard to diabetes but not as a predictor of coronary artery disease. Both BMI in adolescence and adulthood

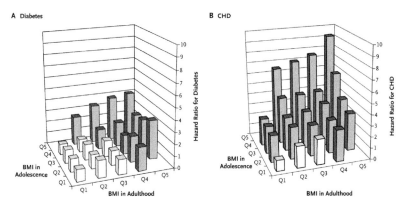

FIGURE 2.—Hazard Ratios for the Risk of Diabetes and Coronary Heart Disease among Apparently Healthy Young Adults, According to BMI in Adolescence and in Adulthood. The joint association of body-mass index (BMI) at 17 years of age (adolescence) and 30 years of age (adulthood) is shown for the incidence of diabetes (Panel A) and the incidence of angiography-proven coronary heart disease (CHD) (Panel B), as calculated with the use of multivariate Cox proportional-hazards models. The gray columns denote significantly elevated hazard ratios as compared with those in the lowest BMI quintile in both adolescence and adulthood (reference group). When BMI was analyzed as a continuous variable with the use of a Cox regression model adjusted for age, triglyceride level, presence or absence of a family history of diabetes, and fasting glucose level, only BMI in adulthood was significantly associated with the risk of diabetes ($\beta = 1.115$, P = 0.003; P = 0.89 for interaction with BMI in adolescence). In contrast, in a regression model adjusted for age, triglyceride level, smoking status, presence or absence of a family history of CHD, and levels of high-density lipoprotein cholesterol and low-density lipoprotein cholesterol, BMI in both adolescence and adulthood was significantly and independently associated with the risk of CHD (BMI in adolescence, $\beta = 1.355$, P = 0.004; BMI in adulthood, $\beta = 1.207$, P = 0.03; P < 0.05 for interaction). (Reprinted from Tirosh A, Shai I, Afek A, et al. Adolescent BMI trajectory and risk of diabetes versus coronary disease. N Engl J Med. 2011;364:1315-1325. © 2011 Massachusetts Medical Society.)

predict coronary disease. These data also support the hypothesis that the processes causing incident coronary heart disease, particularly atherosclerosis, are more gradual than those causing diabetes.

The implications for primary prevention are also far reaching. A decline in funding for sporting activities at schools, the advent of the computer generation, and increasing prosperity among other factors are causing a global epidemic of diabetes and obesity. It is likely that the epidemic of premature coronary artery disease will not lag far behind.

B. J. Gersh, MB, ChB, DPhil, FRCP

References

1. Ford ES, Capewell S. Coronary heart disease mortality among young adults in the U.S. from 1980 through 2002: concealed leveling of mortality rates. *J Am Coll Cardiol.* 2007;50:2128-2132.
2. Gersh BJ, Sliwa K, Myosi BM, Yusuf S. Novel therapeutic concepts: the epidemic of cardiovascular disease in the developing world: global implications. *Eur Heart J.* 2010;31:642-648.

Global Variation in the Relative Burden of Stroke and Ischemic Heart Disease

Kim AS, Johnston SC (Univ of California, San Francisco)
Circulation 124:314-323, 2011

Background.—Although stroke and ischemic heart disease (IHD) have several well-established risk factors in common, the extent of global variation in the relative burdens of these forms of vascular disease and reasons for any observed variation are poorly understood.

Methods and Results.—We analyzed mortality and disability-adjusted life-year loss rates from stroke and IHD, as well as national estimates of vascular risk factors that have been developed by the World Health Organization Burden of Disease Program. National income data were derived from World Bank estimates. We used linear regression for univariable analysis and the Cuzick test for trends. Among 192 World Health Organization member countries, stroke mortality rates exceeded IHD rates in 74 countries (39%), and stroke disability-adjusted life-year loss rates exceeded IHD rates in 62 countries (32%). Stroke mortality ranged from 12.7% higher to 27.2% lower than IHD, and stroke disability-adjusted life-year loss rates ranged from 6.2% higher to 10.2% lower than IHD. Stroke burden was disproportionately higher in China, Africa, and South America, whereas IHD burden was higher in the Middle East, North America, Australia, and much of Europe. Lower national income was associated with higher relative mortality ($P<0.001$) and burden of disease ($P=0.001$) from stroke. Diabetes mellitus prevalence and mean serum cholesterol were each associated with greater relative burdens from IHD even after adjustment for national income.

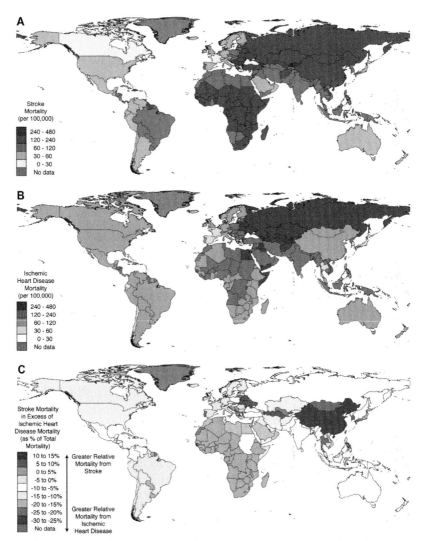

FIGURE 1.—Geographic distribution of relative mortality from stroke and ischemic heart disease (World Health Organization Global Burden of Disease Program, 2004). **A,** Age- and sex-adjusted absolute stroke mortality rates per 100 000, standardized to standard World Health Organization population. The intensity of red shading is proportional to the absolute mortality rates. **B,** Age- and sex-adjusted absolute ischemic heart disease mortality rates per 100 000, standardized to standard World Health Organization population. The intensity of blue shading is proportional to the absolute mortality rates. **C,** Mortality from stroke relative to ischemic heart disease. Countries with more intense blue shading have higher relative mortality rates from stroke than from ischemic heart disease, and countries with more intense red shading have higher relative mortality rates from ischemic heart disease than from stroke. For interpretation of the references to color in this figure legend, the reader is referred to web version of this article. (Reprinted from Kim AS, Johnston SC. Global variation in the relative burden of stroke and ischemic heart disease. *Circulation.* 2011;124:314-323, with permission from American Heart Association.)

Conclusions.—There is substantial global variation in the relative burden of stroke compared with IHD. The disproportionate burden from stroke for many lower-income countries suggests that distinct interventions may be required (Fig 1).

▶ Ischemic heart disease and cardiovascular disease are the 2 leading causes of death in the world, accounting for approximately 20% of all deaths.[1] Both conditions involve overlapping atherosclerotic disease mechanisms and share major modifiable risk factors, although ischemic heart disease is generally considered to have a greater global impact than stroke.

This study used data from the World Health Organization Burden of Disease Program to demonstrate marked global variations in the relative burdens of stroke versus ischemic heart disease on both mortality and morbidity. There was a disproportionately greater stroke burden in China, Africa, and South America, with ischemic heart disease the leader in the Middle East, North America, Australia, and much of Europe. Lower-income countries tend to have a relatively greater relative stroke burden overall, which is likely related to associations with vascular risk factor profiles including hypertension and diets with heavy salt intake. These data exemplify the different stages of the epidemiological transition that provides a framework for understanding the impact of socioeconomic status on the development of cardiovascular disease.[2,3] This could also be a reflection of genetic/ethnic variations in response to the standard risk factors. Because resources are limited, particularly in the developing world, a better understanding of the reasons underlying these striking variations might facilitate the development and maximize the effect of national initiatives and targeted interventions.

B. J. Gersh, MB, ChB, DPhil, FRCP

References

1. Mathers CD, Loncar D. Projections of global mortality and burden of disease from 2002 to 2030. *PLoS Med.* 2006;3:e442.
2. Omran AR. The epidemiologic transition. A theory of the epidemiology of population change. 1971. *Bull World Health Organ.* 2001;79:161-170.
3. Reddy KS. Cardiovascular disease in non-Western countries. *N Engl J Med.* 2004; 350:2438-2440.

Incidence of Cardiovascular Risk Factors in an Indian Urban Cohort: Results From the New Delhi Birth Cohort

Huffman MD, on the behalf of the New Delhi Birth Cohort (Centre for Chronic Disease Control, New Delhi, India; et al)

J Am Coll Cardiol 57:1765-1774, 2011

Background.—The cardiovascular disease (CVD) burden of India is among the highest worldwide. Annual death rate from CVD is expected to increase from 2.26 in 1990 to 4.77 million by 2020. CVD risk factors such as abdominal obesity, hypertension, and diabetes are higher in Indians than other ethnic groups, even at younger ages. The New Delhi

Birth Cohort study allowed the evaluation of the incidence of CVD risk factors in a young, urban Indian population across a 7-year period.

Methods.—Between 1969 and 1972 phase 1 of the study involved 20,755 married women of reproductive age evaluated for pregnancy outcomes and childhood growth. Between 1969 and 1990 (phases 2 through 4) anthropometric and survey data were gathered, then phase 5 (1998 to 2002) focused on the relationship of CVD risk factors to birth and early life anthropometry. For phase 6 (2006 through 2009), 1100 of the phase 5 subjects received home visits to obtain data about personal and family medical history, medication use, material possessions, tobacco use, and alcohol consumption. Measures of subjects' blood pressure, weight, height, and waist and hip circumferences were also noted, as were data on education, diet, alcohol and tobacco use, overweight and obesity, and conditions such as hypertension, metabolic syndrome, diabetes mellitus, and impaired glucose tolerance (IGT). Material possessions were also noted.

Results.—Mean follow-up between phases 5 and 6 was 6.9 years, with subjects' mean age 29 years in phase 5 and 36 years in phase 6. No significant differences were noted with respect to gender, body mass index (BMI), hip circumference, systolic or diastolic blood pressure, fasting and post-load glucose level, low-density lipoprotein (LDL) cholesterol, or the proportions of overweight, obesity, hypertension, IGT, or diabetes. Differences in men between the two phases included age and high-density lipoprotein (HDL) cholesterol levels. Differences in women involved measures of waist circumference, waist-to-hip ratio (WHR), and triglycerides. Statistical analysis showed significant positive relationships between phase 5 BMI, waist circumference, WHR, socioeconomic status, total cholesterol level, triglyceride level, and incident obesity, with a significant inverse relationship to tobacco use. The incidence of obesity was higher in women than in men, but the incidences of hypertension and diabetes were higher in men. Both men and women showed higher rates of central obesity and increased WHR.

Conclusions.—The rapid increase in CVD risk factors may reflect transitions in wealth and lifestyle in these young, urban individuals. Increased urban and socioeconomic development in New Delhi over the period covered by this cohort study is broadly associated with increased caloric intake and diminished physical activity. A life-course approach to risk screening and intervention strategies, specifically targeting health promotion during childhood and adolescence, primary prevention for individuals with CVD risk factors, and secondary prevention for persons with established coronary heart disease and stroke, is suggested (Fig 3).

▶ Cardiovascular disease is a huge problem in India and for much of the developing world and newly industrialized countries. The problem in India is compounded by the large burden of communicable diseases and diseases related to undernutrition as well as a growing but poor elderly population.

The developed world is exposed to multiple nontraditional risk factors, such as air pollution, psychosocial stressors associated with rural to urban migration, overcrowded cities, lack of exercise, and clashes between traditional and

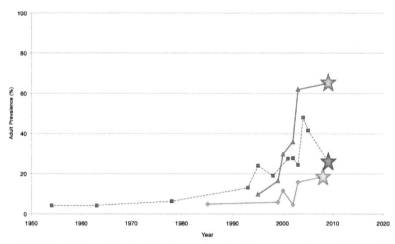

FIGURE 3.—Risk Factor Trends in India. Temporal trends of the prevalence of overweight (**green line**), hypertension (**blue line**), and diabetes (**orange line**) in urban India (diagnosis based on laboratory testing). Each **star** represents the New Delhi Birth Cohort prevalence data during phase 6. Data from World Health Organization (WHO) India (4). *Editor's Note:* Please refer to original journal article for full references. For interpretation of the references to color in this figure legend, the reader is referred to web version of this article. (Reprinted from the Journal of the American College of Cardiology, Huffman MD, on the behalf of the New Delhi Birth. Incidence of cardiovascular risk factors in an Indian urban cohort: results from the New Delhi birth cohort. *J Am Coll Cardiol.* 2011;57:1765-1774. Copyright 2011, with permission from the American College of Cardiology.)

changing cultural values.[1] Nonetheless, we have learned from INTERHEART study that the well-documented "traditional" risk factors, such as abdominal obesity, hypertension, smoking, and diabetes, plus indices of psychosocial stress account for by far most of the attributable risk for premature myocardial infarction and cardiovascular disease.[2] Although the level of risk factors is higher among Indians, whether there is a genetic vulnerability to an interaction with risk factors in the environment is unknown.

This study is very disturbing. Not only is the prevalence of risk factors extremely high at a young age, but the change over a short period of time (7 years) is dramatic. Although India has a large population who are poor, it also has a large middle class, and the cohort in this study was in the middle to upper income groups relative to other Indians. Nonetheless, other data show similar trends in rural India despite the poverty.

Whichever way you look at it, the epidemic of premature cardiovascular disease in India and in many other low- and middle-income countries is rampant and likely to grow at an alarming rate. Getting this under control is a gigantic task, but we do know the main targets—obesity, hypertension, hyperlipidemia, and smoking. Implementation of primary prevention policies is the problem.

B. J. Gersh, MB, ChB, DPhil, FRCP

References

1. Gersh BJ, Sliwa K, Mayosi BM, Yusuf S. Novel therapeutic concepts: the epidemic of cardiovascular disease in the developing world: global implications. *Eur Heart J.* 2010;31:642-648.

2. Yusuf S, Hawken S, Ounpuu S, et al; INTERHEART Study Investigators. Effect of potentially modifiable risk factors associated with myocardial infarction in 52 countries (the INTERHEART study): case-control study. *Lancet.* 2004;364: 937-952.

National, regional, and global trends in body-mass index since 1980: systematic analysis of health examination surveys and epidemiological studies with 960 country-years and 9·1 million participants

Finucane MM, on behalf of the Global Burden of Metabolic Risk Factors of Chronic Diseases Collaborating Group (Body Mass Index) (Harvard School of Public Health, Boston, MA; et al)
Lancet 377:557-567, 2011

Background.—Excess bodyweight is a major public health concern. However, few worldwide comparative analyses of long-term trends of body-mass index (BMI) have been done, and none have used recent national health examination surveys. We estimated worldwide trends in population mean BMI.

Methods.—We estimated trends and their uncertainties of mean BMI for adults 20 years and older in 199 countries and territories. We obtained data from published and unpublished health examination surveys and epidemiological studies (960 country-years and 9·1 million participants). For each sex, we used a Bayesian hierarchical model to estimate mean BMI by age, country, and year, accounting for whether a study was nationally representative.

Findings.—Between 1980 and 2008, mean BMI worldwide increased by 0·4 kg/m² per decade (95% uncertainty interval 0·2—0·6, posterior probability of being a true increase >0·999) for men and 0·5 kg/m² per decade (0·3—0·7, posterior probability >0·999) for women. National BMI change for women ranged from non-significant decreases in 19 countries to increases of more than 2·0 kg/m² per decade (posterior probabilities >0·99) in nine countries in Oceania. Male BMI increased in all but eight countries, by more than 2 kg/m² per decade in Nauru and Cook Islands (posterior probabilities >0·999). Male and female BMIs in 2008 were highest in some Oceania countries, reaching 33·9 kg/m² (32·8—35·0) for men and 35·0 kg/m² (33·6—36·3) for women in Nauru. Female BMI was lowest in Bangladesh (20·5 kg/m², 19·8—21·3) and male BMI in Democratic Republic of the Congo 19·9 kg/m² (18·2—21·5), with BMI less than 21·5 kg/m² for both sexes in a few countries in sub-Saharan Africa, and east, south, and southeast Asia. The USA had the highest BMI of high-income countries. In 2008, an estimated 1·46 billion adults (1·41—1·51 billion) worldwide had BMI of 25 kg/m² or greater, of these 205 million men (193—217 million) and 297 million women (280—315 million) were obese.

Interpretation.—Globally, mean BMI has increased since 1980. The trends since 1980, and mean population BMI in 2008, varied substantially between nations. Interventions and policies that can curb or reverse the

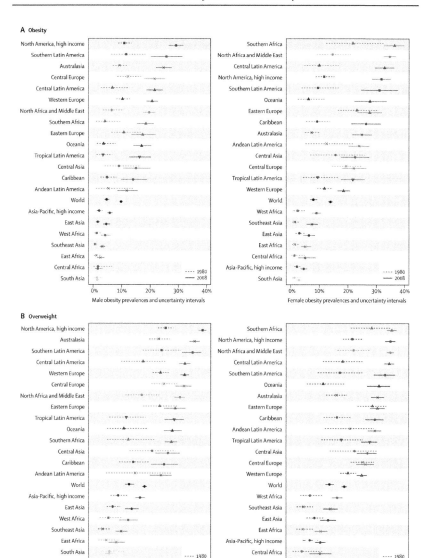

FIGURE 4.—Prevalences of obesity (BMI ≥30 kg/m^2; A) and overweight (BMI ≥25 kg/m^2; B) in 1980 and 2008. BMI=body-mass index. (Reprinted from The Lancet, Finucane MM, on behalf of the Global Burden of Metabolic Risk Factors of Chronic Diseases Collaborating Group (Body Mass Index), National, regional, and global trends in body-mass index since 1980: systematic analysis of health examination surveys and epidemiological studies with 960 country-years and 9·1 million participants. *Lancet.* 2011;377:557-567. © 2011, with permission from Elsevier.)

increase, and mitigate the health effects of high BMI by targeting its metabolic mediators, are needed in most countries (Fig 4).

▶ The findings from this study plus 2 additional articles in the same issue of *Lancet*, which deal with blood pressure and cholesterol levels from the Global Burden of Metabolic Risk Factors of the Chronic Diseases Collaborating Group are stark and alarming in that the consequences of the global increase in risk factors is far reaching. The conclusions are inescapable—a global epidemic of premature cardiovascular disease mortality is already advanced and rapidly expanding. Its impact will be disproportionately born by low- and middle-income countries. On the other hand, there are perhaps some grounds for optimism in that the causes are clear cut and the result of well-established and potentially treatable common cardiovascular risk factors.[1]

The results of this enormous and comprehensive analysis really provide extensive insights into the epidemiology of overweight and obesity throughout the world. The essential findings are that the average population body mass index has increased over time in a large number of low-, middle-, and high-income countries and in both men and women. Although considerable variation in these trends was observed between nations and countries, the trend highlights the growing magnitude of overweight and obesity throughout the world, and implications for the epidemic of diabetes are obvious.

An excellent commentary accompanies this series of articles and illustrates quite strikingly the changing prevalence of risk factors over the last 3 decades stratified by level of income in the United States.[2] The increase in obesity is global and affects both rich and poor. Surprisingly, blood pressure has declined globally after 3 decades, but this has occurred mainly in the high-income countries, is little changed in middle-income countries, and increased in low-income countries, a group comprising a large number of people. Serum cholesterol levels have also declined globally, but not in east and southeast Asia and the Pacific. Notably, serum cholesterol levels have increased in Japan, China, and Thailand.

Although the targets have been identified, implementation of population-level risk factor control is extremely complex and somewhat daunting. As pointed out by Anand and Yusuf,[2] health-related research in these areas cannot be separated from research in multiple diverse areas, ie, policies related to agriculture, trade, education, taxation and tobacco control, pollution, poverty, industrialization, and urban design among other factors. Political stability is another prerequisite.

Hopefully, the forthcoming United Nations General Assembly on chronic noncommunicable diseases in September 2011 will result in a concerted high level and determined commitment from world leaders. The consequences of continuing inactivity are frightening.[3]

B. J. Gersh, MB, ChB, DPhil, FRCP

References

1. An epidemic of risk factors for cardiovascular disease. *Lancet*. 2011;377:527.
2. Anand SS, Yusuf S. Stemming the global tsunami of cardiovascular disease. *Lancet*. 2011;377:529-532.
3. Beaglehole R, Horton R. Chronic diseases: global action must match global evidence. *Lancet*. 2010;376:1619-1621.

Nationwide Cohort Study of Risk of Ischemic Heart Disease in Patients With Celiac Disease

Ludvigsson JF, James S, Askling J, et al (Örebro Univ Hosp, Sweden; Uppsala Univ, Sweden; Karolinska Univ Hosp and Karolinska Institutet, Stockholm, Sweden; et al)
Circulation 123:483-490, 2011

Background.—Studies on ischemic heart disease (IHD) incidence in individuals with celiac disease (CD) are contradictory and do not take small intestinal pathology into account.

Methods and Results.—In this Swedish population-based cohort study, we examined the risk of IHD in patients with CD based on small intestinal histopathology. We defined IHD as death or incident disease in myocardial infarction or angina pectoris in Swedish national registers. In 2006 to 2008, we collected duodenal/jejunal biopsy data on CD (equal to villous atrophy; Marsh 3; n = 28 190 unique individuals) and inflammation without villous atrophy (Marsh 1 to 2; n = 12 598) from all 28 pathology departments in Sweden. A third cohort consisted of 3658 individuals with normal mucosa but positive CD serology (Marsh 0, latent CD). We found an increased risk of incident IHD in patients undergoing small intestinal biopsy that was independent of small intestinal histopathology (CD: hazard ratio [HR], 1.19; 95% confidence interval [CI], 1.11 to 1.28; 991 events; inflammation: HR, 1.28; 95% CI, 1.19 to 1.39; 809 events; and latent CD: HR, 1.14; 95% CI, 0.87 to 1.50; 62 events). Celiac disease (HR, 1.22; 95% CI, 1.06 to 1.40) and inflammation (HR, 1.32; 95% CI, 1.14 to 1.52) were both associated with death resulting from IHD, whereas latent CD was not (HR, 0.71; 95% CI, 0.34 to 1.50).

Conclusions.—Individuals with CD or small intestinal inflammation are at increased risk of incident IHD. We were unable to show a positive association between latent CD and incident IHD (Table 2).

▶ Approximately 1% of the western world suffers from celiac disease, and given the association between chronic inflammation and cardiovascular disease in addition to the frequency of ischemic heart disease deaths, the association between celiac and coronary heart disease and cardiovascular disease is of interest. Celiac disease is characterized by an immune-mediated response in the small intestine following exposure to gluten. Most, but not all, prior studies have shown an increased risk of incident coronary heart disease, death resulting from ischemic heart disease (IHD), or cardiovascular disease in patients with celiac disease.[1] Contradictory results from other studies could be explained by differences in study design and sample sizes.

This study from Sweden was collected from biopsy reports at all of Sweden's 28 regional pathology departments. The patients with celiac disease were divided into those with villous atrophy, those with inflammation on histology but no villous atrophy, and patients with latent celiac disease with normal mucosa on biopsy but positive serology. They found a modest but definitely increased risk in incident coronary heart disease (hazard ratio, 1.19; 95%

TABLE 2.—Any IHD According to Follow-Up

Subgroup and Exposure	Events, n	HR (95% CI)	P	Absolute Risk Rate/100 000 PYAR, n	Excess Risk/100 000 PYAR, n
All					
Reference	8254	1 (Reference)			
CD	991	1.19 (1.11–1.28)	<0.001	375	60
Inflammation	809	1.28 (1.19–1.39)	<0.001	808	179
Latent	62	1.14 (0.87–1.50)	0.340	256	31
Follow-up <1 y					
Reference	785	1 (Reference)			
CD	145	1.77 (1.46–2.14)	<0.001	523	227
Inflammation	106	1.65 (1.33–2.05)	<0.001	892	351
Latent	15	1.63 (0.94–2.85)	0.085	419	162
Follow-up 1–4.99 y					
Reference	2800	1 (Reference)			
CD	284	0.96 (0.85–1.10)	0.561	304	−12
Inflammation	270	1.30 (1.13–1.48)	<0.001	736	168
Latent	23	0.86 (0.56–1.33)	0.506	207	−33
Follow-up ≥5 y					
Reference	4669	1 (Reference)			
CD	562	1.23 (1.12–1.36)	<0.001	393	74
Inflammation	433	1.20 (1.08–1.34)	0.001	840	142
Latent	24	1.31 (0.84–2.04)	0.240	251	59

confidence intervals, 1.11–1.21) in patients undergoing small bowel biopsy, but this was independent of the histopathology (ie, whether villous atrophy was present). In other words, celiac disease and the presence of inflammation were risk factors for ischemic heart disease, but latent celiac disease without any histologic changes was not a predictor of coronary heart disease.

In terms of the clinical implications, this study shows a 19% increased risk of ischemic heart disease in individuals with celiac disease and a 28% increase in risk in those with inflammation but no villous atrophy. Because cardiovascular disease is the most common cause of death in these patients, these data argue for a more comprehensive risk factor assessment than is probably currently practiced. A limitation of this study, however, is the lack of data on blood pressure, smoking, body mass index, lipids, exercise, and other cardiovascular risk factors, all of which could have led to residual confounding.

The case is not proven, but the association with celiac disease and other inflammatory bowel diseases and the risk of cardiovascular disease warrants further study.

B. J. Gersh, MB, ChB, DPhil, FRCP

Reference

1. Peters U, Askling J, Gridley G, Ekbom A, Linet M. Causes of death in patients with celiac disease in a population-based Swedish cohort. *Arch Intern Med.* 2003;163: 1566-1572.

Public health importance of triggers of myocardial infarction: a comparative risk assessment

Nawrot TS, Perez L, Künzli N, et al (Hasselt Univ, Diepenbeek, Belgium; Univ of Basel, Switzerland; et al)
Lancet 377:732-740, 2011

Background.—Acute myocardial infarction is triggered by various factors, such as physical exertion, stressful events, heavy meals, or increases in air pollution. However, the importance and relevance of each trigger are uncertain. We compared triggers of myocardial infarction at an individual and population level.

Methods.—We searched PubMed and the Web of Science citation databases to identify studies of triggers of non-fatal myocardial infarction to calculate population attributable fractions (PAF). When feasible, we did a meta-regression analysis for studies of the same trigger.

Findings.—Of the epidemiologic studies reviewed, 36 provided sufficient details to be considered. In the studied populations, the exposure prevalence for triggers in the relevant control time window ranged from 0·04% for cocaine use to 100% for air pollution. The reported odds ratios (OR) ranged from 1·05 to 23·7. Ranking triggers from the highest to the lowest OR resulted in the following order: use of cocaine, heavy meal, smoking of marijuana, negative emotions, physical exertion, positive emotions, anger, sexual activity, traffic exposure, respiratory infections, coffee consumption, air pollution (based on a difference of 30 μg/m^3 in particulate matter with a diameter <10 μm [PM$_{10}$]). Taking into account the OR and the prevalences of exposure, the highest PAF was estimated for traffic exposure (7·4%), followed by physical exertion (6·2%), alcohol (5·0%), coffee (5·0%), a difference of 30 μg/m^3 in PM$_{10}$ (4·8%), negative emotions (3·9%), anger (3·1%), heavy meal (2·7%), positive emotions (2·4%), sexual activity (2·2%), cocaine use (0·9%), marijuana smoking (0·8%) and respiratory infections (0·6%).

Interpretation.—In view of both the magnitude of the risk and the prevalence in the population, air pollution is an important trigger of myocardial infarction, it is of similar magnitude (PAF 5–7%) as other well accepted triggers such as physical exertion, alcohol, and coffee. Our work shows that ever-present small risks might have considerable public health relevance (Fig 2).

▶ An American Heart Association (AHA) scientific statement in 2004 drew attention to the relationship between air pollution and cardiovascular disease. A subsequent report from the AHA stated that "this body of evidence has grown and been strengthened substantially since the first American Heart Association statement was published."[1]

This interesting assessment from published studies of triggers of myocardial infarction over a 50-year period provides a rather unusual perspective. The use of the population attributable fraction (PAF) is a useful approach to quantifying the importance of a particular trigger from a public health standpoint. For

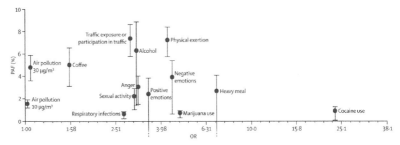

FIGURE 2.—Relation between OR and the PAF for each studies trigger. PAFs were calculated and reported with their 95% CI (error bars). Not significant triggers show 95% CIs that are lower than 0%. X-axis is log scale, and ORs are given as anti-logs. OR=odds ratio. PAF=population attributable fraction. (Reprinted from The Lancet, Nawrot TS, Perez L, Künzli N, et al. Public health importance of triggers of myocardial infarction: a comparative risk assessment. *Lancet.* 2011;377:732-740. Copyright 2011, with permission from Elsevier.)

example, the odds ratio for cocaine as a trigger of myocardial infarction is huge, but because the prevalence of exposure in most countries is low, the PAF is also low. Air pollution and participation in traffic are associated with low odds ratios but a high prevalence, and the public health impact is potentially enormous. To what extent traffic exposure is the result of exposure to air pollutants, stress, noise, or other factors is, however, unknown. As addressed by the authors, they were unable to assess the effects of passive smoking, which is another major cause of air pollution in many parts of the world.

The potential mechanisms whereby air pollution would be a cardiovascular risk factor are many, and it is likely there are complex interactions among factors such as inflammation, oxidative stress, thrombosis and coagulation, vascular function, hypertension, cardiac ischemia, and interactions with traditional risk factors.

The world's most polluted cities are in the low- to middle-income countries, and it would appear that air pollution is yet another evolving risk factor contributing to the global epidemic of cardiovascular disease.

B. J. Gersh, MB, ChB, DPhil, FRCP

Reference

1. Brook RD, Rajagopalan S, Pope CA III, et al. Particulate matter air pollution and cardiovascular disease: an update of the scientific statement from the American Heart Association. *Circulation.* 2010;121:2331-2378.

Using Additional Information on Working Hours to Predict Coronary Heart Disease: A Cohort Study

Kivimäki M, Batty GD, Hamer M, et al (Univ College London, UK; Univ of Turku and Turku Univ Hosp, Finland; Finnish Inst of Occupational Health and Univ of Helsinki, Finland; et al)
Ann Intern Med 154:457-463, 2011

Background.—Long working hours are associated with increased risk for coronary heart disease (CHD). Adding information on long hours to traditional risk factors for CHD may help to improve risk prediction for this condition.

Objective.—To examine whether information on long working hours improves the ability of the Framingham risk model to predict CHD in a low-risk, employed population.

Design.—Cohort study with baseline medical examination performed between 1991 and 1993 and prospective follow-up for incident CHD performed until 2004.

Setting.—Civil service departments in London (the Whitehall II study).

Participants.—7095 adults (2109 women and 4986 men) aged 39 to 62 years working full-time without CHD at baseline.

Measurements.—Working hours and the Framingham risk score were measured at baseline. Coronary death and nonfatal myocardial infarction were ascertained from medical screenings every 5 years, hospital data, and registry linkage.

Results.—192 participants had incident CHD during a median 12.3-year follow-up. After adjustment for their Framingham risk score, participants working 11 hours or more per day had a 1.67-fold (95% CI, 1.10- to 2.55-fold) increased risk for CHD compared with participants working 7 to 8 hours per day. Adding working hours to the Framingham risk score led to a net reclassification improvement of 4.7% ($P = 0.034$) due to better identification of persons who later developed CHD (sensitivity gain).

Limitation.—The findings may not be generalizable to populations with a larger proportion of high-risk persons and were not validated in an independent cohort.

Conclusion.—Information on working hours may improve risk prediction of CHD on the basis of the Framingham risk score in low-risk, working populations (Table 2).

▶ This article will be viewed as a piece of good news for those who champion a shorter workweek on the grounds that it may be beneficial from a coronary heart disease standpoint, although not for the economy as a whole.

Although the Framingham risk score is the most commonly used algorithm for risk predictions[1] and is based on levels of the traditional risk factors, the importance of psychosocial stress is receiving increasing emphasis. This may be particularly relevant in changing urban societies in the developing world.[2] Stress at work has also been implicated as a risk factor, and one such stressor is long working hours. This long-standing study from the United Kingdom of civil servants in London has a median follow-up of 12 years. Patients were aged 39 to 62 years at entry and without prior evidence of coronary heart disease. After adjustment for the Framingham risk score, patients working 11 hours or more per day had a 1.67-fold increased risk for coronary heart disease compared with participants working 7 to 8 hours a day. The net reclassification improvement was, however, modest at 4.7% ($P = .034$).

There are several limitations to these kinds of studies, and one of these relates to the specific population under study; this was a low-risk population. These data may not apply to populations at higher risk or in other nationalities and

TABLE 2.—Comparison of Observed CHD Risk With Predicted Risk, Using 2 Framingham Risk Score Models*

CHD Risk by Framingham Risk Score Alone	CHD Risk by Framingham Risk Score and Working Hours			
	<5.0%	5.0%–9.9%	≥10.0%	Total
<5.0%				
Participants, n	6412	142	0	6554
Reclassified, %	–	2.2	–	2.2
Cases, n	139	11	0	–
Person-years at risk	73 164.7	1531.1	0.0	–
Observed risk, %	1.9	6.9	–	–
Predicted risk, %[†]	1.8 vs. 1.8	4.3 vs. 6.1	–	–
5.0%–9.9%				
Participants, n	86	330	20	436
Reclassified, %	19.7	–	4.6	24.3
Cases, n	4	27	3	–
Person-years at risk	961.0	3515.1	220.4	–
Observed risk, %	4.1	7.4	12.7	–
Predicted risk, %[†]	5.2 vs. 4.7	7.1 vs. 6.9	8.3 vs. 11.7	–
≥10%				
Participants, n	0	17	88	105
Reclassified, %	–	16.2	–	16.2
Cases, n	0	0	8	–
Person-years at risk	–	181.8	836.7	–
Observed risk, %	–	0.0	9.1	–
Predicted risk, %[†]	–	10.6 vs. 9.7	16.8 vs. 16.9	–
Total, n	6498	489	108	7095

CHD = coronary heart disease.
*Calculated by using the Framingham risk score alone and the Framingham risk score plus working hours, according to strata of predicted risk from the 2 models.
[†]Framingham risk score alone vs. Framingham risk score plus working hours.

social systems. In this respect, 2 Japanese studies demonstrated no association,[3] although other studies from Sweden, Netherlands, and the United Kingdom have demonstrated an association between working overtime and acute myocardial infarction or coronary death. Other confounding factors that may not be accounted for include the underlying reasons and implications for working time, (eg, financial stress, domestic stress, lack of exercise). In any event, before we can consider incorporating work hours into risk stratification models, additional prospective validation studies in different populations may be necessary, but this is certainly an avenue worth pursuing.

B. J. Gersh, MB, ChB, DPhil, FRCP

References

1. Grundy SM, Cleeman JI, Merz CN, et al; National Heart, Lung, and Blood Institute, American Heart Association. Implications of recent clinical trials for the National Cholesterol Education Program Adult Treatment Panel III guidelines. *Circulation.* 2004;110:227-239.
2. Yusuf S, Hawken S, Ounpuu S, et al; INTERHEART Study Investigators. Effective of potentially modifiable risk factors associated with myocardial infarction in 52 countries (the INTERHEART study): case-control study. *Lancet.* 2004;364: 937-952.

3. Uchiyama S, Kurasawa T, Sekizawa T, Nakatsuka H. Job strain and risk of cardio-vascular events in treated hypertensive Japanese workers: hypertension follow-up group study. *J Occup Health.* 2005;47:102-111.

Miscellaneous

Clinical Events as a Function of Proton Pump Inhibitor Use, Clopidogrel Use, and Cytochrome P450 2C19 Genotype in a Large Nationwide Cohort of Acute Myocardial Infarction: Results From the French Registry of Acute ST-Elevation and Non—ST-Elevation Myocardial Infarction (FAST-MI) Registry

Simon T, Steg PG, Gilard M, et al (Assistance Publique-Hôpitaux de Paris, France; Université Paris 7—Denis Diderot, France; Centre Hospitalier Universitaire, Brest, France; et al)

Circulation 123:474-482, 2011

Background.—Clopidogrel requires metabolic activation by cyto-chrome P450 2C19 (CYP2C19). Proton pump inhibitors (PPIs) that inhibit CYP2C19 are commonly coadministered with clopidogrel to reduce the risk of gastrointestinal bleeding. This analysis compares treatment outcomes for patients in the French Registry of Acute ST-Elevation and Non—ST-Elevation Myocardial Infarction (FAST-MI) who did or did not receive clopidogrel and/or PPIs.

Methods and Results.—The FAST-MI registry included 3670 patients (2744 clopidogrel- and PPI-naïve patients) presenting with definite MI. Patients were categorized according to use of clopidogrel and/or PPI within 48 hours after hospital admission. PPI use was not associated with an increased risk for any of the main in-hospital events (in-hospital survival, reinfarction, stroke, bleeding, and transfusion). Likewise, PPI treatment was not an independent predictor of 1-year survival (hazard ratio, 0.97; 95% confidence interval [CI], 0.87 to 1.08; $P=0.57$) or 1-year MI, stroke, or death (hazard ratio, 0.98; 95% CI, 0.90 to 1.08; $P=0.72$). No differences were seen when the type of PPI or CYP2C19 genotype was taken into account. In the propensity-matched cohorts, the odds ratios for major in-hospital events in PPI versus no PPI were 0.29 (95% CI, 0.06 to 1.44) and 1.70 (95% CI, 0.10 to 30.3) for patients with 1 and 2 variant alleles, respec-tively. Similarly, the hazard ratio for 1-year events in hospital survivors was 0.68 (95% CI, 0.26 to 1.79) and 0.55 (95% CI, 0.06 to 5.30), respectively.

Conclusion.—PPI use was not associated with an increased risk of cardiovascular events or mortality in patients administered clopidogrel for recent MI, whatever the CYP2C19 genotype, although harm could not be formally excluded in patients with 2 loss-of-function alleles.

Clinical Trial Registration.—URL: http://www.clinicaltrials.gov. Unique identifier: NCT00673036.

▶ Clopidogrel is established as a key antiplatelet agent in patients undergoing acute coronary intervention, and proton pump inhibitors (PPI) are widely used in conjunction to reduce gastrointestinal bleeding, a practice supported by the guidelines. Concerns regarding adverse drug-drug interactions have been raised by in vitro experimental pharmacodynamic studies and by 2 large observational studies.[1,2] Nonetheless, the debate continues on the basis of other studies that show no interaction with regard to clinical outcomes, and the only randomized, controlled trial to address this issue using omeprazole was completely neutral.[3]

Because clopidogrel is a prodrug that requires metabolic activation by cytochrome P450 2C19/CYP2C19, there remains the potential that PPI that inhibit CYP2C19 might increase adverse cardiac events.

This excellent study from a large French registry analyzed outcomes according to clopidogrel use with PPIs stratified by specific cytochrome P450 2C19 genotypes and did not demonstrate any significant interactions. The authors point out that in the relatively few patients with 2 loss-of-function alleles, evidence of harm could not be definitively excluded due to a lack of power.

This is reassuring because other studies have suggested that polymorphisms, which actually confer reduced CYP2C19 enzyme activity, may be associated with an increase in cardiovascular risk in clopidogrel-treated patients. There is now a growing body of evidence to support the clinical use of both clopidogrel and PPIs despite experimental evidence that omeprazole and statins may attenuate the antiplatelet effects of clopidogrel in vitro. Perhaps the effect, however, is too weak to be important clinically. Nonetheless, there remains much to learn to better understand the relationship between in vitro platelet reactivity and outcomes as pointed out in an excellent accompanying editorial.[4] From a clinical standpoint, however, it is important to ask the initial question, and that is, does the patient actually need a proton pump inhibitor?

B. J. Gersh, MB, ChB, DPhil, FRCP

References

1. Bhatt DL, Scheiman J, Abraham NS, et al. ACCF/ACG/AHA 2008 expert consensus document on reducing the gastrointestinal risks of antiplatelet therapy and NSAID use: a report of the American College of Cardiology Foundation Task Force on Clinical Expert Consensus Documents. *J Am Coll Cardiol.* 2008;52:1502-1517.
2. Small DS, Farid NA, Payne CV, et al. Effects of the proton pump inhibitor lansoprazole on the pharmacokinetics and pharmacodynamics of prasugrel and clopidogrel. *J Clin Pharmacol.* 2008;48:475-484.
3. Bhatt DL, Cryer BL, Contant F, et al. Clopidogrel with or without omeprazole in coronary artery disease. *N Eng J Med.* 2010;363:1909-1917.
4. O'Donoghue ML. CYP2C19 genotype and proton pump inhibitors in clopidogrel-treated patients: does it take two to tango? *Circulation.* 2011;123:468-470.

Absolute and Attributable Risks of Atrial Fibrillation in Relation to Optimal and Borderline Risk Factors: The Atherosclerosis Risk in Communities (ARIC) Study

Huxley RR, Lopez FL, Folsom AR, et al (Univ of Minnesota, Minneapolis; et al)
Circulation 123:1501-1508, 2011

Background.—Atrial fibrillation (AF) is an important risk factor for stroke and overall mortality, but information about the preventable burden of AF is lacking. The aim of this study was to determine what proportion of the burden of AF in blacks and whites could theoretically be avoided by the maintenance of an optimal risk profile.

Methods and Results.—This study included 14 598 middle-aged Atherosclerosis Risk in Communities (ARIC) Study cohort members. Previously established AF risk factors, namely high blood pressure, elevated body mass index, diabetes mellitus, cigarette smoking, and prior cardiac disease, were categorized into optimal, borderline, and elevated levels. On the basis of their risk factor levels, individuals were classified into 1 of these 3 groups. The population-attributable fraction of AF resulting from having a nonoptimal risk profile was estimated separately for black and white men and women. During a mean follow-up of 17.1 years, 1520 cases of incident AF were identified. The age-adjusted incidence rates were highest in white men and lowest in black women (7.45 and 3.67 per 1000 person-years, respectively). The overall prevalence of an optimal risk profile was 5.4% but varied according to race and gender: 10% in white women versus 1.6% in black men. Overall, 56.5% of AF cases could be explained by having ≥1 borderline or elevated risk factors, of which elevated blood pressure was the most important contributor.

Conclusion.—As with other forms of cardiovascular disease, more than half of the AF burden is potentially avoidable through the optimization of cardiovascular risk factors levels (Fig 1).

▶ It has been postulated that atrial fibrillation is not simply an electrical disease that belongs solely in the category of arrhythmias but that its etiology is multifactorial and relevant to the epidemic of atherosclerosis in general.[1] In younger patients without structural heart disease and predominantly paroxysmal atrial fibrillation, atrial fibrillation is probably an electrical disease due to triggers in the left atrium and pulmonary veins and probably with a very strong genetic basis. Nonetheless, the major burden of atrial fibrillation is in older patients over the age of 75 to 80 years, and in this setting, the etiology is likely to be very different. It has been postulated with strong supporting evidence that atrial fibrillation may be a vascular disease secondary to aortic atherosclerosis, reduced arterial compliance, and increased stiffness leading to diastolic dysfunction and left atrial volume overload followed by structural and electrical remodeling of the atria, leading to an increased vulnerability to atrial fibrillation.[2] Several studies have shown that left atrial volume is a predictor not only of atrial fibrillation but also of subsequent cardiovascular events. Left atrial volume as such provides a window into the integrity and stiffness of the vascular system[3] and could be considered the equivalent of the HbA1C of vascular disease.

These data from the ARIC study provide additional support of the evidence by demonstrating that more than half of the atrial fibrillation burden in participants aged 45 to 64 years on entry into the study was attributable to the common modifiable cardiovascular risk factors. It is of interest that the incidence was lower in blacks than in whites even within each profile of risk. Moreover, hypertension and obesity is more frequent in blacks so the explanation for

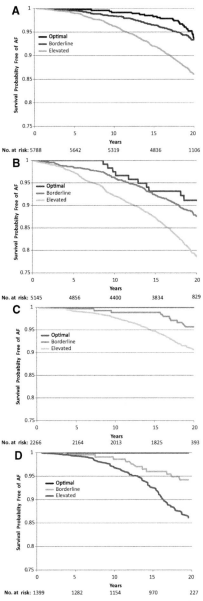

FIGURE 1.—Survival curves adjusted for age, study center, education, and height showing time free from atrial fibrillation (AF) according to risk factor group (optimal, borderline, or elevated) in white women (**A**), white men (**B**), black women (**C**), and black men (**D**). The numbers of subjects at risk throughout the duration of study follow-up are shown on the *x* axis. (Reprinted from Huxley RR, Lopez FL, Folsom AR, et al. Absolute and attributable risks of atrial fibrillation in relation to optimal and borderline risk factors: the Atherosclerosis Risk in Communities (ARIC) Study. *Circulation.* 2011;123:1501-1508, with permission from American Heart Association, Inc.)

the lower rate in blacks may be genetic or other as yet undetermined risk factors that are determinants of atrial fibrillation.[4]

Atrial fibrillation is 1 of the 3 growing epidemics of cardiovascular disease in the United States, in concert with congestive heart failure and the epidemic of obesity, metabolic syndrome, and diabetes. The steady increase in the incidence of atrial fibrillation over the past 20 years is of concern; perhaps the message is that if atrial fibrillation is a vascular disease secondary to modifiable risk factors, the epidemic can be controlled in the future.

B. J. Gersh, MB, ChB, DPhil, FRCP

References

1. Wyse DG, Gersh BJ. Atrial fibrillation: a perspective: thinking inside and outside the box. *Circulation.* 2004;109:3089-3095.
2. Tsang TS, Miyasaka Y, Barnes ME, Gersh BJ. Epidemiological profile of atrial fibrillation: a contemporary perspective. *Prog Cardiovasc Dis.* 2005;48:1-8.
3. Tsang TS, Gersh BJ, Appleton CP, et al. Left ventricular diastolic dysfunction as a predictor of the first diagnosed nonvalvular atrial fibrillation in 840 elderly men and women. *J Am Coll Cardiol.* 2002;40:1636-1644.
4. Christophersen IE, Ravn LS, Budtz-Joergensen E, et al. Familial aggregation of atrial fibrillation: a study in Danish twins. *Circ Arrhythm Electrophysiol.* 2009; 2:378-383.

Atherosclerosis in Ancient Egyptian Mummies: The Horus Study

Allam AH, Thompson RC, Wann LS, et al (Al Azhar Med School, Cairo, Egypt; St. Luke's MidAmerica Heart Inst, Kansas City, MO; Wisconsin Heart Hosp, Milwaukee; et al)

J Am Coll cardial Img 4:315-327, 2011

Objectives.—The purpose of this study was to determine whether ancient Egyptians had atherosclerosis.

Background.—The worldwide burden of atherosclerotic disease continues to rise and parallels the spread of diet, lifestyles, and environmental risk factors associated with the developed world. It is tempting to conclude that atherosclerotic cardiovascular disease is exclusively a disease of modern society and did not affect our ancient ancestors.

Methods.—We performed whole body, multislice computed tomography scanning on 52 ancient Egyptian mummies from the Middle Kingdom to the Greco-Roman period to identify cardiovascular structures and arterial calcifications. We interpreted images by consensus reading of 7 imaging physicians, and collected demographic data from historical and museum records. We estimated age at the time of death from the computed tomography skeletal evaluation.

Results.—Forty-four of 52 mummies had identifiable cardiovascular (CV) structures, and 20 of these had either definite atherosclerosis (defined as calcification within the wall of an identifiable artery, n = 12) or probable atherosclerosis (defined as calcifications along the expected course of an artery, n = 8). Calcifications were found in the aorta as well as the coronary, carotid, iliac, femoral, and peripheral leg arteries. The 20 mummies with definite or probable atherosclerosis were older at time of death (mean age 45.1 ± 9.2 years) than the mummies with CV tissue but no atherosclerosis (mean age 34.5 ± 11.8 years, p < 0.002). Two mummies had evidence of severe arterial atherosclerosis with calcifications in virtually every arterial bed. Definite coronary atherosclerosis was present in 2 mummies, including a princess who lived between 1550 and 1580 BCE. This finding represents the earliest documentation of coronary atherosclerosis in a human. Definite or probable atherosclerosis was present in mummies who lived during virtually every era of ancient Egypt represented in this study, a time span of >2,000 years.

Conclusions.—Atherosclerosis is commonplace in mummified ancient Egyptians (Fig 8).

▶ This is a most unusual article to say the least. The Horus study is rather aptly named after Horus who is thought to be either one of the most important gods in Egypt or else the name is used as a catchall for multiple deities.

Prior autopsy studies have identified histologic evidence of coronary atherosclerosis in Egyptian mummies[1] and arterial calcification as a marker of arteriosclerosis demonstrated in studies using computed x-ray tomography (CT).[2] This extensive study of 44 mummies with detectable cardiovascular structures demonstrates that approximately half had evidence of atherosclerosis including a striking example of left main coronary artery disease and also severe diffuse calcific disease in 2 mummies. Interestingly, 2 others had mitral annulus calcification. We do not know the causes of death, but mummies with atherosclerotic disease are approximately 45.1 years old at the time of death versus 34.5 years old in those without atherosclerosis (*P* < .0002).

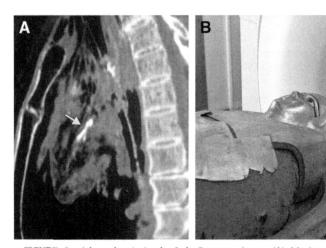

FIGURE 8.—Atherosclerosis in the Left Coronary Artery. (A) Maximum intensity projection computed tomography image showing calcifications of the left coronary artery (**arrow**). (B) Anthropoid mask of the same mummy, a man who lived during the Ptolemaic Period (Djeher, Mummy #12). (Reprinted from JACC, Cardiovascular Imaging, Allam AH, Thompson RC, Wann LS, et al. Atherosclerosis in ancient Egyptian mummies: the horus study. *JACC Cardiovasc Imaging.* 2011;4:315-327. Copyright 2011, with permission of Elsevier.)

From the evidence available, it is likely that the majority was from a higher socioeconomic class and may have had a diet different from that eaten by common farmers and laborers. Ancient Egypt saw the birth of an organized agricultural society, including animal husbandry, and hieroglyphic inscriptions from temples indicated the diet may have been quite atherogenic because of the consumption of beef, sheep, goats, wild fowl, bread, and cake.[3]

It would appear that atherosclerosis has been around for centuries, and in the Ebers papyrus there is a memorable physician's comment "if thy examinst a man for illness in his cardia and he has pains in his arms, in his breasts, and on one side of his cardia... it is death threatening him."[4] Nonetheless, it is noteworthy that the major causes of death in the United States and in Western Europe until the 20th century were still communicable diseases, and the epidemic of cardiovascular disease became rampant. Nonetheless, these findings that atherosclerotic cardiovascular disease was actually present and probably quite common in ancient Egypt really does raise fascinating questions with regard to the nature and extent of the human predisposition to atherosclerosis.

B. J. Gersh, MB, ChB, DPhil, FRCP

References

1. Ruffer MA. On arterial lesions found in Egyptian mummies (1580 BC—535 AD). *J Pathol Bacteriol.* 1911;16:453-462.
2. Allam AH, Thompson RC, Wann LS, Miyamoto MI, Thomas GS. Computed tomographic assessment of atherosclerosis in ancient Egyptian mummies. *JAMA.* 2009;302:2091-2094.
3. David R. The art of medicine—atherosclerosis and diet in ancient Egypt. *Lancet.* 2010;175:718-719.
4. Ebbel B. *The Papyrus TP Ebers.* Copenhagen, Denmark: Levinn and Munksgaard; 1937. 48.

C-reactive protein concentration and the vascular benefits of statin therapy: an analysis of 20536 patients in the Heart Protection Study

Heart Protection Study Collaborative Group (Univ of Oxford, UK; et al)
Lancet 377:469-476, 2011

Background.—It has been suggested that inflammation status, as assessed by C-reactive protein (CRP) concentration, modifies the vascular protective effects of statin therapy. In particular, there have been claims that statins might be more beneficial in people with raised CRP concentrations, and might even be ineffective in people with low concentrations of both CRP and LDL cholesterol. This study aimed to test this hypothesis.

Methods.—In 69 UK hospitals, 20536 men and women aged 40–80 years at high risk of vascular events were randomly assigned to simvastatin 40 mg daily versus matching placebo for a mean of 5·0 years. Patients were categorised into six baseline CRP groups (<1·25, 1·25–1·99, 2·00–2·99, 3·00–4·99, 5·00–7·99, and ≥8·00 mg/L). The primary endpoint for subgroup analyses was major vascular events, defined as the composite of coronary death, myocardial infarction, stroke, or revascularisation.

Analysis was by intention to treat. This study is registered, number ISRCTN48489393.

Findings.—Overall, allocation to simvastatin resulted in a significant 24% (95% CI 19–28) proportional reduction in the incidence of first major vascular event after randomisation (2033 [19·8%] allocated simvastatin *vs* 2585 [25·2%] allocated placebo). There was no evidence that the proportional reduction in this endpoint, or its components, varied with baseline CRP concentration (trend p=0·41). Even in participants with baseline CRP concentration less than 1·25 mg/L, major vascular events were significantly reduced by 29% (99% CI 12–43, p<0·0001; 239 [14·1%] *vs* 329 [19·4%]). No significant heterogeneity in the relative risk reduction was recorded between the four subgroups defined by the combination of low or high baseline concentrations of LDL cholesterol and CRP (p=0·72). In particular, there was clear evidence of benefit in those with both low LDL cholesterol and low CRP (27% reduction, 99% CI 11–40, p<0·0001; 295 [15·6%] *vs* 400 [20·9%]).

Interpretation.—Evidence from this large-scale randomised trial does not lend support to the hypothesis that baseline CRP concentration modifies the vascular benefits of statin therapy materially (Fig 2).

▶ This analysis from the largest of the statin trials (Heart Protection Study) adds more fuel to a healthy debate over the place of C-reactive protein concentrations (CRP) in the galaxy of cardiovascular risk factors and whether it remains a surrogate or a target for therapy.[1]

CRP is a marker of inflammation that has been shown in multiple studies to be strongly associated with the risk of coronary heart disease, ischemic stroke, and both vascular and nonvascular mortality.[2] Nonetheless, these associations have been largely explained by the positive correlations between CRP and other conventional risk factors and as such might not reflect a direct cause-and-effect

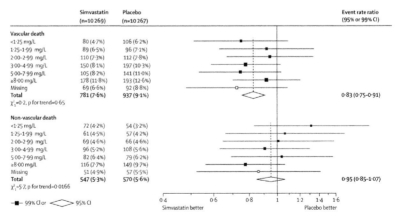

FIGURE 2.—Effect of simvastatin allocation on vascular and non-vascular death by concentration of baseline C-reactive protein. (Reprinted from The Lancet, Heart Protection Study Collaborative Group, C-reactive protein concentration and the vascular benefits of statin therapy: an analysis of 20 536 patients in the Heart Protection Study. *Lancet.* 2011;377:469-476. © 2011, with permission from Elsevier.)

relationship. In addition, there are data to suggest that elevated CRP levels might identify patients who are more likely to experience a benefit from statins and that among patients with a low CRP level and a low low-density lipoprotein cholesterol level, statins might not be of benefit.[3]

This study of more than 20 000 people at a higher risk of vascular events compared with prior studies does not support the hypothesis that baseline CRP levels have any impact on the magnitude of the benefit from statins. Even patients with low baseline CRP and LDL cholesterol levels experienced significant reductions in the risk of cardiovascular events. Moreover, there was no relationship between the extent of benefit in other inflammatory biomarkers, such as lipoprotein-associated phospholipase A or albumin, a liver-derived acute phased reactant.

An extensive accompanying editorial emphasizes that the importance of CRP as a driver of cardiovascular risk may vary among populations at lower risk as in the JUPITER trial and those at higher risk as in the Heart Protection Study. Nonetheless, a subsequent analysis from JUPITER did not demonstrate changes in the relative risk reduction across subgroups of CRP levels. In summary, the CRP story among other biomarkers has not yet been fully written.

B. J. Gersh, MB, ChB, DPhil, FRCP

References

1. Després JP. CRP: star trekking the galaxy of risk markers (editorial). *Lancet.* 2011; 377:441-442.
2. Emerging Risk Factors Collaboration, Kaptoge S, Di Angelantonio E, Lowe G, et al. C-reactive protein concentration and risk of coronary heart disease, stroke, and mortality: an individual participant meta-analysis. *Lancet.* 2010;375: 132-140.
3. Ridker PM, Danielson E, Fonseca FA, et al. Rosuvastatin to prevent vascular events in men and women with elevated C-reactive protein. *N Engl J Med.* 2008;359:2195-2207.

Development and Validation of a Risk Calculator for Prediction of Cardiac Risk After Surgery

Gupta PK, Gupta H, Sundaram A, et al (Creighton Univ, Omaha, NE; et al)
Circulation 124:381-387, 2011

Background.—Perioperative myocardial infarction or cardiac arrest is associated with significant morbidity and mortality. The Revised Cardiac Risk Index is currently the most commonly used cardiac risk stratification tool; however, it has several limitations, one of which is its relatively low discriminative ability. The objective of the present study was to develop and validate a predictive cardiac risk calculator.

Methods and Results.—Patients who underwent surgery were identified from the American College of Surgeons' 2007 National Surgical Quality Improvement Program database, a multicenter (>250 hospitals) prospective database. Of the 211 410 patients, 1371 (0.65%) developed perioperative myocardial infarction or cardiac arrest. On multivariate logistic regression analysis, 5 predictors of perioperative myocardial infarction or cardiac arrest were identified: type of surgery, dependent functional status, abnormal creatinine, American Society of Anesthesiologists' class, and increasing age. The risk model based on the 2007 data set was subsequently validated on the 2008 data set (n = 257 385). The model performance was very similar between the 2007 and 2008 data sets, with C statistics (also known as area under the receiver operating characteristic curve) of 0.884 and 0.874, respectively. Application of the Revised Cardiac Risk Index to the 2008 National Surgical Quality Improvement Program data set yielded a relatively lower C statistic (0.747). The risk model was used to develop an interactive risk calculator.

Conclusions.—The cardiac risk calculator provides a risk estimate of perioperative myocardial infarction or cardiac arrest and is anticipated to simplify the informed consent process. Its predictive performance surpasses that of the Revised Cardiac Risk Index (Fig 1).

▶ The incidence of perioperative myocardial infarction after noncardiac surgery varies widely depending on the nature of the surgical procedure, the presence of underlying coronary artery disease, and the number of cardiac risk factors.[1] The morbidity of perioperative cardiac events, including perioperative myocardial infarction, is high, and these events are a leading cause of death after cardiac surgery,[2] emphasizing the importance of perioperative risk stratification in an attempt to identify patients who may require additional optimization of cardiac status preoperatively. Many of the risk algorithms in place were established many years ago and antedate many developments in the treatment of coronary disease, anesthesia, and perioperative management.

This study, on a very large database of more than 200 000 patients, identified 5 major predictors of myocardial infarction or cardiac arrest on multivariate analysis. This led to the creation of a predictive model amenable to the use of

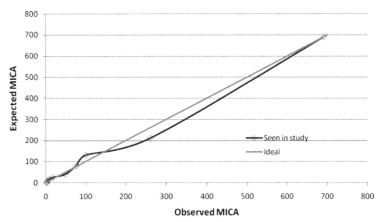

FIGURE 1.—Observed vs expected perioperative myocardial infarction or cardiac arrest (MICA): calibration of predictions in the training set. (Reprinted from Gupta PK, Gupta H, Sundaram A, et al, Development and validation of a risk calculator for prediction of cardiac risk after surgery. *Circulation.* 2011;124:381-387. © American Heart Association.)

a risk index calculator. The model is well validated and allows clinicians to make point-of-care decisions.[3] The use of models to provide objective prognostic information is clearly an advance over more subjective assessment, but as the accompanying editorial points out, what is necessary is for the calculator to be widely used and updated every few years.[3]

B. J. Gersh, MB, ChB, DPhil, FRCP

References

1. Goldman L, Caldera DL, Nussbaum SR, et al. Multifactorial index of cardiac risk in noncardiac surgical procedures. *N Engl J Med.* 1977;297:845-850.
2. Mangano DT. Perioperative cardiac morbidity. *Anesthesiology.* 1990;72:153-184.
3. Grover FL, Edwards FH. Objective assessment of cardiac risk for noncardiac surgical patients: an up-to-date simplified approach. *Circulation.* 2011;124:376-377.

Dose Response Between Physical Activity and Risk of Coronary Heart Disease: A Meta-Analysis
Sattelmair J, Pertman J, Ding EL, et al (Harvard School of Public Health, Boston, MA; et al)
Circulation 124:789-795, 2011

Background.—No reviews have quantified the specific amounts of physical activity required for lower risks of coronary heart disease when assessing the dose-response relation. Instead, previous reviews have used qualitative estimates such as low, moderate, and high physical activity.

Methods and Results.—We performed an aggregate data meta-analysis of epidemiological studies investigating physical activity and primary prevention of CHD. We included prospective cohort studies published in English since 1995. After reviewing 3194 abstracts, we included 33 studies. We used random-effects generalized least squares spline models for trend estimation to derive pooled dose-response estimates. Among the 33 studies, 9 allowed quantitative estimates of leisure-time physical activity. Individuals who engaged in the equivalent of 150 min/wk of moderate-intensity leisure-time physical activity (minimum amount, 2008 US federal guidelines) had a 14% lower coronary heart disease risk (relative risk, 0.86; 95% confidence interval, 0.77 to 0.96) compared with those reporting no leisure-time physical activity. Those engaging in the equivalent of 300 min/wk of moderate-intensity leisure-time physical activity (2008 US federal guidelines for additional benefits) had a 20% (relative risk, 0.80; 95% confidence interval, 0.74 to 0.88) lower risk. At higher levels of physical activity, relative risks were modestly lower. People who were physically active at levels lower than the minimum recommended amount also had significantly lower risk of coronary heart disease. There was a significant interaction by sex ($P=0.03$); the association was stronger among women than men.

Conclusions.—These findings provide quantitative data supporting US physical activity guidelines that stipulate that "some physical activity is

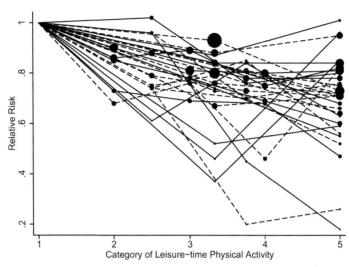

FIGURE 1.—Plot of the relative risks of coronary heart disease by category of leisure-time physical activity. All study categories were standardized to 5 categories for ease of comparison. The size of the data point corresponds to the study size; the larger the dot is, the larger the sample size is. Dashed lines indicate studies with physical activity categorized quantitatively; solid lines, studies with physical activity categorized categorically. (Reprinted from Sattelmair J, Pertman J, Ding EL, et al. Dose response between physical activity and risk of coronary heart disease: a meta-analysis. *Circulation.* 2011;124:789-795. © American Heart Association, Inc.)

better than none" and "additional benefits occur with more physical activity (Fig 1)."

▶ It is well accepted that physical activity plays an important role in the primary prevention of coronary artery disease,[1] and prior reviews suggest that physical activity is associated with a 20% to 30% reduction in the risk of coronary heart disease.[2] The strength of this meta-analysis of 33 studies is the focus on the amount of physical activity and its impact on risk. Of the 33 studies, 9 provided qualitative information about the amount of leisure time regular physical activity. Individuals who engaged in the equivalent of 150 minutes per week of moderate-intensity physical activity had a 14% lower coronary heart disease risk, and for 300 minutes of work per week this was 20% less, with little additional risk reduction as the intensity of exercise increased. Any exercise appeared better than no exercise (even if the amount was less than the US recommended guidelines), and the association was stronger in women. So the results are not surprising, but it is reassuring to know the biggest bang for the primary prevention buck comes at a lower level of the activity spectrum—that is, very modest, easily achievable levels of physical activity.

B. J. Gersh, MB, ChB, DPhil, FRCP

References

1. Pate RR, Pratt M, Blair SN, et al; Physical activity and public health. A recommendation from the Centers for Disease Control and Prevention and the American College of Sports Medicine. *JAMA.* 1995;273:402-407.

2. Sofi F, Capalbo A, Cesari F, Abbate R, Gensini GF. Physical activity during leisure time and primary prevention of coronary heart disease: an updated meta-analysis of cohort studies. *Eur J Cardiovasc Prev Rehabil.* 2008;15:247-257.

Isolated Coronary Artery Bypass Graft Combined With Bone Marrow Mononuclear Cells Delivered Through a Graft Vessel for Patients With Previous Myocardial Infarction and Chronic Heart Failure: A Single-Center, Randomized, Double-Blind, Placebo-Controlled Clinical Trial
Hu S, Liu S, Zheng Z, et al (Fuwai Hosp, Beijing, China)
J Am Coll Cardiol 57:2409-2415, 2011

Objectives.—This study aimed at examining the efficacy of bone marrow mononuclear cell (BMMNC) delivery through graft vessel for patients with a previous myocardial infarction (MI) and chronic heart failure during coronary artery bypass graft (CABG).

Background.—Little evidence exists supporting the practice of BMMNC delivery through graft vessel for patients with a previous MI and chronic heart failure during CABG.

Methods.—From November 2006 to June 2009, a randomized, placebo-controlled trial was conducted to test the efficacy and safety of CABG for multivessel coronary artery disease combined with autologous BMMNCs in patients with congestive heart failure due to severe ischemic cardiomyopathy. Sixty-five patients were recruited, and 60 patients remained in the final trial and were randomized to a CABG + BMMNC group (n = 31) and a placebo-control group (i.e., CABG-only group, n = 29). All patients discharged received a 6-month follow-up. Changes in left ventricular ejection fraction from baseline to 6-month follow-up, as examined by magnetic resonance imaging, were of primary interest.

Results.—The overall baseline age was 59.5 ± 9.2 years, and 6.7% were women. After a 6-month follow-up, compared with the placebo-control group, the CABG + BMMNC group had significant changes in left ventricular ejection fraction (p = 0.029), left ventricular end-systolic volume index (p = 0.017), and wall motion index score (p = 0.011). Also, the changes in the distance on the 6-min walking test as well as B-type natriuretic peptide were significantly greater in the CABG + BMMNC group than in the control group.

Conclusions.—In summary, patients with a previous MI and chronic heart failure could potentially benefit from isolated CABG (i.e., those who received CABG only) combined with BMMNCs delivered through a graft vessel. (Stem Cell Therapy to Improve Myocardial Function in Patients Undergoing Coronary Artery Bypass Grafting [CABG]; NCT00395811) (Table 2).

▶ Although this is one of many small trials of bone marrow mononuclear cell administration in post—myocardial infarction patients,[1] there are several aspects of this trial that I find particularly interesting. Firstly, the trial was not only

TABLE 2.—Change in MRI Indexes After Surgery ($\bar{x} \pm s$)

	Pre-Operative			Post-Operative			Changing Value		
	CABG + BMMNC Group (n = 31)	Placebo-Control Group (n = 29)	p Value	CABG + BMMNC Group (n = 31)	Placebo-Control Group (n = 28)	p Value	CABG + BMMNC Group (n = 31)	Placebo-Control Group (n = 28)	p Value
LVEF, %	22.78 (19.76, 27.46)	24.95 (20.72, 29.15)	0.287	33.80 (26.21,44.99)	31.82 (21.97, 39.93)	0.152	10.62 (4.94, 21.11)	5.69 (1.88, 11.15)	0.029*
LVEDVI, ml/m²	106.20 (90.10, 121.55)	93.33 (83.35, 111.13)	0.116	82.65 (67.07, 94.38)	95.15 (69.11, 106.83)	0.272	−18.71 (−43.28, −1.61)	10.77 (−28.18, 12.88)	0.080
LVESVI, ml/m²	80.13 (67.18, 101.89)	71.51 (62.61 84.11)	0.140	52.70 40.18,66.49)	64.84 (42.66, 87.80)	0.190	−23.38 (−47.65, −6.90)	14.83 (−25.62, 9.03)	0.017*
Beat volume, ml	42.05 (34.35, 55.15)	43.15 (35.00, 47.15)	0.889	50.95 (43.43,61.23)	49.74 (41.75, 58.43)	0.600	8.40 (0.43, 18.53)	6.90 (−1.60, 14.70)	0.507
Cardiac index, l/min/m²	1.70 (1.34, 1.99)	1.70 (1.37, 2.17)	0.640	1.95 (1.48, 2.32)	1.96 (1.76, 2.34)	0.321	0.22 (−0.12, 0.68)	0.09 (−0.16, 0.74)	0.682

Values are median (quartile).
Abbreviations as in Table 1.

randomized but also completely blinded, and secondly, this was a sick population with a preoperative ejection fraction of less than 0.30, chronic heart failure (New York Heart Association Class 2-3), and at least 3 months had elapsed since the last myocardial infarction.

The results are quite impressive in terms of the magnitude of the increase in ejection fraction and improvement in regional wall motion abnormalities and also despite the small sample size and increase in 6-minute walking distance. The imaging techniques that were used were unable to quantify infarct size.

The entire area of cell repair therapy is fascinating.[2] What we have learned to date is that it is safe and feasible with the exception of malignant ventricular arrhythmias after skeletal myoblast implantation. Changes in left ventricular function, including ejection fraction and left ventricular volumes, have been positive, but one should emphasize that these have also been extremely modest, although almost universally in the right direction. Nonetheless, some recent trials have been completely neutral. On the other hand, there has been no documentation of myocyte regeneration and cell survival, and retention rates are very low. This has supported the concept that the benefits are a result of paracrine as opposed to cellular effects. This field has come to "the end of the beginning," and the next phase will focus on different cells and on a variety of cell-based and substrate-based interventions to enhance the survival and retention of transplanted cells.[3] In any event, stay tuned, as this remains an interesting and dynamic area.

B. J. Gersh, MB, ChB, DPhil, FRCP

References

1. Wollert KC, Meyer GP, Lotz J, et al. Intracoronary autologous bone-marrow cell transfer after myocardial infarction: the BOOST randomised controlled clinical trial. *Lancet*. 2004;364:141-148.
2. Gersh BJ, Simari RD, Behfar A, Terzic CM, Terzic A. Cardiac cell repair therapy: a clinical perspective. *Mayo Clin Proc*. 2009;84:876-892.
3. Behfar A, Crespo-Diaz R, Nelson TJ, Terzic A, Gersh BJ. Stem cells: clinical trials results the end of the beginning or the beginning of the end? *Cardiovasc Haematol Disord Drug Targets*. 2010;10:186-201.

Positron Emission Tomography Measurement of Periodontal ^{18}F-Fluorodeoxyglucose Uptake Is Associated With Histologically Determined Carotid Plaque Inflammation

Fifer KM, Qadir S, Subramanian S, et al (Cardiac MR-PET-CT Program at Massachusetts General Hosp and Harvard Med School, Boston)

J Am Coll Cardiol 57:971-976, 2011

Objectives.—This study aimed to test the hypothesis that metabolic activity within periodontal tissue (a possible surrogate for periodontal inflammation) predicts inflammation in a remote atherosclerotic vessel, utilizing ^{18}F-fluorodeoxyglucose (FDG) positron emission tomography (PET) imaging.

Background.—Several lines of evidence establish periodontal disease as an important risk factor for atherosclerosis. FDG-PET imaging is an established method for measuring metabolic activity in human tissues and blood vessels.

Methods.—One hundred twelve patients underwent FDG-PET imaging 92 ± 5 min after FDG administration (13 to 25 mCi). Periodontal FDG uptake was measured by obtaining standardized uptake values from the periodontal tissue of each patient, and the ratio of periodontal to background (blood) activity was determined (TBR). Standardized uptake value measurements were obtained in the carotid and aorta as well as in a venous structure. Localization of periodontal, carotid, and aortic activity was facilitated by PET coregistration with computed tomography or magnetic resonance imaging. A subset of 16 patients underwent carotid endarterectomy within 1 month of PET imaging, during which atherosclerotic plaques were removed and subsequently stained with anti-CD68 antibodies to quantify macrophage infiltration. Periodontal FDG uptake was compared with carotid plaque macrophage infiltration.

Results.—Periodontal FDG uptake (TBR) is associated with carotid TBR (R = 0.64, p < 0.0001), as well as aortic TBR (R = 0.38; p = 0.029). Moreover, a strong relationship was observed between periodontal TBR and histologically assessed inflammation within excised carotid artery plaques (R = 0.81, p < 0.001).

Conclusions.—FDG-PET measurements of metabolic activity within periodontal tissue correlate with macrophage infiltration within carotid plaques. These findings provide direct evidence for an association between periodontal disease and atherosclerotic inflammation (Fig 2).

▶ This is a rather novel and intriguing study from a mechanistic standpoint. Periodontal disease is extremely common, and multiple clinical and epidemiologic studies have demonstrated an association with cardiovascular disease. Nonetheless, whether this is a cause-and-effect relationship or the result of confounders (eg, socioeconomic factors) remains unclear, although a biological association has been postulated.[1] A common denominator linking periodontal disease and atherosclerosis is the presence of inflammation.[2]

This study investigated the relationship between 18F-fluorodeoxyglucose (FDG) uptake in periodontal tissue (a nuclear marker of inflammation) and FDG uptake in atherosclerotic plaques within the carotid arteries and the aorta. The authors clearly demonstrate an association with plaques at both sites and with histologically assessed inflammation in excised carotid tissue.

These findings certainly strengthen the association between the 2 conditions. The mechanisms are likely multifactorial but include an atherogenic role for periodontal pathogens, induction of foam cells secondary to periodontal inflammation, and endothelial cell dysfunction. There is some evidence from prior studies that periodontal treatment resulted in an improvement in carotid intima-medial thickness,[3] and improved oral health may reduce systemic markers of inflammation and improve endothelial function.[4]

These data are hypothesis-generating and need to be followed by prospective trials assessing indices of periodontal activity as predictors of atherosclerotic

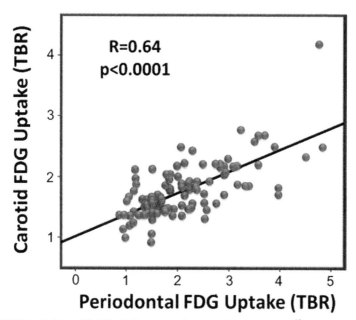

FIGURE 2.—Periodontal FDG Uptake Versus Carotid FDG Uptake. In 112 patients, ^{18}F-fluorodeoxyglucose (FDG) uptake (target-to-background ratio [TBR]) within periodontal tissues was compared with FDG uptake in the carotid arteries of the same patients. A significant relationship was observed between periodontal TBR and carotid artery TBR. (Reprinted from the Journal of the American College of Cardiology, Fifer KM, Qadir S, Subramanian S, et al. Positron emission tomography measurement of periodontal ^{18}F-fluorodeoxyglucose uptake is associated with histologically determined carotid plaque inflammation. *J Am Coll Cardiol.* 2011;57:971-976. Copyright 2011, with permission from the American College of Cardiology.)

plaque formation and the resolution with improved periodontal health. These will be difficult to do, but this is an important and interesting topic.

B. J. Gersh, MB, ChB, DPhil, FRCP

References

1. Espinola-Klein C, Rupprecht HJ, Blankenberg S, et al. Impact of infectious burden on extent and long-term prognosis of atherosclerosis. *Circulation.* 2002;105:15-21.
2. Blum A, Front E, Peleg A. Periodontal care may improve systemic inflammation. *Clin Invest Med.* 2007;30:E114-E117.
3. Piconi S, Trabattoni D, Luraghi C, et al. Treatment of periodontal disease results in improvements in endothelial dysfunction and reduction of the carotid intima-media thickness. *FASEB J.* 2009;23:1196-1204.
4. Blum A, Kryuger K, Mashiach Eizenberg M, et al. Periodontal care may improve endothelial function. *Eur J Intern Med.* 2007;18:295-298.

Predictors of Coronary Heart Disease Events Among Asymptomatic Persons With Low Low-Density Lipoprotein Cholesterol: MESA (Multi-Ethnic Study of Atherosclerosis)

Blankstein R, Budoff MJ, Shaw LJ, et al (Brigham and Women's Hosp, Boston, MA; Harbor-UCLA Med Ctr; Emory Univ School of Medicine, Atlanta, GA; et al)

J Am Coll Cardiol 58:364-374, 2011

Objectives.—Our aim was to identify risk factors for coronary heart disease (CHD) events among asymptomatic persons with low (≤130 mg/dl) low-density lipoprotein cholesterol (LDL-C).

Background.—Even among persons with low LDL-C, some will still experience CHD events and may benefit from more aggressive pharmacologic and lifestyle therapies.

Methods.—The MESA (Multi-Ethnic Study of Atherosclerosis) is a prospective cohort of 6,814 participants free of clinical cardiovascular disease. Of 5,627 participants who were not receiving any baseline lipid-lowering therapies, 3,714 (66%) had LDL-C ≤130 mg/dl and were included in the present study. Unadjusted and adjusted hazard ratios were calculated to assess the association of traditional risk factors and biomarkers with CHD events. To determine if subclinical atherosclerosis markers provided additional information beyond traditional risk factors, coronary artery calcium (CAC) and carotid intima media thickness were each separately added to the multivariable model.

Results.—During a median follow-up of 5.4 years, 120 (3.2%) CHD events were observed. In unadjusted analysis, age, male sex, hypertension, diabetes mellitus, low high-density lipoprotein cholesterol (HDL-C), high triglycerides, and subclinical atherosclerosis markers (CAC >0; carotid intima media thickness ≥1 mm) predicted CHD events. Independent predictors of CHD events included age, male sex, hypertension, diabetes, and low HDL-C. After accounting for all traditional risk factors, the predictive value of CAC was attenuated but remained highly significant. The relationship of all independent clinical predictors remained robust even after accounting for elevated CAC.

Conclusions.—Among persons with low LDL-C, older age, male sex, hypertension, diabetes, and low HDL-C are associated with adverse CHD events. Even after accounting for all such variables, the presence of CAC provided incremental prognostic value. These results may serve as a basis for deciding which patients with low LDL-C may be considered for more aggressive therapies (Fig 3).

▶ This is an interesting article from a large prospective epidemiologic study in the United States. It is well established that low-density lipoprotein (LDL) cholesterol is a risk factor for cardiovascular events and, as such, is the primary target of lipid-lowering therapy.[1] Initial guidelines were amended in 2004 and suggest a target of 100 mg/dL in high-risk persons and LDL cholesterol ≤70 mg/dL in those at very high risk. Other studies have found that the LDL

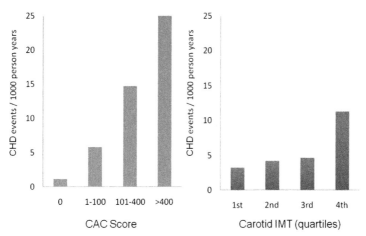

FIGURE 3.—CHD Outcomes Across CAC and Carotid IMT. The rates of incident coronary heart disease (CHD) per 1,000 person-years at risk are displayed by increasing categories of coronary artery calcium (CAC) and carotid intima media thickness (IMT). There was a substantial stepwise increase in event rates across increasing categories of CAC, but a less pronounced relationship between CHD events across increasing quartiles of carotid IMT. (Reprinted from the Journal of the American College of Cardiology, Blankstein R, Budoff MJ, Shaw LJ, et al. Predictors of coronary heart disease events among asymptomatic persons with low low-density lipoprotein cholesterol: MESA (Multi-Ethnic Study of Atherosclerosis). *J Am Coll Cardiol.* 2011;58:364-374. Copyright 2011, with permission from the American College of Cardiology.)

cholesterol can be lowered to less than 60 mg/dL, and the concept that "the lower the better" has taken hold. To date, there is no known threshold LDL cholesterol level below which no further reduction occurs. The purpose of this study was to look for predictors of cardiovascular events in a relatively low-risk group of patients without known coronary artery disease plus an LDL cholesterol of less than 130 mg/dL.

Over the 5-year follow-up there was no difference in events in individuals with an LDL of 100 mg/dL or lower versus those with an LDL cholesterol of 101 to 130 mg/dL and the event rate over the relatively short period was low in both groups (3.2%). Male sex, hypertension, diabetes, and a low level of high-density lipoprotein cholesterol remained powerful independent predictors of events. On multivariate analysis, the hazard ratio for these variables was approximately doubled. In addition, markers of subclinical atherosclerosis, such as carotid intimal medial thickness and coronary artery calcification, were predictive of coronary heart disease events, and after adjustment for all of the traditional risk factors, coronary artery calcification, but not carotid intimal medial thickness, remained independently predictive, although the strength of the association was attenuated.

Because statins do have their own side effects, a policy of statins for all is not feasible as a primary prevention strategy. The results of this study may serve as a basis for selecting which patients with a low LDL cholesterol level should nonetheless still be the target for aggressive therapies, including statins. What we do not know, however, is whether selective treatment of these subgroups would translate into improved clinical outcomes, and this is a great topic for future studies.

B. J. Gersh, MB, ChB, DPhil, FRCP

Reference

1. Grundy SM, Cleeman JI, Merz CN, et al. Implications of recent clinical trials for the National Cholesterol Education Program Adult Treatment Panel III guidelines. *Circulation.* 2004;110:227-239.

Prevalence and Predictors of Concomitant Carotid and Coronary Artery Atherosclerotic Disease

Steinvil A, Sadeh B, Arbel Y, et al (Tel Aviv Univ, Israel; et al)
J Am Coll Cardiol 57:779-783, 2011

Objectives.—The purpose of this research was to evaluate the relationship between coronary and carotid atherosclerotic disease using current guidelines for the definition of carotid artery stenosis (CAS).

Background.—The reported prevalence of concomitant coronary and carotid atherosclerotic disease has varied among studies due to differences in study populations and methodologies used.

Methods.—We performed a retrospective analysis of prospectively collected data obtained between January 2007 and May 2009 from consecutive patients undergoing same-day coronary angiography and carotid Doppler studies. Spearman correlations and multinomial logistic regression models were used to identify independent correlates of CAS.

Results.—The study included 1,405 patients (age 65 ± 11 years, 77.2% male), of whom 12.8% had significant CAS (peak systolic velocity [PSV] >125 cm/s) and 4.6% had severe CAS (PSV >230 cm/s). Mild CAS (PSV <125 cm/s and the presence of a sonographic atherosclerotic lesion) was present in 58%. The severity of CAS and the extent of coronary artery disease (CAD) were significantly correlated (r = 0.255, p < 0.001). Independent predictors of severe CAS defined by PSV were the presence of left-main or 3-vessel CAD, increasing age, a history of stroke, smoking status, and diabetes mellitus.

Conclusions.—The degree of internal carotid artery (ICA) stenosis is related to the extent of CAD, though the prevalence of clinically significant ICA stenosis is lower in specific CAD subsets than previously reported (Table 2).

▶ Atherosclerosis is a systemic inflammatory disease involving multiple arterial beds.[1] In general, the concomitant presence of both coronary artery disease (CAD) and carotid disease (CAS) identifies a group with a worse prognosis after myocardial infarction, cardiac surgery, and carotid surgery. What to do about it is another matter. For example, in the patient undergoing cardiac surgery, the presence of carotid stenosis may be a surrogate of more extensive aortic and cerebrovascular disease and as such an increased risk of stroke, but this will not be alleviated by addressing the carotid stenosis itself.

This is an interesting prospective study from Israel from 1490 patients undergoing nonemergency coronary angiography in addition to cardiac ultrasound

TABLE 2.—Frequencies of CAS Severity by the Degree of CAD Severity

CAD Extent	CAS Severity		
	Normal or Mild	Moderate	Severe or Total Occlusion
Normal or nonobstructive	272 (94.1)	11 (3.8)	6 (2.1)
1-vessel disease	243 (93.5)	9 (3.5)	8 (3.1)
2-vessel disease	335 (87)	36 (9.4)	14 (3.6)
3-vessel disease	319 (82.2)	42 (10.8)	27 (7.0)
Left main disease	57 (68.7)	17 (20.5)	9 (10.8)

Values are n (%). Carotid artery stenosis (CAS) defined as: normal (PSV <125 cm/s with no signs of atherosclerotic lesions); mild CAS (defined as PSV <125 cm/s and the presence of a sonographic atherosclerotic lesion correlating to diameter stenosis of <50%); moderate CAS (defined as PSV between 125 and 230 cm/s correlating to diameter stenosis of 50% to 70%); severe CAS (defined as PSV >230 cm/s correlating to diameter stenosis of >70%); and total or near occlusion (defined as 0 PSV and no visible flow).
CAD = coronary artery disease.

and Doppler. The majority of these patients had symptomatic angina pectoris and other features of coronary artery disease, including a positive stress test in 15.2% and unstable angina in 39.7%. The prevalence of CAS was high in that a lesion was noted on ultrasound scan in 58%, but the severity of CAS was significantly correlated with the extent of coronary disease. Independent predictors of severe CAS on multivariate analysis with a presence of left main and 3-vessel disease are increasing age, a history of stroke, smoking status, and diabetes.

These data are confirmatory of prior studies showing an association between the severity of CAD and CAS. These data also support the current guidelines, which do not recommend screening for CAS among individuals without neurologic symptoms consistent with carotid disease.[2] Whether high-risk patients undergoing cardiac surgery should be routinely screened for CAS is highly controversial. In the event that significant CAS is present, the indications for treatment must be made independently of the fact that the patient is undergoing cardiac surgery. In other words, the carotid disease needs to be treated in its own right based on stenosis, severity, and symptoms, and the role of the proposed cardiac surgical procedure is to influence the timing of cardiac surgery and the neurologic procedure but is not in itself an indication for carotid endarterectomy.

B. J. Gersh, MB, ChB, DPhil, FRCP

References

1. Ross R. Atherosclerosis—an inflammatory disease. *N Engl J Med.* 1999;340: 115-126.
2. Qureshi AI, Alexandrov AV, Tegeler CH, Hobson RW 2nd, Dennis Baker J, Hopkins LN. Guidelines for screening of extracranial carotid artery disease: a statement for healthcare professionals from the multidisciplinary practice guidelines committee of the American Society of Neuroimaging; cosponsored by the Society of Vascular and Interventional Neurology. *J Neuroimaging.* 2007;17:19-47.

Use of Herbal Products and Potential Interactions in Patients With Cardiovascular Diseases

Tachjian A, Maria V, Jahangir A (Mayo Clinic, Rochester, MN; Mayo Clinic, Scottsdale, AZ)

J Am Coll Cardiol 55:515-525, 2010

More than 15 million people in the U.S. consume herbal remedies or high-dose vitamins. The number of visits to providers of complementary and alternative medicine exceeds those to primary care physicians, for annual out of-pocket costs of $30 billion. Use of herbal products forms the bulk of treatments, particularly by elderly people who also consume multiple prescription medications for comorbid conditions, which increases the risk of adverse herb-drug-disease interactions. Despite the paucity of scientific evidence supporting the safety or efficacy of herbal products, their widespread promotion in the popular media and the unsubstantiated health

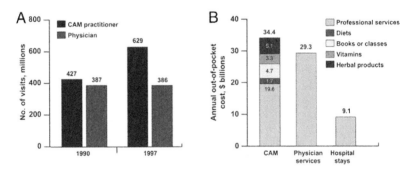

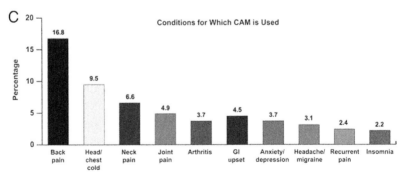

FIGURE 1.—Comparison of Number of Visits, Costs, and Conditions Treated Medically or by CAM. (**A**) Annual visits to physicians versus those to complementary and alternative medicine (CAM) practitioners. Adapted, with permission, from Eisenberg et al. (1). (**B**) The costs of CAM services by type compared with the costs of physician services and hospitalizations. Adapted, with permission, from Eisenberg et al. (1). (**C**) The most common conditions for which CAM therapies are used in the U.S. Data from Barnes PM, Powell-Griner E, McFann K, Nahin RL. Complementary and alternative medicine use among adults: United States, 2002. Advance data from vital and health statistics; no 343. Hyattsville, MD: National Center for Health Statistics, 2004. GI = gastrointestinal. (Reprinted from the Journal of the American College of Cardiology, Tachjian A, Maria V, Jahangir A. Use of herbal products and potential interactions in patients with cardiovascular diseases. *J Am Coll Cardiol.* 2010;55:515-525. Copyright 2010, with permission from the American College of Cardiology.)

TABLE 3.—Commonly Used Herbs That Can Potentiate the Risk of Bleeding of Arrhythmogenesis

Bleeding
  Alfalfa
  Bilberry
  Danshen
  Dong quai
  Fenugreek
  Garlic
  Ginkgo biloba
  Ginseng
  Motherwort
  Saw palmetto
Arrhythmogenesis (QT prolongation)
  Aloe vera
  Bitter orange
  Echinacea
  Ginkgo biloba
  Ginseng
  Guarana
  Hawthorn
  Horny goat weed
  Licorice
  Lily of the valley
  Night-blooming cereus
  Oleander
  Rhodiola
  St. John's wort

care claims about their efficacy drive consumer demand. In this review, we highlight commonly used herbs and their interactions with cardiovascular drugs. We also discuss health-related issues of herbal products and suggest ways to improve their safety to better protect the public from untoward effects (Fig 1, Table 3).

▶ This is a timely review of an important but often neglected topic, namely, the use of herbal products and complementary and alternative medicine (CAM) and their potential interactions with cardiovascular and other medications.

It is a huge problem. Approximately 34 billion dollars in out-of-pocket expenses is spent annually on CAM, and 17.7 billion dollars was for dietary and weight loss supplements.[1] Given the epidemic of obesity, these costs are likely to increase substantially, and herbal products already account for the largest proportion of CAM treatments in the United States.

The authors comprehensively list the potential drug interactions for a wide variety of products, emphasizing the potential interactions with antiplatelet and anticoagulants, which increase the risk of bleeding and the potential for serious arrhythmias via QT interval prolongation. In one study of patients attending a cardiovascular clinic, 58% took supplements that had potential interactions with warfarin, amiodarone, sotalol, or digoxin.[2] In a geriatric clinic, 46% of patients were taking supplements with anticoagulant properties as shown in another study.

The problems related to the use of herbal products are multiple, indicating lack of specific evidence of safety, lack of regulatory oversight, lack of quality control, misinformation due to unethical and aggressive marketing techniques, under-reporting of adverse reactions, and a lack of knowledge about drug-drug interactions among patients and health care providers. This is compounded by a lack of reporting such use by patients and health care providers not remembering to ask the question. The authors make a strong and appropriate argument that manufacturers should be required to register with the US Food and Drug Administration and to provide evidence of good manufacturing practices with regard to preparation, storage, and standardization techniques. Clinical trials are needed and sorely lacking. We need to be far more aware of the problem—patients are being placed at increased risk. Furthermore, large amounts of money are being spent on questionable products, and the entire field is characterized by lack of evidence-based practice.

B. J. Gersh, MB, ChB, DPhil, FRCP

References

1. Eisenberg DM, Davis RB, Ettner SL, et al. Trends in alternative medicine use in the United States, 1990-1997: results of a follow-up national survey. *JAMA.* 1998; 280:1569-1575.
2. Cohen RJ, Ek K, Pan CX. Complementary and alternative medicine (CAM) use by older adults: a comparison of self-report and physician chart documentation. *J Gerontol A Biol Sci Med Sci.* 2002;57:M223-M227.

Non-ST Elevation Acute Coronary Syndromes

3-Year Follow-Up of Patients With Coronary Artery Spasm as Cause of Acute Coronary Syndrome: The CASPAR (Coronary Artery Spasm in Patients With Acute Coronary Syndrome) Study Follow-Up
Ong P, Athanasiadis A, Borgulya G, et al (Robert-Bosch-Krankenhaus, Stuttgart, Germany; St. George's Univ of London, UK)
J Am Coll Cardiol 57:147-152, 2011

Objectives.—We sought to determine the prognosis of patients with acute coronary syndrome without culprit lesion and proof of coronary spasm during 3 years of follow-up.

Background.—Coronary artery spasm has been identified as an alternative cause for acute coronary syndrome (ACS) in patients without culprit lesion. In the CASPAR (Coronary Artery Spasm as a Frequent Cause for Acute Coronary Syndrome) study, we recently showed that ~50% of ACS patients without culprit lesion, in whom intracoronary acetylcholine provocation was performed, had coronary spasm. However, data on prognosis in these patients are sparse.

Methods.—After 3 years of follow-up, data regarding the following end points were obtained: death (cardiac and noncardiac), nonfatal myocardial infarction, and recurrent angina leading to repeated coronary angiography. The analysis focused on patients with a culprit lesion (n = 270) and patients without a culprit lesion (n = 76) but with acetylcholine provocation (total n = 346).

Results.—In patients without culprit lesion, there was no cardiac death or nonfatal myocardial infarction during follow-up; 1 patient died due to a noncardiac cause. However, 38 of 76 patients reported persistent angina requiring repeated angiography in 3 cases (3.9%). Thirty of 270 patients with culprit lesion died due to a cardiac cause (11.1%) and 13 due to a noncardiac cause (4.8%). Eleven patients had nonfatal myocardial infarction (4.1%) and 27 repeated angiography due to persistent or

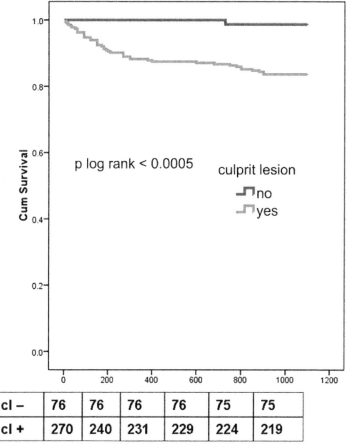

| cl − | 76 | 76 | 76 | 76 | 75 | 75 |
| cl + | 270 | 240 | 231 | 229 | 224 | 219 |

FIGURE 2.—Kaplan-Meier Survival Curves: All-Cause Mortality. Kaplan-Meier survival curves (cumulative survival) for all-cause mortality showing significantly more deaths in the group with culprit lesion (cl +, **green**) than in the group without (cl −, **blue**) (p < 0.0005, log-rank test) during follow-up (1,095 days). The number of patients alive during follow-up is given **below the graph**. Cum = cumulative. For interpretation of the references to color in this figure legend, the reader is referred to web version of this article. (Reprinted from the Journal of the American College of Cardiology, Ong P, Athanasiadis A, Borgulya G, et al. 3-year follow-up of patients with coronary artery spasm as cause of acute coronary syndrome: the CASPAR (Coronary Artery Spasm in Patients with Acute Coronary Syndrome) study follow-up. *J Am Coll Cardiol.* 2011;57:147-152. Copyright 2011, with permission from the American College of Cardiology.)

recurrent angina (10%). Patients with a culprit lesion had a higher mortality and more coronary events compared with those without (p < 0.0005, log-rank test).

Conclusions.—ACS patients without culprit lesion and proof of coronary spasm have an excellent prognosis for survival and coronary events after 3 years compared with patients with obstructive ACS. However, persistent angina represents a challenging problem in these patients, leading in some cases to repeated coronary angiography (Figs 2 and 3).

▶ This is a rather unusual and interesting study of patients with an acute coronary syndrome, among whom 28% did not have a culprit lesion on angiography.

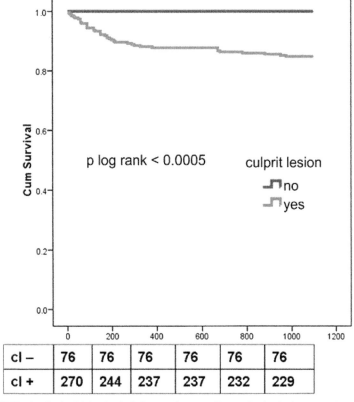

FIGURE 3.—Kaplan-Meier Survival Curves: Coronary Events. Kaplan-Meier curves (cumulative survival) comparing coronary events in patients with and without culprit lesion. The culprit lesion group (cl +, **green**) had significantly more events than the group without culprit lesion (cl −, **blue**) (p < 0.0005, log-rank test) during follow-up (1,095 days). The number of patients without coronary events during follow-up is given **below the graph.** Cum = cumulative. For interpretation of the references to color in this figure legend, the reader is referred to web version of this article. (Reprinted from the Journal of the American College of Cardiology, Ong P, Athanasiadis A, Borgulya G, et al. 3-year follow-up of patients with coronary artery spasm as cause of acute coronary syndrome: the CASPAR (Coronary Artery Spasm in Patients with Acute Coronary Syndrome) study follow-up. *J Am Coll Cardiol.* 2011;57:147-152. Copyright 2011, with permission from the American College of Cardiology.)

Among the 86 patients undergoing intracoronary acetylcholine provocation for the detection of coronary spasm, the result was positive in 49%.[1] A prior study from Japan described the late follow-up in 93 patients,[2] but since racial differences have been described between Asian and white patients with coronary spasm,[3] this study provides new information on outcomes in a group of white patients.

The prognosis in terms of mortality and nonfatal myocardial infarctions is excellent, as was the case in the prior Japanese study, although other studies have described a higher rate of events such as nonfatal infarction, but in some of the studies, these included patients with spasm at the site of an obstructed lesion. It is interesting that the proportion of smokers in this study was low, and smoking may predispose to spasm-related myocardial infarction, which might also account for the relatively benign prognosis.

Nonetheless, a significant proportion of patients continue to experience angina, perhaps because of underlying abnormal coronary vasoreactivity and microvascular dysfunction. From a clinical perspective, such patients need careful follow-up with attention to adjustment of antianginal therapy and control of risk factors.

B. J. Gersh, MB, ChB, DPhil, FRCP

References

1. Ong P, Athanasiadis A, Hill S, Vogelsberg H, Voehringer M, Sechtem U. Coronary artery spasm as a frequent cause of acute coronary syndrome: the CASPAR (Coronary Artery Spasm in Patients with Acute Coronary Syndrome) Study. *J Am Coll Cardiol.* 2008;52:523-527.
2. Wang CH, Kuo LT, Hung MJ, Cherng WJ. Coronary vasospasm as a possible cause of elevated cardiac troponin I in patients with acute coronary syndrome and insignificant coronary artery disease. *Am Heart J.* 2002;144:275-281.
3. Beltrame JF, Sasayama S, Maseri A. Racial heterogeneity in coronary artery vasomotor reactivity: differences between Japanese and Caucasian patients. *J Am Coll Cardiol.* 1999;33:1442-1452.

Optimal timing of coronary angiography and potential intervention in non-ST-elevation acute coronary syndromes

Katritsis DG, Siontis GCM, Kastrati A, et al (Athens Euroclinic, Greece; Univ of Ioannina School of Medicine, Greece; Technische Universität München, Munich, Germany; et al)
Eur Heart J 32:32-40, 2011

Aims.—An invasive approach is superior to medical management for the treatment of patients with acute coronary syndromes without ST-segment elevation (NSTE-ACS), but the optimal timing of coronary angiography and subsequent intervention, if indicated, has not been settled.

Methods and Results.—We conducted a meta-analysis of randomized trials addressing the optimal timing (early vs. delayed) of coronary angiography in NSTE-ACS. Four trials with 4013 patients were eligible (ABOARD, ELISA, ISAR-COOL, TIMACS), and data for longer follow-up periods than those published became available for this meta-analysis by the ELISA and ISAR-COOL investigators. The median time from admission or randomization to coronary angiography ranged from 1.16 to 14 h in the early and 20.8−86 h in the delayed strategy group. No statistically significant difference of risk of death [random effects risk ratio (RR) 0.85, 95% confidence interval (CI) 0.64−1.11] or myocardial infarction (MI) (RR 0.94, 95% CI 0.61−1.45) was detected between the two strategies. Early intervention significantly reduced the risk for recurrent ischaemia (RR 0.59, 95% CI 0.38−0.92, $P = 0.02$) and the duration of hospital stay (by 28%, 95% CI 22−35%, $P < 0.001$). Furthermore, decreased major bleeding events (RR 0.78, 95% CI 0.57−1.07, $P = 0.13$), and less major events (death, MI, or stroke) (RR 0.91, 95% CI 0.82−1.01, $P = 0.09$) were observed with the early strategy but these differences were not nominally significant.

Conclusion.—Early coronary angiography and potential intervention reduces the risk of recurrent ischaemia, and shortens hospital stay in patients with NSTE-ACS (Fig 1).

▶ Non-ST-segment elevation acute coronary syndromes (NSTE-ACS) represent a major burden of cardiovascular care, and the literature to some extent has been dominated by trials of antiplatelet and anticoagulant therapies in

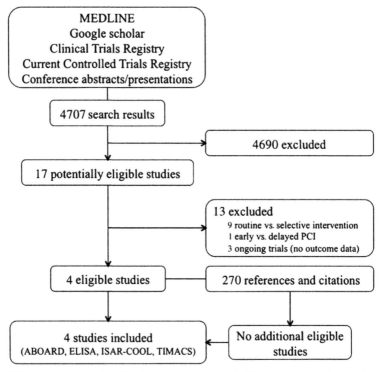

FIGURE 1.—Selection of studies. (Reprinted from Katritsis DG, Siontis GCM, Kastrati A, et al. Optimal timing of coronary angiography and potential intervention in non-ST-elevation acute coronary syndromes. *Eur Heart J.* 2011;32:32-40, by permission of The European Society of Cardiology.)

this patient subset. In addition, the role of an aggressive strategy of early intervention as opposed to a more conservative ischemia-driven strategy has been the focus of several randomized controlled trials in what appears to be a barrage of meta-analyses.[1] A prevailing consensus, however, is that the superior strategy for NSTE-ACS in centers with the requisite facilities and expertise is an invasive approach. The evidence is particularly strong in high-risk patients on the basis of elevated troponin, prior angina, diabetes, older age, ST-segment depression, and transient heart failure, among other variables, and a variety of risk scores are being developed for this purpose.[2]

A different issue is the optimal timing of angiography, which is addressed by this meta-analysis of 4 trials that enrolled 4300 patients. The conclusion is that early angiography reduces the risk of recurrent ischemia and shortens the duration of hospital stay.

Personally, I am not sure that a meta-analysis is needed because the trials all addressed slightly different questions. ABOARD demonstrated no benefit from emergency primary percutaneous coronary intervention (PCI) versus waiting for up to 24 hours, and in the "delayed" group, the time to angiography was 20.8 hours (median range 17.5—24.6 hours). This conclusion probably created a sense of relief among many interventionists given the exigencies of emergency primary PCI 24 hours around the clock. The TIMACS supported a policy of angiography within 24 hours but not as an emergency, and the ISAR-COOL trial showed no advantage in waiting for several days for "plaque passivation."

In summary, early catheterization with a view to coronary revascularization within the first 24 hours is superior to a conservative strategy, but emergency primary PCI is not necessary in patients with NSTE-ACS.

B. J. Gersh, MB, ChB, DPhil, FRCP

References

1. Bavry AA, Kumbhani DJ, Rassi AN, Bhatt DL, Askari AT. Benefit of early invasive therapy in acute coronary syndromes: a meta-analysis of contemporary randomized clinical trials. *J Am Coll Cardiol.* 2006;48:1319-1325.
2. Eagle KA, Lim MJ, Dabbous OH, et al; GRACE Investigators. A validated prediction model for all forms of acute coronary syndrome: estimating the risk of 6-month postdischarge death in an international registry. *JAMA.* 2004;291:2727-2733.

5 Non-Coronary Heart Disease in Adults

Congestive Heart Failure Therapy and Technology

Dose-dependent augmentation of cardiac systolic function with the selective cardiac myosin activator, omecamtiv mecarbil: a first-in-man study

Teerlink JR, Clarke CP, Saikali KG, et al (Univ of California, San Francisco; Univ of Manchester, UK; Cytokinetics Inc, South San Francisco, CA; et al)
Lancet 378:667-675, 2011

Background.—Decreased systolic function is central to the pathogenesis of heart failure in millions of patients worldwide, but mechanism-related adverse effects restrict existing inotropic treatments. This study tested the hypothesis that omecamtiv mecarbil, a selective cardiac myosin activator, will augment cardiac function in human beings.

Methods.—In this dose-escalating, crossover study, 34 healthy men received a 6-h double-blind intravenous infusion of omecamtiv mecarbil or placebo once a week for 4 weeks. Each sequence consisted of three ascending omecamtiv mecarbil doses (ranging from $0 \cdot 005$ to $1 \cdot 0$ mg/kg per h) with a placebo infusion randomised into the sequence. Vital signs, blood samples, electrocardiographs (ECGs), and echocardiograms were obtained before, during, and after each infusion. The primary aim was to establish maximum tolerated dose (the highest infusion rate tolerated by at least eight participants) and plasma concentrations of omecamtiv mecarbil; secondary aims were evaluation of pharmacodynamic and pharmacokinetic characteristics, safety, and tolerability. This study is registered at ClinicalTrials.gov, number NCT01380223.

Findings.—The maximum tolerated dose of omecamtiv mecarbil was $0 \cdot 5$ mg/kg per h. Omecamtiv mecarbil infusion resulted in dose-related and concentration-related increases in systolic ejection time (mean increase from baseline at maximum tolerated dose, 85 [SD 5] ms), the most sensitive indicator of drug effect ($r^2=0 \cdot 99$ by dose), associated with increases in stroke volume (15 [2] mL), fractional shortening (8% [1]), and ejection fraction (7% [1]; all $p<0 \cdot 0001$). Omecamtiv mecarbil increased atrial contractile function, and there were no clinically relevant changes in diastolic function. There were no clinically significant dose-related adverse effects on vital signs, serum chemistries, ECGs, or adverse events up to a dose of 0·625 mg/kg per h. The dose-limiting toxic effect was myocardial ischaemia due to excessive prolongation of systolic ejection time.

Interpretation.—These first-in-man data show highly dose-dependent augmentation of left ventricular systolic function in response to omecamtiv mecarbil and support potential clinical use of the drug in patients with heart failure (Figs 1 and 3).

▶ There have been phenomenal advances in the pharmacologic and device treatment of heart systolic heart failure (HF) in the last 20 years.[1] The first drug that increased cardiac contractility to be used was digitalis in the 18th century. Since then, there have been a number of positive inotropic drugs starting with adrenalin more than 120 years ago. We have a number of positive inotropes including dopamine, dobutamine, and milrinone that improve contractility by increasing cardiac myocyte intracellular calcium. This increase in intracellular calcium is responsible

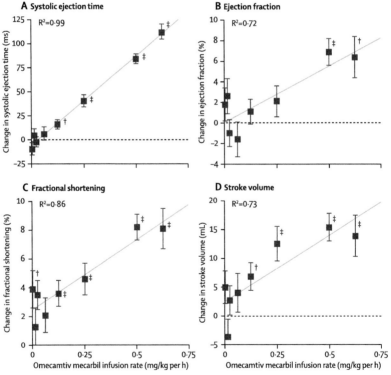

FIGURE 1.—Dose-dependent changes in echocardiogram measures by omecamtiv mecarbil dose*. Placebo-corrected change in (A) systolic ejection time, (B) ejection fraction, (C) fractional shortening, and (D) stroke volume by omecamtiv mecarbil dose (mg/kg per h after 6 h of infusion). Error bars show SEM. *p<0·0001 for all associations. †p<0·01. ‡p<0·0001. (Reprinted from The Lancet, Teerlink JR, Clarke CP, Saikali KG, et al. Dose-dependent augmentation of cardiac systolic function with the selective cardiac myosin activator, omecamtiv mecarbil: a first-in-man study. *Lancet.* 2011;378:667-675. © 2011, with permission from Elsevier.)

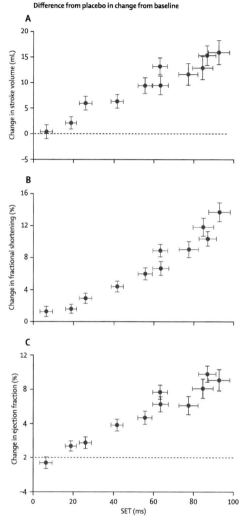

FIGURE 3.—Relation between changes in systolic ejection time and changes in selected echocardiogram variables. Placebo-corrected change in (A) stroke volume, (B) fractional shortening, and (C) ejection fraction by change in systolic ejection time. SET=systolic ejection time. Error bars show SEM. (Reprinted from The Lancet, Teerlink JR, Clarke CP, Saikali KG, et al. Dose-dependent augmentation of cardiac systolic function with the selective cardiac myosin activator, omecamtiv mecarbil: a first-in-man study. *Lancet.* 2011;378:667-675. © 2011, with permission from Elsevier.)

for the limitations these drugs have when used chronically: exacerbating myocardial ischemia, promoting atrial and ventricular arrhythmias, and increasing mortality.[2,3] Therefore, they are only useful in the acute setting. Another inodilator, levosimendan, showed potential clinical benefits but has failed to demonstrate survival benefit and has shown significant adverse effects compared with placebo.[4,5] Recently, a small-molecule, cardiac myosin activator, omecamtiv mecarbil, has been developed that increases contractility without affecting the intramyocyte calcium transient.[6] In a dog HF model, it increases left ventricular (LV) performance and cardiac output and decreases heart rate without increasing myocardial O_2 demand.[6] Unlike other inotropes, it does not increase LV dP/dt and prolongs systolic ejection time. This drug directly activates cardiac myosin, increasing the probability of transition to a strongly actin-bound, force-producing state.[6] A detailed explanation of the mechanism by which contractility is increased is presented in an article by Fady and colleagues.[6] The current article describes the first human use that establishes the maximum-tolerated dose and plasma concentration of omecamtiv mecarbil, administered as a 6-hour intravenous infusion in healthy volunteers in a crossover, placebo-controlled study. There was an 8 to 10 percentage-point increase in LV ejection fraction and decreased end-systolic volume, consistent with clinically beneficial direct improvements in end-systolic elastance.[7] There was also a 13% increase in stroke volume without an increase in heart rate. The limitation is the increase in systolic ejection time, which in doses above the maximum increase in contractility can result in decreased diastolic filling and myocardial ischemia. This study is important because it presents the first member of a novel class of drugs that can improve cardiac function by directly modulating the contractile apparatus, independent of second messenger systems, such as intracellular calcium or cyclic AMP that can cause unacceptable adverse events.

M. D. Cheitlin, MD

References

1. Dickstein K, Cohen-Solal A, Filippatos G, et al. ESC Guidelines for the diagnosis and treatment of acute and chronic heart failure 2008: the Task force for the diagnosis and treatment of acute and chronic heart failure 2008 of the European Society of Cardiology. Developed in collaboration with the Heart Failure Association of the ESC (HFA) and endorsed by the European Society of Intensive Care Medicine (ESICM). *Eur Heart J.* 2008;29:2388-2442.
2. Felker GM, Benza RL, Chandler AB, et al. Heart failure etiology and response to milrinone in decompensated heart failure: results from the OPTIME-CHF study. *J Am Coll Cardiol.* 2003;41:997-1003.
3. Cohn JN, Goldstein SO, Greenberg BH, et al. A dose-dependent increase in mortality with vesnarinone among patients with severe heart failure. Vesnarinone Trial Investigators. *N Engl J Med.* 1998;339:1810-1816.
4. Cleland JG, Freemantle N, Coletta AP, Clark AL. Clinical trials update from the American Heart Association: REPAIR-AMI, ASTAMI, JELIS, MEGA, REVIVE-II, SURVIVE, and PROACTIVE. *Eur J Heart Fail.* 2006;8:105-110.
5. Mebazaa A, Nieminen MS, Packer M, et al. Levosimendan vs dobutamine for patients with acute decompensated heart failure: the SURVIVE randomized trial. *JAMA.* 2007;297:1883-1891.
6. Malik FI, Hartman JJ, Elias KA, et al. Cardiac myosin activation: a potential therapeutic approach for systolic heart failure. *Science.* 2011;331:1439-1443.
7. Thomas JD, Popović ZB. Assessment of left ventricular function by cardiac ultrasound. *J Am Coll Cardiol.* 2006;48:2012-2025.

Cardiac Resynchronization Therapy as a Therapeutic Option in Patients With Moderate-Severe Functional Mitral Regurgitation and High Operative Risk

van Bommel RJ, Marsan NA, Delgado V, et al (Leiden Univ Med Ctr, the Netherlands)
Circulation 124:912-919, 2011

Background.—Functional mitral regurgitation (MR) is a common finding in heart failure patients with dilated cardiomyopathy and has important prognostic implications. However, the increased operative risk of these patients may result in low referral or high denial rate for mitral valve surgery. Cardiac resynchronization therapy (CRT) has been shown to have a favorable effect on MR. Aims of this study were to (1) evaluate CRT as a therapeutic option in heart failure patients with functional MR and high operative risk and (2) investigate the effect of MR improvement after CRT on prognosis.

Methods and Results.—A total of 98 consecutive patients with moderate-severe functional MR and high operative risk underwent CRT according to current guidelines. Echocardiography was performed at baseline and 6-month follow-up; severity of MR was graded according to a multiparametric approach. Significant improvement of MR was defined as a reduction ≥ 1 grade. All-cause mortality was assessed during follow-up (median 32 [range 6.0 to 116] months). Thirteen patients (13%) died before 6-months follow-up. In the remaining 85 patients, significant reduction in MR was observed in all evaluated parameters. In particular, 42 patients (49%) improved ≥ 1 grade of MR and were considered MR improvers. Survival was superior in MR improvers compared to MR nonimprovers (log rank $P<0.001$). Mitral regurgitation improvement was an independent prognostic factor for survival (hazard ratio 0.35, confidence interval 0.13 to 0.94; $P=0.043$).

Conclusions.—Cardiac resynchronization therapy is a potential therapeutic option in heart failure patients with moderate-severe functional MR and high risk for surgery. Improvement in MR results in superior survival after CRT.

▶ With ischemic and nonischemic cardiomyopathy, functional mitral regurgitation (FMR) is common and has negative prognostic implications.[1,2] After good medical management, if significant FMR persists, a recommended approach is for surgical restrictive mitral annuloplasty, but many patients are considered too high a surgical risk for valve surgery.[3] There is also some question as to whether mitral valve surgery improves prognosis in this group of heart failure (HF) patients.[4] Cardiac resynchronization therapy (CRT) has been found to decrease FMR in patients with mild-moderate MR and with a follow-up of only 6 months.[5-8] This study was designed to examine the effect of CRT in patients with HF, a wide QRS, decreased left ventricular ejection fraction (LVEF), and moderate-severe FMR. All the patients were classified as high risk for surgery. Thirteen patients died in the first 6 months. Follow-up time was a median of

32 months, and improvement of FMR was defined as improvement of ≥1 grade at 6 months of CRT. FMR improved in 49% of the surviving patients. In the entire group, FMR improved by all measurements, as did New York Heart Association (NYHA) class and LV remodeling by decrease in LV systolic and diastolic volumes. LVEF also increased. Comparing responders with nonresponders, ischemic cardiomyopathy was more frequent among the nonresponders, and improved NYHA class was more frequent in the responders, as was significant LV volume decrease. Most significant were the long-term survival rates at 22-year follow-up: 92% in responders and 67% in nonresponders. After correction for other significant variables, FMR improvement was a strong independent predictor of survival after CRT with a hazard ratio of 0.35. These findings show a sustained increased survival benefit of CRT for patients in HF with moderate to severe FMR who otherwise qualify for CRT.

M. D. Cheitlin, MD

References

1. Trichon BH, Felker GM, Shaw LK, Cabell CH, O'Connor CM. Relation of frequency and severity of mitral regurgitation to survival among patients with left ventricular systolic dysfunction and heart failure. *Am J Cardiol.* 2003;91: 538-543.
2. Robbins JD, Maniar PB, Cotts W, Parker MA, Bonow RO, Gheorghiade M. Prevalence and severity of mitral regurgitation in chronic systolic heart failure. *Am J Cardiol.* 2003;91:360-362.
3. Bach DS, Awais M, Gurm HS, Kohnstamm S. Failure of guideline adherence for intervention in patients with severe mitral regurgitation. *J Am Coll Cardiol.* 2009;54:860-865.
4. Calafiore AM, Iacò AL, Tash A, Abukudair W, Di Mauro M. Mitral valve surgery for functional mitral regurgitation in patients with chronic heart failure—update of the results. *Thorac Cardiovasc Surg.* 2010;58:131-135.
5. Breithardt OA, Sinha AM, Schwammenthal E, et al. Acute effects of cardiac resynchronization therapy on functional mitral regurgitation in advanced systolic heart failure. *J Am Coll Cardiol.* 2003;41:765-770.
6. Lancellotti P, Melon P, Sakalihasan N, et al. Effect of cardiac resynchronization therapy on functional mitral regurgitation in heart failure. *Am J Cardiol.* 2004; 94:1462-1465.
7. Solis J, McCarty D, Levine RA, et al. Mechanism of decrease in mitral regurgitation after cardiac resynchronization therapy: optimization of the force-balance relationship. *Circ Cardiovasc Imaging.* 2009;2:444-450.
8. Sitges M, Vidal B, Delgado V, et al. Long-term effect of cardiac resynchronization therapy on functional mitral valve regurgitation. *Am J Cardiol.* 2009;104: 383-388.

Cardiac resynchronization therapy in patients with left ventricular systolic dysfunction and right bundle branch block: A systematic review
Nery PB, Ha AC, Keren A, et al (Univ of Ottawa Heart Inst, Ontario, Canada)
Heart Rhythm 8:1083-1087, 2011

Background.—Whether patients with right bundle branch block (RBBB) benefit from cardiac resynchronization therapy (CRT) is unclear.

Objective.—The purpose of this study was to systematically review the published data from randomized clinical trials of CRT on the outcomes in patients with baseline RBBB.

Methods.—Randomized controlled trials of CRT in heart failure and left ventricular systolic dysfunction were identified from MEDLINE (1950–2010), EMBASE (1980–2010, week 45), Cochrane Controlled Trials Register (2009), Cochrane Database of Systematic Reviews, National Institutes of Health Clinical Trials.gov database.

Results.—A total of 112 references were retrieved. Four publications from five studies reported data on patients with RBBB and were included in this investigation, with 259 patients randomized to CRT and 226 randomized to non-CRT. None of the available data showed more favorable outcomes (soft or hard) in patients with CRT.

Conclusion.—None of the available data showed more favorable outcomes with CRT in patients with RBBB. A meta-analysis of RBBB patients from the major CRT trials is urgently needed. Results of the meta-analysis can direct further research, perhaps indicating a need for randomized trials in RBBB. Physicians and patients should be aware of the likely reduced benefit form CRT in patients with RBBB, and this should be factored into decision making. However, until more data are available it is too early to change guidelines (Table 1).

▶ Cardiac resynchronization therapy (CRT) has been shown to decrease symptoms and prolong life in patients with heart failure (HF) and a prolonged QRS (>120 msec) and reduced left ventricular ejection fraction (LVEF).[1-4] Most of these patients with prolonged QRS have had left bundle branch block (LBBB), and it is uncertain that patients with right bundle branch block (RBBB) would benefit from CRT. Current guidelines state that all patients with QRS >2120 msec fulfill the requirement for CRT[5] but emphasize that there is a lack of evidence to provide specific recommendations for RBBB. Small observational studies concerning this problem have been inconclusive.[6-9] This study is a report of an extensive literature search of all randomized, controlled trials of CRT in patients with HF, a prolonged QRS and reduced LVEF. A quality scoring scale was developed citing 13 criteria that constituted a high-quality study. Five publications included patients with RBBB and were included in this study with a quality score of ≥10 of 13, but only 4 reported details of outcomes. Of all the enrolled patients in these 5 studies, only between 4.3% and 12.5% were patients with RBBB. The primary endpoints were slightly different among the 4 studies but included hard endpoints, such as all-cause and cardiac death, hospitalization for worsening HF, development of malignant arrhythmias requiring an ICD, and soft endpoints, such as 6-minute walk test, quality-of-life scores, and change in New York Heart Association class. None of the available data suggest more favorable soft or hard outcomes with CRT in these trials. This is the first systematic review of randomized trials of CRT use in patients with HF, reduced LVEF, and RBBB. There was insufficient detail in these studies to perform a formal meta-analysis, but if an evidence-based recommendation about patients with prolonged QRS

TABLE 1.—Inclusion Criteria and Demographics of Selected Studies

Study	Inclusion Criteria	Randomization	Primary Endpoint	Enrolled Patients with RBBB (% of Total Cohort)	Quality Assessment Score
MIRACLE[12]	NYHA III–IV, LVEF ≤35%, LVEDD ≥55 mm, QRS ≥130 ms, 6-MW ≤450 m	CRT-P vs no CRT	1. NYHA class 2. QoL 3. 6-MW	28 (6.2)	12/13
CONTAK CD[13]	NYHA II–IV, LVEF ≤35%, QRS ≥120 ms, ICD indication	CRT-D vs ICD	Composite of all-cause mortality, hospitalization for HF, and VT/VF requiring ICD therapy	33 (5.7)	10/13
CARE-HF[2]	NYHA III–IV, LVEF ≤35%, QRS ≥120 ms	CRT-P vs no CRT	Composite of death from any cause or unplanned hospitalization for a cardiovascular event	35 (4.3)	11/13
MADIT-CRT[14]	NYHA I–II, LVEF ≤30%, QRS >130 ms	CRT-D vs ICD	Death from any cause or nonfatal HF events	228 (12.5)	12/13
RAFT[4]	NYHA II–III, LVEF <30%, QRS ≥120, ms	CRT-D vs ICD	Death from any cause or hospitalization for HF	161 (9)	13/13

6-MW = 6-minute walk distance; CRT = cardiac resynchronization therapy; HF = heart failure; ICD = implantable cardioverter-defibrillator; LVEDD = left ventricular end-diastolic diameter; LVEF = left ventricular ejection fraction; NYHA = New York Heart Association; QoL = quality of life; RBBB = right bundle branch block; VF = ventricular fibrillation; VT = ventricular tachycardia.
Editor's Note: Please refer to original journal article for full references.

of the RBBB configuration should be made, it will require more studies of patients with RBBB and enough details of outcomes to allow a formal meta-analysis.

M. D. Cheitlin, MD

References

1. Bristow MR, Saxon LA, Boehmer J, et al. Cardiac-resynchronization therapy with or without an implantable defibrillator in advanced chronic heart failure. *N Engl J Med.* 2004;350:2140-2150.
2. Cleland JG, Daubert JC, Erdmann E, et al. The effect of cardiac resynchronization on morbidity and mortality in heart failure. *N Engl J Med.* 2005;352:1539-1549.
3. Bradley DJ, Bradley EA, Baughman KL, et al. Cardiac resynchronization and death from progressive heart failure: a meta-analysis of randomized controlled trials. *JAMA.* 2003;289:730-740.
4. Tang AS, Wells GA, Talajic M, et al. Cardiac-resynchronization therapy for mild-to-moderate heart failure. *N Engl J Med.* 2010;363:2385-2395.
5. Epstein AE, DiMarco JP, Ellenbogen KA, et al. ACC/AHA/HRS 2008 Guidelines for Device-Based Therapy of Cardiac Rhythm Abnormalities: a report of the American College of Cardiology/American Heart Association Task Force on Practice Guidelines (Writing Committee to Revise the ACC/AHA/NASPE 2002 Guideline Update for Implantation of Cardiac Pacemakers and Antiarrhythmia Devices): developed in collaboration with the American Association for Thoracic Surgery and Society of Thoracic Surgeons. *Circulation.* 2008;117:e350-e408.
6. Adelstein EC, Saba S. Usefulness of baseline electrocardiographic QRS complex pattern to predict response to cardiac resynchronization. *Am J Cardiol.* 2009; 103:238-242.
7. Garrigue S, Reuter S, Labeque JN, et al. Usefulness of biventricular pacing in patients with congestive heart failure and right bundle branch block. *Am J Cardiol.* 2001;88:1436-1441.
8. Sturdivant JL, Robert BL, Ron Ben S, et al. Comparison of acute hemodynamic effects of cardiac resynchronization therapy in patients with right and left bundle branch block. *Heart Rhythm.* 2005;2:S129.
9. Rickard J, Kumbhani DJ, Gorodeski EZ, et al. Cardiac resynchronization therapy in non-left bundle branch block morphologies. *Pacing Clin Electrophysiol.* 2010; 33:590-595.

Defining potential to benefit from implantable cardioverter defibrillator therapy: the role of biomarkers

Scott PA, Townsend PA, Ng LL, et al (Southampton Univ Hosps NHS Trust, UK; Univ of Southampton, UK; Univ Hosps of Leicester, UK)
Europace 13:1419-1427, 2011

Aims.—Implantable cardioverter defibrillator (ICD) therapy improves survival in patients at high sudden cardiac death (SCD) risk. However, some patient groups fulfilling indications for ICD therapy may not gain significant benefit: patients whose absolute risk of SCD is low and patients whose risk of death even with an ICD is high. The value of biomarkers in identifying patients' potential for survival benefit from ICD therapy is unknown. We performed a pilot study to investigate this.

Methods and Results.—Five established cardiovascular biomarkers were measured in patients with ICDs on the background of left ventricular dysfunction: N-terminal pro-brain natriuretic peptide [NT-proBNP], soluble ST2 [sST2], growth differentiation factor-15, C-reactive protein, and interleukin-6. The endpoints were all-cause mortality and survival with appropriate ICD therapy. One hundred and fifty-six patients were enrolled (age 69 years [Q1–Q3 62–77], 85% male, 76% ischaemic aetiology). During a follow-up of 15 ± 3 months, 12 patients died and 43 survived with appropriate ICD therapy. In a Cox proportional hazards model, the strongest predictors of death were Log sST2 ($P < 0.001$), serum creatinine ($P < 0.001$), and Log NT-proBNP ($P = 0.002$). The strongest predictor of survival with appropriate ICD therapy was Log NT-proBNP ($P = 0.01$).

Conclusion.—The biomarkers NT-proBNP and sST2 are promising biomarkers for identifying patients with little potential to gain significant survival benefit from ICD therapy. However, their incremental benefit, in addition to currently available clinical risk prediction models, remains

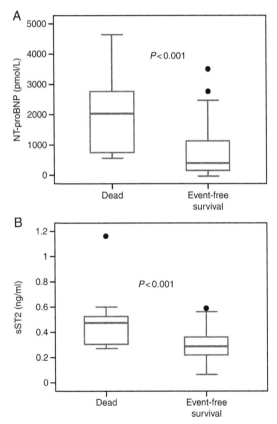

FIGURE 1.—Box plots showing the baseline concentrations of N-terminal pro-brain natriuretic peptide (A) and soluble ST2 (B) in patients who died and patients with event-free survival. Biomarker levels are presented as box (25th percentile, median, 75th percentile) and whisker (10th and 90th percentiles) plots. (Reprinted from Scott PA, Townsend PA, Ng LL, et al. Defining potential to benefit from implantable cardioverter defibrillator therapy: the role of biomarkers. *Europace.* 2011;13:1419-1427, by permission of the European Society of Cardiology and the European Heart Rhythm Association.)

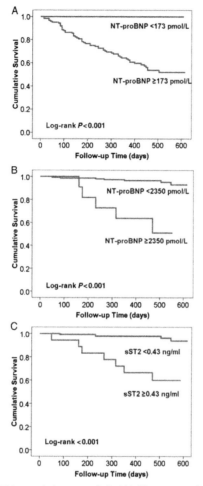

FIGURE 2.—Kaplan—Meier survival curve analysis. (A) All-cause mortality or appropriate implant-able cardioverter defibrillator therapy (reflecting event-free survival) in groups stratified by N-terminal pro-brain natriuretic peptide level (cut-off 173 pmol/L); (B) death in groups stratified N-terminal pro-brain natriuretic peptide level (cut-off 2350 pmol/L); and (C) death in groups stratified by soluble ST2 (cut-off 0.43 ng/mL). (Reprinted from Scott PA, Townsend PA, Ng LL, et al. Defining potential to benefit from implantable cardioverter defibrillator therapy: the role of biomarkers. *Europace.* 2011;13:1419-1427, by permission of the European Society of Cardiology and the European Heart Rhythm Association.)

unclear. These results demand a confirmatory prospective cohort study, designed and powered to derive and validate prediction algorithms incor-porating these markers (Figs 1 and 2, Table 4).

▶ Implantable cardioverter defibrillators (ICD) improve survival in patients at high risk of sudden cardiac death (SCD).[1] However, not all patients implanted with an ICD die, implying that they were not truly at high risk, and patients with ICD die with a workable ICD in place that did not discharge, indicating

TABLE 4.—Combining Biomarkers to Identify Groups of Patients Unlikely to Gain Significant Benefit From Implantable Cardioverter-Defibrillator Therapy

	Group 1 Low Risk of ICD Therapy and Death	Group 2 High Risk of ICD Therapy and Low Risk of Death	Group 3 High Risk of Death
Model 1	NT-proBNP < 173 pmol/L	NT-proBNP ≥ 173 pmol/L and <2350 pmol/L	NT-proBNP ≥ 2350 pmol/L
Total Patients in Group	31	114	11
Death	0	7	5
Survival with any appropriate ICD therapy	0	41	2
Model 2	NT-proBNP < 173 pmol/L	NT-proBNP ≥ 173 pmol/L and sST2 < 0.43 ng/mL	sST2 ≥ 0.43 ng/mL
Total Patients in Group	31	107	18
Death	0	5	7
Survival with any appropriate ICD therapy	0	38	5

that death was probably not due to a fatal arrhythmia.[2-4] The ability to identify more accurately those high-risk patients who would benefit from an ICD would be extremely valuable. Biomarkers reflect myocardial injury, inflammation, collagen turnover, and myocardial stretch independent of left ventricular ejection fraction[5] and may predict appropriate discharge for malignant arrhythmias in patients with ICDs.[6-8] In this study, 5 biomarkers were selected reflecting a range of pathophysiologic processes: N-terminal pro-brain natriuretic peptide (NT-proBNP) and serum ST2 as markers of myocardial stretch,[6,10] growth differentiation factor-15 as a marker for multiple cardiac stress pathways,[10] and C-reactive protein (CRP) and interleukin-6 (IL-6) as markers for inflammation.[8] Previous studies in patients with left ventricular systolic dysfunction with these markers demonstrated an independent association with mortality,[6,8-10] SCD,[6,9] and occurrence of ventricular arrhythmias.[6,8] The 156 patients with ICDs were a mean of 4 years after implantation and were followed for a mean of 15 months. Twelve patients (8%) died and 47 (30%) experienced appropriate ICD therapy, 4 of whom later died leaving 43 (28%) of patients who experienced appropriate ICD therapy and survived. Of the biomarkers on univariate analyses, all but CRP were significant predictors of all-cause mortality and only NT-proBNP significantly predicted survival with appropriate ICD therapy versus event-free survival. Using the best cut-off values of ST2 and NT-proBNP, models were developed that divided patients into 3 groups: those with low risk of death or appropriate ICD therapy, those with a high risk of appropriate ICD therapy but low risk of death, and those with a high risk of death (Table). The major limitations of this pilot study are the small size, the limited number of deaths, and the short follow-up time. There are other more complex risk scores using clinical variables that examined the relationship between the score and benefit from ICD therapy.[4,11] How the use of these biomarkers compares with these other risk scores or whether they would add incremental accuracy to these scores is unclear and deserves further larger studies.

M. D. Cheitlin, MD

References

1. Epstein AE, Dimarco JP, Ellenbogen KA, et al. ACC/AHA/HRS 2008 guidelines for device-based therapy of cardiac rhythm abnormalities: executive summary. *Heart Rhythm.* 2008;5:934-955.
2. Germano JJ, Reynolds M, Essebag V, Josephson ME. Frequency and causes of implantable cardioverter-defibrillator therapies: is device therapy proarrhythmic? *Am J Cardiol.* 2006;97:1255-1261.
3. Cuculich PS, Sánchez JM, Kerzner R, et al. Poor prognosis for patients with chronic kidney disease despite ICD therapy for the primary prevention of sudden death. *Pacing Clin Electrophysiol.* 2007;30:207-213.
4. Goldenberg I, Vyas AK, Hall WJ, et al. Risk stratification for primary implantation of a cardioverter-defibrillator in patients with ischemic left ventricular dysfunction. *J Am Coll Cardiol.* 2008;51:288-296.
5. Braunwald E. Biomarkers in heart failure. *N Engl J Med.* 2008;358:2148-2596.
6. Scott PA, Barry J, Roberts PR, Morgan JM. Brain natriuretic peptide for the prediction of sudden cardiac death and ventricular arrhythmias: a meta-analysis. *Eur J Heart Fail.* 2009;11:958-966.
7. Kanoupakis EM, Manios EG, Kallergis EM, et al. Serum markers of collagen turnover predict future shocks in implantable cardioverter-defibrillator recipients with dilated cardiomyopathy on optimal treatment. *J Am Coll Cardiol.* 2010;55: 2753-2759.
8. Streitner F, Kuschyk J, Veltmann C, et al. Role of proinflammatory markers and NT-proBNP in patients with an implantable cardioverter-defibrillator and an electrical storm. *Cytokine.* 2009;47:166-172.
9. Pascual-Figal DA, Ordoñez-Llanos J, Tornel PL, et al. Soluble ST2 for predicting sudden cardiac death in patients with chronic heart failure and left ventricular systolic dysfunction. *J Am Coll Cardiol.* 2009;54:2174-2179.
10. Khan SQ, Ng K, Dhillon O, et al. Growth differentiation factor-15 as a prognostic marker in patients with acute myocardial infarction. *Eur Heart J.* 2009;30: 1057-1065.
11. Levy WC, Lee KL, Hellkamp AS, et al. Maximizing survival benefit with primary prevention implantable cardioverter-defibrillator therapy in a heart failure population. *Circulation.* 2009;120:835-842.

Mortality Reduction of Cardiac Resynchronization and Implantable Cardioverter-Defibrillator Therapy in Heart Failure: An Updated Meta-Analysis. Does Recent Evidence Change the Standard of Care?

Bertoldi EG, Polanczyk CA, Cunha V, et al (Federal Univ of Rio Grande do Sul, Porto Alegre, Brazil; et al)
J Card Fail 17:860-866, 2011

Background.—The recent publication of the MADIT-CRT and RAFT trials has more than doubled the number of patients in which a direct comparison of the combination of cardiac resynchronization therapy (CRT) and implantable cardioverter-defibrillator (ICD) versus ICD alone was carried out. The present meta-analysis aims to assess the impact of combined CRT and ICD therapy on survival of heart failure (HF) patients.

Methods and Results.—Medline, Embase, and the Cochrane Library databases were searched, and all randomized controlled trials of CRT alone or combined with ICDs in HF resulting from left ventricular systolic dysfunction were included. Main outcome was all-cause mortality. Summary relative risk (RR) and 95% confidence interval (CI) were calculated employing random-effects models. Twelve studies were included, with a total of 8,284 randomized patients. For the comparison of CRT alone versus medical therapy, pooled analysis of 5 available trials demonstrated a significant reduction in all-cause mortality with CRT (RR 0.76, 95% CI: 0.64−0.9). Pooled analysis of 6 trials that compared the combination of CRT and ICD therapy to ICD alone also showed a statistically significant reduction in all-cause mortality (RR 0.83, 95% CI: 0.72−0.96). Stratified analysis showed significant mortality reductions in all New York Heart Association class subgroups, with greater effect in classes III−IV (RR 0.70; 95% CI: 0.57−0.88). Pooled estimates of implant-related risks were 0.6% for death and 8% for implant failure.

Conclusion.—Combined CRT and ICD therapy reduces overall mortality in HF patients when compared with ICD alone (Figs 2B, 3, and 4).

▶ The introduction of implantable cardioverter-defibrillators (ICD) and cardiac resynchronization therapy (CRT) has been a major advance in the treatment of patients with advanced heart failure (HF).[1] There is good evidence that both of these devices in appropriate patients with HF prolong life and, in the case of CRT when added to optimal medical therapy, reduce symptoms.[2,3] Most previous trials compared the use of either ICD or CRT with optimal medical therapy.[4-6] Earlier studies are not convincing that the combination added significant improvement in all-cause mortality. Recently, the MADIT-CRT and the RAFT trials compared the combination of CRT and ICD with ICD alone.[7,8] Because these studies more than doubled the number of patients involved in this comparison, this study does a combined analysis of all trials allowing greater reliability to whether the combination of the 2 devices brings incremental benefit over either treatment alone. To be included, the studies had to be randomized controlled trials of more than 2 weeks duration that included HF patients with left ventricular (LV)

Study or Subgroup	CRT+ICD Events	Total	ICD Events	Total	Weight	Risk Ratio IV, Random, 95% CI	Year	Risk Ratio IV, Random, 95% CI
CONTAK CD	11	245	16	245	3.7%	0.69 [0.33, 1.45]	2003	
MIRACLE ICD	14	187	15	182	4.2%	0.91 [0.45, 1.83]	2003	
MIRACLE ICD II	2	85	2	101	0.5%	1.19 [0.17, 8.26]	2004	
REVERSE	9	419	3	191	1.2%	1.37 [0.37, 4.99]	2008	
MADIT-CRT	74	1089	53	731	17.8%	0.94 [0.67, 1.32]	2009	
RAFT	186	894	236	904	72.5%	0.80 [0.67, 0.94]	2010	
Total (95% CI)		2919		2354	100.0%	0.83 [0.72, 0.96]		
Total events	296		325					

Heterogeneity: Tau² = 0.00; Chi² = 1.72, df = 5 (P = 0.89); I² = 0%
Test for overall effect: Z = 2.58 (P = 0.010)

0.2 0.5 1 2 5
Favours CRT + ICD   Favours ICD

FIGURE 2.—All-cause mortality—CRT + ICD versus ICD alone. CRT, cardiac resynchronization therapy; ICD, implantable cardioverter defibrillator therapy; IV, inverse variance method. (Reprinted from the Journal of Cardiac Failure, Bertoldi EG, Polanczyk CA, Cunha V, et al. Mortality reduction of cardiac resynchronization and implantable cardioverter-defibrillator therapy in heart failure: an updated meta-analysis. Does recent evidence change the standard of care? *J Card Fail.* 2011;17:860-866. Copyright 2011 with permission from Elsevier.)

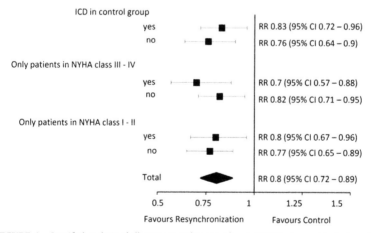

FIGURE 3.—Cumulative meta-analysis of all-cause mortality with CRT+ICD versus ICD alone. CRT, cardiac resynchronization therapy; ICD, implantable cardioverter defibrillator therapy; IV, inverse variance method. Note that the point estimate suggests a reduction in mortality since the earlier trials, but statistical significance only appears after addition of the RAFT trial. (Reprinted from the Journal of Cardiac Failure, Bertoldi EG, Polanczyk CA, Cunha V, et al. Mortality reduction of cardiac resynchronization and implantable cardioverter-defibrillator therapy in heart failure: an updated meta-analysis. Does recent evidence change the standard of care? *J Card Fail.* 2011;17:860-866. Copyright 2011 with permission from Elsevier.)

FIGURE 4.—Stratified analysis of all-cause mortality according to NYHA class and inclusion of ICD therapy. CI, confidence interval; ICD, implantable cardioverter-defibrillator; NYHA, New York Heart Association; RR, relative risk. (Reprinted from the Journal of Cardiac Failure, Bertoldi EG, Polanczyk CA, Cunha V, et al. Mortality reduction of cardiac resynchronization and implantable cardioverter-defibrillator therapy in heart failure: an updated meta-analysis. Does recent evidence change the standard of care? *J Card Fail.* 2011;17:860-866. Copyright 2011 with permission from Elsevier.)

systolic dysfunction and evaluated CRT, either alone or with an ICD, versus ICD therapy alone. The primary outcome was all-cause mortality. Twelve trials met the criteria, all with prolonged QRS interval and, most commonly, ischemic etiology of the HF, and follow-up time in various series was from 6 to 40 months. The pooled analysis of trials found that when comparing CRT with medical therapy, CRT reduced all-cause mortality by 24% and with CRT + ICD versus ICD alone, CRT + ICD reduced all-cause mortality 17%, both highly significant reductions. Implant failure rate of CRT in the pooled studies was 8%, and risk of major peri-implant complication was 13.2%. These complication rates declined progressively from earlier to more recent studies. Earlier trials that found no difference in mortality were either too small in number or with too short a follow-up time.

M. D. Cheitlin, MD

References

1. Jessup M, Abraham WT, Casey DE, et al. 2009 focused update: ACCF/AHA Guidelines for the Diagnosis and Management of Heart Failure in Adults: a report of the American College of Cardiology Foundation/American Heart Association Task Force on Practice Guidelines: developed in collaboration with the International Society for Heart and Lung Transplantation. *Circulation*. 2009;119: 1977-2016.
2. Ezekowitz JA, Armstrong PW, McAlister FA. Implantable cardioverter defibrillators in primary and secondary prevention: a systematic review of randomized, controlled trials. *Ann Intern Med*. 2003;138:445-452.
3. Bradley DJ, Bradley EA, Baughman KL, et al. Cardiac resynchronization and death from progressive heart failure: a meta-analysis of randomized controlled trials. *JAMA*. 2003;289:730-740.
4. Freemantle N, Tharmanathan P, Calvert MJ, Abraham WT, Ghosh J, Cleland JG. Cardiac resynchronisation for patients with heart failure due to left ventricular systolic dysfunction—a systematic review and meta-analysis. *Eur J Heart Fail*. 2006;8:433-440.
5. McAlister FA, Ezekowitz JA, Wiebe N, et al. Systematic review: cardiac resynchronization in patients with symptomatic heart failure. *Ann Intern Med*. 2004;141: 381-390.
6. Lam SK, Owen A. Combined resynchronisation and implantable defibrillator therapy in left ventricular dysfunction: Bayesian network meta-analysis of randomised controlled trials. *BMJ*. 2007;335:925.
7. Moss AJ, Hall WJ, Cannom DS, et al. Cardiac-resynchronization therapy for the prevention of heart-failure events. *N Engl J Med*. 2009;361:1329-1338.
8. Tang AS, Wells GA, Talajic M, et al. Cardiac-resynchronization therapy for mild-to-moderate heart failure. *N Engl J Med*. 2010;363:2385-2395.

Prognostic value of cardiac troponin T in patients with moderate to severe heart failure scheduled for cardiac resynchronization therapy

Aarones M, Gullestad L, Aakhus S, et al (Univ of Oslo, Norway; Oslo Univ Hosp-Rikshospitalet, Norway; et al)

Am Heart J 161:1031-1037, 2011

Background.—Predicting response to cardiac resynchronization therapy (CRT) is challenging. Highly sensitive cardiac troponin T (hsTnT) might predict response to CRT and identify patients at a high risk of experiencing severe cardiovascular events. We investigated whether baseline levels of hsTnT were associated with response to CRT and with severe cardiovascular events after long-term follow-up.

Methods.—Eighty-one consecutive patients were included according to the current guidelines for CRT. Biochemical, functional, and clinical parameters were assessed at baseline and at 3, 6, and 12 months of follow-up; and mortality/cardiac transplantation after 46 ± 6 months of follow-up was investigated. Cardiac magnetic resonance imaging and echocardiography were used to assess left ventricular function including viability and remodeling.

Results.—Seventy-five patients completed 12 months of follow-up; and after a follow-up of 46 ± 6 months, a total of 15 patients died, 13 of these from cardiovascular causes, and 7 underwent heart transplantation. Baseline hsTnT <15 ng/L predicted response to CRT and was associated with a more favorable outcome with regard to severe cardiovascular events. Multivariate analysis found that presence of transmural scar tissue/fibrosis on magnetic resonance imaging and use of statins were independently associated with higher concentrations of hsTnT at baseline. There was a strong correlation between hsTnT and N-terminal pro—B-type natriuretic peptide levels.

Conclusions.—Highly sensitive TnT levels were elevated in the majority of heart failure patients who were scheduled for CRT. The HsTnT levels predicted response to CRT as well as long-time survival (Figs 1 and 2).

▶ Cardiac resynchronization therapy (CRT) in congestive heart failure (CHF) patients with wide QRS and decreased ejection fraction has been shown to improve ventricular function, improve the New York Heart Association class, and increase survival. However, with the present criteria for selection, only 60% to 70% of patients respond with improved cardiac function,[1,2] so more accurate predictors of success with CRT are needed. Cardiac troponins are sensitive and specific serum markers for myocardial necrosis,[3] and elevated

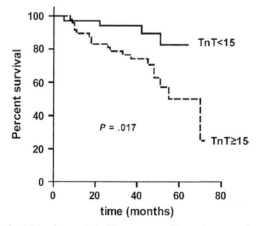

FIGURE 1.—Kaplan-Meier plot: survival without severe cardiovascular events of patients with baseline hsTnT < or ≥15 ng/L. (Reprinted from the American Heart Journal, Aarones M, Gullestad L, Aakhus S, et al. Prognostic value of cardiac troponin T in patients with moderate to severe heart failure scheduled for cardiac resynchronization therapy. *Am Heart J*. 2011;161:1031-1037. Copyright 2011, with permission from Elsevier.)

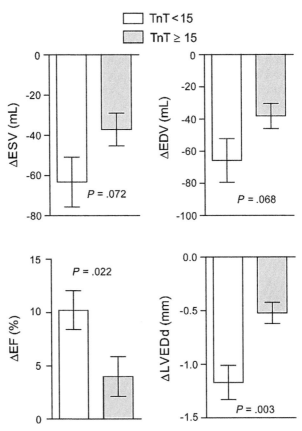

FIGURE 2.—Effect on echocardiographic parameters on patients with baseline hsTnT < or ≥15 ng/L. (Reprinted from the American Heart Journal, Aarones M, Gullestad L, Aakhus S, et al. Prognostic value of cardiac troponin T in patients with moderate to severe heart failure scheduled for cardiac resynchronization therapy. *Am Heart J.* 2011;161:1031-1037. Copyright 2011, with permission from Elsevier.)

troponin blood levels have been found in patients with chronic CHF.[4,5] Presumably elevated Tnt is a marker for progression of the CHF. Recently, a highly sensitive assay for troponin T (hsTnT) has been developed.[6] With the traditional assay, 10% of CHF patients had detectable TnT, but with the hsTnT assay, TnT was detectable in 92% of CHF patients, and the levels of hsTnT were highly associated with the severity of the CHF and with worse outcomes.[6] This study shows that patients with an hsTnT < 15 ng/L had greater decrease in LVend-diastolic and end-systolic diameter and more increase in left ventricular ejection fraction than those with hsTnT ≥15 ng/L. At 1 year, multiple logistic regression analysis showed that hsTnT was the only independent predictor of survival from cardiovascular events with patents with baseline hsTnT < 15 ng/L having a significantly lower cardiovascular mortality. Larger studies will be necessary to define a particular cutoff value that can be used clinically to predict survival and response to CRT. Other important questions need to be answered. Whether a decrease in hsTnT during CRT will predict better cardiac remodeling response, decreased incidence of severe cardiovascular events, or longer survival needs to be shown.

M. D. Cheitlin, MD

References

1. Cazeau S, Bordachar P, Jauvert G, et al. Echocardiographic modeling of cardiac dyssynchrony before and during multisite stimulation: a prospective study. *Pacing Clin Electrophysiol.* 2003;26:137-143.
2. Yu CM, Bax JJ, Gorcsan J III. Critical appraisal of methods to assess mechanical dyssynchrony. *Curr Opin Cardiol.* 2009;24:18-28.
3. Olivetti G, Abbi R, Quaini F, et al. Apoptosis in the failing human heart. *N Engl J Med.* 1997;336:1131-1141.
4. Wallace TW, Abdullah SM, Drazner MH, et al. Prevalence and determinants of troponin T elevation in the general population. *Circulation.* 2006;113:1958-1965.
5. Sato Y, Yamada T, Taniguchi R, et al. Persistently increased serum concentrations of cardiac troponin T in patients with idiopathic dilated cardiomyopathy are predictive of adverse outcomes. *Circulation.* 2001;103:369-374.
6. Latini R, Masson S, Anand IS, et al; Val-HeFT Investigators. Prognostic value of very low plasma concentrations of troponin T in patients with stable chronic heart failure. *Circulation.* 2007;116:1242-1249.

Relationship between improvement in left ventricular dyssynchrony and contractile function and clinical outcome with cardiac resynchronization therapy: the MADIT-CRT trial

Pouleur A-C, for the MADIT-CRT Investigators (Brigham and Women's Hosp, Boston, MA; et al)

Eur Heart J 32:1720-1729, 2011

Aims.—To assess long-term effects of cardiac resynchronization therapy (CRT) on left ventricular (LV) dyssynchrony and contractile function, by two-dimensional speckle-tracking echocardiography, compared with implantable cardioverter defibrillator (ICD) only in MADIT-CRT.

Methods and Results.—We studied 761 patients in New York Heart Association I/II, ejection fraction $\leq 30\%$, and QRS <130 ms [$n = 434$, CRT-defibrillator (CRT-D), $n = 327$, ICD] with echocardiographic studies available at baseline and 12 months. Dyssynchrony was determined as the standard deviation of time to peak transverse strain between 12 segments of apical four- and two-chamber views, and contractile function as global longitudinal strain (GLS) by averaging longitudinal strain over these 12 segments. We compared changes in LV dyssynchrony and contractile function between treatment groups and assessed relationships between these changes over the first year and subsequent outcomes (median post 1-year follow-up = 14.9 months). Mean changes in LV dyssynchrony and contractile function measured by GLS in the overall population were, respectively, -29 ± 83 ms and $-1 \pm 2.9\%$. However, both LV dyssynchrony (CRT-D: -47 ± 83 ms vs. ICD: -6 ± 76 ms, $P < 0.001$) and contractile function (CRT-D: $-1.4 \pm 3.1\%$ vs. ICD: $-0.4 \pm 2.5\%$, $P < 0.001$) improved to a greater extent in the CRT-D group compared with the ICD-only group.

A greater improvement in dyssynchrony and contractile function at 1 year was associated with lower rates of the subsequent primary outcome of death or heart failure, adjusting for baseline dyssynchrony and contractile function, treatment arm, ischaemic status, and change in LV end-systolic volume. Each 20 ms decrease in LV dyssynchrony was associated with a 7% reduction in the primary outcome ($P = 0.047$); each 1% improvement in GLS over the 12-month period was associated with a 24% reduction in the primary outcome ($P < 0.001$).

Conclusion.—Cardiac resynchronization therapy resulted in a significant improvement in both LV dyssynchrony and contractile function measured by GLS compared with ICD only and these improvements were associated with better subsequent outcomes (Figs 4 and 5).

▶ Cardiac resynchronization therapy (CRT) has been shown to reduce the risk of death and improve functional status in patients with advanced systolic heart failure (SHF), wide QRS and decreased left ventricular ejection fraction (LVEF).[1-3] The Multicenter Automatic Defibrillator Implantation Trial-Cardiac Resynchronization Therapy (MADIT-CRT) trial and the REVERSE and RAFT trials have broadened the indications for CRT to mildly symptomatic patients.[4-6] The response to CRT varies with approximately 30% of patients not responding symptomatically or by favorable echocardiographic remodeling. Previous studies suggest that both improvement in LV size and performance are the most important contributors to improved outcomes in heart failure (HF) patients receiving CRT.[7-9] More recent studies suggest that both LV mechanical dyssynchrony and contractile function are important determinants of CRT benefit.[10-12] Speckle tracking strain analysis permits assessment of both LV dyssynchrony and contractile function in an angle-independent manner.[13,14] When including patients from the MADIT-CRT trial, they were New York Heart Association (NYHA) Class I-II with LVEF ≤30% and QRS ≥0.13 seconds. After 1 year they found that there was improvement in both ventricular dyssynchrony and LV contractile function in the CRT-defibrillator group compared with the ICD-only group in the total

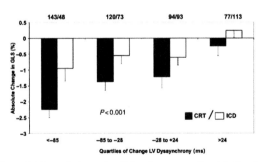

FIGURE 4.—Change in left ventricular contractile function measured by global longitudinal strain according to quartiles of change in dyssynchrony within-treatment group. Data are expressed as mean ± SEM. *Note:* the greater the absolute per cent reduction in left ventricular strain, the greater the improvement in left ventricular contractile function. (Reprinted from Pouleur A-C, for the MADIT-CRT Investigators. Relationship between improvement in left ventricular dyssynchrony and contractile function and clinical outcome with cardiac resynchronization therapy: the MADIT-CRT trial. *Eur Heart J.* 2011;32:1720-1729, by permission from The European Society of Cardiology.)

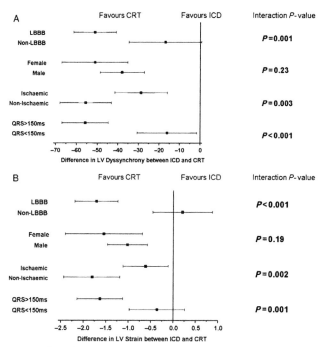

FIGURE 5.—(A) Effect of treatment on left ventricular dyssynchrony in subgroups. (B) Effect of treatment on left ventricular contractile function in subgroups. (Reprinted from Pouleur A-C, for the MADIT-CRT Investigators. Relationship between improvement in left ventricular dyssynchrony and contractile function and clinical outcome with cardiac resynchronization therapy: the MADIT-CRT trial. *Eur Heart J.* 2011;32:1720-1729, by permission of The European Society of Cardiology.)

study and in all subgroups. However, the improvement in dyssynchrony and LV contractile function was significantly greater in those with left bundle branch block, nonischemic cardiomyopathy, and wider QRS. These changes were related to the outcomes of death from any cause or nonfatal HF event, consistent with the possibility that improvements in synchrony and LV contractile function account for a considerable amount of the benefit from CRT in these patients. Moreover, the changes in synchrony may result in the improved LV contractile function.

M. D. Cheitlin, MD

References

1. Abraham WT, Fisher WG, Smith AL, et al; MIRACLE Study Group. Cardiac resynchronization in chronic heart failure. *N Engl J Med.* 2002;346:1845-1853.
2. Cleland JG, Daubert JC, Erdmann E, et al; Cardiac Resynchronization-Heart Failure (CARE-HF) Study Investigators. The effect of cardiac resynchronization on morbidity and mortality in heart failure. *N Engl J Med.* 2005;352:1539-1549.
3. Bristow MR, Saxon LA, Boehmer J, et al; Comparison of Medical Therapy, Pacing, and Defibrillation in Heart Failure (COMPANION) Investigators. Cardiac-resynchronization therapy with or without an implantable defibrillator in advanced chronic heart failure. *N Engl J Med.* 2004;350:2140-2150.

4. Moss AJ, Hall WJ, Cannom DS, et al; MADIT-CRT Trial Investigators. Cardiac-resynchronization therapy for the prevention of heart-failure events. *N Engl J Med.* 2009;361:1329-1338.

5. Linde C, Abraham WT, Gold MR, et al; REVERSE (REsynchronization reVErses Remodeling in Systolic left vEntricular dysfunction) Study Group. Randomized trial of cardiac resynchronization in mildly symptomatic heart failure patients and in asymptomatic patients with left ventricular dysfunction and previous heart failure symptoms. *J Am Coll Cardiol.* 2008;52:1834-1843.

6. Tang AS, Wells GA, Talajic M, et al; Resynchronization-Defibrillation for Ambulatory Heart Failure Trial Investigators. Cardiac-resynchronization therapy for mild-to-moderate heart failure. *N Engl J Med.* 2010;363:2385-2395.

7. Solomon SD, Foster E, Bourgoun M, et al; MADIT-CRT Investigators. Effect of cardiac resynchronization therapy on reverse remodeling and relation to outcome: multicenter automatic defibrillator implantation trial: cardiac resynchronization therapy. *Circulation.* 2010;122:985-992.

8. Yu CM, Bleeker GB, Fung JW, et al. Left ventricular reverse remodeling but not clinical improvement predicts long-term survival after cardiac resynchronization therapy. *Circulation.* 2005;112:1580-1586.

9. Ypenburg C, van Bommel RJ, Borleffs CJ, et al. Long-term prognosis after cardiac resynchronization therapy is related to the extent of left ventricular reverse remodeling at midterm follow-up. *J Am Coll Cardiol.* 2009;53:483-490.

10. White JA, Yee R, Yuan X, et al. Delayed enhancement magnetic resonance imaging predicts response to cardiac resynchronization therapy in patients with intraventricular dyssynchrony. *J Am Coll Cardiol.* 2006;48:1953-1960.

11. Marsan NA, Westenberg JJ, Ypenburg C, et al. Magnetic resonance imaging and response to cardiac resynchronization therapy: relative merits of left ventricular dyssynchrony and scar tissue. *Eur Heart J.* 2009;30:2360-2367.

12. Delgado V, Ypenburg C, van Bommel RJ, et al. Assessment of left ventricular dyssynchrony by speckle tracking strain imaging comparison between longitudinal, circumferential, and radial strain in cardiac resynchronization therapy. *J Am Coll Cardiol.* 2008;51:1944-1952.

13. Amundsen BH, Helle-Valle T, Edvardsen T, et al. Noninvasive myocardial strain measurement by speckle tracking echocardiography: validation against sonomicrometry and tagged magnetic resonance imaging. *J Am Coll Cardiol.* 2006;47: 789-793.

14. Stanton T, Leano R, Marwick TH. Prediction of all-cause mortality from global longitudinal speckle strain: comparison with ejection fraction and wall motion scoring. *Circ Cardiovasc Imaging.* 2009;2:356-364.

Impact of Remote Telemedical Management on Mortality and Hospitalizations in Ambulatory Patients With Chronic Heart Failure: The Telemedical Interventional Monitoring in Heart Failure Study

Koehler F, on behalf of the Telemedical Interventional Monitoring in Heart Failure Investigators (Charité- Universitätsmedizin Berlin, Germany; et al)
Circulation 123:1873-1880, 2011

Background.—This study was designed to determine whether physician-led remote telemedical management (RTM) compared with usual care would result in reduced mortality in ambulatory patients with chronic heart failure (HF).

Methods and Results.—We enrolled 710 stable chronic HF patients in New York Heart Association functional class II or III with a left ventricular ejection fraction ≤35% and a history of HF decompensation within the previous 2 years or with a left ventricular ejection fraction ≤25%. Patients were randomly assigned (1:1) to RTM or usual care. Remote telemedical management used portable devices for ECG, blood pressure, and body weight measurements connected to a personal digital assistant that sent automated encrypted transmission via cell phones to the telemedical centers. The primary end point was death from any cause. The first secondary end point was a composite of cardiovascular death and hospitalization for HF. Baseline characteristics were similar between the RTM (n=354) and control (n=356) groups. Of the patients assigned to RTM, 287 (81%) were at least 70% compliant with daily data transfers and no break for >30 days (except during hospitalizations). The median follow-up was 26 months (minimum 12), and was 99.9% complete. Compared with usual care, RTM had no significant effect on all-cause mortality (hazard ratio, 0.97; 95% confidence interval, 0.67 to 1.41; P=0.87) or on cardiovascular death or HF hospitalization (hazard ratio, 0.89; 95% confidence interval, 0.67 to 1.19; P=0.44).

Conclusions.—In ambulatory patients with chronic HF, RTM compared with usual care was not associated with a reduction in all-cause mortality.

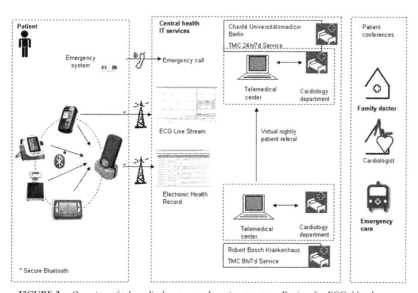

FIGURE 2.—Overview of telemedical system and service structure. Devices for ECG, blood pressure, and body weight measurements are connected via Bluetooth at the patient's home. A personal digital assistant transmits the data via its integrated cell phone module to the central servers. In the Telemedical Interventional Monitoring in Heart Failure trial, there were 2 telemedical centers, the first located in Berlin and the second in Stuttgart, that communicated via electronic patient records. A home emergency call system enables the patient to have direct contact with the healthcare specialist. IT indicates information technology; TMC, telemedical center. (Reprinted from Koehler F, on behalf of the Telemedical Interventional Monitoring in Heart Failure Investigators. Impact of remote telemedical management on mortality and hospitalizations in ambulatory patients with chronic heart failure: the telemedical interventional monitoring in heart failure study. *Circulation.* 2011;123:1873-1880. © American Heart Association, Inc.)

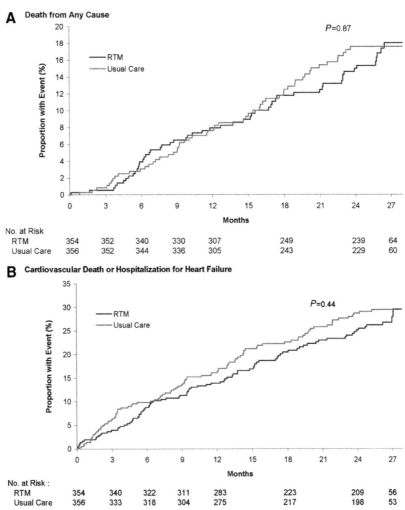

A Death from Any Cause

No. at Risk

RTM	354	352	340	330	307	249	239	64
Usual Care	356	352	344	336	305	243	229	60

B Cardiovascular Death or Hospitalization for Heart Failure

No. at Risk :

RTM	354	340	322	311	283	223	209	56
Usual Care	356	333	318	304	275	217	198	53

FIGURE 3.—Shown are the cumulative incidence of the primary outcome (death from any cause) (**A**) and the composite secondary outcome (hospitalization for heart failure or cardiovascular death) (**B**) during follow-up. RTM indicates remote telemedical management. (Reprinted from Koehler F, on behalf of the Telemedical Interventional Monitoring in Heart Failure Investigators. Impact of remote telemedical management on mortality and hospitalizations in ambulatory patients with chronic heart failure: the telemedical interventional monitoring in heart failure study. *Circulation.* 2011;123:1873-1880. © American Heart Association, Inc.)

Clinical Trial Registration.—URL: http://www.ClinicalTrials.gov. Unique identifier: NCT00543881. (Figs 2 and 3).

▶ Heart failure (HF) has many etiologies but is a common pathway to increasing disabling symptoms, progressive ventricular dysfunction, and eventual death. In many patients on this downward spiraling pathway, there are a series of expensive hospitalizations. The idea that this dismal course could be altered and rehospitalizations prevented by close and frequent contact with the medical team so that early signs of progression could be recognized and treated was intuitively correct. Patients could have symptoms reviewed and daily weights recorded and, if progression was suspected, the patient could be seen as an outpatient, medications could be adjusted, and hospitalization could be prevented. There were many reports and 2 recent meta-analyses that suggested that telemonitoring of chronic HF patients could improve survival by 17% to 47% within a 6- to 12-month period.[1,2] This study is the largest randomized, prospective trial of what intuitively should work: contact 24 hours a day, 7 days a week. Unfortunately, comparing telemonitoring with usual care in a follow-up of more than 2 years demonstrated no difference in all-cause mortality or the combined endpoint of cardiovascular death or rehospitalization. These findings are similar to those of another recent study, Telemonitoring to Improve Heart Failure Outcomes (Tele-HF), that found that compared with usual care, there was no decrease in rehospitalization or all-cause mortality.[3] Although there are differences in the severity of the HF and time of follow-up between the 2 studies, the findings confirmed the overall negative results. Why the differences from the 2 meta-analyses? The meta-analyses combined many dissimilar small telemonitoring studies of HF patients of varying profiles, not prospectively designed, and followed up for different durations where different interventions were used between the studies.

This study does not have statistical power to rule out with a larger study followed for a longer time a clinically relevant difference in mortality between the pared treatment groups, so we probably have not heard the last of this concept.

M. D. Cheitlin, MD

References

1. Klersy C, De Silvestri A, Gabutti G, Regoli F, Auricchio A. A meta-analysis of remote monitoring of heart failure patients. *J Am Coll Cardiol.* 2009;54:1683-1694.
2. Inglis SC, Clark RA, McAlister FA, et al. Structured telephone support or telemonitoring programmes for patients with chronic heart failure. *Cochrane Database Syst Rev.* 2010;(8):CD007228. 10.1002/14651858.CD007228.pub2.
3. Chaudhry SI, Mattera JA, Curtis JP, et al. Telemonitoring in patients with heart failure. *N Engl J Med.* 2010;363:2301-2309.

Clinical Strategies and Outcomes in Advanced Heart Failure Patients Older Than 70 Years of Age Receiving the HeartMate II Left Ventricular Assist Device: A Community Hospital Experience
Adamson RM, Stahovich M, Chillcott S, et al (Sharp Memorial Hosp, San Diego, CA)
J Am Coll Cardiol 57:2487-2495, 2011

Objectives.—The primary objective of this study was to determine outcomes in left ventricular assist device (LVAD) patients older than age 70 years.

Background.—Food and Drug Administration approval of the HeartMate II (Thoratec Corporation, Pleasanton, California) LVAD for destination therapy has provided an attractive option for older patients with advanced heart failure.

Methods.—Fifty-five patients received the HeartMate II LVAD between October 5, 2005, and January 1, 2010, as part of either the bridge to transplantation or destination therapy trials at a community hospital. Patients were divided into 2 age groups: ≥70 years of age (n = 30) and <70 years of age (n = 25). Outcome measures including survival, length of hospital stay, adverse events, and quality of life were compared between the 2 groups.

Results.—Pre-operatively, all patients were in New York Heart Association functional class IV refractory to maximal medical therapy. Kaplan-Meier survival for patients ≥70 years of age (97% at 1 month, 75% at 1 year, and 70% at 2 years) was not statistically different from patients <70 years of age (96% 1 month, 72% at 1 year, and 65% at 2 years, p = 0.806). Average length of hospital stay for the ≥70-year age group was 24 ± 15 days, similar to that of the <70-year age group (23 ± 14 days, p = 0.805). There were no differences in the incidence of adverse events between the 2 groups. Quality of life and functional status improved significantly in both groups.

Conclusions.—The LVAD patients ≥70 years of age have good functional recovery, survival, and quality of life at 2 years. Advanced age should not be used as an independent contraindication when selecting a patient for LVAD therapy at experienced centers (Fig 2, Table 1).

▶ The REMATCH (Randomized Evaluation of Mechanical Assistance for the Treatment of Congestive Heart Failure) trial that showed superiority of a left ventricular assist device (LVAD) over optimal medical therapy proved the value of a new technology in the treatment of patients with end-stage heart failure (HF).[1] Mechanical circulatory support (MCS) was further enhanced with the development of second-generation devices, such as the HeartMate II continuous flow LVAD, that are durable with fewer adverse events than the first-generation devices.[2-5] These devices have been shown to increase survival and improve the quality of life and are used as a bridge to transplantation or as destination therapy for patients who are refractory to optimal medical management.[2-4] With HF a common condition in the elderly population, affecting up to 10% of people over age 70 with as many as 150 000 patients with New York Heart Association class IV symptoms,[5] the possible utilization of these devices could be extensive and expensive. Although cardiac transplantation is the gold standard for patients with end-stage HF, the limited number of donor hearts (~ 2000 per year in the United States), the contraindication for serious other comorbid conditions and the arbitrary restriction to patients < 70 years old, are the limitations. This study found that advanced HF patients refractory to optimal medical management who were older than 70 years of age and had acceptable hospital stays, adverse events, and functional recovery are candidates for MCS. Their results were similar to those seen with patients less than 70 years of age. The limitations of the study are the small numbers of patients from a single center who participated in

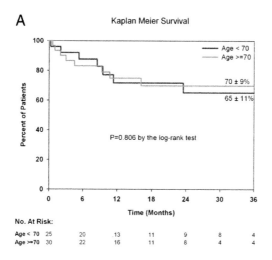

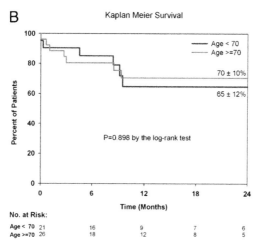

FIGURE 2.—Kaplan-Meier Survival Analysis. (A) Survival of patients, including those who had a HeartMate XVE replaced with a HeartMate II (HMII). (B) Survival of patients with the HMII as their first device, excluding patients who had a HeartMate XVE replaced with an HMII. Red lines indicate age <70 years; blue lines indicate age ≥70 years. For interpretation of the references to color in this figure legend, the reader is referred to web version of this article. (Reprinted from the Journal of the American College of Cardiology, Adamson RM, Stahovich M, Chillcott S, et al. Clinical strategies and outcomes in advanced heart failure patients older than 70 years of age receiving the HeartMate II left ventricular assist device: a community hospital experience. *J Am Coll Cardiol.* 2011;57:2487-2495. Copyright © 2011, with permission from the American College of Cardiology.)

a multicenter trial and the retrospective review of the patients referred for terminal HF evaluation. Therefore, as in all such studies, a larger trial randomized to optimal therapy and MCS compared with optimal therapy alone with evaluation of factors that predict adverse event—free MCS is necessary.

M. D. Cheitlin, MD

TABLE 1.—Criteria for Selecting Patients as LVAD Candidates

Characteristics of Patients Selected for LVAD Therapy	High-Risk LVAD Patient But Not Absolute Contraindications	Contraindications to LVAD Support
Intolerable congestive heart failure symptoms and/or lifestyle limitations despite maximal medical/surgical therapies	Severe chronic obstructive pulmonary disease	Patient refusal
Meets national standardized inclusion criteria	History of stroke with worsened defect secondary to congestive heart failure	Insufficient significant other support, home environment, or financial resources
Adequate mental, psychological, social, and financial support to comply with the complex LVAD management protocols	Primary right-side heart failure (i.e., hypertrophic myopathy, arrhythmogenic right ventricular dysplasia, or post-transplant constrictive/restrictive disease	Irreversible neurocognitive defects that preclude routine LVAD care
A strong desire to have an LVAD implanted held by both the patient and his/her significant other caregivers.	Fixed pulmonary artery hypertension	Ongoing cardiogenic shock refractory to all resuscitation measures including peripheral cardiopulmonary bypass resuscitation
	Active infections	End-stage pulmonary disease out of proportion to congestive heart failure
		Fungemia
	Hepatic fibrosis or cirrhosis	Ongoing drug or alcohol addiction or recent history of noncompliance to medical therapy
	Blood dyscrasias (heparin-induced thrombocytopenia, hypercoagulable states, current 2B3A drug use)	
	Renal failure including chronic dialysis dependence	
	Patient or significant other ambivalence regarding the LVAD implant	

References

1. Rose EA, Gelijns AC, Moskowitz AJ, et al. Long-term use of a left ventricular assist device for end-stage heart failure. *N Engl J Med.* 2001;345:1435-1443.
2. Pagani FD, Miller LW, Russell SD, et al. Extended mechanical circulatory support with a continuous-flow rotary left ventricular assist device. *J Am Coll Cardiol.* 2009;54:312-321.
3. Slaughter MS, Rogers JG, Milano CA, et al. Advanced heart failure treated with continuous-flow left ventricular assist device. *N Engl J Med.* 2009;361:2241-2251.
4. Rogers JG, Aaronson KD, Boyle AJ, et al. Continuous flow left ventricular assist device improves functional capacity and quality of life of advanced heart failure patients. *J Am Coll Cardiol.* 2010;55:1826-1834.
5. Lloyd-Jones D, Adams R, Carnethon M, et al. Heart disease and stroke statistics—2009 update: a report from the American Heart Association Statistics Committee and Stroke Statistics Subcommittee. *Circulation.* 2009;119:e21-e181.

Isolated Coronary Artery Bypass Graft Combined With Bone Marrow Mononuclear Cells Delivered Through a Graft Vessel for Patients With Previous Myocardial Infarction and Chronic Heart Failure: A Single-Center, Randomized, Double-Blind, Placebo-Controlled Clinical Trial

Hu S, Liu S, Zheng Z, et al (Fuwai Hosp, Beijing, China)
J Am Coll Cardiol 57:2409-2415, 2011

Objectives.—This study aimed at examining the efficacy of bone marrow mononuclear cell (BMMNC) delivery through graft vessel for patients with a previous myocardial infarction (MI) and chronic heart failure during coronary artery bypass graft (CABG).

Background.—Little evidence exists supporting the practice of BMMNC delivery through graft vessel for patients with a previous MI and chronic heart failure during CABG.

Methods.—From November 2006 to June 2009, a randomized, placebo-controlled trial was conducted to test the efficacy and safety of CABG for multivessel coronary artery disease combined with autologous BMMNCs in patients with congestive heart failure due to severe ischemic cardiomyopathy. Sixty-five patients were recruited, and 60 patients remained in the final trial and were randomized to a CABG + BMMNC group (n = 31) and a placebo-control group (i.e., CABG-only group, n = 29). All patients discharged received a 6-month follow-up. Changes in left ventricular ejection fraction from baseline to 6-month follow-up, as examined by magnetic resonance imaging, were of primary interest.

Results.—The overall baseline age was 59.5 ± 9.2 years, and 6.7% were women. After a 6-month follow-up, compared with the placebo-control group, the CABG + BMMNC group had significant changes in left ventricular ejection fraction (p = 0.029), left ventricular end-systolic volume index (p = 0.017), and wall motion index score (p = 0.011). Also, the changes in the distance on the 6-min walking test as well as B-type natriuretic peptide were significantly greater in the CABG + BMMNC group than in the control group.

Conclusions.—In summary, patients with a previous MI and chronic heart failure could potentially benefit from isolated CABG (i.e., those who received CABG only) combined with BMMNCs delivered through a graft vessel. (Stem Cell Therapy to Improve Myocardial Function in Patients Undergoing Coronary Artery Bypass Grafting [CABG]; NCT00395811).

▶ There is continued interest in stem cell therapy and evidence for its effect on cardiac function in patients with severe left ventricular (LV) dysfunction. A number of randomized studies of stem cell injection in patients with acute myocardial infarction have shown improved LV function and limited reversal of ventricular remodeling.[1-3] This is the first randomized, placebo-controlled study to show improvement in LV function and decrease in wall motion abnormalities in patients with severe ischemic cardiomyopathy undergoing bypass surgery compared with bypass surgery alone with injection of bone marrow monocyte cells (BMMNCs) directly into the grafts supplying the infarcted areas. There was no evidence of surviving myocardium by single-photon emission computed tomography scanning and LV angiography, but this does not rule out hibernating myocardium. There was also at 6 months of follow-up, evidence of increased functional capacity by the 6-minute walk test. Compared with other studies of stem cell injection during CABG,[4-6] this study selected only patients with 3-vessel disease with a previous myocardial infarction, LV ejection fraction < 30%, and chronic heart failure. BMMNCs are an ideal source for stem cell therapy in that bone marrow is reasonably accessible and contains endothelial progenitor cells, mesenchymal stem cells, and hematopoietic progenitor cells, each capable of improving ventricular function.[5-8] The delivery of the BMMNCs by coronary perfusion is also probably better than direct myocardial injection because there is probably more even delivery throughout the scarred myocardium with possibly greater retention of the cells in the target area.[9] The major problem with the study is the small number of patients, but the results are quite impressive and demand larger, placebo-controlled studies for confirmation.

M. D. Cheitlin, MD

References

1. Wollert KC, Meyer GP, Lotz J, et al. Intracoronary autologous bone marrow cell transfer after myocardial infarction: the BOOST randomised controlled clinical trial. *Lancet.* 2004;364:141-148.
2. Schächinger V, Assmus B, Erbs S, et al. Intracoronary infusion of bone marrowderived mononuclear cells abrogates adverse left ventricular remodelling postacute myocardial infarction: insights from the reinfusion of enriched progenitor cells and infarct remodelling in acute myocardial infarction (REPAIR-AMI) trial. *Eur J Heart Fail.* 2009;11:973-979.
3. Martin-Rendon E, Brunskill SJ, Hyde CJ, Stanworth SJ, Mathur A, Watt SM. Autologous bone marrow stem cells to treat acute myocardial infarction: a systematic review. *Eur Heart J.* 2008;29:1807-1818.
4. Eagle KA, Guyton RA, Davidoff R, et al. ACC/AHA 2004 guideline update for coronary artery bypass graft surgery: a report of the American College of Cardiology/American Heart Association Task Force on Practice Guidelines. *J Am Coll Cardiol.* 2004;44:e213-e311.

5. Stamm C, Kleine HD, Choi YH, et al. Intramyocardial delivery of CD133+ bone marrow cells and coronary artery bypass grafting for chronic ischemic heart disease: safety and efficacy studies. *J Thorac Cardiovasc Surg.* 2007;133:717-725.
6. Zhao Q, Sun Y, Xia L, Chen A, Wang Z. Randomized study of mononuclear bone marrow cell transplantation in patients with coronary surgery. *Ann Thorac Surg.* 2008;86:1833-1840.
7. Hu S, Liu S, Song Y, et al. Coronary artery bypass graft combined with intracoronary infusion autologous stem cell transplant treatment in heart failure patients. *Chinese J Thoracic Cardiovasc Surg.* 2009;25:321-323.
8. Korf-Klingebiel M, Kempf T, Sauer T, et al. Bone marrow cells are a rich source of growth factors and cytokines: implications for cell therapy trials after myocardial infarction. *Eur Heart J.* 2008;29:2851-2858.
9. Zhang H, Song P, Tang Y, et al. Injection of bone marrow mesenchymal stem cells in the borderline area of infarcted myocardium: heart status and cell distribution. *J Thorac Cardiovasc Surg.* 2007;134:1234-1240.

Medical Treatment of Congestive Heart Failure

Factors associated with improvement in ejection fraction in clinical practice among patients with heart failure: Findings from IMPROVE HF

Wilcox JE, Fonarow GC, Yancy CW, et al (Northwestern Univ Feinberg School of Medicine, Chicago, IL; UCLA Med Ctr; et al)
Am Heart J 163:49-56.e2, 2012

Background.—Available data suggest that improvement in left ventricular ejection fraction (LVEF) is a major predictor of improved survival in heart failure (HF). Although certain factors are associated with improvements in LVEF in select patients with HF enrolled in clinical trials, relatively little is known about such factors among patients in clinical practice. This study evaluated changes in LVEF and associated factors in outpatients with systolic HF or post-myocardial infarction with reduced LVEF during 24 months of follow-up.
Methods.—IMPROVE HF is a prospective evaluation of a practice-based performance improvement intervention implemented at outpatient cardiology/multispecialty practices to increase use of guideline-recommended care for eligible patients. Data were analyzed by patient groups based on absolute improvement in LVEF (<0%, 0−≤10%, and >10%) from baseline to 24 months and by change in LVEF as a continuous variable.
Results.—A total of 3,994 patients from 155 of 167 practices were eligible for analysis. The overall mean LVEF increased from 25.8% at baseline to 32.3% (+6.4%) at 24 months (*P* < .001), and 28.6% of patients had a >10% improvement in ejection fraction (from 24.5% to 46.2%, 92% relative improvement). Age, race, and practice setting were similar between the 3 LVEF improvement groups. Multivariate analysis revealed female sex, no prior myocardial infarction, nonischemic HF etiology, and no digoxin use were associated with >10% improvement in LVEF.
Conclusions.—Among patients with HF receiving care in cardiology/multispecialty practices participating in a performance measure intervention, surviving, and having repeat LVEF assessment, close to one third of patients had a >10% improvement in LVEF at 24 months. These

findings indicate that HF is not always a progressive disease and that differentiation of the heterogeneous HF phenotypes may set the stage for future research and therapeutic targets (Fig 2).

▶ There are many effective therapies for patients with heart failure (HF) and reduced left ventricular ejection fraction (LVEF) including beta-blockers, angiotensin-converting enzyme inhibitors (ACEI), angiotensin receptor blockers (ARBs), aldosterone antagonists, and cardiac resynchronization therapy that have been shown to improve clinical outcomes.[1] Improved LVEF with therapy has been found to be a major predictor of improved survival in these patients.[2-4] Clinical factors have been found to be associated with improved LVEF in select patients enrolled in clinical trials followed and treated systematically, but it may be different in such patients treated in outpatient clinical practices. The Registry to Improve the Use of Evidence-Based Heart Failure Therapies in the Outpatient Setting (IMPROVE-HF) provides data to measure the influence of the use of guideline-recommended therapies for patients with HF managed in cardiology outpatient practices.[5,6] The goal of this study was to evaluate changes in LVEF from baseline to 24 months in 15 177 HF patients with LVEF ≤35% entered into IMPROVE-HF and to assess the baseline treatment factors associated with improvement in LVEF. After 24 months, they found in those with baseline and follow-up LVEFs an increase from 25.8% at baseline to 32.3% at follow-up ($P < .001$). There were 39.2% in the lowest tertile (< 0% improvement) experiencing an average of 4.4% decrease in LVEF, and 60.8% had no change or an increase in LVEF. There were 28.6% who had a considerable increase in LVEF (> 10% tertile). Among these, the LVEF doubled from 24.5% at baseline to 46.2% at 24 months. HF medications and target dosing were similar across the LVEF improvement tertiles. The practice characteristics, such as university based versus hospital based, and a number of other surprising factors, such as age, diabetes, and renal insufficiency, also were not associated with improvement in LVEF. The patients who had less than 10% improvement were more likely to be women, to have a nonischemic etiology, to have no prior myocardial infarction, and not to be taking digoxin. These findings suggest

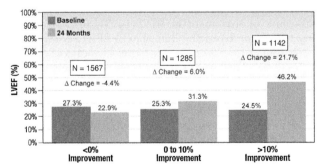

FIGURE 2.—Left ventricular ejection fraction at baseline and 24 months according to tertile of LVEF improvement. (Reprinted from the American Heart Journal, Wilcox JE, Fonarow GC, Yancy CW, et al. Factors associated with improvement in ejection fraction in clinical practice among patients with heart failure: findings from IMPROVE HF. *Am Heart J.* 2012;163:49-56.e2. Copyright 2012, with permission from Elsevier.)

that some patients have viable myocardium capable of improving function, possibly from other causes unrelated to ischemia. Because many of these patients were already taking beta-blockers and ACEI/ARB at the time of entry into the study, the baseline LVEF may have reflected improved LVEF at the time of entry. During the study period, further substantial improvements in the use and dosage of these HF medications occurred over time. This study shows that HF is not always a progressive disease, that guideline-recommended therapy can improve LV function, and that viable but dysfunctional myocardium may be the next target therapy in patients with HF.

M. D. Cheitlin, MD

References

1. Hunt SA, Abraham WT, hin MH, et al; American College of Cardiology; American Heart Association Task Force on Practice Guidelines; American College of Chest Physicians; International Society for Heart and Lung Transplantation; Heart Rhythm Society. ACC/AHA 2005 guideline update for the diagnosis and management of chronic heart failure in the adult: a report of the American College of Cardiology/American Heart Association Task Force on Practice Guidelines (Writing committee to update the 2001 guidelines for the evaluation and management of heart failure): developed in collaboration with the American College of Chest Physicians and the International Society for Heart and Lung Transplantation: endorsed by the heart rhythm society. *Circulation.* 2005;112:e154-235.
2. St John Sutton M, Pfeffer MA, Moye L, et al. Cardiovascular death and left ventricular remodeling two years after myocardial infarction: baseline predictors and impact of long-term use of captopril: information from the Survival and Ventricular Enlargement (SAVE) trial. *Circulation.* 1997;96:3294-3299.
3. Solomon SD, Skali H, Anavekar NS, et al. Changes in ventricular size and function in patients treated with valsartan, captopril, or both after myocardial infarction. *Circulation.* 2005;111:3411-3419.
4. Gula LJ, Klein GJ, Hellkamp AS, et al. Ejection fraction assessment and survival: an analysis of the Sudden Cardiac Death in Heart Failure Trial (SCD-HeFT). *Am Heart J.* 2008;156:1196-1200.
5. Fonarow GC, Albert NM, Curtis AB, et al. Improving evidence-based care for heart failure in outpatient cardiology practices: primary results of the Registry to Improve the Use of Evidence-Based Heart Failure Therapies in the Outpatient Setting (IMPROVE HF). *Circulation.* 2010;122:585-596.
6. Fonarow GC, Heywood JT, Heidenreich PA, Lopatin M, Yancy CW; ADHERE Scientific Advisory Committee and Investigators. Temporal trends in clinical characteristics, treatments, and outcomes for heart failure hospitalizations, 2002 to 2004: findings from Acute Decompensated Heart Failure National Registry (ADHERE). *Am Heart J.* 2007;153:1021-1028.

Intensive glycemic control has no impact on the risk of heart failure in type 2 diabetic patients: Evidence from a 37,229 patient meta-analysis
Castagno D, Baird-Gunning J, Jhund PS, et al (Univ of Turin, Italy; Univ of Glasgow, UK; et al)
Am Heart J 162:938-948, 2011

Background.—More intensive glycemic control reduces the risk of microvascular disease in patients with diabetes mellitus but has not been proven to reduce the risk of macrovascular events such as myocardial infarction and stroke. Poorer glycemic control, as indicated by glycated hemoglobin level concentration, is associated with an increased risk of heart failure (HF), but it is not known whether improved glycemic control reduces this risk. We conducted a meta-analysis of randomized controlled trials comparing strategies of more versus less intensive glucose-lowering that reported HF events.

Methods.—Two investigators independently searched PubMed, the Cochrane CENTRAL register of controlled trials, metaRegister, pre-MEDLINE, and CINAHL from January 1970 to October 2010 for prospective controlled randomized trials comparing a more intensive glucose-lowering regimen to a standard regimen. The outcome of interest was HF-related events (both fatal and nonfatal). Odds ratios (ORs) were calculated from published data from relevant trials and pooled with a random-effects meta-analysis.

Results.—A total of 37,229 patients from 8 randomized trials were included in the analysis. Follow-up ranged from 2.3 to 10.1 years, and the overall number of HF-related events was 1469 (55% in the intensive treatment arm). The mean difference in glycated hemoglobin level between patients given standard treatment and those allocated to a more intensive regimen was 0.9%. Overall, the risk of HF-related events did not differ significantly between intensive glycemic control and standard treatment

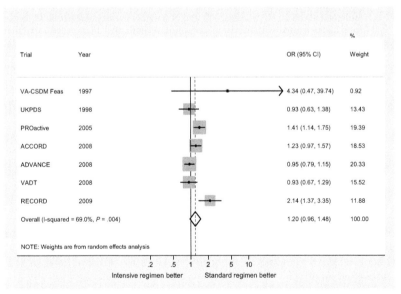

FIGURE 3.—Probability of HF-related events with intensive glucose-lowering versus standard treatment. The size of the markers (squares) is approximately proportional to the statistical weight of each trial. (Reprinted from the American Heart Journal, Castagno D, Baird-Gunning J, Jhund PS, et al. Intensive glycemic control has no impact on the risk of heart failure in type 2 diabetic patients: Evidence from a 37,229 patient meta-analysis. *Am Heart J.* 2011;162:938-948. Copyright 2011, with permission from Elsevier.)

(OR 1.20, 95% CI 0.96-1.48), but the effect estimate was highly hetero-geneous ($I^2 = 69\%$). At subgroup analysis, intensive glycemic control achieved with high thiazolidinediones use significantly increased HF risk (OR 1.33, 95% CI 1.02-1.72).

Conclusions.—More intensive glycemic control in patients with type 2 diabetes mellitus did not reduce the occurrence of HF events. Furthermore, intensive glycemic control with thiazolidinediones increased the risk of HF. These findings question a direct mechanistic link between hypergly-cemia and HF (Figs 3 and 5).

▶ There is an increased risk of heart failure (HF) in patients with diabetes mel-litus (DM) that is independent of the other major HF risk factors of coronary disease and hypertension.[1-5] For instance, in the Kaiser Permanente cohort study of almost 50 000 patients with type II DM, with each 1% increase in glycated hemoglobin (HbA1c) level, there was an 8% increased risk of HF, suggesting a graded association.[3] Certain population-based studies and clinical trials have suggested a direct relationship between strict glycemic control as measured by HbA1c levels and the risk of HF.[5,6] However, many studies have found that although strict glycemic control decreases the incidence of micro-vascular complications, the evidence that it reduces the incidence of

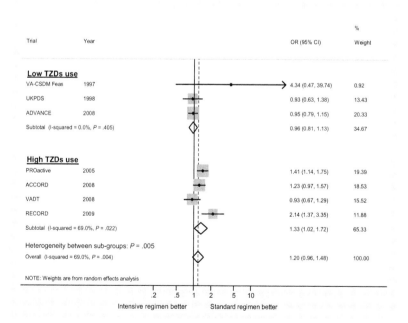

FIGURE 5.—Sensitivity analysis demonstrating the effect of low- versus high-TZD use in the glucose-lowering regimen on probability of HF-related events. (Reprinted from the American Heart Journal, Castagno D, Baird-Gunning J, Jhund PS, et al. Intensive glycemic control has no impact on the risk of heart failure in type 2 diabetic patients: Evidence from a 37,229 patient meta-analysis. *Am Heart J.* 2011;162:938-948.e2. Copyright 2011, with permission from Elsevier.)

macrovascular events, including HF, is mixed at best and inconclusive.[7-10] To examine the possibility that the studies showing lack of effect of strict glycemic control on macrovascular events are related to small numbers of HF events, short follow-up time, late start of glycemic control, or to the medications, such as thiazolidinediones (TZDs), this study did a meta-analysis of all randomized, controlled studies of patients with type II DM that compared the degree and strategy of glycemic control with that reported in HF events. The number of randomized patients to the 2 treatment strategies was very large, with more than 37 000 patients with over two thirds randomized to tight glycemic control. There were also in the follow-up period a large number of HF events (1469) over a mean of 5 years. There was no difference in the incidence of HF events between the group treated with intensive glycemic control and those with standard treatment. The finding that TZDs increased the incidence of HF (odds ratio, 1.33 [95% confidence interval, 1.02–1.72]) was probably, at least in part, by promoting fluid retention in patients with compromised left ventricular function. The limitations of this meta-analysis include the fact that the studies included spanned 13 years and the management controlling hyperglycemia changed during this time, and the problems of a lack of information about the duration of DB before the treatment-control study and left ventricular function at baseline and follow-up remain. Why the strict control of DM does not decrease the incidence of HF over standard control is uncertain. Possibilities are that the follow-up of the studies is too short, that the duration of the intensive therapy is too short or too late in the course of the disease, or that therapy used increases the risk of HF. Currently, the conclusion is that there is no direct causal link between the degree of glycemic control and the development of HF.

M. D. Cheitlin, MD

References

1. Gottdiener JS, Arnold AM, Aurigemma GP, et al. Predictors of congestive heart failure in the elderly: the Cardiovascular Health Study. *J Am Coll Cardiol.* 2000;35:1628-1637.
2. He J, Ogden LG, Bazzano LA, Vupputuri S, Loria C, Whelton PK. Risk factors for congestive heart failure in US men and women: NHANES I epidemiologic follow-up study. *Arch Intern Med.* 2001;161:996-1002.
3. Iribarren C, Karter AJ, Go AS, et al. Glycemic control and heart failure among adult patients with diabetes. *Circulation.* 2001;103:2668-2673.
4. Nichols GA, Gullion CM, Koro CE, Ephross SA, Brown JB. The incidence of congestive heart failure in type 2 diabetes: an update. *Diabetes Care.* 2004;27:1879-1884.
5. Thrainsdottir IS, Aspelund T, Thorgeirsson G, et al. The association between glucose abnormalities and heart failure in the population-based Reykjavik study. *Diabetes Care.* 2005;28:612-616.
6. Stratton IM, Adler AI, Neil HA, et al. Association of glycaemia with macrovascular and microvascular complications of type 2 diabetes (UKPDS 35): prospective observational study. *BMJ.* 2000;321:405-412.
7. Intensive blood-glucose control with sulphonylureas or insulin compared with conventional treatment and risk of complications in patients with type 2 diabetes (UKPDS 33). UK Prospective Diabetes Study (UKPDS) Group. *Lancet.* 1998;352:837-853.

8. Action to Control Cardiovascular Risk in Diabetes Study Group, Gerstein HC, Miller ME, Byington RP, et al. Effects of intensive glucose lowering in type 2 diabetes. *N Engl J Med.* 2008;358:2545-2559.
9. ADVANCE Collaborative Group, Patel A, MacMahon S, Chalmers J, et al. Intensive blood glucose control and vascular outcomes in patients with type 2 diabetes. *N Engl J Med.* 2008;358:2560-2572.
10. Duckworth W, Abraira C, Moritz T, et al. Glucose control and vascular complications in veterans with type 2 diabetes. *N Engl J Med.* 2009;360:129-139.

Effects of selective heart rate reduction with ivabradine on left ventricular remodelling and function: results from the SHIFT echocardiography substudy

Tardif J-C, on behalf of the SHIFT Investigators (Université de Montréal, Quebec, Canada; et al)

Eur Heart J 32:2507-2515, 2011

Aims.—The SHIFT echocardiographic substudy evaluated the effects of ivabradine on left ventricular (LV) remodelling in heart failure (HF).

Methods and Results.—Eligible patients had chronic HF and systolic dysfunction [LV ejection fraction (LVEF) ≤35%], were in sinus rhythm, and had resting heart rate ≥70 bpm. Patients were randomly allocated to ivabradine or placebo, superimposed on background therapy for HF. Complete echocardiographic data at baseline and 8 months were available for 411 patients (ivabradine 208, placebo 203). Treatment with ivabradine reduced LVESVI (primary substudy endpoint) vs. placebo [−7.0 ± 16.3 vs. −0.9 ± 17.1 mL/m^2; difference (SE), −5.8 (1.6), 95% CI −8.8 to −2.7, $P < 0.001$]. The reduction in LVESVI was independent of beta-blocker use, HF aetiology, and baseline LVEF. Ivabradine also improved LV end-diastolic volume index (−7.9 ± 18.9 vs. −1.8 ± 9.0 mL/m^2, $P = 0.002$) and LVEF (+2.4 ± 7.7 vs. −0.1 ± 8.0%, $P < 0.001$). The incidence of the SHIFT primary composite outcome (cardiovascular mortality or hospitalization for worsening HF) was higher in patients with LVESVI above the median (59 mL/m^2) at baseline (HR 1.62, 95% CI 1.03−2.56, $P = 0.04$). Patients with the largest relative reductions in LVESVI had the lowest event rates.

Conclusion.—Ivabradine reverses cardiac remodelling in patients with HF and LV systolic dysfunction (Figs 2 and 3).

▶ In 2010, the Systolic Heart Failure Treatment with the If Inhibitor Ivabradine Trial (SHIFT) investigators reported that provoking slowing of sinus rhythm in heart failure (HF) patients with a heart rate ≥70 beats per minute, and with an ejection fraction ≤35% by ivabradine, a specific inhibitor of the If current in the sinoatrial node, there was an 18% reduction in the primary composite endpoint of cardiovascular death or hospitalization for worsening HF.[1] Left ventricular (LV) enlargement predicts adverse cardiovascular events,[2] and reduced LV ejection fraction is a powerful predictor of cardiovascular outcomes and all-cause mortality.[3] This substudy of the SHIFT using echocardiography evaluates the

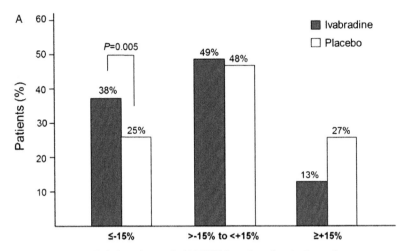

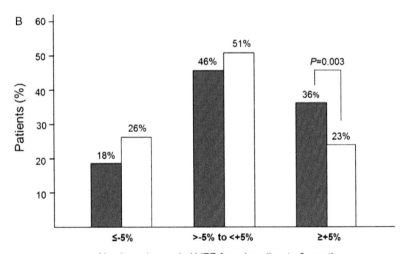

FIGURE 2.—(A) Relative change in left ventricular end-systolic volume index (LVESVI) and (B) absolute change in left ventricular ejection fraction (LVEF) from baseline to 8 months. The grey and white bars represent percentages of patients reaching echocardiographic criteria for the ivabradine and placebo groups, respectively. (Reprinted from Tardif J-C, on behalf of the SHIFT Investigators. Effects of selective heart rate reduction with ivabradine on left ventricular remodelling and function: results from the SHIFT echocardiography substudy. *Eur Heart J*. 2011;32:2507-2515, by permission of The European Society of Cardiology.)

effects of ivabradine versus placebo on left ventricular remodeling (LVR). Because ivabradine affects only the heart rate and has no effect on myocardial contractility and intracardiac conduction, ivabradine's effect is related to isolated heart rate reduction. After 8 months from the baseline echocardiogram, the finding of a significantly greater reduction in LV end-systolic and end-diastolic

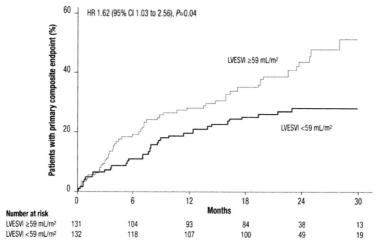

FIGURE 3.—Kaplan—Meier cumulative event curves for the SHIFT primary composite endpoint of cardiovascular death or hospitalization for worsening heart failure in the placebo group split by median left ventricular end-systolic volume index (LVESVI) ≥59 vs. <59 mL/m². (Reprinted from Tardif J-C, on behalf of the SHIFT Investigators. Effects of selective heart rate reduction with ivabradine on left ventricular remodelling and function: results from the SHIFT echocardiography substudy. *Eur Heart J.* 2011;32:2507-2515, by permission of The European Society of Cardiology.)

volumes and increase in LV ejection fraction with ivabradine compared with placebo shows a positive effect of ivabradine on LVR. Larger decreases in heart rate were associated with greater increases in LV ejection fraction. In contrast, there was no significant relationship between changes in heart rate and changes in LV volumes for all patients. However, when split by baseline median heart rate of 77 beats per minute, those patients with higher heart rates had larger LV end volumes and lower ejection fractions at baseline. In evaluating the impact of the baseline values of the echocardiographic parameters of LV function, they divided the LV end-systolic volume index in the placebo group by the median baseline of 59 mL/m² and found the incidence of the combined endpoint of hospitalization for worsening HF or CV mortality was greater in those with the higher values. There were too few composite endpoints in the echocardiographic SHIFT substudy to evaluate the effect of treatment on outcomes according to the effect of ivabradine on LV volumes. However, when dividing the ivabradine and placebo groups into tertiles of change in LV end-systolic volume indices and determining the incidence of composite endpoints after 8 months of therapy for each third, those with the greatest relative reductions in LV end-systolic volume index had lower event rates than those with smaller reductions or increases. This study shows reversal of LVR with ivabradine over 8 months of therapy in patients, 90% of whom were on beta-blockers and renin-angiotensin-aldosterone system (RAAS) antagonists. These findings are supported by studies in animal models of HF showing effects of ivabradine on reduction of fibrosis, RAAS and sympathetic stimulation, and improvement in endothelial function.[4-6] How important these findings of the effect of ivabradine in patients with heart failure will be is questionable. First, it is possible that the same effects can be accomplished by pushing beta-blockers to the same level of heart rate reduction.

Second, Cullington and colleagues[7] evaluated more than 2200 patients with systolic dysfunction (LV ejection fraction < 50%) attending an HF clinic and reported that if a high resting heart rate greater than 70 beats per minute in patients on optimum HF therapy is necessary for ivabradine's use, then only about 5% would be suitable candidates.

M. D. Cheitlin, MD

References

1. Swedberg K, Komajda M, Böhm M, et al; SHIFT Investigators. Ivabradine and outcomes in chronic heart failure (SHIFT): a randomised placebo-controlled study. *Lancet*. 2010;376:875-885.
2. St John Sutton M, Pfeffer MA, Plappert T, et al. Quantitative two-dimensional echocardiographic measurements are major predictors of adverse cardiovascular events after acute myocardial infarction. The protective effects of captopril. *Circulation*. 1994;89:68-75.
3. Solomon SD, Anavekar N, Skali H, et al; Candesartan in Heart Failure Reduction in Mortality (CHARM) Investigators. Influence of ejection fraction on cardiovascular outcomes in a broad spectrum of heart failure patients. *Circulation*. 2005; 112:3738-3744.
4. Dedkov EI, Zheng W, Christensen LP, Weiss RM, Mahlberg-Gaudin F, Tomanek RJ. Preservation of coronary reserve by ivabradine-induced reduction in heart rate in infarcted rats is associated with decrease in perivascular collagen. *Am J Physiol Heart Circ Physiol*. 2007;293:H590-H598.
5. Milliez P, Messaoudi S, Nehme J, Rodriguez C, Samuel JL, Delcayre C. Beneficial effects of delayed ivabradine treatment on cardiac anatomical and electrical remodeling in rat severe chronic heart failure. *Am J Physiol Heart Circ Physiol*. 2009;296: H435-H441.
6. Vercauteren M, Favre J, Mulder P, Mahlberg-Gaudin F, Thuillez C, Richard V. Protection of endothelial function by long-term heart rate reduction induced by ivabradine in a rat model of chronic heart failure. *Eur Heart J*. 2007;28:48. P468.
7. Cullington D, Goode KM, Cleland JG, Clark AL. Limited role for ivabradine in the treatment of chronic heart failure. *Heart*. 2011;97:1961-1966.

Efficacy of statin therapy in chronic systolic cardiac insufficiency: A meta-analysis

Zhang S, Zhang L, Sun A, et al (Fudan Univ, Shanghai, China)
Eur J Intern Med 22:478-484, 2011

Background.—Conflicting results currently exist on the clinical use of statins in patients with chronic systolic heart failure (CHF). This study aimed to investigate the effect of statins on clinical outcomes of CHF by a meta-analysis based on randomized controlled trials (RCTs).

Methods.—We searched PubMed, MEDLINE, EMBASE, and Cochrane databases through 2010 and renewed in February 2011. We included RCTs of subjects who underwent statin or placebo treatment for established CHF, and provided data on clinical outcomes. Risk ratios (RR) were calculated using a random effects model.

Results.—Thirteen trials involving 10,447 CHF patients were included in the meta-analysis. The pooling analysis showed that statin treatment

TABLE 2.—Subgroup Analysis of All-Cause Mortality, Cardiovascular Mortality, and Rehospitalization for Worsening Heart Failure

Subgroup	All-Cause Mortality			Cardiovascular Mortality			Rehospitalization for Worsening Heart Failure		
	RR (95% CI)	p Value	I^2	RR (95% CI)	p Value	I^2	RR (95% CI)	p Value	I^2
Age<65 years	0.48 [0.29, 0.77]	0.003	0%	0.30 [0.09, 1.02]	0.05	0%	0.52 [0.33, 0.82]	0.004	0%
Age≥65 years	0.98 [0.92, 1.05]	0.66	17%	0.98 [0.91, 1.05]	0.54	0%	0.96 [0.90, 1.02]	0.20	0%
Simvastatin 40 mg/day	0.26 [0.06, 1.22]	0.09	—	0.26 [0.06, 1.22]	0.09	—	1.13 [0.07, 17.02]	0.93	—
Atorvastatin 10 mg/day	0.49 [0.29, 0.84]	0.009	0%	0.38 [0.05, 2.85]	0.35	0%	0.51 [0.33, 0.81]	0.005	0%
Rosuvastatin 10 mg/day	0.98 [0.92, 1.05]	0.61	0%	0.98 [0.91, 1.05]	0.54	0%	0.96 [0.88, 1.04]	0.30	23%
Non-Ischemic etiology	0.92 [0.28, 3.06]	0.90	0%	0.66 [0.04, 10.09]	0.76	—	0.73 [0.40, 1.33]	0.31	0%
Mixed etiology	0.67 [0.34, 1.33]	0.25	61%	0.98 [0.87, 1.09]	0.70	0%	0.65 [0.29, 1.44]	0.29	30%
Ischemic etiology	0.63 [0.29, 1.38]	0.25	51%	0.63 [0.19, 2.14]	0.46	64%	0.61 [0.23, 1.60]	0.32	82%
LVEF<32%*	0.60 [0.34, 1.07]	0.08	47%	0.70 [0.34, 1.44]	0.33	24%	0.88 [0.69, 1.14]	0.33	5%
LVEF≥32%	1.02 [0.93, 1.11]	0.71	0%	0.98 [0.88, 1.10]	0.74	—	0.66 [0.38, 1.17]	0.16	53%

*32% indicated the mean value of LVEF in the overall populations. CI=confidence interval; LVEF=left ventricular ejection fraction; RR=risk ratios.

did not significantly reduce the risk of all-cause death (RR=0.93, 95% CI: 0.81−1.07, p=0.31), death for cardiovascular cause or pump failure (p>0.10), and rehospitalization for heart failure (RR=0.90, 95% CI: 0.78−1.04, p=0.15). In addition, statin therapy had a non-significant trend towards reduced risk of nonfatal myocardial infarction (RR=0.84, 95% CI: 0.68−1.02, p=0.08). When restricted to various statins and patients' age, the analysis demonstrated that atorvastatin was associated with reduced all-cause mortality (p=0.009) and readmission rate for heart failure (p=0.005), and the superiority of statin therapy was significant in CHF patients less than 65 years (both p<0.01).

Conclusions.—Although statin has little impact on clinical outcomes in overall CHF patients, statin administration if needed is feasible to CHF patients, and the treatment might be effective when restricted to specific statins or populations (Table 2).

▶ Hydroxymethylglutaryl-coenzyme A reductase inhibitors, or "statins," in addition to their beneficial effect on lipids, have pleiotropic actions including antifibrotic, anti-inflammatory, antioxidant, and antineurohormonal activation effects that would be valuable in patients with heart failure (HF).[1-3] Post hoc analysis of several randomized, placebo-controlled trials and several observational trials have indicated that statins are related to improved long-term outcomes in patients with HF.[4,5] However, because HF has multiple etiologies and not all studies have shown benefit in HF patients,[6,7] the value of statins in HF has been questioned.[5,6] This meta-analysis of pooled randomized, placebo-controlled trials has shown that overall, in patients with HF statins did not reduce the incidence of death from any cause, death from cardiac cause or pump failure, or rehospitalization. When analysis was restricted to atorvastatin, there was a significant 51% reduction in all-cause mortality and a 49% reduction in rehospitalization for HF that was not seen with rosuvastatin. Also, statins were beneficial in patients with HF aged younger than 65 years. The 2 largest trials, the CORONA study[6] and the GISSI-HF study,[7] both using rosuvastatin and comprising more than 90% of the patients, were negative, and because of their size, determined the negative outcome of this meta-analysis. When these 2 trials are removed, statin treatment is significant in improving survival and reducing rehospitalization for HF. One possibility is the differences in lipophilicity and hydrophilicity among statins, with atorvastatin and simvastatin being lipophilic and rosuvastatin being hydrophilic.[8,9] There is greater uptake in myocardium of lipophilic statins that might give atorvastatin an advantage over rosuvastatin in patients in HF. Also, patient age might be important regarding whether statins are effective in reducing mortality with patients younger than 65 years having a 52% reduction in all-cause mortality and those 65 and older only a 2% reduction. Since, with the pleiotropic effects of statins, there is intuitively a strong basis for beneficial effects in patients with HF, this meta-analysis should not put the issue at rest. A large, randomized study using a lipophilic statin in patients with HF aged younger than 65 is needed.

M. D. Cheitlin, MD

References

1. Jain MK, Ridker PM. Anti-inflammatory effects of statins: clinical evidence and basic mechanisms. *Nat Rev Drug Discov.* 2005;4:977-987.
2. Dilaveris P, Giannopoulos G, Riga M, Synetos A, Stefanadis C. Beneficial effects of statins on endothelial dysfunction and vascular stiffness. *Curr Vasc Pharmacol.* 2007;5:227-237.
3. Krum H, McMurray JJ. Statins and chronic heart failure: do we need a large-scale outcome trial? *J Am Coll Cardiol.* 2002;39:1567-1573.
4. Mozaffarian D, Nye R, Levy WC. Statin therapy is associated with lower mortality among patients with severe heart failure. *Am J Cardiol.* 2004;93:1124-1129.
5. Roik M, Starczewska MH, Huczek Z, Kochanowski J, Opolski G. Statin therapy and mortality among patients hospitalized with heart failure and preserved left ventricular function—a preliminary report. *Acta Cardiol.* 2008;63:683-692.
6. Kjekshus J, Apetrei E, Barrios V, et al. Rosuvastatin in older patients with systolic heart failure. *N Engl J Med.* 2007;357:2248-2261.
7. Gissi-HF Investigators, Tavazzi L, Maggioni AP, Marchioli R, et al. Effect of rosuvastatin in patients with chronic heart failure (the GISSI-HF trial): a randomised, double-blind, placebo-controlled trial. *Lancet.* 2008;372:1231-1239.
8. Nezasa K, Higaki K, Matsumura T, et al. Liver-specific distribution of rosuvastatin in rats: comparison with pravastatin and simvastatin. *Drug Metab Dispos.* 2002; 30:1158-1163.
9. Ford JS, Tayek JA. Lipophilicity and cardiovascular outcome in patients with CHF. *Am Heart J.* 2008;156:e7.

Eplerenone Survival Benefits in Heart Failure Patients Post-Myocardial Infarction Are Independent From its Diuretic and Potassium-Sparing Effects: Insights From an EPHESUS (Eplerenone Post-Acute Myocardial Infarction Heart Failure Efficacy and Survival Study) Substudy

Rossignol P, Ménard J, Fay R, et al (INSERM, Nancy, France; INSERM, Paris, France; et al)
J Am Coll Cardiol 58:1958-1966, 2011

Objectives.—The purpose of this study was to determine whether a diuretic effect may be detectable in patients treated with eplerenone, a mineralocorticoid receptor antagonist, as compared with placebo during the first month of EPHESUS (Eplerenone Post-Acute Myocardial Infarction Heart Failure Efficacy and Survival study) (n = 6,080) and whether this was associated with eplerenone's beneficial effects on cardiovascular outcomes.

Background.—The mechanism of the survival benefit of eplerenone in patients with heart failure post-myocardial infarction remains uncertain.

Methods.—A diuretic effect was indirectly estimated by changes at 1 month that was superior to the median changes in the placebo group in body weight (-0.05 kg) and in the estimated plasma volume reduction ($+1.4\%$). A potassium-sparing effect was defined as a serum potassium increase greater than the median change in the placebo group: $+0.11$ mmol/l.

Results.—In the eplerenone group, body weight ($p < 0.0001$) and plasma volume ($p = 0.047$) decreased, whereas blood protein and serum potassium increased (both, $p < 0.0001$), as compared with the placebo group, suggesting a diuretic effect induced by eplerenone, associated with a potassium-sparing effect. A diuretic effect, as defined by an estimated plasma volume reduction, was independently associated with 11% to 19% better outcomes (lower all-cause death, cardiovascular death or cardiovascular hospitalization, all-cause death or hospitalization, hospitalization for heart failure). Potassium sparing was also independently associated with 12% to 34% better outcomes. There was no statistically significant interaction between the observed beneficial effects of eplerenone (9% to 17%) on cardiovascular outcomes and potassium-sparing or diuretic effects.

Conclusions.—Eplerenone's beneficial effects on long-term survival and cardiovascular outcomes are independent from early potassium-sparing or diuretic effects, suggesting that mineralocorticoid receptor antagonism provides cardiovascular protection beyond its diuretic and potassium-sparing properties (Figs 2 and 3).

▶ Congestion in patients with heart failure (HF) is associated with a poor outcome.[1,2] Diuretics in patients with HF are valuable in that they reduce symptoms and improve the quality of life. However, diuretic use is associated with a worse prognosis and is not supported by large clinical, randomized placebo-controlled

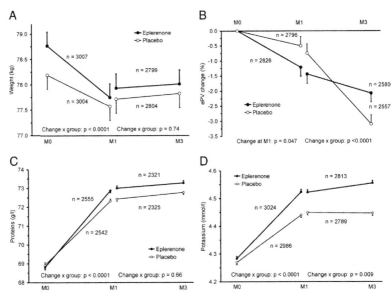

FIGURE 2.—Eplerenone Exerts Early (1-Month) Diuretic-Like and K-Sparing Effects. Diuretic-like (A to C) and K-sparing (D) effects are shown. As a result of missing data, frequencies did not sum to 6,080 (M1) nor 5,692 (M3). M0-M1 and M1-M3 mean values are those for patients with available data at both ends of the period. Change at M1: single comparison of plasma volume change (Mann-Whitney test). Baseline values were set to zero for the graphical presentation. Change × group: interaction between change from M1 to M3 and study group (repeated measures analysis of variance). ePV = estimated plasma volume; M0 = inclusion; M1 = month 1; M3 = month 3. (Reprinted from the Journal of the American College of Cardiology, Rossignol P, Ménard J, Fay R, et al. Eplerenone survival benefits in heart failure patients post-myocardial infarction are independent from its diuretic and potassium-sparing effects: insights from an EPHESUS (Eplerenone Post-Acute Myocardial Infarction Heart Failure Efficacy and Survival Study) substudy. *J Am Coll Cardiol.* 2011;58:1958-1966. Copyright 2011, with permission from the American College of Cardiology.)

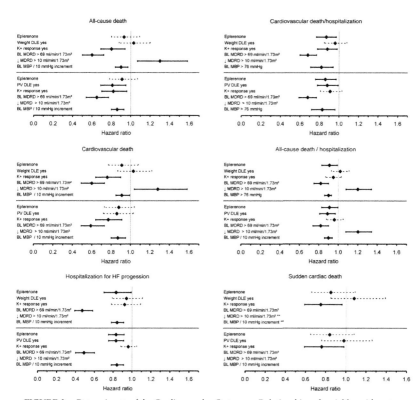

FIGURE 3.—Determinants of the Cardiovascular Outcomes. Relationships of variables with outcomes are shown with the assessment of a diuretic effect either by body weight changes (**upper half of each plot**) or by estimated plasma volume changes (**lower half of each plot**) added into the model. Weight DLE indicates weight-based diuretic-like effect (included in the **upper panels**); ePV DLE indicates estimated plasma volume—based diuretic-like effect (included in the **lower panels**). Potassium response indicates the potassium-sparing effect; ↓MDRD (Modification of Diet in Renal Disease) >10 ml/min/1.73 m^2 indicates a decrease between inclusion and month 1 in estimated glomerular filtration rate using the MDRD formula >10 ml/min/1.73 m^2. Covariables were removed from the models when they did not reach significance or have to be used as stratification factors in order to meet the models validity assumptions. BL = baseline; MBP = mean blood pressure. (Reprinted from the Journal of the American College of Cardiology, Rossignol P, Ménard J, Fay R, et al. Eplerenone survival benefits in heart failure patients post-myocardial infarction are independent from its diuretic and potassium-sparing effects: insights from an EPHESUS (Eplerenone Post-Acute Myocardial Infarction Heart Failure Efficacy and Survival Study) substudy. *J Am Coll Cardiol.* 2011;58:1958-1966. Copyright 2011, with permission from the American College of Cardiology.)

studies. Furthermore, diuretics stimulate the renin-angiotensin and sympathetic nervous systems and are associated with a decrease in glomerular filtration rate. The EPHESUS (Eplerenone Post-Acute Myocardial Infarction Heart Failure Efficacy and Survival) study showed that eplerenone, a mineralocorticoid receptor blocker, added to standard optimal therapy that included diuretic use, in more than 6000 patients with an acute myocardial infarction and HF with systolic dysfunction improved survival by 15% and significantly reduced cardiovascular deaths, sudden deaths, and hospitalization for HF.[3] Because eplerenone is a diuretic, spares potassium loss, and has other pleiotropic effects,[5] this study was done to examine which of these effects could be detected and whether these effects related to cardiovascular outcomes. This substudy of the EHESUS trial showed an early diuretic and potassium-sparing effect of eplerenone compared with the control group and, independent of eplerenone use, that plasma volume depletion was significantly associated with a 11% to 19% improvement in all-cause death, cardiovascular death or cardiovascular hospitalization, and hospitalization for HF, but not for sudden death. Furthermore, plasma volume depletion, across the spectrum of cardiovascular outcomes except for sudden death, showed a significant linear trend in the crude event rates in the whole study population. This was not true with the weight-based definition of diuretic effect, representing intracellular and extracellular volume depletion that was not associated with any of the assessed outcomes. Multivariate analysis of the main cardiovascular outcomes confirmed that the effect of eplerenone on outcomes was independent from early diuretic and potassium-sparing effects. This is the first time in patients with systolic dysfunction and HF after an acute myocardial infarction that an initial and short-term diuretic-like effect as defined by plasma volume depletion after 1 month is associated with better cardiovascular outcomes, independent of potassium-sparing effect. Also the benefit of eplerenone on outcomes was independent of the diuretic and potassium-sparing effects. Another important finding of this study is the independent early potassium-sparing effect, consistent with eplerenone's mineralocorticoid receptor antagonism, which was associated with improved long-term cardiovascular outcomes. The conclusions of the authors is that this study supports the hypothesis that pleiotropic effects of the eplerenone may involve left ventricular and vascular remodeling, including effects on collagen synthesis and endothelial and immune function. It remains to be seen whether the same effects are seen in patients with HF not caused by acute myocardial infarction.

M. D. Cheitlin, MD

References

1. Drazner MH, Rame JE, Stevenson LW, Dries DL. Prognostic importance of elevated jugular venous pressure and a third heart sound in patients with heart failure. *N Engl J Med.* 2001;345:574-581.
2. Lucas C, Johnson W, Hamilton MA, et al. Freedom from congestion predicts good survival despite previous class iv symptoms of heart failure. *Am Heart J.* 2000;140:840-847.
3. Pitt B, Remme W, Zannad F, et al. Eplerenone, a selective aldosterone blocker, in patients with left ventricular dysfunction after myocardial infarction. *N Engl J Med.* 2003;348:1309-1321.

Erythropoietin as a treatment of anemia in heart failure: Systematic review of randomized trials

Kotecha D, Ngo K, Walters JA, et al (Imperial College, London, UK; Univ of Tasmania, Hobart, Australia; et al)
Am Heart J 161:822-831.e2, 2011

Background.—Anemia in heart failure is both common and associated with worse symptoms and increased mortality. Several small randomized controlled trials (RCTs) have assessed erythropoiesis-stimulating agents (ESAs), but definitive evaluation and clinical guidance are required. We sought to systematically review the effects of ESAs in chronic heart failure.

Methods.—An extensive search strategy identified 11 RCTs with 794 participants comparing any ESA with control over 2 to 12 months of follow-up. Published and additionally requested data were incorporated into a Cochrane systematic review (CD007613).

Results.—Nine studies were placebo controlled, and 5, double blinded. Erythropoiesis-stimulating agent treatment significantly improved exercise duration by 96.8 seconds (95% CI 5.2-188.4, $P = .04$) and 6-minute walk distance by 69.3 m (95% CI 17.0-121.7, $P = .009$) compared with control. Benefit was also noted for peak oxygen consumption (+2.29 mL/kg per minute, $P = .007$), New York Heart Association class (-0.73, $P < .001$), ejection fraction ($+5.8\%$, $P < .001$), B-type natriuretic peptide (-226.99 pg/mL, $P < .001$), and quality-of-life indicators with a mean increase in hemoglobin level of 2 g/dL. There was a significantly lower rate of heart failure—related hospitalizations with ESA therapy (odds ratio 0.56, 95% CI 0.37-0.84, $P = .005$). No associated increase in adverse events or mortality (odds ratio 0.58, 95% CI 0.34-0.99, $P = .047$) was observed, although the number of events was limited.

Conclusion.—Meta-analysis of small RCTs suggests that ESA treatment can improve exercise tolerance, reduce symptoms, and have benefits on clinical outcomes in anemic patients with heart failure. Confirmation requires larger, well-designed studies with careful attention to dose, attained hemoglobin level, and long-term outcomes (Figs 2 and 6).

▶ Anemia is common in a variety of chronic diseases, including congestive heart failure (HF).[1] Groenvelt and colleagues reported a meta-analysis of more than 150 000 patients with HF and found that a low hemoglobin level increased the risk in patients with either systolic or diastolic HF of all-cause mortality almost 2-fold over a 6-month to 5-year follow-up period.[2] Erythropoeitin-stimulating agents (ESAs) have been shown to improve the quality of life in chronically ill patients.[3] There have been a few small, randomized, controlled trials of the treatment of anemia with a variety of ESAs that showed some benefit for reduced hospitalization[4]; the mechanism for this reduction is not yet clear. Also, there are conflicting data on ESA's effect on activity capacity, functional level, and mortality in patients with HF. This reports the result of a systematic review of the literature and meta-analysis for ESAs in HF patients in randomized trials, controlled with either placebo or no treatment. Eleven such studies were identified. The patients had symptomatic HF with an ejection fraction of less than 40%. The use of HF medications was similar in the ESA and the control groups. There was an almost 2-g/dL increase in hemoglobin over the period of follow-up. The treatment increased left ventricular ejection fraction (LVEF) and reduced B-type natriuretic peptide, improved symptoms and exercise capacity, and significantly reduced HF-related hospitalizations and all-cause mortality compared with the control patients. Unlike other ESA therapy in other conditions, there was no significant increase in adverse events. The mechanism by which these

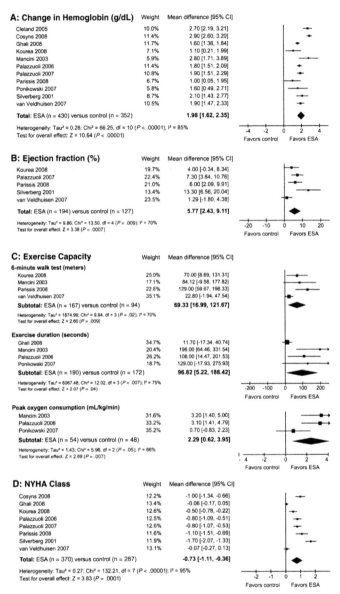

A: Change in Hemoglobin (g/dL)

	Weight	Mean difference [95% CI]
Cleland 2005	10.0%	2.70 [2.19, 3.21]
Cosyns 2008	11.4%	2.90 [2.60, 3.20]
Ghali 2008	11.7%	1.60 [1.36, 1.84]
Kourea 2008	7.1%	1.10 [0.21, 1.99]
Mancini 2003	5.9%	2.80 [1.71, 3.89]
Palazzuoli 2006	11.4%	1.80 [1.51, 2.09]
Palazzuoli 2007	10.8%	1.90 [1.51, 2.29]
Parissis 2008	6.7%	1.00 [0.05, 1.95]
Ponikowski 2007	5.8%	1.60 [0.49, 2.71]
Silverberg 2001	8.7%	2.10 [1.43, 2.77]
van Veldhuisen 2007	10.5%	1.90 [1.47, 2.33]
Total: ESA (n = 430) versus control (n = 352)		**1.98 [1.62, 2.35]**

Heterogeneity: Tau² = 0.28; Chi² = 66.25, df = 10 (P < .00001); I² = 85%
Test for overall effect: Z = 10.64 (P < .00001)

B: Ejection fraction (%)

	Weight	Mean difference [95% CI]
Kourea 2008	19.7%	4.00 [-0.34, 8.34]
Palazzuoli 2007	22.4%	7.30 [3.84, 10.76]
Parissis 2008	21.0%	6.00 [2.09, 9.91]
Silverberg 2001	13.4%	13.30 [6.56, 20.04]
van Veldhuisen 2007	23.5%	1.29 [-1.80, 4.38]
Total: ESA (n = 194) versus control (n = 127)		**5.77 [2.43, 9.11]**

Heterogeneity: Tau² = 9.86; Chi² = 13.50, df = 4 (P = .009); I² = 70%
Test for overall effect: Z = 3.38 (P = .0007)

C: Exercise Capacity

	Weight	Mean difference [95% CI]
6-minute walk test (meters)		
Kourea 2008	25.0%	70.00 [8.69, 131.31]
Mancini 2003	17.1%	84.12 [-9.58, 177.82]
Parissis 2008	22.8%	129.00 [59.67, 198.33]
van Veldhuisen 2007	35.1%	22.80 [-1.94, 47.54]
Subtotal: ESA (n = 167) versus control (n = 94)		**69.33 [16.99, 121.67]**

Heterogeneity: Tau² = 1874.99; Chi² = 9.94, df = 3 (P = .02); I² = 70%
Test for overall effect: Z = 2.60 (P = .009)

	Weight	Mean difference [95% CI]
Exercise duration (seconds)		
Ghali 2008	34.7%	11.70 [-17.34, 40.74]
Mancini 2003	20.4%	198.00 [64.46, 331.54]
Palazzuoli 2006	26.2%	108.00 [14.47, 201.53]
Ponikowski 2007	18.7%	129.00 [-17.93, 275.93]
Subtotal: ESA (n = 190) versus control (n = 172)		**96.82 [5.22, 188.42]**

Heterogeneity: Tau² = 6067.48; Chi² = 12.02, df = 3 (P = .007); I² = 75%
Test for overall effect: Z = 2.07 (P = .04)

	Weight	Mean difference [95% CI]
Peak oxygen consumption (mL/kg/min)		
Mancini 2003	31.6%	3.20 [1.40, 5.00]
Palazzuoli 2006	33.2%	3.10 [1.41, 4.79]
Ponikowski 2007	35.2%	0.70 [-0.83, 2.23]
Subtotal: ESA (n = 54) versus control (n = 48)		**2.29 [0.62, 3.95]**

Heterogeneity: Tau² = 1.43; Chi² = 5.96, df = 2 (P = .05); I² = 66%
Test for overall effect: Z = 2.89 (P = .007)

D: NYHA Class

	Weight	Mean difference [95% CI]
Cosyns 2008	12.2%	-1.00 [-1.34, -0.66]
Ghali 2008	13.4%	-0.06 [-0.17, 0.05]
Kourea 2008	12.6%	-0.50 [-0.78, -0.22]
Palazzuoli 2006	12.5%	-0.80 [-1.09, -0.51]
Palazzuoli 2007	12.6%	-0.80 [-1.07, -0.53]
Parissis 2008	11.6%	-1.10 [-1.51, -0.69]
Silverberg 2001	11.9%	-1.70 [-2.07, -1.33]
van Veldhuisen 2007	13.1%	-0.07 [-0.27, 0.13]
Total: ESA (n = 370) versus control (n = 287)		**-0.73 [-1.11, -0.36]**

Heterogeneity: Tau² = 0.27; Chi² = 132.21, df = 7 (P < .00001); I² = 95%
Test for overall effect: Z = 3.83 (P = .0001)

FIGURE 2.—Effect of ESA therapy on hemoglobin level, ejection fraction, and functional outcomes. Weighted mean differences are shown on a logarithmic scale; the size of each square is proportional to the weight of the individual study, and the diamond represents the pooled difference using a random effects model. I^2 is the percentage of total variation across studies due to heterogeneity. (Reprinted from the American Heart Journal, Kotecha D, Ngo K, Walters JA, et al. Erythropoietin as a treatment of anemia in heart failure: Systematic review of randomized trials. Am Heart J. 2011;161:822-831.e2. Copyright © 2011, with permission from Elsevier.)

A. Left-ventricular ejection fraction

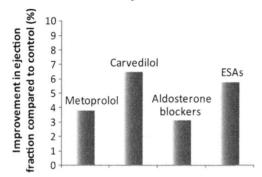

B. B-type natriuretic peptide

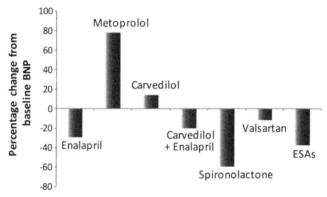

FIGURE 6.—Indirect comparison of heart failure therapies with ESAs (when added to standard treatment). Graphs represent the effect of evidence-based treatments on heart failure measures and are indicative only as head-to-head comparisons have not been made and studies vary according to baseline demographics and follow-up. Graph A depicts left ventricular ejection fraction compared with control.[24,36] Graph **B** depicts BNP change from baseline; note that values for spironolactone, valsartan, and ESAs are an addition to ACE inhibitors (most participants) and β-blockers (substantial minority).[43-46] *Editor's Note*: Please refer to original journal article for full references. (Reprinted from the American Heart Journal, Kotecha D, Ngo K, Walters JA, et al. Erythropoietin as a treatment of anemia in heart failure: Systematic review of randomized trials. *Am Heart J.* 2011;161:822-831.e2. Copyright © 2011, with permission from Elsevier.)

beneficial effects occur is speculative and may be the result of an increase in LVEF as a result of the increased hemoglobin level. The anemia in HF can be the result of multiple factors, including inadequate erythropoietin production caused by reduced renal blood flow, bone marrow depression as a result of inflammation, and effects of medications such as ACE inhibitors on erythropoiesis.[5] Anemia may affect cardiovascular function by increasing neurohormonal activity and salt and water retention.[6] The compensatory LV remodeling eventually results in worsened LV function and a cycle of renal impairment and reduced erythropoiesis (the cardiorenal syndrome). This meta-analysis provides evidence for the safety and efficacy of erythropoietin therapy in patients with HF and anemia.

M. D. Cheitlin, MD

References

1. Mitchell JE. Emerging role of anemia in heart failure. *Am J Cardiol.* 2007;99: 15D-20D.
2. Groenveld HF, Januzzi JL, Damman K, et al. Anemia and mortality in heart failure patients a systematic review and meta-analysis. *J Am Coll Cardiol.* 2008;52:818-827.
3. Kimel M, Leidy NK, Mannix S, Dixon J. Does epoetin alfa improve health-related quality of life in chronically ill patients with anemia? Summary of trials of cancer, HIV/AIDS, and chronic kidney disease. *Value Health.* 2008;11:57-75.
4. van der Meer P, Groenveld HF, Januzzi JL Jr, van Veldhuisen DJ. Erythropoietin treatment in patients with chronic heart failure: a meta-analysis. *Heart.* 2009; 95:1309-1314.
5. Okonko D, Anker SD. Anemia in chronic heart failure: pathogenetic mechanisms. *J Card Fail.* 2004;10:S5-S9.
6. Anand IS. Anemia and chronic heart failure implications and treatment options. *J Am Coll Cardiol.* 2008;52:501-511.

Pulmonary Hypertension in Heart Failure With Preserved Ejection Fraction: A Target of Phosphodiesterase-5 Inhibition in a 1-Year Study
Guazzi M, Vicenzi M, Arena R, et al (Univ of Milan, Italy; Virginia Commonwealth Univ, Richmond)
Circulation 124:164-174, 2011

Background.—The prevalence of heart failure with preserved ejection fraction is increasing. The prognosis worsens with pulmonary hypertension and right ventricular (RV) failure development. We targeted pulmonary hypertension and RV burden with the phosphodiesterase-5 inhibitor sildenafil.

Methods and Results.—Forty-four patients with heart failure with preserved ejection fraction (heart failure signs and symptoms, diastolic dysfunction, ejection fraction ≥50%, and pulmonary artery systolic pressure >40 mm Hg) were randomly assigned to placebo or sildenafil (50 mg thrice per day). At 6 months, there was no improvement with placebo, but sildenafil mediated significant improvements in mean pulmonary artery pressure (−42.0 ± 13.0%) and RV function, as suggested by leftward shift of the RV Frank-Starling relationship, increased tricuspid annular systolic excursion (+69.0 ± 19.0%) and ejection rate (+17.0 ± 8.3%), and reduced right atrial pressure (−54.0 ± 7.2%). These effects may have resulted from changes within the lung (reduced lung water content and improved alveolar-capillary gas conductance, +15.8 ± 4.5%), the pulmonary vasculature (arteriolar resistance, −71.0 ± 8.2%), and left-sided cardiac function (wedge pulmonary pressure, −15.7 ± 3.1%; cardiac index, +6.0 ± 0.9%; deceleration time, −13.0 ± 1.9%; isovolumic relaxation time, −14.0 ± 1.7%; septal mitral annulus velocity, −76.4 ± 9.2%). Results were similar at 12 months.

Conclusions.—The multifaceted response to phosphodiesterase-5 inhibition in heart failure with preserved ejection fraction includes improvement in pulmonary pressure and vasomotility, RV function and dimension, left ventricular relaxation and distensibility (structural changes and/or ventricular interdependence), and lung interstitial water metabolism (wedge pulmonary pressure decrease improving hydrostatic balance and right atrial pressure reduction facilitating lung lymphatic drainage). These results enhance our understanding of heart failure with preserved ejection fraction and offer new directions for therapy.

▶ Heart failure with preserved ejection fraction (HFpEF) accounts for almost half of patients seen in HF and is associated with a prognosis similar to that of systolic dysfunction HF.[1,2] Pulmonary hypertension (PH) in left-sided HF is common, often severe, and places an afterload burden of the right ventricle resulting in right ventricular failure and increased right atrial and central venous pressure, all associated with increased mortality.[3,4] Attempts to decrease the pulmonary artery pressure and thus improve right heart hemodynamics have involved endothelin receptor antagonists[5] and prostacyclin analogs[6] and in general have been without success. With elevation of left atrial and pulmonary venous pressure, there is both passive elevation in pulmonary artery pressure[7] and a reactive increase in pulmonary vascular resistance due to increase in pulmonary vascular tone or intrinsic arterial remodeling.[8] There is evidence in HF that there is pulmonary endothelial dysfunction and that nitric oxide (NO) vasodilatation is impaired.[7,9] For this reason, phosphodiesterase-5 (PDE-5) inhibitors, such as sildenafil, that increase cyclic GMP and prolong NO vasodilatation have been used in patients with HF.[10,11] PDE-5 inhibitors have the advantage of selectively dilating the pulmonary vessels without producing tachyphylaxis.[12] This study, using 50 mg of sildenafil 3 times a day over 1 year compared with placebo resulted in a significant decrease in pulmonary artery pressure, pulmonary arteriolar resistance, improved right ventricular function, and hemodynamics as well as left-sided cardiac function. By decreasing the right atrial and superior vena cava pressure, improvement in pulmonary lymphatic drainage occurs, decreasing pulmonary interstitial fluid and improving pulmonary function. The improvement in left-sided hemodynamics may be in part explained by the cardiac antihypertrophic and antifibrotic properties of PDE-5 inhibitors seen in animal and human studies.[13] This study is evidence that decreasing PH in patients with HFpEF is a reasonable target and that PDE-5 inhibitors can achieve this goal. Given the favorable effects on both right and left heart hemodynamics, there might even be favorable prognostic implications.

M. D. Cheitlin, MD

References

1. Owan TE, Hodge DO, Herges RM, Jacobsen SJ, Roger VL, Redfield MM. Trends in prevalence and outcome of heart failure with preserved ejection fraction. *N Engl J Med.* 2006;355:251-259.
2. Bhatia RS, Tu JV, Lee DS, et al. Outcome of heart failure with preserved ejection fraction in a population-based study. *N Engl J Med.* 2006;355:260-269.
3. Ghio S, Gavazzi A, Campana C, et al. Independent and additive prognostic value of right ventricular systolic function and pulmonary artery pressure in patients with chronic heart failure. *J Am Coll Cardiol.* 2001;37:183-188.
4. Lam CS, Roger VL, Rodeheffer RJ, Borlaug BA, Enders FT, Redfield MM. Pulmonary hypertension in heart failure with preserved ejection fraction: a community-based study. *J Am Coll Cardiol.* 2009;53:1119-1126.

5. Gottlieb SS. The impact of finally publishing a negative study: new conclusions about endothelin antagonists. *J Card Fail.* 2005;11:21-22.
6. Califf RM, Adams KF, McKenna WJ, et al. A randomized controlled trial of epoprostenol therapy for severe congestive heart failure: the Flolan International Randomized Survival Trial (FIRST). *Am Heart J.* 1997;134:44-54.
7. Guazzi M, Arena R. Pulmonary hypertension with left-sided heart disease. *Nat Rev Cardiol.* 2010;7:648-659.
8. Delgado JF, Conde E, Sánchez V, et al. Pulmonary vascular remodeling in pulmonary hypertension due to chronic heart failure. *Eur J Heart Fail.* 2005;7:1011-1016.
9. Moraes DL, Colucci WS, Givertz MM. Secondary pulmonary hypertension in chronic heart failure: the role of the endothelium in pathophysiology and management. *Circulation.* 2000;102:1718-1723.
10. Guazzi M, Samaja M, Arena R, Vicenzi M, Guazzi MD. Long-term use of sildenafil in the therapeutic management of heart failure. *J Am Coll Cardiol.* 2007;50:2136-2144.
11. Lewis GD. The role of the pulmonary vasculature in heart failure with preserved ejection fraction. *J Am Coll Cardiol.* 2009;53:1127-1129.
12. Guazzi M. Clinical use of phoshodiesterase-5 inhibitors in chronic heart failure. *Circ Heart Fail.* 2008;1:272-280.
13. Guazzi M, Vicenzi M, Arena R, Guazzi MD. PDE5 inhibition with sildenafil improves left ventricular diastolic function, cardiac geometry and clinical status in patients with stable systolic heart failure: results of a 1-year prospective, randomized, placebo-controlled study. *Circ Heart Fail.* 2011;4:8-17.

Cardiac resynchronisation therapy in patients with heart failure and a normal QRS duration: the RESPOND study

Foley PWX, Patel K, Irwin N, et al (Univ of Birmingham, UK; Sandwell and City Hosps NHS Trust, Birmingham, UK; Good Hope Hosp, Sutton Coldfield, West Midlands, UK; et al)
Heart 97:1041-1047, 2011

Objectives.—To evaluate the clinical response to cardiac resynchronisation therapy (CRT) in patients with heart failure and a normal QRS duration (<120 ms).

Setting.—Single centre.

Patients.—60 patients with heart failure and a normal QRS duration receiving optimal pharmacological treatment (OPT).

Interventions.—Patients were randomly assigned to CRT (n=29) or to a control group (OPT, n=31). Cardiovascular magnetic resonance was used in order to avoid scar at the site of left ventricular (LV) lead deployment.

Main Outcome Measures.—The primary end point was a change in 6 min walking distance (6-MWD). Other measures included a change in quality of life scores (Minnesota Living with Heart Failure questionnaire) and New York Heart Association class.

Results.—In 93% of implantations, the LV lead was deployed over non-scarred myocardium. At 6 months, the 6-MWD increased with CRT compared with OPT (p<0.0001), with more patients reaching a ≥25% increase (51.7% vs 12.9%, p=0.0019). Compared with OPT, CRT led to an improvement in quality-of-life scores (p=0.0265) and a reduction in NYHA class (p<0.0001). The composite clinical score (survival for

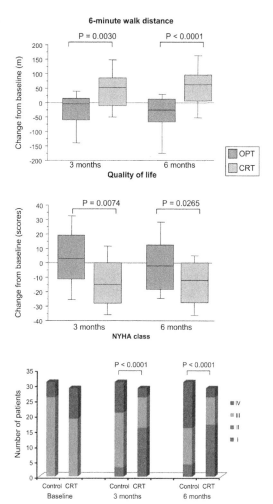

FIGURE 1.—Effect of cardiac resynchronisation therapy (CRT) on clinical variables. The change from baseline for 6 min walking distance and quality of life scores (Minnesota Living with Heart Failure questionnaire) at 3 and 6 months are shown in box-and-whisker plots, in which the five horizontal lines represent the 10th, 25th, 50th, 75th and 90th centiles, from bottom to top. For quality of life, scores range from 0 to 105, with high scores denoting the poorest quality of life. A reduction denotes improvement in quality of life. For New York Heart Association (NYHA) class, the distribution of classes at baseline, 3 months and 6 months is shown. p Values refer to differences in NYHA class, expressed as a continuous variable. OPT, optimal pharmacological treatment. (Reproduced from Heart, Foley PWX, Patel K, Irwin N, et al. Cardiac resynchronisation therapy in patients with heart failure and a normal QRS duration: the RESPOND study. *Heart*. 2011;97:1041-1047. Copyright © 2011, with permission from the BMJ Publishing Group Ltd.)

6 months free of heart failure hospitalisations plus improvement by one or more NYHA class or by ≥25% in 6-MWD) was better in CRT than in OPT (83% vs 23%, respectively; p<0.0001). Although no differences in total or cardiovascular mortality emerged between OPT and CRT, patients

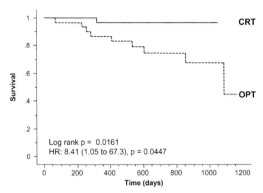

FIGURE 2.—Kaplan—Meier estimates of the time to death from pump failure. Results of univariate Cox proportional hazards analyses are expressed as hazards ratio (HR) and 95% confidence limits (in parentheses). (Reproduced from Heart, Foley PWX, Patel K, Irwin N, et al. Cardiac resynchronisation therapy in patients with heart failure and a normal QRS duration: the RESPOND study. *Heart.* 2011;97:1041-1047. Copyright © 2011, with permission from the BMJ Publishing Group Ltd.)

receiving OPT had a higher risk of death from pump failure than patients assigned to CRT (HR=8.41, p=0.0447) after a median follow-up of 677.5 days.

Conclusions.—CRT leads to an improvement in symptoms, exercise capacity and quality of life in patients with heart failure and a normal QRS duration. (ClinicalTrials.gov number, NCT00480051.) (Figs 1 and 2).

▶ Cardiac resynchronization therapy (CRT) in patients with heart failure (HF) has been shown to decrease symptoms, increase exercise capacity, improve the quality of life (QOL), and reduce all-cause mortality.[1-3] Initially, a wide QRS was the marker for ventricular dyssynchrony, so in most studies, a QRS ≥ 120 msec has been adopted and appears in the treatment guidelines.[1-3] There is increasing recognition that mechanical dyssynchrony can be present in patients with heart failure and a QRS less than 120 msec,[4-6] and this observation has led to evaluating the effect of CRT in these patients[7] where several observational studies have shown a benefit.[8-10] The only randomized study in patients with a QRS less than 130 msec did not show a benefit for peak O_2 uptake on exercise.[11] This study includes patients with New York Heart Association (NYHA) class III—IV HF, a left ventricular ejection fraction (LVEF) less than 35% and a QRS less than 120 msec on optimal medical therapy. The patients were randomly assigned to CRT versus optimal therapy alone and followed for a median of almost 2 years. They found that the CRT patients had the primary endpoint of a 6-minute walking distance (6-MWD) significantly increased, as well as the QOL score significantly improved, and a better composite score of freedom from HF hospitalizations, lower NYHA class, and improvement by ≥25% of 6-MWD compared with the patients on optimal therapy alone. Also, there was a significant reduction time of death from heart failure in the CRT patients. Since symptomatic patients with HF and a reduced LVEF and a QRS less than 120 msec are far more prevalent than those with QRS greater than 120 msec, this observation is potentially very important in that it expands the population of HF patients who might benefit from CRT (and the cost) enormously. The key to narrowing the field to those patients with narrow QRS to those who actually will benefit from CRT is probably to focus on the patients with mechanical dyssynchrony.

M. D. Cheitlin, MD

References

1. Cleland JG, Daubert JC, Erdmann E, et al; Cardiac Resynchronization-Heart Failure (CARE-HF) Study Investigators. The effect of cardiac resynchronization on morbidity and mortality in heart failure. *N Engl J Med.* 2005;352:1539-1549.
2. Abraham WT, Fisher WG, Smith AL, et al. Cardiac resynchronization in chronic heart failure. *N Engl J Med.* 2002;346:1845-1853.
3. Bristow MR, Saxon LA, Boehmer J, et al; Comparison of Medical Therapy, Pacing, and Defibrillation in Heart Failure (COMPANION) Investigators. Cardiac-resynchronization therapy with or without an implantable defibrillator in advanced chronic heart failure. *N Engl J Med.* 2004;350:2140-2150.
4. Bleeker GB, Schalij MJ, Molhoek SG, et al. Relationship between QRS duration and left ventricular dyssynchrony in patients with end-stage heart failure. *J Cardiovasc Electrophysiol.* 2004;15:544-549.
5. Haghjoo M, Bagherzadeh A, Fazelifar AF, et al. Prevalence of mechanical dyssynchrony in heart failure patients with different QRS durations. *Pacing Clin Electrophysiol.* 2007;30:616-622.
6. Yu CM, Lin H, Zhang Q, Sanderson JE. High prevalence of left ventricular systolic and diastolic asynchrony in patients with congestive heart failure and normal QRS duration. *Heart.* 2003;89:54-60.
7. Kashani A, Barold SS. Significance of QRS complex duration in patients with heart failure. *J Am Coll Cardiol.* 2005;46:2183-2192.
8. Yu CM, Chan YS, Zhang Q, et al. Benefits of cardiac resynchronization therapy for heart failure patients with narrow QRS complexes and coexisting systolic asynchrony by echocardiography. *J Am Coll Cardiol.* 2006;48:2251-2257.
9. Achilli A, Sassara M, Ficili S, et al. Long-term effectiveness of cardiac resynchronization therapy in patients with refractory heart failure and "narrow" QRS. *J Am Coll Cardiol.* 2003;42:2117-2124.
10. Bleeker GB, Holman ER, Steendijk P, et al. Cardiac resynchronization therapy in patients with a narrow QRS complex. *J Am Coll Cardiol.* 2006;48:2243-2250.
11. Beshai JF, Grimm RA, Nagueh SF, et al. Cardiac-resynchronization therapy in heart failure with narrow QRS complexes. *N Engl J Med.* 2007;357:2461-2471.

Pathogenesis and Prognosis

Comparison of Mortality and Morbidity in Patients With Atrial Fibrillation and Heart Failure With Preserved Versus Decreased Left Ventricular Ejection Fraction

Badheka AO, Rathod A, Kizilbash MA, et al (Wayne State Univ School of Medicine, Detroit, MI)
Am J Cardiol 108:1283-1288, 2011

Almost 50% of patients with congestive heart failure (HF) have preserved ejection fraction (PEF). Data on the effect of HF-PEF on atrial fibrillation outcomes are lacking. We assessed the prognostic significance of HF-PEF in an atrial fibrillation population compared to a systolic heart failure (SHF) population. A post hoc analysis of the National Heart, Lung, and Blood Institute-limited access data set of the Atrial Fibrillation Follow-up

Investigation of Rhythm Management (AFFIRM) trial was carried out. The patients with a history of congestive HF and a preserved ejection fraction (EF >50%) were classified as having HF-PEF (n = 320). The patients with congestive HF and a qualitatively depressed EF (EF <50%) were classified as having SHF (n = 402). Cox proportional hazards analysis was performed. The mean follow-up duration was 1,181 ± 534 days/patient. The patients with HF-PEF had lower all-cause mortality (hazard ratio [HR] 0.62, 95% confidence interval [CI] 0.46 to 0.85, p = 0.003) and cardiovascular mortality (HR 0.56, 95% CI 0.38 to 0.84, p = 0.006), with a possible decreased arrhythmic end point (HR 0.39, 95% CI 0.16 to 1.006, p = 0.052) than did the patients with SHF. No differences were observed for ischemic stroke (HR 1.08, 95% CI 0.48 to 2.39, p = 0.86), rehospitalization (HR 0.89, 95% CI 0.75 to 1.07, p = 0.24), or progression to New York Heart Association class III-IV (odds ratio 0.80, 95% CI 0.42 to 1.54, p = 0.522). In conclusion, although patients with HF-PEF have better mortality outcomes than those with SHF, the morbidity appears to be similar (Figs 2, 3, 5 and 6).

▶ Most risk stratification scores for stroke in patients with atrial fibrillation (AF) including the CHADS2 score take into account either a history of congestive heart

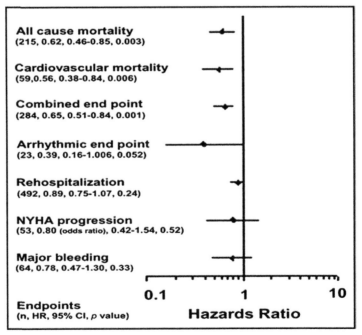

FIGURE 2.—HF-PEF versus SHF for outcomes. (Reprinted from the American Journal of Cardiology, Badheka AO, Rathod A, Kizilbash MA, et al. Comparison of mortality and morbidity in patients with atrial fibrillation and heart failure with preserved versus decreased left ventricular ejection fraction. *Am J Cardiol.* 2011;108:1283-1288. Copyright 2011, with permission from Elsevier.)

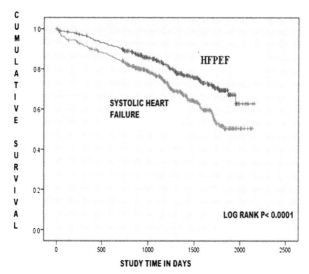

FIGURE 3.—Kaplan-Meier (K-M) curves for all-cause mortality for HF-PEF versus SHF. (Reprinted from the American Journal of Cardiology, Badheka AO, Rathod A, Kizilbash MA, et al. Comparison of mortality and morbidity in patients with atrial fibrillation and heart failure with preserved versus decreased left ventricular ejection fraction. *Am J Cardiol.* 2011;108:1283-1288. Copyright 2011, with permission from Elsevier.)

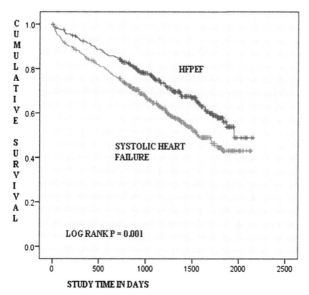

FIGURE 5.—Kaplan-Meier (K-M) curves for combined end point for HF-PEF versus SHF. (Reprinted from the American Journal of Cardiology, Badheka AO, Rathod A, Kizilbash MA, et al. Comparison of mortality and morbidity in patients with atrial fibrillation and heart failure with preserved versus decreased left ventricular ejection fraction. *Am J Cardiol.* 2011;108:1283-1288. Copyright 2011, with permission from Elsevier.)

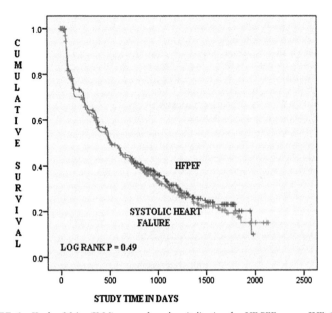

FIGURE 6.—Kaplan-Meier (K-M) curves for rehospitalization for HF-PEF versus SHF. (Reprinted from the American Journal of Cardiology, Badheka AO, Rathod A, Kizilbash MA, et al. Comparison of mortality and morbidity in patients with atrial fibrillation and heart failure with preserved versus decreased left ventricular ejection fraction. *Am J Cardiol.* 2011;108:1283-1288. Copyright 2011, with permission from Elsevier.)

failure or decreased ejection fraction (EF). There is an independent association of a history of heart failure (HF) and left ventricular systolic dysfunction with poor outcomes in patients with AF.[1-3] Unclear is whether the risk is the same for patients with heart failure and preserved EF (HF-PEF) as it is for those with systolic heart failure (SHF), and because HF-PEF accounts for half of the patients with heart failure, this question is important.[3-5] Using the data from the Atrial Fibrillation Follow-up Investigation of Rhythm Management (AFFIRM) trial, this study found over a duration of greater than 3 years that there was a lower all-cause and cardiovascular mortality in patients with HF-PEF than in SHF but no difference in ischemic stroke, progression to New York Heart Association (NYHA) III/IV, or rehospitalization. Arrhythmic risk trended to be lower in patients with HF-PEF. Parkash and colleagues found no difference in mortality between HF-PEF and SHF at 5 years, but their study (compared with this study) was single center and smaller, and fewer had warfarin use; NYHA class, a strong predictor of mortality independent of left ventricular (LV) ejection fraction, was lacking.[4,6] This study had similar findings as the Candesartan in Heart Failure Assessment of Reduction in Mortality and Morbidity (CHARM) study[5] and the Irbesartan in Heart Failure With Preserved Ejection Fraction Study (I-Preserve) trial.[7] The reason for the similar morbidity between the patients with HF with or without LV dysfunction is extensively discussed, but the explanation remains unclear. Because this is a substudy of the AFFIRM trial, it is hypothesis generating only and should not change the risk scores for stroke in patients with AF.

M. D. Cheitlin, MD

References

1. Gage BF, Waterman AD, Shannon W, Boechler M, Rich MW, Radford MJ. Validation of clinical classification schemes for predicting stroke: results from the National Registry of Atrial Fibrillation. *JAMA.* 2001;285:2864-2870.
2. Wyse DG, Waldo AL, DiMarco JP, et al; Atrial Fibrillation Follow-up Investigation of Rhythm Management (AFFIRM) Investigators. A comparison of rate control and rhythm control in patients with atrial fibrillation. *N Engl J Med.* 2002;347: 1825-1833.
3. Fung JW, Sanderson JE, Yip GW, Zhang Q, Yu CM. Impact of atrial fibrillation in heart failure with normal ejection fraction: a clinical and echocardiographic study. *J Card Fail.* 2007;13:649-655.
4. Parkash R, Maisel WH, Toca FM, Stevenson WG. Atrial fibrillation in heart failure: high mortality risk even if ventricular function is preserved. *Am Heart J.* 2005;150:701-706.
5. Olsson LG, Swedberg K, Ducharme A, et al; CHARM Investigators. Atrial fibrillation and risk of clinical events in chronic heart failure with and without left ventricular systolic dysfunction: results from the Candesartan in Heart Failure-Assessment of Reduction in Mortality and morbidity (CHARM) program. *J Am Coll Cardiol.* 2006;47:1997-2004.
6. Parkash R, Stevenson WG. Atrial fibrillation and clinical events in chronic heart failure. *J Am Coll Cardiol.* 2007;49:376-377.
7. Zile MR, Gaasch WH, Anand IS, et al; I-Preserve Investigators. Mode of death in patients with heart failure and a preserved ejection fraction: results from the Irbesartan in Heart Failure With Preserved Ejection Fraction Study (I-Preserve) trial. *Circulation.* 2010;121:1393-1405.

Disordered Iron Homeostasis in Chronic Heart Failure: Prevalence, Predictors, and Relation to Anemia, Exercise Capacity, and Survival

Okonko DO, Mandal AKJ, Missouris CG, et al (Imperial College London, UK; Wexham Park Hosp, Slough, UK)

J Am Coll Cardiol 58:1241-1251, 2011

Objectives.—The aim of this study was to comprehensively delineate iron metabolism and its implications in patients with chronic heart failure (CHF).

Background.—Iron deficiency is an emerging therapeutic target in CHF.

Methods.—Iron and clinical indexes were quantified in 157 patients with CHF.

Results.—Several observations were made. First, iron homeostasis was deranged in anemic and nonanemic subjects and characterized by diminished circulating (transferrin saturation) and functional (mean cell hemoglobin concentration) iron status in the face of seemingly adequate stores (ferritin). Second, while iron overload and elevated iron stores were rare (1%), iron deficiency (transferrin saturation <20%) was evident in 43% of patients. Third, disordered iron homeostasis related closely to worsening inflammation and disease severity and strongly predicted lower hemoglobin levels independently of age, sex, erythrocyte sedimentation rate, New York Heart Association (NYHA) functional class, and creatinine. Fourth, the etiologies of anemia varied with disease severity, with an iron-deficient substrate (anemia of chronic disease and/or iron-deficiency anemia) evident in 16%, 72%, and 100% of anemic NYHA functional class I or II, III, and IV patients, respectively. Although anemia of chronic disease was more prevalent than iron-deficiency anemia, both conditions coexisted in 17% of subjects. Fifth, iron deficiency was associated with lower peak oxygen consumption and higher ratios of ventilation to carbon dioxide production and identified those at enhanced risk for death (hazard ratio: 3.38; 95% confidence interval: 1.48 to 7.72; p = 0.004) independently of hemoglobin. Nonanemic iron-deficient patients had a 2-fold greater risk for death than anemic iron-replete subjects.

Conclusions.—Disordered iron homeostasis in patients with CHF relates to impaired exercise capacity and survival and appears prognostically more ominous than anemia (Figs 4 and 5).

▶ Many patients with chronic heart failure (CHF), even on optimal medications, can remain exercise intolerant and have a high mortality rate, suggesting that some risk factors for disease progression are not being addressed by current therapy. Many patients with chronic disease have a derangement of systemic iron homeostasis,[1-3] and this is probably true of CHF, but the integrity of iron metabolism is poorly characterized in CHF and is mainly reported in anemic

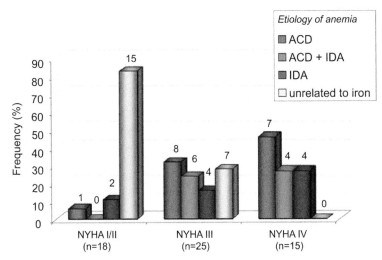

FIGURE 4.—Etiology of Anemia Stratified by NYHA Functional Class. Figures above bars correspond to numbers of patients. ACD = anemia of chronic disease; IDA = iron-deficiency anemia; NYHA = New York Heart Association. (Reprinted from the Journal of the American College of Cardiology, Okonko DO, Mandal AKJ, Missouris CG, et al. Disordered iron homeostasis in chronic heart failure: prevalence, predictors, and relation to anemia, exercise capacity, and survival. *J Am Coll Cardiol*. 2011;58:1241-1251. Copyright 2011, with permission from the American College of Cardiology.)

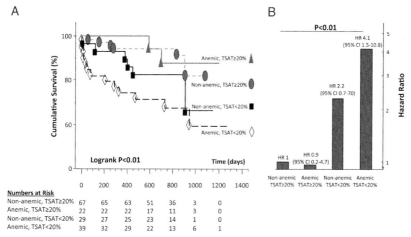

FIGURE 5.—Prognostic Association of Varying Hematological Groups. Kaplan-Meier survival curves for hematological subsets (**A**) with corresponding hazard ratios (HRs) and 95% confidence intervals (CIs) depicted (**B**). TSAT = transferrin saturation. (Reprinted from the Journal of the American College of Cardiology, Okonko DO, Mandal AKJ, Missouris CG, et al. Disordered iron homeostasis in chronic heart failure: prevalence, predictors, and relation to anemia, exercise capacity, and survival. *J Am Coll Cardiol.* 2011;58:1241-1251. Copyright 2011, with permission from the American College of Cardiology.)

patients[4,5] or based entirely on serum iron and ferritin levels.[6,7] Iron is quantitatively the most important biocatalyst in the human physiology with multiple roles other than hemoglobin synthesis.[8-10] Iron deficiency plays an important role in exercise intolerance and dyspnea[11,12] and in the general population identifies those with a higher risk for mortality.[13] Transferrin saturation (TSAT) is a more reliable marker for iron depletion than ferritin in inflammatory cohorts and also correlates with decreased survival.[14,15] It is not clear in CHF whether lower TSAT relates to higher risk of mortality independently and more powerfully than anemia in uremia. Total body iron is distributed across several circulating and functional iron compartments that can be altered independently of one another.[16,17] Therefore, a patient may be iron deficient without anemia. For this reason, multiple biomarkers are needed to assess the total state of iron homeostasis,[16] and there is no study that has done this in patients with CHF. This study, in a diverse group of 157 systolic CHF patients and 22 normal control subjects, in which iron metabolism and its predictors are characterized, emphasizes the differences between anemia of chronic disease and iron deficiency anemia and its combination. Also, the etiologies of anemia vary with New York Heart Association (NYHA) class, and the relation of iron deficiency to the ability to exercise and to survival are examined. Iron deficiency is defined as TSAT less than 29%, and diminished circulating iron status is a feature of both absolute (TSAT < 20%, low ferritin) and functional (TSAT < 20%, normal or high ferritin) iron deficiency. From this study, the 5 observations cited in the abstract are made. The study finds that iron metabolism is deranged in CHF, characterized by a diminished circulating and functional iron status in spite of adequate iron stores. This disordered iron homeostasis correlates to worsening inflammation and NYHA functional class and increasingly underlies anemia with CHF progression. Iron deficiency as measured by TSAT less than 20% correlates to exercise intolerance and increased mortality. Future trials should target TSAT levels to determine whether exercise tolerance and mortality can be altered.

M. D. Cheitlin, MD

References

1. Goyal R, Das R, Bambery P, Garewal G. Serum transferrin receptor-ferritin index shows concomitant iron deficiency anemia and anemia of chronic disease is common in patients with rheumatoid arthritis in north India. *Indian J Pathol Microbiol.* 2008;51:102-104.
2. Darveau M, Denault AY, Blais N, Notebaert E. Bench-to-bedside review: iron metabolism in critically ill patients. *Crit Care.* 2004;8:356-362.
3. Andrews NC. Disorders of iron metabolism. *N Engl J Med.* 1999;341:1986-1995.
4. Nanas JN, Matsouka C, Karageorgopoulos D, et al. Etiology of anemia in patients with advanced heart failure. *J Am Coll Cardiol.* 2006;48:2485-2489.
5. Opasich C, Cazzola M, Scelsi L, et al. Blunted erythropoietin production and defective iron supply for erythropoiesis as major causes of anaemia in patients with chronic heart failure. *Eur Heart J.* 2005;26:2232-2237.
6. Adlbrecht C, Kommata S, Hülsmann M, et al. Chronic heart failure leads to an expanded plasma volume and pseudoanaemia, but does not lead to a reduction in the body's red cell volume. *Eur Heart J.* 2008;29:2343-2350.
7. Witte KK, Desilva R, Chattopadhyay S, Ghosh J, Cleland JG, Clark AL. Are hematinic deficiencies the cause of anemia in chronic heart failure? *Am Heart J.* 2004;147:924-930.
8. Oexle H, Gnaiger E, Weiss G. Iron-dependent changes in cellular energy metabolism: influence on citric acid cycle and oxidative phosphorylation. *Biochim Biophys Acta.* 1999;1413:99-107.
9. Dhur A, Galan P, Hercberg S. Effects of different degrees of iron deficiency on cytochrome P450 complex and pentose phosphate pathway dehydrogenases in the rat. *J Nutr.* 1989;119:40-47.
10. Lederman HM, Cohen A, Lee JW, Freedman MH, Gelfand EW. Deferoxamine: a reversible S-phase inhibitor of human lymphocyte proliferation. *Blood.* 1984; 64:748-753.
11. Brownlie T 4th, Utermohlen V, Hinton PS, Haas JD. Tissue iron deficiency without anemia impairs adaptation in endurance capacity after aerobic training in previously untrained women. *Am J Clin Nutr.* 2004;79:437-443.
12. Verdon F, Burnand B, Stubi CL, et al. Iron supplementation for unexplained fatigue in non-anaemic women: double blind randomised placebo controlled trial. *BMJ.* 2003;326:1124.
13. Corti MC, Guralnik JM, Salive ME, et al. Serum iron level, coronary artery disease, and all-cause mortality in older men and women. *Am J Cardiol.* 1997; 79:120-127.
14. Kovesdy CP, Estrada W, Ahmadzadeh S, Kalantar-Zadeh K. Association of markers of iron stores with outcomes in patients with nondialysis-dependent chronic kidney disease. *Clin J Am Soc Nephrol.* 2009;4:435-441.
15. Cunietti E, Chiari MM, Monti M, et al. Distortion of iron status indices by acute inflammation in older hospitalized patients. *Arch Gerontol Geriatr.* 2004;39: 35-42.
16. Brittenham GM. Disorders of iron metabolism: iron deficiency and overload. In: Hoffman R, Shattil SJ, Furie B, Cohen HJ, Silberstein LE, McGlave P, eds. *Hematology: Basic Principles and Practice.* 3rd ed. London, UK: Churchill Livingstone; 2000:397-428.
17. Besarab A, Hörl WH, Silverberg D. Iron metabolism, iron deficiency, thrombocytosis, and the cardiorenal anemia syndrome. *Oncologist.* 2009;14:22-33.

Mortality and Readmission of Patients With Heart Failure, Atrial Fibrillation, or Coronary Artery Disease Undergoing Noncardiac Surgery: An Analysis of 38 047 Patients

van Diepen S, Bakal JA, McAlister FA, et al (Univ of Alberta, Edmonton, Canada)

Circulation 124:289-296, 2011

Background.—The postoperative risks for patients with coronary artery disease (CAD) undergoing noncardiac surgery are well described. However, the risks of noncardiac surgery in patients with heart failure (HF) and atrial fibrillation (AF) are less well known. The purpose of this study is to compare the postoperative mortality of patients with HF, AF, or CAD undergoing major and minor noncardiac surgery.

Methods and Results.—Population-based data were used to create 4 cohorts of consecutive patients with either nonischemic HF (NIHF; n=7700), ischemic HF (IHF; n=12 249), CAD (n=13 786), or AF (n= 4312) who underwent noncardiac surgery between April 1, 1999, and September 31, 2006, in Alberta, Canada. The main outcome was 30-day postoperative mortality. The unadjusted 30-day postoperative mortality was 9.3% in NIHF, 9.2% in IHF, 2.9% in CAD, and 6.4% in AF (each versus CAD, *P*<0.0001). Among patients undergoing minor surgical procedures, the 30-day postoperative mortality was 8.5% in NIHF, 8.1% in IHF, 2.3% in CAD, and 5.7% in AF (*P*<0.0001). After multivariable adjustment, postoperative mortality remained higher in NIHF, IHF, and AF patients than in those with CAD (NIHF versus CAD: odds ratio 2.92; 95% confidence interval 2.44 to 3.48; IHF versus CAD: odds ratio 1.98; 95% confidence interval 1.70 to 2.31; AF versus CAD: odds ratio 1.69; 95% confidence interval 1.34 to 2.14).

Conclusions.—Although current perioperative risk prediction models place greater emphasis on CAD than HF or AF, patients with HF or AF have a significantly higher risk of postoperative mortality than patients

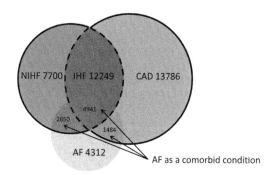

FIGURE 2.—Overlap between nonischemic heart failure (NIHF), ischemic heart failure (IHF), coronary artery disease (CAD), and atrial fibrillation/flutter (AF) cohorts. (Reprinted from van Diepen S, Bakal JA, McAlister FA, et al. Mortality and readmission of patients with heart failure, atrial fibrillation, or coronary artery disease undergoing noncardiac surgery: an analysis of 38 047 patients. *Circulation.* 2011;124:289-296. © American Heart Association, Inc.)

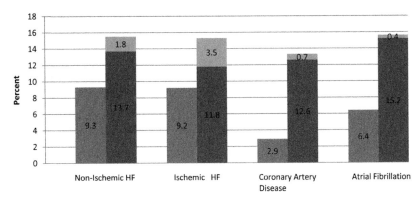

FIGURE 3.—Unadjusted 30-day perioperative mortality (blue), rehospitalization (red), and cardiac rehospitalization (green). HF indicates heart failure. For interpretation of the references to color in this figure legend, the reader is referred to web version of this article. (Reprinted from van Diepen S, Bakal JA, McAlister FA, et al. Mortality and readmission of patients with heart failure, atrial fibrillation, or coronary artery disease undergoing noncardiac surgery: an analysis of 38 047 patients. *Circulation.* 2011;124:289-296. © American Heart Association, Inc.)

TABLE 3.—Unadjusted 30-Day Perioperative Mortality for In-Patient and Out-Patient Minor Procedures

Minor Procedure Category	HF Cohorts		CAD Cohort, n (%)	AF, n (%)
	Nonischemic HF, n (%)	Ischemic HF, n (%)		
All	511 (8.5)	782 (8.1)	266 (2.3)	177 (5.7)
In-patient	367 (14.7)	429 (13.2)	191 (8.5)	131 (13.4)
Out-patient	144 (4.1)	278 (4.8)	75 (0.8)	46 (2.2)

HF indicates heart failure; CAD, coronary artery disease; and AF, atrial fibrillation and flutter.

with CAD, and even minor procedures carry a risk higher than previously appreciated (Figs 2 and 3, Table 3).

▶ Most perioperative risk-stratification models for noncardiac surgery find heart failure (HF) as a predictor of adverse cardiac complications but emphasize coronary artery disease (CAD) as the main impetus of perioperative risk.[1-6] Most of these studies were single center with few clinical events and were developed before the wide use of life-prolonging medications such as beta-blockers, angiotensin-converting enzyme inhibitors. Perioperative risks of cardiac events in patients with a history of HF undergoing noncardiac surgery vary from 5%[6] to 10%.[4] In 2 Medicare studies of patients older than 65 years, the rates were 8% and 12% after major noncardiac surgery.[7,8] None of the currently used risk models for perioperative cardiac events after noncardiac surgery list atrial fibrillation (AF) as an independent risk factor, and the perioperative risk of AF remains ill defined.[1,6] The current large unselected population-based study of patients undergoing major and minor noncardiac surgery linking 3 Canadian databases created 4 mutually exclusive study cohorts: (1) HF with CAD (ischemic HF);

(2) HF without CAD (NIHF); (3) patients hospitalized for the first time with CAD without HF (CAD); (4) AF without HF or CAD (AF). They found that patients with HF or AF are at a significantly higher risk of death and rehospitalization than patients with CAD. Furthermore, HF patients undergoing minor surgical procedures (undefined in this article) do not have a low postoperative risk as suggested by current guidelines in which patients undergoing planned minor surgery have a combined morbidity and mortality of less than 1%.[9] Finally, patients after an index hospitalization for HF or AF undergoing surgery within 4 weeks have a significantly higher mortality than those undergoing surgery at a later date. Future research should focus on identifying perioperative risk factors and prediction models in patients with HF and AF.

M. D. Cheitlin, MD

References

1. Goldman L, Caldera DL, Nussbaum SR, et al. Multifactorial index of cardiac risk in noncardiac surgical procedures. *N Engl J Med.* 1977;297:845-850.
2. Detsky AS, Abrams HB, McLaughlin JR, et al. Predicting cardiac complications in patients undergoing non-cardiac surgery. *J Gen Intern Med.* 1986;1:211-219.
3. Mangano DT, Browner WS, Hollenberg M, London MJ, Tubau JF, Tateo IM. Association of perioperative myocardial ischemia with cardiac morbidity and mortality in men undergoing noncardiac surgery. The Study of Perioperative Ischemia Research Group. *N Engl J Med.* 1990;323:1781-1788.
4. Kumar R, McKinney WP, Raj G, et al. Adverse cardiac events after surgery: assessing risk in a veteran population. *J Gen Intern Med.* 2001;16:507-518.
5. Larsen SF, Olesen KH, Jacobsen E, et al. Prediction of cardiac risk in non-cardiac surgery. *Eur Heart J.* 1987;8:179-185.
6. Lee TH, Marcantonio ER, Mangione CM, et al. Derivation and prospective validation of a simple index for prediction of cardiac risk of major noncardiac surgery. *Circulation.* 1999;100:1043-1049.
7. Hernandez AF, Whellan DJ, Stroud S, Sun JL, O'Connor CM, Jollis JG. Outcomes in heart failure patients after major noncardiac surgery. *J Am Coll Cardiol.* 2004; 44:1446-1453.
8. Hammill BG, Curtis LH, Bennett-Guerrero E, et al. Impact of heart failure on patients undergoing major noncardiac surgery. *Anesthesiology.* 2008;108:559-567.
9. Fleisher LA, Beckman JA, Brown KA, et al. 2009 ACCF/AHA focused update on perioperative beta blockade incorporated into the ACC/AHA 2007 guidelines on perioperative cardiovascular evaluation and care for noncardiac surgery. *J Am Coll Cardiol.* 2009;54:e13-e118.

Prognostic value of serial measurements of highly sensitive cardiac troponin I in stable outpatients with nonischemic chronic heart failure

Kawahara C, Tsutamoto T, Sakai H, et al (Shiga Univ of Med Science, Seta, Otsu, Japan; Toyosato Hosp, Hachime, Japan)

Am Heart J 162:639-645, 2011

Background.—Cardiac troponin I (cTnI) is a useful biomarker in patients with chronic heart failure (CHF), and a highly sensitive cTnI (hs-cTnI) commercial assay has become available. However, the prognostic role of serial measurements of hs-cTnI in stable outpatients with CHF remains unknown.

Methods.—At entry to the study, we evaluated 95 stable outpatients with nonischemic CHF showing a serum hs-cTnI (Centaur TnI-Ultra [Siemens Medical Solution Diagnostics, New York, NY], lower limit of detection 0.006 ng/mL) value ≥0.006 ng/mL. To evaluate the role of repetitive measurements of hs-cTnI, we performed echocardiography and measured serum levels of cTnI and N-terminal proBNP at baseline and 6 months later and then prospectively followed up these patients for 4.25 years.

Results.—During long-term follow-up, there were 27 cardiac deaths. On multivariate analyses, high plasma N-terminal pro–brain natriuretic peptide (≥711 pg/mL, *P* =.0008), high serum hs-cTnI at baseline (≥0.03 ng/mL, *P* =.0011), and an increase in hs-cTnI (Δhs-cTnI ≥0 ng/mL, *P* =.022) after 6 months were independent significant prognostic predictors. The hazard ratio for mortality of patients with high hs-cTnI (≥0.03 ng/mL) and an increase in hs-cTnI (Δhs-cTnI ≥0 ng/mL) was 3.59 (95% CI 1.3-9.9, *P* =.014) compared with that of those with high hs-cTnI (≥0.03 ng/mL) and a decrease in hs-cTnI (Δhs-cTnI <0 ng/mL).

Conclusions.—These findings indicated that not only the serum concentration of hs-cTnI at baseline but also an increase in hs-cTnI were independent and useful prognostic predictors in patients with nonischemic CHF (Figs 2-4).

▶ Cardiac troponins (cTn), both cTnI and cTnT, are important and useful biomarkers in acute coronary syndromes and chronic heart failure (HF).[1-6] The

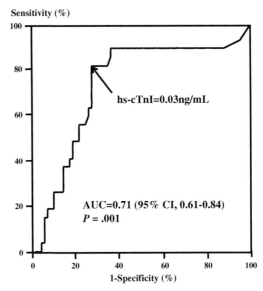

FIGURE 2.—The cutoff level for hs-cTnI at baseline calculated by receiver operating characteristics analysis to detect cardiac death in patients with NICHF. AUC indicates area under curve. (Reprinted from the American Heart Journal, Kawahara C, Tsutamoto T, Sakai H, et al. Prognostic value of serial measurements of highly sensitive cardiac troponin I in stable outpatients with nonischemic chronic heart failure. *Am Heart J.* 2011;162:639-645. Copyright 2011, with permission from Elsevier.)

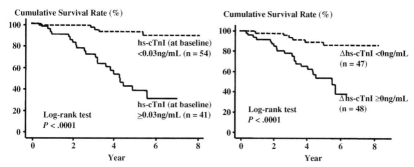

FIGURE 3.—Kaplan-Meier survival curves according to cutoff values for hs-cTnI at baseline (0.03 ng/mL) and change in hs-cTnI after 6 months in patients with NICHF. (Reprinted from the American Heart Journal, Kawahara C, Tsutamoto T, Sakai H, et al. Prognostic value of serial measurements of highly sensitive cardiac troponin I in stable outpatients with nonischemic chronic heart failure. *Am Heart J*. 2011;162:639-645. Copyright 2011, with permission from Elsevier.)

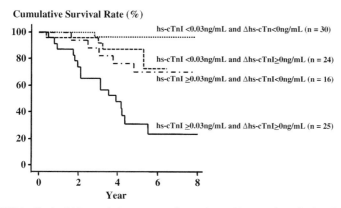

FIGURE 4.—Kaplan-Meier survival curves according to the combination of cutoff values for hs-cTnI at baseline (0.03 ng/mL) and change in hs-cTnI after 6 months in patients with NICHF. (Reprinted from the American Heart Journal, Kawahara C, Tsutamoto T, Sakai H, et al. Prognostic value of serial measurements of highly sensitive cardiac troponin I in stable outpatients with nonischemic chronic heart failure. *Am Heart J*. 2011;162:639-645. Copyright 2011, with permission from Elsevier.)

clinical use of cTn is limited by the low sensitivity of the conventional assay system.[7] A highly sensitive assay of cTnI (hs-cTnI) has recently been developed and a high serum concentration shown to be an independent prognostic indicator in patients with chronic HF.[8] This study evaluated the prognostic value of serial measurements of hs-cTnI in patients with stable nonischemic chronic HF (NICHF) in 138 consecutive outpatients who were New York Heart Association class I to III. After 6 months, 95 had hs-cTnI ≥0.006 ng/mL, a value greater than the lower detection limit of the assay. The patients were taking the usual guideline recommended therapy and were followed up for 6 months, and the baseline biomarkers of hs-cTnI and NT-proBNP changes baseline to 6 months correlated with the endpoint of cardiac death. On multivariate analysis, hs-cTnI at baseline ≥0.03 ng/mL, change in hs-cTnI (Δ hs-cTnI) ≥0 ng/mL, and NT-proBNP at baseline ≥711 pg/mL were significant independent predictors of cardiac death. Because the changes in hs-cTnI were probably not ischemic, they were most likely caused by subclinical ongoing leaking from permeable plasma membranes of viable injured myocardium.[9] The mechanism of cTn release in HF is unknown, but multiple contributing mechanisms proposed have been neurohormonal activation, oxidative stress, and apoptosis.[10,11] This study for the first time showed the prognostic value of serial measurements of hs-cTnI in stable outpatients with nonischemic chronic HF.

M. D. Cheitlin, MD

References

1. Sato Y, Yamada T, Taniguchi R, et al. Persistently increased serum concentrations of cardiac troponin T in patients with idiopathic dilated cardiomyopathy are predictive of adverse outcomes. *Circulation.* 2001;103:369-374.
2. Ishii J, Nomura M, Nakamura Y, et al. Risk stratification using a combination of cardiac troponin T and brain natriuretic peptide in patients hospitalized for worsening chronic heart failure. *Am J Cardiol.* 2002;89:691-695.
3. Setsuta K, Seino Y, Ogawa T, Arao M, Miyatake Y, Takano T. Use of cytosolic and myofibril markers in the detection of ongoing myocardial damage in patients with chronic heart failure. *Am J Med.* 2002;113:717-722.
4. Horwich TB, Patel J, MacLellan WR, Fonarow GC. Cardiac troponin I is associated with impaired hemodynamics, progressive left ventricular dysfunction, and increased mortality rates in advanced heart failure. *Circulation.* 2003;108:833-838.
5. Ishii J, Cui W, Kitagawa F, et al. Prognostic value of combination of cardiac troponin T and B-type natriuretic peptide after initiation of treatment in patients with chronic heart failure. *Clin Chem.* 2003;49:2020-2026.
6. Latini R, Masson S, Anand IS, et al. Prognostic value of very low plasma concentrations of troponin T in patients with stable chronic heart failure. *Circulation.* 2007;116:1242-1249.
7. Tsutamoto T, Kawahara C, Yamaji M, et al. Relationship between renal function and serum cardiac troponin T in patients with chronic heart failure. *Eur J Heart Fail.* 2009;11:653-658.
8. Tsutamoto T, Kawahara C, Nishiyama K, et al. Prognostic role of highly sensitive cardiac troponin I in patients with systolic heart failure. *Am Heart J.* 2010;159:63-67.
9. Sato Y, Kita T, Takatsu Y, Kimura T. Biochemical markers of myocyte injury in heart failure. *Heart.* 2004;90:1110-1113.
10. Braunwald E. Biomarkers in heart failure. *N Engl J Med.* 2008;358:2148-2159.
11. Kociol RD, Pang PS, Gheorghiade M, Fonarow GC, O'Connor CM, Felker GM. Troponin elevation in heart failure prevalence, mechanisms, and clinical implications. *J Am Coll Cardiol.* 2010;56:1071-1078.

Myocarditis and Cardiomyopathy

Long-Term Survival in Patients With Resting Obstructive Hypertrophic Cardiomyopathy: Comparison of Conservative Versus Invasive Treatment

Ball W, Ivanov J, Rakowski H, et al (Univ of Toronto, Ontario, Canada)
J Am Coll Cardiol 58:2313-2321, 2011

Objectives.—The aim of this study was to compare the survival of patients with hypertrophic cardiomyopathy (HCM) and resting left ventricular outflow tract (LVOT) obstruction managed with an invasive versus a conservative strategy.

Background.—In patients with resting obstructive HCM, clinical benefit can be achieved after invasive septal reduction therapy. However, it remains controversial whether invasive treatment improves long-term survival.

Methods.—We studied a consecutive cohort of 649 patients with resting obstructive HCM. Total and HCM-related mortality were compared in 246 patients who were conservatively managed with 403 patients who were invasively managed by surgical myectomy, septal ethanol ablation, or dual-chamber pacing.

Results.—Multivariable analyses (with invasive therapy treated as a time-dependent covariate) showed that an invasive intervention was a significant determinant of overall mortality (hazard ratio: 0.6, 95% confidence interval: 0.4 to 0.97, p = 0.04). Overall survival rates were greater in the invasive (99.2% 1-year, 95.7% 5-year, and 87.8% 10-year survival) than in the conservative (97.3% 1-year, 91.1% 5-year, and 75.8% 10-year survival, p = 0.008) cohort. However, invasive therapy was not found to be a significant independent predictor of HCM-related mortality (hazard ratio: 0.7, 95% confidence interval: 0.4 to 1.3, p = 0.3). The HCM-related survival was 99.5% (1 year), 96.3% (5 years), and 90.2% (10 years) in the invasive cohort, and 97.8% (1 year), 94.6% (5 years), and 86.9% (10 years) in the conservative cohort (p = 0.3).

Conclusions.—Patients treated invasively have an overall survival advantage compared with conservatively treated patients, with the latter group more likely to die from noncardiac causes. The HCM-related mortality is similar, regardless of a conservative versus invasive strategy (Figs 1-3).

▶ Hypertrophic cardiomyopathy can be obstructive (HOCM) with a resting left ventricular outflow tract (LVOT) gradient or nonobstructive. Studies in the past have consistently shown worsened survival in those with compared to those without LVOT obstruction.[1-3] Whether the magnitude of the gradient is associated with increased mortality is an unresolved issue. Current management in symptomatic patients (New York Heart Association [NYHA] class III-IV) is beta-blockers, disopyramide, or calcium channel blockers (conservative managed) and those who remain symptomatic or are intolerant of medication have surgical septal myectomy or septal ethanol ablation (SEA). Although dual chamber pacing (DDD) was used and reduces symptoms, it is not often used currently. Although all of these therapies can reduce symptoms, it is not clear whether there is a survival advantage of invasive over medical therapy in patients with HOCM.[4] There are no randomized trials of medical versus invasive therapy, and most retrospective cohort studies were done before the modern era. One study found that surgical myectomy patients had a better survival than conservatively medically treated patients; however, the invasive patients and medical patients were treated in different institutions, raising the possibility of referral bias. Also, there was an unusually low 10-year survival rate of 61% in the conservatively treated patients.[5] This study from 1 tertiary care center compared survival of 246 patients with HOCM who were treated conservatively with 403 patients treated invasively with surgical septal myectomy, SEA, or a small number with DDD. Also, factors predicting long-term survival in patients with HOCM were evaluated. Mean

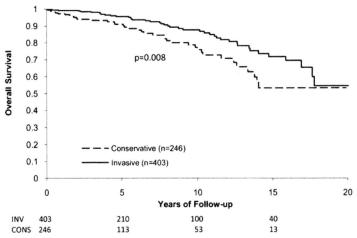

FIGURE 1.—Comparison of Overall Survival in Patients With Resting Obstructive HCM. Kaplan-Meier plots of overall survival in patients with hypertrophic cardiomyopathy (HCM) and resting left ventricular outflow tract obstruction managed with either invasive (INV) or conservative (CONS) therapy (p = 0.008). (Reprinted from the Journal of the American College of Cardiology, Ball W, Ivanov J, Rakowski H, et al. Long-term survival in patients with resting obstructive hypertrophic cardiomyopathy: comparison of conservative versus invasive treatment. *J Am Coll Cardiol.* 2011;58:2313-2321. Copyright 2011, with permission from the American College of Cardiology.)

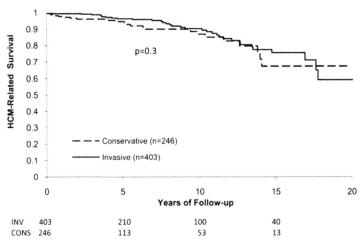

FIGURE 2.—Comparison of HCM-Related Survival in Patients With Resting Obstructive HCM. Kaplan-Meier plots of HCM-related survival in patients with HCM and resting left ventricular outflow tract obstruction managed with either invasive or conservative therapy (p = NS). Abbreviations as in Figure 1. (Reprinted from the Journal of the American College of Cardiology, Ball W, Ivanov J, Rakowski H, et al. Long-term survival in patients with resting obstructive hypertrophic cardiomyopathy: comparison of conservative versus invasive treatment. *J Am Coll Cardiol.* 2011;58:2313-2321. Copyright 2011, with permission from the American College of Cardiology.)

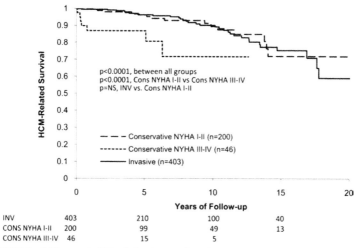

FIGURE 3.—Differences in HCM-Related Survival on the Basis of Management Strategy and Functional Class. Kaplan-Meier survival curves of HCM-related survival in HCM patients with left ventricular outflow tract obstruction managed with INV therapy or CONS therapy. Conservatively treated New York Heart Association (NYHA) functional class I/II patients had similar HCM-related survival to patients treated invasively. Abbreviations as in Figure 1. (Reprinted from the Journal of the American College of Cardiology, Ball W, Ivanov J, Rakowski H, et al. Long-term survival in patients with resting obstructive hypertrophic cardiomyopathy: comparison of conservative versus invasive treatment. *J Am Coll Cardiol.* 2011;58:2313-2321. Copyright 2011, with permission from the American College of Cardiology.)

follow-up time was 7.2 ± 5.5 years. They found that the long-term survival of conservatively treated patients was much better than in other studies[3,5,6] with excellent symptom control. The medically treated NYHA class I-II HOCM patients had an all-cause and HCM-related mortality similar to patients treated invasively. Although the all-cause mortality was higher in the conservative than the invasive patients, the HCM-related mortality was the same in the 2 groups. The difference was that the subset of conservatively treated patients who die prematurely are those very symptomatic patients who refuse surgery or who have serious comorbidities that preclude invasive therapy. The results were the same when the DDD patients were excluded. On multivariate analysis, there were 4 independent determinants of HCM-related mortality: age greater than 50 years, female gender, septal thickness ≥20 mm, and a resting gradient ≥64 mm Hg. Finally, the excellent 5-year survival with SEA was similar to that with surgery. This is the largest study from a single institution available with much support for the existing recommended criteria for septal myectomy or SEA.

M. D. Cheitlin, MD

References

1. Maron MS, Olivotto I, Betocchi S, et al. Effect of left ventricular outflow tract obstruction on clinical outcome in hypertrophic cardiomyopathy. *N Engl J Med.* 2003;348:295-303.
2. Autore C, Bernabò P, Barillà CS, Bruzzi P, Spirito P. The prognostic importance of left ventricular outflow obstruction in hypertrophic cardiomyopathy varies in relation to the severity of symptoms. *J Am Coll Cardiol.* 2005;45:1076-1080.

3. Elliott PM, Gimeno JR, Tomé MT, et al. Left ventricular outflow tract obstruction and sudden death risk in patients with hypertrophic cardiomyopathy. *Eur Heart J.* 2006;27:1933-1941.
4. Woo A, Rakowski H. Does myectomy convey survival benefit in hypertrophic cardiomyopathy? *Heart Fail Clin.* 2007;3:275-288.
5. Ommen SR, Maron BJ, Olivotto I, et al. Long-term effects of surgical septal myectomy on survival in patients with obstructive hypertrophic cardiomyopathy. *J Am Coll Cardiol.* 2005;46:470-476.
6. Shah PM, Adelman AG, Wigle ED, et al. The natural (and unnatural) history of hypertrophic obstructive cardiomyopathy. *Circ Res.* 1974;35:179-195.

Comparison of Prevalence, Clinical Course, and Pathological Findings of Left Ventricular Systolic Impairment Versus Normal Systolic Function in Patients With Hypertrophic Cardiomyopathy

Fernández A, Vigliano CA, Casabé JH, et al (Univ Hosp, Buenos Aires, Argentina)
Am J Cardiol 108:548-555, 2011

Impaired left ventricular systolic function (ILVSF) in hypertrophic cardiomyopathy (HC) is a risk factor for sudden death and a determinant of high mortality. We determined its prevalence, clinical parameters, long-term outcome, and pathologic findings of explanted hearts. We retrospectively analyzed 382 patients with HC; ILVSF was characterized by LV ejection fraction <50% at rest and was identified in 24 patients (6.3%). Patients with ILVSF were younger than patients with normal SF (43.5 ± 14.1 vs 55.3 ± 20.4 years, p = 0.001) and had larger LV end-diastolic cavity diameter (53.2 ± 12.2 vs 43.8 ± 6.2 mm, p = 0.001), larger left atrium (51.2 ± 6.5 vs 44.3 ± 8 mm, p <0.001), and lower fractional shortening (30.7 ± 11.1% vs 45.5% ± 10.3%, p <0.001). A combined end point (heart failure death or heart transplantation) was considered. Median follow-up was 3 years (1.2 to 6.3). Fourteen patients with ILVSF (58.3%) had the end point compared to 3 (0.8%) with normal SF (p <0.001). In explanted hearts, fibrosis represented 30.5 ± 12.5% of the left ventricle; we observed a direct correlation between fibrosis and ventricular dilation (r = 0.794, p = 0.001) and an inverse correlation between fibrosis and ejection fraction (r = −0.623, p = 0.023). Number and length density of small arterioles (<50 μm in diameter) were significantly decreased. In conclusion, ILVSF in HC has a poor prognosis and is associated with fibrosis and selective decreased development of small arterioles (Figs 2 and 3).

▶ Hypertrophic cardiomyopathy (HC) is characterized by unexplained left ventricular (LV) hypertrophy that can be concentric or regional, for instance, in the base of the interventricular septum. It can be obstructive in the LV outflow tract with a systolic gradient that mimics aortic stenosis. The majority of the time, the LV function as manifested by the LV ejection fraction (LVEF) is normal or even supernormal, but about 5% of the time, LVEF can be decreased.[1] This study attempts to determine the differences in clinical course and pathologic

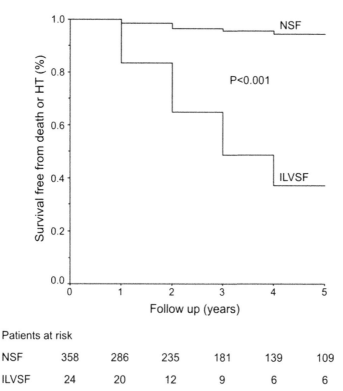

FIGURE 2.—Kaplan–Meier survival estimates for freedom from death from heart failure or heart transplantation in 382 patients with hypertrophic cardiomyopathy according to systolic function. (Reprinted from the American Journal of Cardiology, Fernández A, Vigliano CA, Casabé JH, et al. Comparison of prevalence, clinical course, and pathological findings of left ventricular systolic impairment versus normal systolic function in patients with hypertrophic cardiomyopathy. *Am J Cardiol*. 2011;108:548-555. Copyright 2011, with permission from Elsevier.)

findings in these patients and compare them with those patients with hypertrophic obstructive cardiomyopathy (HOCM) and normal LVEF. In 382 patients with HOCM, they identified retrospectively 24 (6.3%) with an LVEF less than 50% at rest. Comparing the patients with impaired left ventricular systolic function (ILVSF) with those with normal function (NF), the patients with ILVSF were younger, had more NYHA class III-IV dyspnea, and a greater prevalence of malignant ventricular arrhythmias and sudden death. In the median follow-up time of 3 (range, 1.2—6.3) years, there were 25 deaths in those with NF and 16 in those with ILVSF and heart failure (HF), death, or transplantation in 3 with NF and in 14 with ILVSF. The reason for the decreased LV function has been unclear, but in the explanted hearts, there were more fibrosis and fewer small arterioles measuring less than 50 μm in diameter in the hearts of the patients with ILVSF. Maron and colleagues[2] found that in HC, arterioles have a thickened wall and a narrow lumen. Cecchi and colleagues,[3] using positron emission tomography evaluated the vasodilator effect of dipyridamole and showed that the degree of

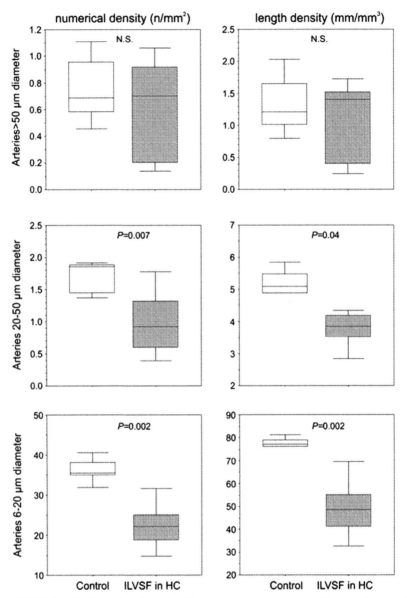

FIGURE 3.—Morphometric analyses of small arteries expressed as median and interquartile range of numerical and length density of small, medium, and large coronary arterioles. Explanted hearts affected by hypertrophic cardiomyopathy presented a significant decrease in the numerical and length densities of small arteries (6 to 50 μm in diameter) compared to control hearts. (Reprinted from the American Journal of Cardiology, Fernández A, Vigliano CA, Casabé JH, et al. Comparison of prevalence, clinical course, and pathological findings of left ventricular systolic impairment versus normal systolic function in patients with hypertrophic cardiomyopathy. *Am J Cardiol.* 2011;108:548-555. Copyright 2011, with permission from Elsevier.)

microvascular dysfunction is a potent independent predictor of clinical worsening and death. The fibrosis is probably related to the loss of myocytes. One explanation for the decreased density of small arterioles is that in ILVSF with an increase in LV hypertrophy, the smaller arterioles could not remodel to keep pace with the increased myocardial mass. The decrease in LVEF in patients with HC is premonitory to the end stage of the disease.

M. D. Cheitlin, MD

References

1. Harris KM, Spirito P, Maron MS, et al. Prevalence, clinical profile, and significance of left ventricular remodeling in the end-stage phase of hypertrophic cardiomyopathy. *Circulation.* 2006;114:216-225.
2. Maron BJ, Wolfson JK, Epstein SE, Roberts WC. Intramural ("small vessel") coronary artery disease in hypertrophic cardiomyopathy. *J Am Coll Cardiol.* 1986;8:545-557.
3. Cecchi F, Olivotto I, Gistri R, Lorenzoni R, Chiriatti G, Camici PG. Coronary microvascular dysfunction and prognosis in hypertrophic cardiomyopathy. *N Engl J Med.* 2003;349:1027-1035.

Alcohol Septal Ablation for the Treatment of Hypertrophic Obstructive Cardiomyopathy: A Multicenter North American Registry

Nagueh SF, Groves BM, Schwartz L, et al (Methodist DeBakey Heart Ctr, Houston, TX; Univ of Colorado Hosp, Aurora; Univ of Toronto, Ontario, Canada; et al)
J Am Coll Cardiol 58:2322-2328, 2011

Objectives.—The purpose of the study is to identify the predictors of clinical outcome (mortality and survival without repeat septal reduction procedures) of alcohol septal ablation for the treatment of patients with hypertrophic obstructive cardiomyopathy.

Background.—Alcohol septal ablation is used for treatment of medically refractory hypertrophic obstructive cardiomyopathy patients with severe outflow tract obstruction. The existing literature is limited to single-center results, and predictors of clinical outcome after ablation have not been determined. Registry results can add important data.

Methods.—Hypertrophic obstructive cardiomyopathy patients (N = 874) who underwent alcohol septal ablation were enrolled. The majority (64%) had severe obstruction at rest, and the remaining had provocable obstruction. Before ablation, patients had severe dyspnea (New York Heart Association [NYHA] functional class III or IV: 78%) and/or severe angina (Canadian Cardiovascular Society angina class III or IV: 43%).

Results.—Significant improvement (p < 0.01) occurred after ablation (~5% in NYHA functional classes III and IV, and 8 patients in Canadian Cardiovascular Society angina class III). There were 81 deaths, and survival estimates at 1, 5, and 9 years were 97%, 86%, and 74%, respectively. Left anterior descending artery dissections occurred in 8 patients and arrhythmias in 133 patients. A lower ejection fraction at baseline, a smaller number of septal arteries injected with ethanol, a larger number of ablation procedures per patient, a higher septal thickness post-ablation, and the use beta-blockers post-ablation predicted mortality.

Conclusions.—Variables that predict mortality after ablation include baseline ejection fraction and NYHA functional class, the number of septal arteries injected with ethanol, post-ablation septal thickness, beta-blocker use, and the number of ablation procedures (Fig 1).

▶ This article reports the data concerning alcohol septal ablation in symptomatic patients with hypertrophic obstructive cardiomyopathy (HOCM), the most common inherited cardiomyopathy. Fifteen years after the first report of alcohol septal ablation, most articles in the literature reporting outcomes and complications of septal ablation are single-center, retrospective, relatively small studies. This multicenter registry, collected prospectively, reports on 874 HOCM patients with advanced symptoms who had alcohol septal ablation regarding the outcomes, safety, and predictors of survival after ablation. The indications for ablation were patients with angina or exertional dyspnea in spite of medical management. Patients with concomitant coronary artery disease or valve disease were treated surgically and not included, and there were no patients with poor left ventricle (LV) function or dilated LV included. Patients had a resting gradient ≥30 mm Hg or provoked gradient ≥60 mm Hg.

Ablation resulted in marked alleviation of symptoms but was accompanied with a number of complications, chief among which were heart block requiring a pacemaker and malignant ventricular arrhythmias requiring an implanted cardioverter defibrillator (ICD). There were also injuries to the left anterior descending coronary artery caused by the stiff guide wires initially used. Comparisons with

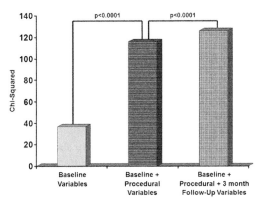

FIGURE 1.—Chi-Square Test Results for the Prediction of Mortality: 3 Models. Model 1 includes baseline variables (New York Heart Association functional class, ejection fraction, and maximum left ventricular outflow tract gradient; chi-square = 36.73). Model 2 includes baseline and procedural variables (the number of procedures and volume of ethanol injected; chi-square = 116.15). Model 3 includes baseline, procedural, and 3-month follow-up variables (use of negative inotropic drugs after ablation and maximum septal thickness at 3-month follow-up; chi-square = 126.06). (Reprinted from the Journal of the American College of Cardiology, Nagueh SF, Groves BM, Schwartz L, et al. Alcohol septal ablation for the treatment of hypertrophic obstructive cardiomyopathy: a multicenter North American registry. *J Am Coll Cardiol.* 2011;58: 2322-2328. Copyright 2011, with permission from the American College of Cardiology.)

the single-center reports and with surgical myomectomy were cited, but since the indications for surgery and comorbidities differ among the various studies, a direct comparison is invalid. Given that, the first year survival rate of 97% in the registry is similar to that of the disease-free general population of previous studies, but the 5- and 9-year survival rates are lower, but higher in the alcohol ablation group at 10 years than in those patients with HOCM without septal reduction (74% vs 61%).[1] Compared with reports of surgical septal myomectomy, the residual gradient is higher than that in the registry patients as is the incidence of heart block and malignant ventricular arrhythmias. The 9- to 10-year survival is also higher in the myomectomy groups (83%—90% vs 74%).[1,2]

The value of the registry is the numbers of patients with data collected prospectively, which allowed the defining of multivariable predictors of death and the need for repeat septal ablation therapy.

M. D. Cheitlin, MD

References

1. Ommen SR, Maron BJ, Olivotto I, et al. Long-term effects of surgical septal myectomy on survival in patients with obstructive hypertrophic cardiomyopathy. *J Am Coll Cardiol.* 2005;46:470-476.
2. Smedira NG, Lytle BW, Lever HM, et al. Current effectiveness and risks of isolated septal myectomy for hypertrophic obstructive cardiomyopathy. *Ann Thorac Surg.* 2008;85:127-133.

Chemical Cardiomyopathies: The Negative Effects of Medications and Nonprescribed Drugs on the Heart

Figueredo VM (Jefferson Med College, Philadelphia, PA)
Am J Med 124:480-488, 2011

The heart is a target of injury for many chemical compounds, both medically prescribed and not medically prescribed. Pathophysiologic mechanisms underlying the development of chemical-induced cardiomyopathies vary depending on the inciting agent, including direct toxic effects, neurohormonal activation, altered calcium homeostasis, and oxidative stress. Numerous chemicals and drugs are implicated in cardiomyopathy. This article discusses examples of medication and nonprescribed drug-induced cardiomyopathies and reviews their pathophysiologic mechanisms (Figs 1, 3 and 7, Table 1).

▶ One etiology of dilated cardiomyopathies consists of chemicals, the commonest of which is alcohol. Currently, cocaine and amphetamines are a major problem, as are the antineoplastic drugs epitomized by anthracycline. This review article is a valuable resource for information about this group of cardiomyopathies, with a short discussion of the mechanisms by which these drugs damage the heart and with a useful bibliography that will enable the reader who seeks more information to easily find it. Although not covering all the drugs known to cause cardiomyopathy, the article includes the most frequent and important

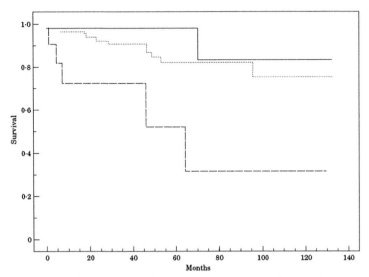

FIGURE 1.—Survival curves of cardiac deaths in patients with alcoholic dilated cardiomyopathy: with (—) and without (− −) abstinence) and idiopathic dilated cardiomyopathy (··). Idiopathic dilated cardiomyopathy versus alcoholic dilated cardiomyopathy with abstinence, P = not significant; idiopathic dilated cardiomyopathy versus alcoholic dilated cardiomyopathy without abstinence, P =.002; alcoholic dilated cardiomyopathy with abstinence versus alcoholic dilated cardiomyopathy without abstinence, P =.003. Reprinted with permission from Fauchier L, Babuty D, Poret P, et al. Comparison of long-term outcome of alcoholic and idiopathic dilated cardiomyopathy. *Eur Heart J.* 2000;21:306-314. (Reprinted from The American Journal of Medicine, Figueredo VM. Chemical cardiomyopathies: the negative effects of medications and nonprescribed drugs on the heart. *Am J Med.* 2011;124:480-488. Copyright 2011, with permission from Elsevier.)

chemicals. This article is a useful reference to many of the less-often-encountered etiologies of cardiomyopathy.

M. D. Cheitlin, MD

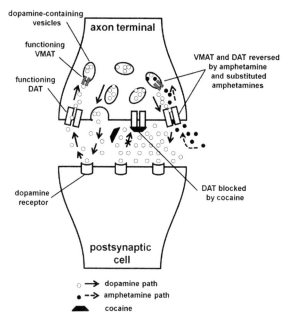

FIGURE 3.—Effects of various drugs on the presynaptic axon terminal and postsynaptic cells in the heart. *Left*: normal functioning dopamine transporter (and norepinephrine and serotonin transporters) and vesicular monoamine transporter in the presynaptic axon terminal, and dopamine uptake in the postsynaptic cell. *Center*: Cocaine, a transporter antagonist, increases extracellular dopamine (and neuroepinephrine) by binding to dopamine transporter and blocking neurotransmitter uptake. *Right*: amphetamine and substituted amphetamines, including methamphetamine, methylphenidate (Ritalin, Novartis Pharmaceuticals Corporation, East Hanover, NJ), methylenedioxymethamphetamine (ecstasy), and ephedra (ma huang), reverse the action of the dopamine transporter and vesicular monoamine transporter, increasing neurotransmitter available in the synapse. DAT = dopamine transporter; VMAT = vesicular monoamine transporter. (Reprinted from The American Journal of Medicine, Figueredo VM. Chemical cardiomyopathies: the negative effects of medications and nonprescribed drugs on the heart. *Am J Med*. 2011;124: 480-488. Copyright 2011, with permission from Elsevier.)

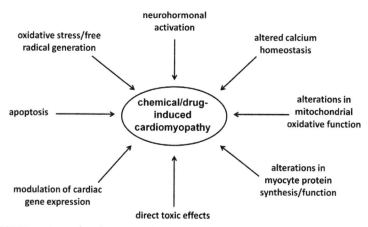

FIGURE 7.—Potential mechanisms involved in chemical-induced cardiomyopathies. (Reprinted from The American Journal of Medicine, Figueredo VM. Chemical cardiomyopathies: the negative effects of medications and nonprescribed drugs on the heart. *Am J Med*. 2011;124:480-488. Copyright 2011, with permission from Elsevier.)

TABLE 1.—Medications, Nonprescribed Drugs, and Chemicals Implicated in Cardiomyopathy

Amphetamine	Ethanol
Anabolic/androgenic steroids	Idarubicin
Anthraquinone	Imatinib
Arnica herb	Isoproterenol
Arsenic	Ma huang (ephedra)
Azidothymidine	Melarsoprol
Anagrelide	Methamphetamine
Catecholamines	Methylphenidate
Chloroquine	Minoxidil
Clozapine	Mitomycin
Cobalt	Mitoxantrone
Cocaine	Paclitaxel
Chloroquine	Pentamidine
Cyclophosphamide	Stibogluconate
Daunorubicin	Sunitinib
Diazoxide	Trastuzumab
Doxorubicin (Adriamycin, Bedford Laboratories, Bedford, OH)	Zidovudine

Clinical Characteristics and Cardiovascular Magnetic Resonance Findings in Stress (Takotsubo) Cardiomyopathy

Eitel I, von Knobelsdorff-Brenkenhoff F, Bernhardt P, et al (Univ of Leipzig, Germany; Charité Univ Medicine Berlin, Germany; Univ of Ulm, Germany; et al)
JAMA 306:277-286, 2011

Context.—Stress cardiomyopathy (SC) is a transient form of acute heart failure triggered by stressful events and associated with a distinctive left ventricular (LV) contraction pattern. Various aspects of its clinical profile have been described in small single-center populations, but larger, multi-center data sets have been lacking so far. Furthermore, it remains difficult to quickly establish diagnosis on admission.

Objectives.—To comprehensively define the clinical spectrum and evolution of SC in a large population, including tissue characterization data from cardiovascular magnetic resonance (CMR) imaging; and to establish a set of CMR criteria suitable for diagnostic decision making in patients acutely presenting with suspected SC.

Design, Setting, and Patients.—Prospective study conducted at 7 tertiary care centers in Europe and North America between January 2005 and October 2010 among 256 patients with SC assessed at the time of presentation as well as 1 to 6 months after the acute event.

Main Outcome Measures.—Complete recovery of LV dysfunction.

Results.—Eighty-one percent of patients (n = 207) were postmenopausal women, 8% (n = 20) were younger women (aged ≤50 years), and 11% (n = 29) were men. A stressful trigger could be identified in 182 patients (71%). Cardiovascular magnetic resonance imaging data (available for 239 patients [93%]) revealed 4 distinct patterns of regional ventricular ballooning: apical (n = 197 [82%]), biventricular (n = 81 [34%]), midventricular (n = 40 [17%]), and basal (n = 2 [1%]). Left ventricular ejection fraction was reduced (48% [SD, 11%]; 95% confidence interval [CI], 47%-50%) in all patients. Stress cardiomyopathy was accurately identified by CMR using specific criteria: a typical pattern of LV dysfunction, myocardial edema, absence of significant necrosis/fibrosis, and markers for myocardial inflammation. Follow-up CMR imaging showed complete normalization of LV ejection fraction (66% [SD, 7%]; 95% CI, 64%-68%) and inflammatory markers in the absence of significant fibrosis in all patients.

Conclusions.—The clinical profile of SC is considerably broader than reported previously. Cardiovascular magnetic resonance imaging at the time of initial clinical presentation may provide relevant functional and tissue information that might aid in the establishment of the diagnosis of SC.

▶ Takotsubo or stress cardiomyopathy (SC) is characterized by acute segmental left ventricular (LV) myocardial stunning and dysfunction in the absence of significant coronary disease, precipitated by acute emotional stress.[1] Most often, the patient presents with an acute coronary syndrome. Although the exact mechanism by which SC occurs is not known, there is evidence that enhanced sympathetic activity plays a pathogenic role.[2,3] Complications are rare, and the prognosis in this disease is considered to be favorable.[4,5] Cardiovascular magnetic resonance (CMR) imaging[6] is ideal for evaluating this disease because it allows visualization of regional wall motion and LV function and provides markers for inflammation (inflammation, ischemic edema) and irreversible myocardial necrosis/fibrosis injury that differentiates SC from myocardial infarction and myocarditis.[4,5,7,8] Although small, single-center series are reported,[4,9,10] this study is a large, multicenter study using a CMR imaging protocol to define the clinical spectrum in detail, tissue characteristics, and evolution of SC. While confirmatory of findings in other series of patients with SC, there are interesting findings in this study that demonstrate that the clinical profile of these patients is broader than previously reported. Inflammation with hyperemia, myocardial edema, and absence of fibrosis are markers of reversible myocardial injury and provide insight into the pathogenesis of SC, and this study indicates that CMR imaging may be very useful in making a diagnosis of SC at the time of the acute clinical presentation. Men comprised 11% of the patients, and there were a number of younger women (17% ≤ age 55). Also, despite a careful history, only two-thirds of patients had a clearly identifiable preceding stressor compared with previous reports where up to 89% had emotional or physical preceding triggers.[4] Although more than 80% had apical ballooning, 17% of patients had a mid-ventricular variant with apical sparing, and 34% had right ventricular involvement that might augment more severe patient morbidity and poorer outcome. Late gadolinium enhancement (T2-weighted signal intensity [SI] > 5 SD) was universally negative, although with SI > 3 SD, 9% had evidence of minute focal or patchy myocardial scarring, indicating that the pathogenesis of the disease creates severe enough injury to create myocardial dysfunction but reverses in time to prevent myocardial necrosis and allow full recovery of function. In the absence of elevated circulating catecholamines and contraction band necrosis on myocardial biopsy,[11] together with absence of precipitating stressors, although elevated sympathetic tone may be important in the pathogenesis of this disease, other factors must also be involved, such as abnormal vasoreactivity or endothelial and microcirculatory dysfunction.

M. D. Cheitlin, MD

References

1. Maron BJ, Towbin JA, Thiene G, et al. Contemporary definitions and classification of the cardiomyopathies: an American Heart Association Scientific Statement from the Council on Clinical Cardiology, Heart Failure and Transplantation Committee; Quality of Care and Outcomes Research and Functional Genomics and Translational Biology Interdisciplinary Working Groups; and Council on Epidemiology and Prevention. *Circulation.* 2006;113:1807-1816.
2. Wittstein IS, Thiemann DR, Lima JA, et al. Neurohumoral features of myocardial stunning due to sudden emotional stress. *N Engl J Med.* 2005;352:539-548.
3. Abraham J, Mudd JO, Kapur NK, Klein K, Champion HC, Wittstein IS. Stress cardiomyopathy after intravenous administration of catecholamines and beta-receptor agonists. *J Am Coll Cardiol.* 2009;53:1320-1325.
4. Sharkey SW, Windenburg DC, Lesser JR, et al. Natural history and expansive clinical profile of stress (tako-tsubo) cardiomyopathy. *J Am Coll Cardiol.* 2010; 55:333-341.
5. Hurst RT, Prasad A, Askew JW III, Sengupta PP, Tajik AJ. Takotsubo cardiomyopathy: a unique cardiomyopathy with variable ventricular morphology. *JACC Cardiovasc Imaging.* 2010;3:641-649.
6. Eitel I, Behrendt F, Schindler K, et al. Differential diagnosis of suspected apical ballooning syndrome using contrast-enhanced magnetic resonance imaging. *Eur Heart J.* 2008;29:2651-2659.
7. Abdel-Aty H, Cocker M, Friedrich MG. Myocardial edema is a feature of takotsubo cardiomyopathy and is related to the severity of systolic dysfunction: insights from T2-weighted cardiovascular magnetic resonance. *Int J Cardiol.* 2009;132:291-293.
8. Eitel I, Lücke C, Grothoff M, et al. Inflammation in takotsubo cardiomyopathy: insights from cardiovascular magnetic resonance imaging. *Eur Radiol.* 2010;20: 422-431.
9. Eshtehardi P, Koestner SC, Adorjan P, et al. Transient apical ballooning syndrome—clinical characteristics, ballooning pattern, and long-term follow-up in a Swiss population. *Int J Cardiol.* 2009;135:370-375.
10. Singh NK, Rumman S, Mikell FL, Nallamothu N, Rangaswamy C. Stress cardiomyopathy: clinical and ventriculographic characteristics in 107 North American subjects. *Int J Cardiol.* 2010;141:297-303.
11. Madhavan M, Borlaug BA, Lerman A, Rihal CS, Prasad A. Stress hormone and circulating biomarker profile of apical ballooning syndrome (takotsubo cardiomyopathy): insights into the clinical significance of B-type natriuretic peptide and troponin levels. *Heart.* 2009;95:1436-1441.

Isolated Noncompaction of the Left Ventricular Myocardium in Adults: A Systematic Overview

Bhatia NL, Tajik AJ, Wilansky S, et al (Mayo Clinic Arizona, Scottsdale)
J Card Fail 17:771-778, 2011

Background.—Owing to inconsistent diagnostic criteria and small heterogeneous cohorts, little is known about the long-term outcomes of adult left ventricular noncompaction (LVNC), a rare cardiomyopathy with potentially

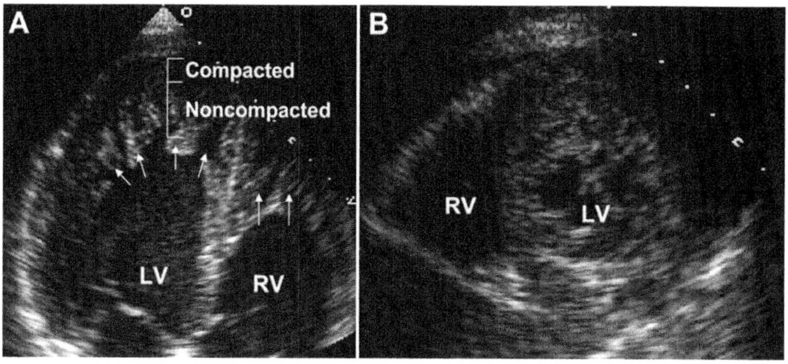

FIGURE 1.—Transthoracic echocardiography. (A) 4-chamber view. Arrows indicate inferolateral apical trabeculations in left ventricle (LV) as well as in the right ventricle (RV). Note that the ratio of noncompacted to compacted LV myocardium is greater than 2:1. (B) Shortaxis view. Trabeculations project into the LV cavity. (Reprinted from the Journal of Cardiac Failure, Bhatia NL, Tajik AJ, Wilansky S, et al. Isolated noncompaction of the left ventricular myocardium in adults: a systematic overview. *J Card Fail.* 2011;17: 771-778. Copyright 2011, with permission from Elsevier.)

serious outcomes. This systematic overview aimed to better delineate the natural history of adult LVNC.

Method and Results.—A comprehensive computerized search using "noncompaction" and its synonyms initially identified 206 articles, with reference lists subsequently hand scanned. These searches yielded 5 studies that were eligible for this systematic overview, identifying adult cohorts with isolated LVNC diagnosed by similar echocardiographic criteria. This combined cohort (n = 241) was followed for a mean duration of 39 months. The annualized event rate was 4% for cardiovascular deaths, 6.2% for cardiovascular death and its surrogates (heart transplantation and appropriate implantable cardioverter-defibrillator shocks), and 8.6% for all cardiovascular events (death, stroke, implantable cardioverter-defibrillator shocks, and heart transplantation.) Familial occurrence of LVNC in first-degree relatives was identified by echocardiography in 30% of index cases who were screened.

Conclusion.—LVNC is an increasingly recognized cardiomyopathy diagnosed by echocardiography and is associated with familial tendencies, arrhythmias, thromboembolism, advanced heart failure, and death (Figs 1 and 2).

▶ The rare cardiomyopathy of adult left ventricular noncompaction (LVNC), described as recently as 1997,[1] with a prevalence of less than 0.14% of adults referred for echocardiography, will probably increase as it is more frequently recognized.[2,3] As with other cardiomyopathies, LVNC has serious complications including arrhythmias, heart failure (HF), and death. LVNC most likely begins in the fetus. The fetal myocardium is perfused through intracardiac sinusoids, and as the coronary arteries develop, the sinusoids should compact to form the LV cavity walls. Failure to do so results in LVNC.[4,5] Although both acquired and familial noncompaction have been reported, cardiac abnormalities associated with LVNC are linked to a number of genetic disorders.[2,6,7]

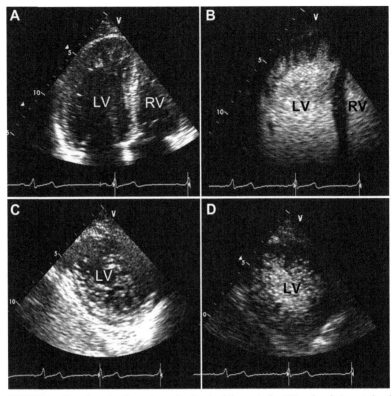

FIGURE 2.—Transthoracic echocardiography showing left ventricular (LV) trabeculations. 4-chamber view without (A) and with (B) contrast. Short-axis view without (C) and with (D) contrast. (Reprinted from the Journal of Cardiac Failure, Bhatia NL, Tajik AJ, Wilansky S, et al. Isolated noncompaction of the left ventricular myocardium in adults: a systematic overview. *J Card Fail*. 2011;17:771-778. Copyright 2011, with permission from Elsevier.)

Echocardiography is the usual way in which the diagnosis is made (Fig 1). Jenni et al[8] proposed these criteria that have now been widely accepted:

1. Excessively thickened LV wall with 2 layers of differing structure.
2. Noncompacted to compacted wall thickness ratio greater than 2:1 at end-systole.
3. Communication of deep intertrabecular recesses with the ventricular cavity, identified by color Doppler echocardiography.
4. Absence of coexisting cardiac abnormalities.
5. Presence of multiple prominent trabeculations.

This article is a report of the subject of LVNC as a result of a comprehensive literature search and serves as an excellent review of this unusual cardiomyopathy.

M. D. Cheitlin, MD

References

1. Ritter M, Oechslin E, Sütsch G, Attenhofer C, Schneider J, Jenni R. Isolated non-compaction of the myocardium in adults. *Mayo Clin Proc.* 1997;72:26-31.
2. Maron BJ, Towbin JA, Thiene G, et al. Contemporary definitions and classification of the cardiomyopathies: an American Heart Association Scientific Statement from the Council on Clinical Cardiology, Heart Failure and Transplantation Committee; Quality of Care and Outcomes Research and Functional Genomics and Translational Biology Interdisciplinary Working Groups; and Council on Epidemiology and Prevention. *Circulation.* 2006;113:1807-1816.
3. Aras D, Tufekcioglu O, Ergun K, et al. Clinical features of isolated ventricular noncompaction in adults long-term clinical course, echocardiographic properties, and predictors of left ventricular failure. *J Card Fail.* 2006;12:726-733.
4. Sedmera D, McQuinn T. Embryogenesis of the heart muscle. *Heart Fail Clin.* 2008;4:235-245.
5. Dusek J, Ostádal B, Duskova M. Postnatal persistence of spongy myocardium with embryonic blood supply. *Arch Pathol.* 1975;99:312-317.
6. Klaassen S, Probst S, Oechslin E, et al. Mutations in sarcomere protein genes in left ventricular noncompaction. *Circulation.* 2008;117:2893-2901.
7. Hoedemaekers YM, Caliskan K, Michels M, et al. The importance of genetic counseling, DNA diagnostics, and cardiologic family screening in left ventricular noncompaction cardiomyopathy. *Circulation.* 2010;3:232e-239e.
8. Jenni R, Oechslin E, Schneider J, et al. Echocardiographic and pathoanatomical characteristics of isolated left ventricular noncompaction: a step toward classification as a distinct cardiomyopathy. *Heart.* 2001;86:666-671.

Valvular Heart Disease and Infective Endocarditis

Anticoagulant therapy in pregnant women with mechanical prosthetic heart valves: no easy option
McLintock C (Auckland City Hosp, New Zealand)
Thromb Res 127:S56-S60, 2011

The choice of anticoagulant agent for pregnant women with mechanical prosthetic heart valves introduces a clinical dilemma for women and the clinicians caring for them. Options include continuing oral anticoagulants (OAC) such as warfarin throughout pregnancy, switching from warfarin to unfractionated heparin or low molecular weight heparin (LMWH) in the first trimester then back to warfarin until close to delivery or taking unfractionated heparin or LMWH throughout pregnancy. The dilemma is that warfarin is the most effective a preventing maternal thromboembolic complications but causes significant fetal morbidity and mortality; unfractionated heparin and in particular LMWH have good fetal outcomes but the risk of thromboembolic complications is high. What is considered to be an "acceptable level" of risk to mother and infant may differ from one clinician to another and of equal importance, it may also differ from one woman to the next. An unbiased discussion of the pros and cons of each

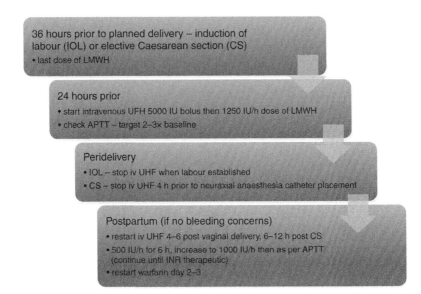

FIGURE 1.—Suggested regimen for peripartum anticoagulation in women with mechanical prosthetic heart valves. APTT: activated partial thromboplastin time; LMWH: low molecular weight heparin; UFH: unfractionated heparin. (Reprinted from Thrombosis Research, McLintock C. Anticoagulant therapy in pregnant women with mechanical prosthetic heart valves: no easy option. *Thromb Res.* 2011;127:S56-S60. Copyright 2011, with permission from Elsevier.)

option is required to allow women to make and informed and confident choice in this very difficult clinical situation (Fig 1).

▶ The first Starr-Edwards mechanical valve was inserted in 1960.[1] Since then, there has been a difficult dilemma when a patient with a mechanical prosthetic heart valve (MPHV) becomes pregnant. These valves have such a high incidence of thromboembolism without anticoagulation (over 70% in 10 years) that anticoagulation almost always with warfarin is mandatory. Even with anticoagulation, the annual risk of thromboembolic events is about 1%.[2] Pregnancy is associated with changes that produce a prothrombotic environment, so anticoagulation is even more essential in patients with MPHV. Oral anticoagulants like warfarin have small molecules that cross the placenta and are teratogenic. Unfractionated heparin and low-molecular-weight heparin don't cross the placenta and avoid the danger of teratogenicity but may be less effective than warfarin in preventing thromboembolism in patients with MPHV. Thus, the dilemma. This article discusses the problems associated with pregnancy in patients with MPHV, the various alternative approaches to keeping the patient on warfarin after the first trimester as long as possible, and the possible bridges for maintaining a reasonable state of anticoagulation during the time of the pregnancy that warfarin should not be used. There are discussions of the arguments for and against unfractionated and low-molecular-weight heparin, the peridelivery management of anticoagulation, and the emergency reversal of anticoagulation in the event of overanticoagulation or frank hemorrhage.

Pregnant women with an MPHV are at great risk. The only greater risk is to be go through the pregnancy unanticoagulated. The physician must inform the patient with the MPHV of the risks of anticoagulation with warfarin and heparin and recommend a program of anticoagulation throughout the pregnancy.

Ultimately, the decision of which drug to take must be made by the informed woman and her family.

M. D. Cheitlin, MD

References

1. Starr A, Edwards ML. Mitral replacement: clinical experience with a ball-valve prosthesis. *Ann Surg.* 1961;154:726-740.
2. McLintock C. Prosthetic heart valves. In: Pavord S, Hunt B, eds. *The Obstetric Haematology Manual.* Cambridge University Press; 2010:109-119.

Changes in mitral regurgitation and left ventricular geometry during exercise affect exercise capacity in patients with systolic heart failure
Izumo M, Suzuki K, Moonen M, et al (St Marianna Univ School of Medicine, Kawasaki, Japan; Univ Hosp of Liège, Belgium)
Eur J Echocardiogr 12:54-60, 2011

Aims.—Exercise may dramatically change the extent of functional mitral regurgitation (MR) and left ventricular (LV) geometry in patients with chronic heart failure (CHF). We hypothesized that dynamic changes in MR and LV geometry would affect exercise capacity.

Methods and Results.—This study included 30 CHF patients with functional MR who underwent symptom-limited bicycle exercise stress echocardiography and cardiopulmonary exercise testing for quantitative assessment of MR (effective regurgitant orifice; ERO), and pulmonary artery systolic pressure (PASP). LV sphericity index was obtained from real-time three-dimensional echocardiograms. The patients were stratified into exercised-induced MR (EMR; $n = 10$, an increase in ERO by ≥ 13 mm^2) or non-EMR (NEMR; $n = 20$, an increase in ERO by < 13 mm^2) group. At rest, no differences in LV volume and function, ERO, and PASP were found between the two groups. At peak exercise, PASP and sphericity index were significantly greater (all $P < 0.01$) in the EMR group. The EMR group revealed lower peak oxygen uptake (peak VO$_2$; $P = 0.018$) and greater minute ventilation/carbon dioxide production slope (VE/VCO$_2$ slope; $P = 0.042$) than the NEMR group. Peak VO$_2$ negatively correlated with changes in ERO ($r = -0.628$) and LV sphericity index ($r = -0.437$); meanwhile, VE/VCO$_2$ slope was well correlated with these changes ($r = 0.414$ and 0.364, respectively). A multivariate analysis identified that the change in ERO was the strongest predictor of peak VO$_2$ ($P = 0.001$).

Conclusion.—Dynamic changes in MR and LV geometry contributed to the limitation of exercise capacity in patients with CHF (Figs 1 and 2).

▶ Patients in stable chronic heart failure (HR) with functional mitral regurgitation (FMR) secondary to changes in the left ventricular (LV) geometry and contractility have been shown to have FMR worsened by exercise.[1] The presence of FMR in patients with HF adversely effects LV function and prognosis.[2-5] Exercise intolerance is one result of LV systolic dysfunction, which is eventually almost universal in patients with HF and is in part related to the maximal stroke volume and cardiac output. This study, which used three-dimensional (3D) echocardiography, examines the determinants of exercise capacity, quantifying the changes in LV geometry, hemodynamics, and exercise gas exchange from rest to peak exercise. The authors divided the patients with chronic stable HF into 2 groups, those with an increase in effective regurgitant orifice area (ERO) of 13 mm^2 or more and those with less than 13 mm^2 and included a control group of 15 healthy age-matched patients. Echocardiography was done at rest and with bicycle exercise. The authors found that an increase in FMR during exercise contributed to exercise intolerance and exercise capacity in patients with systolic HF. They showed with 3D echocardiography that with exercise, the geometry of the LV changes, with the LV becoming more spherical, displacing the papillary muscles, and tethering the mitral leaflets, interfering with leaflet coaptation and worsening the FMR. In the failing heart, the stroke volume with exercise is maintained by the Frank-Starling mechanism, further increasing

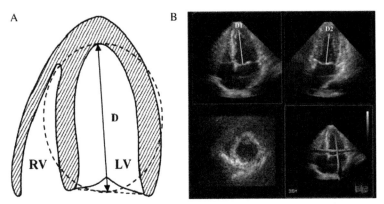

FIGURE 1.—(A) Three-dimensional sphericity index. This figure shows the left ventricular cavity, where D is the left ventricular end-systolic major long axis. The formula: $4/3 \times \pi \times (D/2)^3$. The spherical volumes in millilitres can be calculated, where D is the diameter (cm). The three-dimensional sphericity index is calculated by ESV/[$4/3 \times \pi \times (D/2)^3$], a modification of the equation used in Mannaerts *et al.*[10] (B) Four-tile image display of the dynamic three-dimensional data set with two near perpendicular long axes (top left and right), a short axis (bottom left), and a cubical display with the corresponding cutplanes (bottom right). The measurements of D are shown. The left ventricular long axis (D1 or D2) was obtained from the three-dimensional echocardiographic data set as the longest distance between the centre of the mitral annulus and the endocardial apex. The longest Ds were used in the four-chamber view (D1) and two-chamber view (D2). *Editor's Note:* Please refer to original journal article for full references. (Reprinted from Izumo M, Suzuki K, Moonen M, et al. Changes in mitral regurgitation and left ventricular geometry during exercise affect exercise capacity in patients with systolic heart failure. *Eur J Echocardiogr.* 2011;12:54-60, by permission of the European Society of Cardiology.)

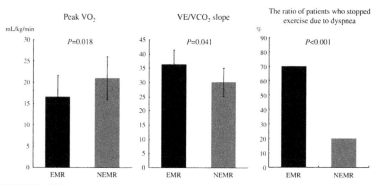

FIGURE 2.—The exercised-induced mitral regurgitation group revealed significantly lower exercise capacity than the non-exercised-induced mitral regurgitation group. The number of patients who stopped exercise because of dyspnoea ws greater in the exercised-induced mitral regurgitation group. (Reprinted from Izumo M, Suzuki K, Moonen M, et al. Changes in mitral regurgitation and left ventricular geometry during exercise affect exercise capacity in patients with systolic heart failure. *Eur J Echocardiogr.* 2011;12:54-60, by permission of the European Society of Cardiology.)

LV end-diastolic volume and increasing LV filling pressure, resulting in dyspnea and pulmonary congestion. With increased FMR during exercise, there is limited ability to increase or even decrease in forward stroke volume, resulting in a decrease in cardiac output for the degree of exercise and an increase in left atrial pressure, further promoting dyspnea. In this study, by multivariate analysis, dynamic changes in the ERO rather than changes in LV sphericity predicted exercise capacity. The increase in ERO and FMR with exercise may explain the observed benefit in HF patients who are still very symptomatic on optimal medications, with almost normal LV ejection fraction, who have markedly reduced exercise capacity.

M. D. Cheitlin, MD

References

1. Lancellotti P, Gérard PL, Piérard LA. Long-term outcome of patients with heart failure and dynamic functional mitral regurgitation. *Eur Heart J.* 2005;26: 1528-1532.
2. Stevenson LW, Brunken RC, Belil D, et al. Afterload reduction with vasodilators and diuretics decreases mitral regurgitation during upright exercise in advanced heart failure. *J Am Coll Cardiol.* 1990;15:174-180.
3. Mollema SA, Nucifora G, Bax JJ. Prognostic value of echocardiography after acute myocardial infarction. *Heart.* 2009;95:1732-1745.
4. Koelling TM, Aaronson KD, Cody RJ, Bach DS, Armstrong WF. Prognostic significance of mitral regurgitation and tricuspid regurgitation in patients with left ventricular systolic dysfunction. *Am Heart J.* 2002;144:524-529.
5. Kwan J, Gillinov MA, Thomas JD, Shiota T. Geometric predictor of significant mitral regurgitation in patients with severe ischemic cardiomyopathy, undergoing Dor procedure: a real-time 3D echocardiographic study. *Eur J Echocardiogr.* 2007; 8:195-203.

Do statins improve outcomes and delay the progression of non-rheumatic calcific aortic stenosis?

Parolari A, Tremoli E, Cavallotti L, et al (Univ of Milan, Italy; et al)
Heart 97:523-529, 2011

Context.—It is not known whether statin treatment improves clinical outcomes and reduces aortic stenosis progression in non-rheumatic calcific aortic stenosis.

Objective.—A meta-analysis of studies was performed comparing statin therapy with placebo or no treatment on outcomes and on aortic stenosis progression echocardiographic parameters.

Data Sources.—The authors searched Medline and Pubmed up to January 2010.

Data Extraction.—Two independent reviewers independently abstracted information on study design (prospective vs retrospective or randomised vs nonrandomised), study and participant characteristics. Fixed and random effects models were used. A-priori subanalyses assessed the effect of statins on low-quality (retrospective or non-randomised) and on high-quality (prospective or randomised) studies separately.

Results.—Meta-analysis identified 10 studies with a total of 3822 participants (2214 non-statin-treated and 1608 statin-treated); five studies were classified as prospective and five as retrospective; concerning randomisation, three trials were randomised whereas seven were not. No significant differences were found in all-cause mortality, cardiovascular mortality or in the need for aortic valve surgery. Lower-quality (retrospective or non-randomised) studies showed that, in statin-treated patients, the annual increase in peak aortic jet velocity and the annual decrease in aortic valve area were lower, but this was not confirmed by the analysis in high-quality (prospective or randomised) studies. Statins did not significantly affect the progression over time of peak and mean aortic gradient.

Conclusions.—Currently available data do not support the use of statins to improve outcomes and to reduce disease progression in non-rheumatic calcific aortic valve stenosis (Fig 1).

▶ Nonrheumatic calcific aortic stenosis (AS) is the most common valve disease in adults and the third most common cardiovascular diagnosis after hypertension and the need for coronary bypass surgery.[1] Studies of the etiology of calcific AS and its progression find it an active process with biochemical similarities to atherosclerosis, provoking the idea that hydroxymethylglutaryl coenzyme-A reductase inhibitors (statins) might be useful in retarding the progression of AS[2,3] with their effect on lipids, platelet aggregation, and inflammation.[4,5] There have been a number of small, observational studies that suggested that statin therapy was successful in delaying the progression as assessed by echocardiography or computed tomography. However, there have been 3 more recent prospective, randomized trials that fail to confirm the effectiveness of statins in preventing progressive obstruction.[6-8] To further evaluate whether statins prevent AS progression, this meta-analysis was done. The requirement for

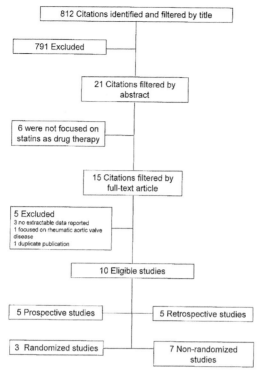

FIGURE 1.—Flow chart of the meta-analysis. (Reproduced from Heart, Parolari A, Tremoli E, Cavallotti L, et al. Do statins improve outcomes and delay the progression of non-rheumatic calcific aortic stenosis? *Heart*. 2011;97:523-529. Copyright © 2011 with permission from the BMJ Publishing Group Ltd.)

inclusion was a study of statins compared with either no statins or placebo, with follow-up ≥1 year and data concerning mid- or long-term hard outcomes (all-cause and cardiac death, need for aortic valve replacement) and AS progression. The literature search yielded 10 studies that were finally selected: 5 prospective and 5 retrospective, with 3 randomized and 7 not randomized. Data for hard outcomes were available only in the prospective studies. The follow-up time averaged 4 years. There were no significant differences between the statin-treated and non–statin-treated patients either in all-cause mortality, cardiac mortality, or need for aortic valve surgery. Data concerning Doppler-echocardiographic progression of AS over time gave support for delaying progression only in the low-quality retrospective or non-randomized studies and not in the high-quality, prospective, randomized studies. The average jet velocity in all studies was greater than 3 m/sec, and the average aortic valve area was between 1.0 and 1.4 cm², so the AS was already advanced by the time they entered the study. Statins may be more effective in the early stages of calcific AS, as suggested by a post-hoc analysis of the SEAS trial data showing that in patients with calcific AS, protection against progression by statins was greatest in patients with a mild degree of AS.[9] This meta-analysis refutes the concept that statins may reduce the progression of calcific AS, but there is still need for a randomized controlled study in patients in the earlier stage of AS.

M. D. Cheitlin, MD

References

1. Carabello BA, Paulus WJ. Aortic stenosis. *Lancet.* 2009;373:956-966.
2. Helske S, Otto CM. Lipid lowering in aortic stenosis: still some light at the end of the tunnel? *Circulation.* 2009;119:2653-2655.
3. Parolari A, Loardi C, Mussoni L, et al. Nonrheumatic calcific aortic stenosis: an overview from basic science to pharmacological prevention. *Eur J Cardiothorac Surg.* 2009;35:493-504.
4. Gelosa P, Cimino M, Pignieri A, Tremoli E, Guerrini U, Sironi L. The role of HMG-CoA reductase inhibition in endothelial dysfunction and inflammation. *Vasc Health Risk Manag.* 2007;3:567-577.
5. Greenwood J, Mason JC. Statins and the vascular endothelial inflammatory response. *Trends Immunol.* 2007;28:88-98.
6. Cowell SJ, Newby DE, Prescott RJ, et al. A randomized trial of intensive lipid-lowering therapy in calcific aortic stenosis. *N Engl J Med.* 2005;352:2389-2397.
7. Rossebø AB, Pedersen TR, Boman K, et al. Intensive lipid lowering with simvastatin and ezetimibe in aortic stenosis. *N Engl J Med.* 2008;359:1343-1356.
8. Chan KL, Teo K, Dumesnil JG, Ni A, Tam J; ASTRONOMER Investigators. Effect of lipid lowering with rosuvastatin on progression of aortic stenosis: results of the aortic stenosis progression observation: measuring effects of rosuvastatin (ASTRONOMER) trial. *Circulation.* 2010;121:306-314.
9. Holme I, Boman K, Brudi P, et al. Observed and predicted reduction of ischemic cardiovascular events in the simvastatin and ezetimibe in aortic stenosis trial. *Am J Cardiol.* 2010;105:1802-1808.

Independent prognostic value of functional mitral regurgitation in patients with heart failure. A quantitative analysis of 1256 patients with ischaemic and non-ischaemic dilated cardiomyopathy

Rossi A, Dini FL, Faggiano P, et al (Universitá di Verona, Italy; Universitá di Pisa, Italy; Universitá di Brescia, Italy; et al)

Heart 97:1675-1680, 2011

Background.—Functional mitral regurgitation (FMR) is a common finding in patients with heart failure (HF), but its effect on outcome is still uncertain, mainly because in previous studies sample sizes were relatively small and semiquantitative methods for FMR grading were used.

Objective.—To evaluate the prognostic value of FMR in patients with HF.

Methods and results.—Patients with HF due to ischaemic and non-ischaemic dilated cardiomyopathy (DCM) were retrospectively recruited. The clinical end point was a composite of all-cause mortality and hospitalisation for worsening HF. FMR was quantitatively determined by measuring vena contracta (VC) or effective regurgitant orifice (ERO) or regurgitant volume (RV). Severe FMR was defined as ERO >0.2 cm^2 or RV >30 ml or VC >0.4 cm. Restrictive mitral filling pattern (RMP) was defined as E-wave deceleration time <140 ms. The study population comprised 1256 patients (mean age 67 ± 11; 78% male) with HF due to DCM: 27% had no FMR, 49% mild to moderate FMR and 24% severe FMR. There was a powerful association between severe FMR and prognosis (HR=2.0, 95% CI 1.5 to 2.6; p<0.0001) after adjustment of left ventricular ejection fraction and RMP. The independent association of severe FMR with prognosis was confirmed in patients with ischaemic DCM (HR=2.0, 95% CI 1.4 to 2.7; p<0.0001) and non-ischaemic DCM (HR=1.9, 95% CI 1.3 to 2.9; p=0.002).

Conclusion.—In a large patient population it was shown that a quantitatively defined FMR was strongly associated with the outcome of patients with HF, independently of LV function (Figs 1, 2 and 4).

▶ In patients with heart failure (HF), functional mitral regurgitation (FMR) frequently occurs because of the distortion of the mitral valvular apparatus with ventricular dilatation and remodeling.[1] In the failing left ventricle (LV), the superimposition of FMR results in further LV dilatation and diastolic wall stress, which is associated with an increase in extracellular matrix turnover, neurohormonal and cytokine activation accelerating concentric ventricular hypertrophy, dilatation, and increasing HF.[2,3] Despite this pathophysiology, some studies indicate that FMR when adjusted for LV ejection fraction is not associated with prognosis and is simply a consequence of LV dysfunction.[4,5] However, if the above scenario is correct, FMR is a potent risk factor in patients with HF, and correction of the FMR would have a beneficial effect on prognosis. This study examines the prognostic effect of FMR in patients with dilated ischemic and nonischemic cardiomyopathy (DCM) and corrects several of the failings of previous studies in that the sample size is large and uses the best objective methods for quantification of the FMR severity. The primary endpoint of the study was all-cause mortality or hospitalization for worsening HF. They found that severe FMR is associated with double the risk of adverse events

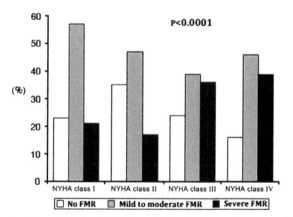

FIGURE 1.—Prevalence of functional mitral regurgitation (FMR) according New York Heart Association class. (Reproduced from Heart, Rossi A, Dini FL, Faggiano P, et al. Independent prognostic value of functional mitral regurgitation in patients with heart failure. A quantitative analysis of 1256 patients with ischaemic and non-ischaemic dilated cardiomyopathy. *Heart.* 2011;97:1675-1680. Copyright © 2011 with permission from the BMJ Publishing Group Ltd.)

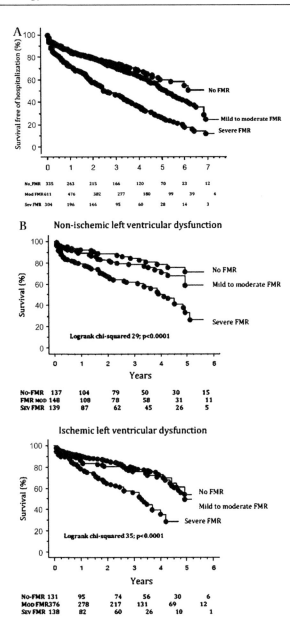

FIGURE 2.—(A) Kaplane–Meier plots showing time to the combined end point of all-cause mortality and heart failure hospitalisation for patients without functional mitral regurgitation (FMR), with mild to moderate FMR and with severe FMR. (B) Kaplane–Meier plots showing time to allcause mortality alone in patients with ischaemic dilated cardiomyopathy and non-ischaemic cardiomyopathy. (Reproduced from Heart, Rossi A, Dini FL, Faggiano P, et al. Independent prognostic value of functional mitral regurgitation in patients with heart failure. A quantitative analysis of 1256 patients with ischaemic and non-ischaemic dilated cardiomyopathy. *Heart.* 2011;97:1675-1680. Copyright © 2011 with permission from the BMJ Publishing Group Ltd.)

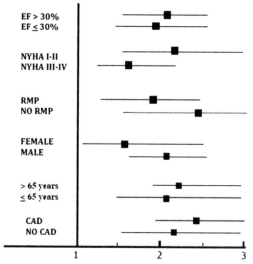

FIGURE 4.—Hazard ratio and interval confidence of severe functional mitral regurgitation (FMR) in different subgroups of patients. CAD, coronary artery disease; EF, ejection fraction, NYHA, New York Heart Association; RMP, restrictive mitral filling. (Reproduced from Heart, Rossi A, Dini FL, Faggiano P, et al. Independent prognostic value of functional mitral regurgitation in patients with heart failure. A quantitative analysis of 1256 patients with ischaemic and non-ischaemic dilated cardiomyopathy. *Heart.* 2011;97:1675-1680. Copyright © 2011 with permission from the BMJ Publishing Group Ltd.)

after adjustment for LV ejection fraction and restrictive mitral filling in patients with HF caused by DCM. Therefore, FMR is not merely a consequence of LV dysfunction but a major predictor for the outcome of patients with HF,[6] suggesting that treatment of the FMR should be considered. Consistent with this is the fact that ACE inhibitors, beta-blockers, and resynchronization therapy increase survival and concomitantly decrease the severity of FMR.[7-9] The trouble with linking these observations to the effect of simply decreasing FMR is that all these therapies have potent antiremodeling effects. Surgically correcting only the FMR and having the same result would settle the question, and so far, surgical correction of FMR reduces symptoms, but there is no evidence that it improves long-term outcome compared with medical treatment.[10,11]

M. D. Cheitlin, MD

References

1. Yiu SF, Enriquez-Sarano M, Tribouilloy C, Seward JB, Tajik AJ. Determinants of the degree of functional mitral regurgitation in patients with systolic left ventricular dysfunction: a quantitative clinical study. *Circulation.* 2000;102:1400-1406.
2. Carabello BA. Mitral valve regurgitation. *Curr Probl Cardiol.* 1998;23:202-241.
3. Spinale FG, Ishihra K, Zile M, DeFryte G, Crawford FA, Carabello BA. Structural basis for changes in left ventricular function and geometry because of chronic mitral regurgitation and after correction of volume overload. *J Thorac Cardiovasc Surg.* 1993;106:1147-1157.

4. Patel JB, Borgenson DD, Barnes M, Rihal CS, Daly RC, Redfield MM. Mitral regurgitation in patients with advanced systolic heart failure. *J Card Fail.* 2004;10:285-291.

5. Giannuzzi P, Temporelli PL, Bosimini E, et al. Independent and incremental prognostic value of Doppler-derived mitral deceleration time of early filling in both symptomatic and asymptomatic patients with left ventricular dysfunction. *J Am Coll Cardiol.* 1996;28:383-390.

6. Persson A, Hartford M, Herlitz J, Karlsson T, Omland T, Caidahl K. Long-term prognostic value of mitral regurgitation in acute coronary syndromes. *Heart.* 2010;96:1803-1808.

7. Seneviratne B, Moore GA, West PD. Effect of captopril on functional mitral regurgitation in dilated heart failure: a randomised double blind placebo controlled trial. *Br Heart J.* 1994;72:63-68.

8. Capomolla S, Febo O, Gnemmi M, et al. Beta-blockade therapy in chronic heart failure: diastolic function and mitral regurgitation improvement by carvedilol. *Am Heart J.* 2000;139:596-608.

9. Breithardt OA, Sinha AM, Schwammnenthal E, et al. Acute effects of cardiac resynchronization therapy on functional mitral regurgitation in advance systolic heart failure. *J Am Coll Cardiol.* 2003;41:765-770.

10. De Bonis M, Lapenna E, La Canna G, et al. Mitral valve repair for functional mitral regurgitation in end-stage dilated cardiomyopathy: role of the "edge-to-edge" technique. *Circulation.* 2005;112:I402-I408.

11. Wu AH, Aaronson KD, Bolling SF, Pagani FD, Welch K, Koelling TM. Impact of mitral valve annuloplasty on mortality risk in patients with mitral regurgitation and left ventricular systolic dysfunction. *J Am Coll Cardiol.* 2005;45:381-387.

Internal and external validation of a model to predict adverse outcomes in patients with left-sided infective endocarditis

López J, Fernández-Hidalgo N, Revilla A, et al (Univ Clinic Hosp, Valladolid, Spain; Hospital Universitari Vall d'Hebron, Barcelona, Spain; et al)
Heart 97:1138-1142, 2011

Introduction.—Early identification of prognostic factors is essential to improve the grim prognosis associated with left-sided infective endocarditis. This group identified three independent risk factors obtained within 72 h of admission, (*Staphylococcus aureus*, heart failure and periannular complications) for inhospital mortality or urgent surgery in a series of 317 patients diagnosed at five tertiary centres (derivation sample). A stratification score was constructed for the test cohort by a simple arithmetic sum of the number of variables present. The goal was to validate this model internally and externally in a prospective manner with two different cohorts of patients.

Methods.—The appropriateness of the model was tested prospectively on predicting events in two cohorts of patients with left-sided endocarditis: internally with the 263 consecutive patients diagnosed at the same centres where the model was derived (internal validation sample), and externally with 264 patients admitted at another hospital (external validation sample).

Results.—The discriminatory power of the model, expressed as the area under the receiver operating characteristic curve was similar between derivation and both validation samples (internal 0.67 vs 0.68, p=0.79; external 0.67 vs p=0.74, p=0.09). There was a progressive, significant pattern of increasing event rates as the risk stratification score increased in both validation cohorts (p<0.001 by χ^2 for trend).

Conclusions.—The early risk stratification model derived, based on variables obtained within 72 h of admission, is applicable to different populations with left-sided endocarditis. A simple bedside assessment tool is provided to clinicians that identifies patients at high risk of having an adverse event (Fig 1, Table 4).

▶ In spite of advances in diagnosis and therapy, the mortality of left-sided infective endocarditis (IE) remains high.[1-3] In 2007, these authors identified

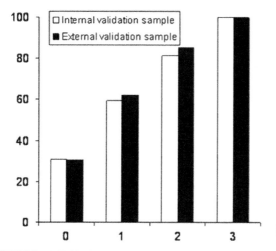

	Internal validation sample	External validation sample
0 variables	31%	30%
Perivalvular complication	65%	58%
Staphylococcus aureus	64%	41%
Heart failure	56%	78%
1 variable overall	60%	62%
Staphylococcus aureus + perivalvular complication	80%	25%
Heart failure + perivalvular complication	71%	95%
Staphylococcus aureus + heart failure	100%	88%
2 variables overall	82%	85%
3 variables	100%	100%

FIGURE 1.—Rate of events depending on the number and type of variables present. (Reproduced from Heart, López J, Fernández-Hidalgo N, Revilla A, et al. Internal and external validation of a model to predict adverse outcomes in patients with left-sided infective endocarditis. *Heart.* 2011;97:1138-1142. Copyright © 2011 with permission from the BMJ Publishing Group Ltd.)

TABLE 4.—Accuracy of the Prognostic Model to Predict Urgent Surgery or Inhospital Mortality Among the Three Groups

| | Parameter (95% CI) | | |
	Derivation Sample	Internal Validation Sample	External Validation Sample
Sensitivity (%)	78 (71 to 85)	73 (64 to 81)	79 (72 to 86)
Specificity (%)	49 (41 to 56)	61 (52 to 69)	57 (47 to 66)
Positive predictive value (%)	51 (44 to 58)	65 (57 to 73)	68 (60 to 75)
Negative predictive value (%)	76 (68 to 84)	69 (60 to 78)	70 (60 to 79)
Positive likelihood ratio	1.53 (1.29 to 1.8)	1.84 (1.4 to 2.3)	1.82 (1.46 to 2.26)
Negative likelihood ratio	0.44 (0.31 to 0.63)	0.45 (0.33 to 0.62)	0.37 (0.26 to 0.53)

3 independent prognostic factors within 72 hours of admission that predicted in-hospital mortality or urgent surgery before completing the course of antibiotics (events) and developed a stratification model based on the variables that predicted the probability of an event.[4] In this study, they prospectively validate their model in 2 different comparable cohorts of patients with left-sided IE, 1 from the same institution as the derivation group (the internal cohort), and 1 from a different institution (the external cohort). Since there are marked differences in the approach to treatment and indications and timing of surgery and the characteristics of the patients among populations,[5] it is important to validate the stratification score in different institutions. With regret as DiSesa wrote "there is still as much art as science in the care of patients with infective endocarditis."[6] The sensitivity, specificity, positive and negative likelihoods ratios, and predictive values for all cohorts are given in the Table, and the discriminatory power of the model, as expressed in the area under the receiver operating characteristic curves, was similar between the derivation and both validation cohorts. There was a progressive, significant pattern of increasing event rates as the risk score increased in the derivation and both validation groups.

The importance of this risk stratification score is that it is easily observed early in the patient's hospitalization so that interventions can be done possibly altering bad outcomes. In other risk stratification, prognostic variables are obtained late in the course so that when it is realized that the patient is at high risk, it may be too late for aggressive management. The next step must be a prospective study to investigate, in patients found to be at increased risk by this stratification score, whether aggressive therapy will beneficially modify the grim outcome in these patients. Delahaye has reviewed 9 observational studies examining the influence of surgery on prognosis in patients with IE by performing a propensity score analysis.[7] There is one ongoing randomized study, the ENDOVAL trial, that addresses this important question.[8]

M. D. Cheitlin, MD

References

1. Leblebicioglu H, Yilmaz H, Tasova Y, et al. Characteristics and analysis of risk factors for mortality in infective endocarditis. *Eur J Epidemiol.* 2006;21:25-31.

2. Thuny F, Di Salvo G, Belliard O, et al. Risk of embolism and death in infective endocarditis: prognostic value of echocardiography: a prospective multicenter study. *Circulation.* 2005;112:69-75.
3. Heiro M, Helenius H, Mäkilä S, et al. Infective endocarditis in a Finnish teaching hospital: a study on 326 episodes treated during 1980-2004. *Heart.* 2006;92: 1457-1462.
4. San Román JA, López J, Vilacosta I, et al. Prognostic stratification of patients with left-sided endocarditis determined at admission. *Am J Med.* 2007;120:e1-e7.
5. Tornos P, Iung B, Permanyer-Miralda G, et al. Infective endocarditis in Europe: lessons from the Euro heart survey. *Heart.* 2005;91:571-575.
6. DiSesa VJ. Art and science in the management of endocarditis. *Ann Thorac Surg.* 1991;51:6-7.
7. Delahaye F. Is early surgery beneficial in infective endocarditis? A systematic review. *Arch Cardiovasc Dis.* 2011;104:35-44.
8. San Román JA, López J, Revilla A, et al. Rationale, design, and methods for the early surgery in infective endocarditis study (ENDOVAL 1): a multicenter, prospective, randomized trial comparing the state-of-the-art therapeutic strategy versus early surgery strategy in infective endocarditis. *Am Heart J.* 2008;156:431-436.

Long-term outcome of combined valve repair and maze procedure for nonrheumatic mitral regurgitation

Fujita T, Kobayashi J, Toda K, et al (Natl Cardiovascular Ctr, Osaka, Japan)
J Thorac Cardiovasc Surg 140:1332-1337, 2010

Objective.—The long-term outcomes of combined mitral repair and maze procedure for patients with nonrheumatic mitral regurgitation and chronic atrial fibrillation were evaluated.

Methods.—Between June 1992 and December 2008, 187 patients underwent a combined mitral repair and maze procedure. The mean follow-up period was 7.4 ± 4.3 years. Chordal reconstruction was performed in 69 patients, leaflet resection in 91, edge-to-edge leaflet suture in 30, and ring annuloplasty in 156. In addition, a cryo-maze procedure was applied in 110, and a Cox—Kosakai maze and radiofrequency maze were applied in the others.

Results.—There were 2 operative deaths and the 15-year survival was 71%. The 15-year freedom from greater than grade 3 mitral regurgitation was 61%; rates of freedom from heart failure (New York Heart Association class ≥III) and reoperations were 79% and 91%, respectively. Cardiac function was improved and left ventricular size was decreased significantly postoperatively. Multivariate analysis showed that a large left ventricular diastolic diameter (≥65 mm) was an independent risk factor for recurrent mitral regurgitation. Eleven thromboembolic episodes (0.79%/patient-year) were detected during follow-up examinations, of which 7 occurred in patients with recurrent atrial fibrillation. Sinus rhythm was regained in 86% after 6 months and in 63% after 15 years. Multivariate analysis showed that a small-voltage f wave was an independent risk factor for AF recurrence.

Conclusions.—A combined mitral valve repair and maze procedure provided low rates of morbidity and mortality and led to well-preserved

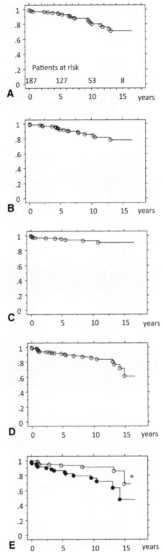

FIGURE 1.—A, Actuarial survival after the operation. B, Rate of freedom from NYHA class III heart failure or greater. C, Rate of freedom from reoperation. D, Rate of freedom from greater than moderate (≥3) MR. E, Rates of freedom for small LV (*line with white circle*; LV diastolic diameter<65 mm, n = 125) and large LV (*line with black circle*; LV diastolic diameter ≥65 mm, n = 62) groups. *P < .01. (Reprinted from the Journal of Thoracic and Cardiovascular Surgery, Fujita T, Kobayashi J, Toda K, et al. Long-term outcome of combined valve repair and maze procedure for nonrheumatic mitral regurgitation. *J Thorac Cardiovasc Surg.* 2010;140:1332-1337. Copyright © 2010 with permission from The American Association for Thoracic Surgery.)

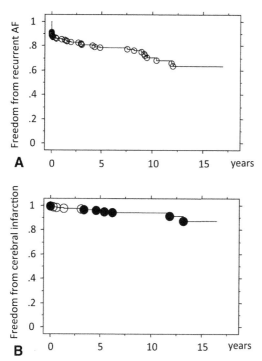

FIGURE 3.—A, Rate of freedom from recurrence of atrial fibrillation *(AF)*. B, Rate of freedom from cerebral infarction. *Open circle*, Cerebral infarction in patient with sinus rhythm. *Closed circle*, Cerebral infarction in patient with recurrent AF. (Reprinted from the Journal of Thoracic and Cardiovascular Surgery, Fujita T, Kobayashi J, Toda K, et al. Long-term outcome of combined valve repair and maze procedure for nonrheumatic mitral regurgitation. *J Thorac Cardiovasc Surg.* 2010;140:1332-1337. Copyright © 2010 with permission from The American Association for Thoracic Surgery.)

cardiac function. Left ventricular diastolic diameter and f-wave voltage can be accurate predictors of good long-term outcome (Figs 1 and 3).

▶ Atrial fibrillation (AF) in patients with severe nonrheumatic mitral regurgitation (MR) occurring in 30% to 40% of patients needing operative repair presents a risk for thromboembolism, especially stroke.[1] Mitral valve repair has been successful in eliminating or reducing the severity of the MR,[2-4] and the maze procedure at the same time has been done to revert the AF to normal sinus rhythm (NSR).[5] The question of how successful in the long term these procedures in patients with long-standing AF are in preventing recurrence of severe MR and AF is addressed in this study. After surgery, there was a decrease in left ventricular (LV) and left atrial diastolic diameter, improved LV function, and return to NSR in 86% in a follow-up of a mean of 7.4 ± 4.3 years. Recurrence of grade 3 MR occurred in 13% of the survivors with a rate of freedom from severe MR of 86% at 10 years postsurgery. The most important risk factor for AF recurrence was the presence of small f-wave voltage (≤0.1 mV) in lead

V1. The implication is that those patients with small f-waves in V1 may not benefit from the maze procedure at the time of MR repair.

M. D. Cheitlin, MD

References

1. Ngaage DL, Schaff HV, Mullany CJ, et al. Influence of preoperative atrial fibrillation on late results of mitral repair: is concomitant ablation justified? *Ann Thorac Surg.* 2007;84:434-442.
2. Kasegawa H, Shimokawa T, Horai T, et al. Long-term echocardiography results of mitral valve repair for mitral valve prolapse. *J Heart Valve Dis.* 2008;17:162-167.
3. David TE, Omran A, Armstrong S, Sun Z, Ivanov J. Long-term results of mitral valve repair for myxomatous disease with and without chordal replacement with expanded polytetrafluoroethylene sutures. *J Thorac Cardiovasc Surg.* 1998; 115:1279-1285.
4. David TE, Ivanov J, Armstrong S, Christie D, Rakowski H. A comparison of outcomes of mitral valve repair for degenerative disease with posterior, anterior, and bileaflet prolapse. *J Thorac Cardiovasc Surg.* 2005;130:1242-1249.
5. Nakajima H, Kobayashi J, Bando K, et al. The effect of cryo-maze procedure on early and intermediate term outcome in mitral valve disease: case matched study. *Circulation.* 2002;106:I46-I50.

Midwall Fibrosis Is an Independent Predictor of Mortality in Patients With Aortic Stenosis

Dweck MR, Joshi S, Murigu T, et al (Royal Brompton Hosp, London, UK; et al)
J Am Coll Cardiol 58:1271-1279, 2011

Objectives.—The goal of this study was to assess the prognostic significance of midwall and infarct patterns of late gadolinium enhancement (LGE) in aortic stenosis.

Background.—Myocardial fibrosis occurs in aortic stenosis as part of the hypertrophic response. It can be detected by LGE, which is associated with an adverse prognosis in a range of other cardiac conditions.

Methods.—Between January 2003 and October 2008, consecutive patients with moderate or severe aortic stenosis undergoing cardiovascular magnetic resonance with administration of gadolinium contrast were enrolled into a registry. Patients were categorized into absent, midwall, or infarct patterns of LGE by blinded independent observers. Patient follow-up was completed using patient questionnaires, source record data, and the National Strategic Tracing Service.

Results.—A total of 143 patients (age 68 ± 14 years; 97 male) were followed up for 2.0 ± 1.4 years. Seventy-two underwent aortic valve replacement, and 27 died (24 cardiac, 3 sudden cardiac deaths). Compared with those with no LGE (n = 49), univariate analysis revealed that patients with midwall fibrosis (n = 54) had an 8-fold increase in all-cause mortality despite similar aortic stenosis severity and coronary artery disease burden. Patients with an infarct pattern (n = 40) had a 6-fold increase. Midwall fibrosis (hazard ratio: 5.35; 95% confidence interval: 1.16 to 24.56; p = 0.03) and ejection fraction (hazard ratio: 0.96; 95% confidence interval:

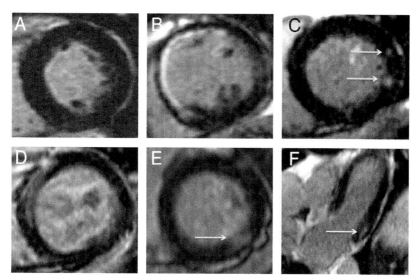

FIGURE 1.—Patterns of LGE in Aortic Stenosis. Images showing the different patterns of late gadolinium enhancement (LGE) observed in patients with aortic stenosis. (**A**) No LGE. (**B**) Infarct LGE with a subendocardial pattern observed in the septum and anterior wall. (**C**) Two focal areas of midwall LGE in the lateral wall of the left ventricle (**red arrows**); (**D**) Midwall LGE in a more linear pattern affecting the septum. (**E**) Short- and (**F**) long-axis views of midwall LGE (**red arrows**) of the inferolateral wall in the same patient. For interpretation of the references to color in this figure legend, the reader is referred to web version of this article. (Reprinted from the Journal of the American College of Cardiology, Dweck MR, Joshi S, Murigu T, et al. Midwall fibrosis is an independent predictor of mortality in patients with aortic stenosis. *J Am Coll Cardiol.* 2011;58:1271-1279. Copyright 2011, with permission from the American College of Cardiology.)

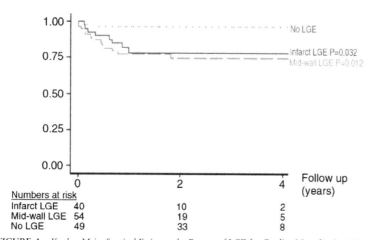

FIGURE 4.—Kaplan-Meier Survival Estimates by Pattern of LGE for Cardiac Mortality in 143 Patients with Moderate or Severe Aortic Stenosis. There was a significant increase in cardiac mortality in the midwall (**orange dashed line**) and infarct groups (**green solid line**) compared with the no late gadolinium enhancement (LGE) group (**blue dotted line**). Among patients followed up for more than 4 years, there were no further deaths. For interpretation of the references to color in this figure legend, the reader is referred to web version of this article. (Reprinted from the Journal of the American College of Cardiology, Dweck MR, Joshi S, Murigu T, et al. Midwall fibrosis is an independent predictor of mortality in patients with aortic stenosis. *J Am Coll Cardiol.* 2011;58:1271-1279. Copyright 2011, with permission from the American College of Cardiology.)

0.94 to 0.99; p = 0.01) were independent predictors of all-cause mortality by multivariate analysis.

Conclusions.—Midwall fibrosis was an independent predictor of mortality in patients with moderate and severe aortic stenosis. It has incremental prognostic value to ejection fraction and may provide a useful method of risk stratification (Figs 1 and 4).

▶ Aortic stenosis (AS) has a course characterized by a long duration without symptoms followed by a short symptomatic period and relatively rapid demise.[1] The 3 major symptom onsets—angina, syncope related to malignant arrhythmias, including sudden death, and heart failure (HF)—are reflective of the pathophysiology of severe AS. The primary problem is that of increased left ventricular (LV) afterload causing increased wall stress, LV myocyte hypertrophy that becomes maladaptive leading to progressive decreased function as manifested by a decreased LV ejection fraction (LVEF), apoptosis, and HF.[2,3] The increased afterload and LV hypertrophy sets the stage for myocardial ischemia, myocardial fibrosis, and malignant arrhythmias. With aortic valve replacement, afterload is immediately normalized and improvement in LVEF is usually seen. However, in some patients, reduced LVEF, HF, and malignant arrhythmias are still seen in spite of the normalized wall stress. This study used cardiovascular magnetic resonance (CMR) imaging with late gadolinium enhancement (LGE) to detect and localize myocardial fibrosis in consecutive patients with moderate (40%) to severe (60%) AS over a 5-year period. The presence and pattern of LGE was assessed, and the primary endpoint was all-cause mortality with a secondary endpoint of cardiac mortality. AS valve replacement was also recorded, and the patients were followed for a mean of 2 years. Three patterns of LGE were observed: no LGE, localized enhancement consistent with prior myocardial infarction, and midwall pattern of LGE, and on follow-up, there was increased all-cause and cardiac morality in the midwall LGE compared with the absent LGE that was comparable with the mortality seen with localized LGE of prior myocardial infarction. Compared with no LGE, those with midwall LGE had an 8-fold increase in mortality. By multivariate analysis, the presence of midwall LGE was an independent predictor of mortality. Left ventricular LGE has been associated with adverse events in a variety of cardiac conditions, including hypertrophic cardiomyopathy, dilated cardiomyopathy, and myocardial infarction.[4-7] It is unlikely that the midwall fibrosis was a consequence of coronary artery disease because coronary disease was present to the same extent in both those with and those without LGE. In AS, midwall LGE represents replacement fibrosis as a sequel to areas of myocyte apoptosis. CMR with LGE may prove to be useful in risk stratification in patients with advanced aortic valve disease and as a future target for antifibrotic therapy.

M. D. Cheitlin, MD

References

1. Otto CM, Burwash IG, Legget ME, et al. Prospective study of asymptomatic valvular aortic stenosis. Clinical, echocardiographic, and exercise predictors of outcome. *Circulation.* 1997;95:2262-2270.

2. Carabello BA. The relationship of left ventricular geometry and hypertrophy to left ventricular function in valvular heart disease. *J Heart Valve Dis.* 1995;4:S132-S138.
3. Grossman W, Jones D, McLaurin LP. Wall stress and patterns of hypertrophy in the human left ventricle. *J Clin Invest.* 1975;56:56-64.
4. Kwong RY, Chan AK, Brown KA, et al. Impact of unrecognized myocardial scar detected by cardiac magnetic resonance imaging on event-free survival in patients presenting with signs or symptoms of coronary artery disease. *Circulation.* 2006; 113:2733-2743.
5. Assomull RG, Prasad SK, Lyne J, et al. Cardiovascular magnetic resonance, fibrosis, and prognosis in dilated cardiomyopathy. *J Am Coll Cardiol.* 2006;48:1977-1985.
6. Moon JC, McKenna WJ, McCrohon JA, Elliott PM, Smith GC, Pennell DJ. Toward clinical risk assessment in hypertrophic cardiomyopathy with gadolinium cardio-vascular magnetic resonance. *J Am Coll Cardiol.* 2003;41:1561-1567.
7. Cheong BY, Muthupillai R, Wilson JM, et al. Prognostic significance of delayed-enhancement magnetic resonance imaging: survival of 857 patients with and without left ventricular dysfunction. *Circulation.* 2009;120:2069-2076.

Percutaneous Repair or Surgery for Mitral Regurgitation

Feldman T, for the EVEREST II Investigators (NorthShore Univ Health System, Evanston, IL; et al)

N Engl J Med 364:1395-1406, 2011

Background.—Mitral-valve repair can be accomplished with an investigational procedure that involves the percutaneous implantation of a clip that grasps and approximates the edges of the mitral leaflets at the origin of the regurgitant jet.

Methods.—We randomly assigned 279 patients with moderately severe or severe (grade 3+ or 4+) mitral regurgitation in a 2:1 ratio to undergo either percutaneous repair or conventional surgery for repair or replacement of the mitral valve. The primary composite end point for efficacy was freedom from death, from surgery for mitral-valve dysfunction, and from grade 3+ or 4+ mitral regurgitation at 12 months. The primary safety end point was a composite of major adverse events within 30 days.

Results.—At 12 months, the rates of the primary end point for efficacy were 55% in the percutaneous-repair group and 73% in the surgery group (P = 0.007). The respective rates of the components of the primary end point were as follows: death, 6% in each group; surgery for mitral-valve dysfunction, 20% versus 2%; and grade 3+ or 4+ mitral regurgitation, 21% versus 20%. Major adverse events occurred in 15% of patients in the percutaneous-repair group and 48% of patients in the surgery group at 30 days (P<0.001). At 12 months, both groups had improved left ventricular size, New York Heart Association functional class, and quality-of-life measures, as compared with baseline.

Conclusions.—Although percutaneous repair was less effective at reducing mitral regurgitation than conventional surgery, the procedure was associated with superior safety and similar improvements in clinical outcomes. (Funded by Abbott Vascular; EVEREST II ClinicalTrials.gov number, NCT00209274.) (Fig 2).

▶ Severe mitral regurgitation (MR) in symptomatic patients treated medically has an annual mortality of 5% or higher.[1,2] The American College of Cardiology/American Heart Association guidelines recommend surgery in patients with moderate-to-severe MR who are symptomatic or have evidence of left ventricular (LV) dysfunction.[3] One surgical approach has been to create a double mitral orifice by suturing the middle of the 2 leaflets together and applying an annuloplasty ring,[4,5] a procedure that in selected patients had successful results for up to 12 years.[6] A device has been developed that is capable of being delivered percutaneously through a catheter technique called a MitraClip that is introduced into the left atrium transseptally and passed through the mitral valve. The MitraClip is able to catch and clip together the anterior and posterior mitral valve leaflets.[7,8] Mitral repair using this device in 107 patients has been shown to

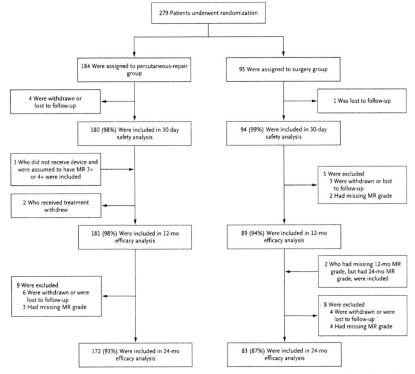

FIGURE 2.—Enrollment and Follow-up in the Intention-to-Treat Group. Data are shown for patients who were available for analysis at 30 days (safety analysis) and at both 12 months and 24 months (efficacy analysis). Since the efficacy end point required echocardiographic assessment of mitral regurgitation (MR), patients who did not undergo implantation of a device, but were known to be alive, were presumed to have retained their baseline grade of mitral regurgitation and thus are included among patients in whom treatment failed. (Reprinted from Feldman T, for the EVEREST II Investigators. Percutaneous repair or surgery for mitral regurgitation. *N Engl J Med.* 2011;364:1395-1406. © 2011 Massachusetts Medical Society.)

significantly decrease the severity of the MR.[9,10] This EVEREST II study randomly assigned patients with indications for repair of moderate-to-severe MR to surgery or percutaneous mitral repair (PMR). Eighty-five percent in the PMR group and 76% in the surgical group were New York Heart Association (NYHA) class II/III. After a follow-up of 1 year, the composite endpoint of freedom from death, surgery for mitral valve dysfunction, or the presence of persistent 3+ or 4+ MR was 55% in the PMR group and 73% in the surgical group, but the reasons for the differences were the higher incidence of surgery for mitral valve dysfunction in the PMR group and the higher incidence of major adverse events in the surgical group.

The study shows that patients with MR who are candidates for mitral valve repair can have PMR as a alternative to surgery. Although PMR was effective in reducing the degree of MR, surgery was more often effective, but clinical results as measured by quality of life, heart failure status, and LV function were similar, and PMR had fewer major adverse events than surgery, a significant advantage in patients who are high risk for surgery. Recently, Rudolph and colleagues[6] reported 104 consecutive patients with grade 3 and 4+ MR, all with NYHA class III/IV symptoms, all not amenable to surgery, who had PMR and were followed for 1 year. At follow-up, 69% were in NYHA class I/II, and three-quarters of the patients improved in the 6-minute walk test and quality of life.

M. D. Cheitlin, MD

References

1. Trichon BH, Felker GM, Shaw LK, Cabell CH, O'Connor CM. Relation of frequency and severity of mitral regurgitation to survival among patients with left ventricular systolic dysfunction and heart failure. *Am J Cardiol.* 2003;91: 538-543.
2. Carabello BA. The current therapy for mitral regurgitation. *J Am Coll Cardiol.* 2008;52:319-326.
3. Bonow RO, Carabello BA, Chatterjee K, et al; American College of Cardiology/American Heart Association Task Force on Practice Guidelines. 2008 Focused update incorporated into the ACC/AHA 2006 guidelines for the management of patients with valvular heart disease: a report of the American College of Cardiology/American Heart Association Task Force on Practice Guidelines (Writing Committee to revise the 1998 guidelines for the management of patients with valvular heart disease). Endorsed by the Society of Cardiovascular Anesthesiologists, Society for Cardiovascular Angiography and Interventions, and Society of Thoracic Surgeons. *J Am Coll Cardiol.* 2008;52:e1-e142.
4. Alfieri O, Maisano F, De Bonis M, et al. The double-orifice technique in mitral valve repair: a simple solution for complex problems. *J Thorac Cardiovasc Surg.* 2001;122:674-681.
5. Maisano F, Schreuder JJ, Oppizzi M, Fiorani B, Fino C, Alfieri O. The double-orifice technique as a standardized approach to treat mitral regurgitation due to severe myxomatous disease: surgical technique. *Eur J Cardiothorac Surg.* 2000; 17:201-205.
6. Rudolph V, Knap M, Franzen O, et al. Echocardiographic and clinical outcomes of mitraclip therapy in patients not amenable to surgery. *J Am Coll Cardiol.* 2011;58:2190-2195.
7. Fann JI, St Goar FG, Komtebedde J, et al. Beating heart catheter-based edge-to-edge mitral valve procedure in a porcine model: efficacy and healing response. *Circulation.* 2004;110:988-993.

8. St Goar FG, Fann JI, Komtebedde J, et al. Endovascular edge-to-edge mitral valve repair: short-term results in a porcine model. *Circulation.* 2003;108:1990-1993.

9. Feldman T, Wasserman HS, Herrmann HC, et al. Percutaneous mitral valve repair using the edge-to-edge technique: six-month results of the EVEREST Phase I Clinical Trial. *J Am Coll Cardiol.* 2005;46:2134-2140.

10. Feldman T, Kar S, Rinaldi M, et al; EVEREST Investigators. Percutaneous mitral repair with the MitraClip system: safety and midterm durability in the initial EVEREST (Endovascular Valve Edge-to-Edge REpair Study) cohort. *J Am Coll Cardiol.* 2009;54:686-694.

Prospective Validation of the Prognostic Usefulness of B-Type Natriuretic Peptide in Asymptomatic Patients With Chronic Severe Aortic Regurgitation

Pizarro R, Bazzino OO, Oberti PF, et al (Hosp Italiano de Buenos Aires, Argentina)

J Am Coll Cardiol 58:1705-1714, 2011

Objectives.—The purpose of this study was to determine the independent and additive prognostic value of B-type natriuretic peptide (BNP) in patients with severe asymptomatic aortic regurgitation and normal left ventricular function.

Background.—Early surgery could be advisable in selected patients with chronic severe aortic regurgitation, but there are no uniform criteria to identify candidates who could benefit from this strategy. Assessment of BNP has not been studied for this purpose.

Methods.—We prospectively evaluated 294 consecutive patients with severe asymptomatic organic aortic regurgitation and left ventricular ejection fraction above 55%. The first 160 consecutive patients served as the derivation cohort and the next 134 patients served as a validation cohort. The combined endpoint was the occurrence of symptoms of congestive heart failure, left ventricular dysfunction, or death at follow-up.

Results.—The endpoint was reached in 45 patients (28%) of the derivation set and in 35 patients (26%) of the validation cohort. Receiver-operator characteristic curve analysis yielded an optimal cutoff point of 130 pg/ml for BNP that was able to discriminate between patients at higher risk in both cohorts. BNP was the strongest independent predictor by multivariate analysis in the derivation set (odds ratio: 6.9 [95% confidence interval: 2.52 to 17.57], p < 0.0001) and the validation set (odds ratio: 6.7 [95% confidence interval: 2.9 to 16.9], p = 0.0001).

Conclusions.—Among patients with severe asymptomatic aortic regurgitation and normal left ventricular function, BNP ≥ 130 pg/ml categorizes a subgroup of patients at higher risk. Because of its incremental prognostic value, we believe BNP assessment should be used in the routine clinical evaluation of these patients (Figs 1 and 3).

▶ Severe aortic regurgitation (AR) results in left ventricular (LV) dilatation and LV remodeling (eccentric hypertrophy) such that normal LV function and

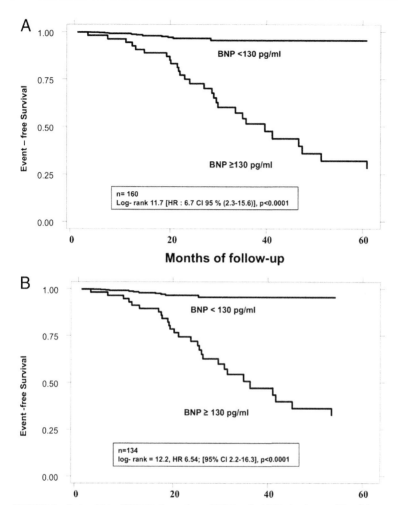

FIGURE 1.—Patient Risk of LVDSD According to BNP Levels. (A) Derivation set; (B) validation set. BNP = B-type natriuretic peptide; CI = confidence interval; HR = hazard ratio; LVDSD = left ventricular systolic dysfunction symptoms or death. (Reprinted from the Journal of the American College of Cardiology, Pizarro R, Bazzino OO, Oberti PF, et al. Prospective validation of the prognostic usefulness of B-type natriuretic peptide in asymptomatic patients with chronic severe aortic regurgitation. *J Am Coll Cardiol.* 2011;58:1705-1714. Copyright 2011, with permission from the American College of Cardiology.)

effective stroke volume is maintained and the patient can have a long asymptomatic period with no limitation of exercise capacity.[1-5] The indications for valve replacement are the development of symptoms of heart failure (HF) or the development of LV dysfunction as manifested by a decrease in LV ejection fraction (LVEF).[1,2,6,7] Although there have been studies to show benefit from "early" surgery before the onset of symptoms or decrease in LV function such as serial echocardiography evaluating end-systolic and end-diastolic LV diameter volumes as well as effective regurgitant orifice (ERO),[1-5,7] there are no

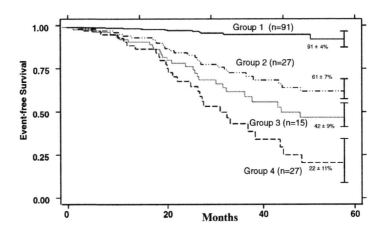

Group 1: EROA<50 mm2 & BNP < 130pg/ml
Group 2: EROA ≥ 50 mm2 & BNP < 130pg/ml : p<0.02 vs. group 1
Group 3: EROA< 50 mm2 & BNP ≥ 130pg/ml : p<0.001 vs. group 1; p<0.015 vs. group 2
Group 4: EROA ≥ 50 mm2 & BNP ≥ 130pg/ml : p<0.0001 vs. group 1; p<0.001 vs. group 2 ; p<0.01 vs. group 3

FIGURE 3.—Survival Free of LVDSD According to BNP in Combination With EROA Levels. Patients' survival free of LVDSD in the derivation set (n = 160). Abbreviations as in Figure 2. (Reprinted from the Journal of the American College of Cardiology, Pizarro R, Bazzino OO, Oberti PF, et al. Prospective validation of the prognostic usefulness of B-type natriuretic peptide in asymptomatic patients with chronic severe aortic regurgitation. *J Am Coll Cardiol.* 2011;58:1705-1714. Copyright 2011, with permission from the American College of Cardiology.)

strong indicators for "early" surgery.[1,2,8] In patients with HF of various etiologies, B-type natriuretic peptide (BNP) and N-Terminal pro-B-type natriuretic peptide are hormones released with increased LV myocardial wall stress that have vasodilator and diuretic action, are adrenergic and renin-angiotensin system antagonists,[1] and have proved prognostic value.[9-11] This study of a large number of asymptomatic patients with severe AR and normal LVEF was divided into a derivation and a validation cohort, followed up for a mean of 46 months in the derivation group and 38 months in the validation cohort. The combined endpoint was the appearance of HF symptoms, LV dysfunction, or death. In addition to BNP measurement, a number of echocardiographic parameters were also measured. By multivariate analysis in the derivation set, the independent predictors were BNP (OR 6.89), end systolic/body surface area ratio (OR 3.14) and ERO (OR 3.87). BNP ≥130 pg/mL was the strongest predictor of the combined endpoint and of isolated LV dysfunction. Because of its strong independent and incremental prognostic value, BNP assessment should be added to serial echocardiographic evaluation of LV parameters in following up with patients with asymptomatic severe AR.

M. D. Cheitlin, MD

References

1. Bonow RO, Carabello BA, Chatterjee K, et al; American College of Cardiology/American Heart Association Task Force on Practice Guidelines. 2008 focused update incorporated into the ACC/AHA 2006 guidelines for the management

of patients with valvular heart disease: a report of the American College of Cardiology/American Heart Association Task Force on Practice Guidelines (Writing Committee to revise the 1998 guidelines for the management of patients with valvular heart disease). Endorsed by the Society of Cardiovascular Anesthesiologists, Society for Cardiovascular Angiography and Interventions, and Society of Thoracic Surgeons. *J Am Coll Cardiol.* 2008;52:e1-142.

2. Dujardin KS, Enriquez-Sarano M, Schaff HV, Bailey KR, Seward JB, Tajik AJ. Mortality and morbidity of aortic regurgitation in clinical practice. A long-term follow-up study. *Circulation.* 1999;99:1851-1857.
3. Vahanian A, Baumgartner H, Bax J, et al. Guidelines on the management of valvular heart disease: the task force on the management of valvular heart disease of the European Society of Cardiology. *Eur Heart J.* 2007;28:230-268.
4. Turina J, Milincic J, Seifert B, Turina M. Valve replacement in chronic aortic regurgitation. True predictors of survival after extended follow-up. *Circulation.* 1998;98:II100-II106.
5. Corti R, Binggeli C, Turina M, Jenni R, Lüscher TF, Turina J. Predictors of long-term survival after valve replacement for chronic aortic regurgitation: is M-mode echocardiography sufficient? *Eur Heart J.* 2001;22:866-873.
6. Scognamiglio R, Negut C, Palisi M, Fasoli G, Dalla-Volta S. Long-term survival and functional results after aortic valve replacement in asymptomatic patients with chronic severe aortic regurgitation and left ventricular dysfunction. *J Am Coll Cardiol.* 2005;45:1025-1030.
7. Detaint D, Messika-Zeitoun D, Maalouf J, et al. Quantitative echocardiographic determinants of clinical outcome in asymptomatic patients with aortic regurgitation: a prospective study. *JACC Cardiovasc Imaging.* 2008;1:1-11.
8. Tornos P, Sambola A, Permanyer-Miralda G, Evangelista A, Gomez Z, Soler-Soler J. Long-term outcome of surgically treated aortic regurgitation: influence of guideline adherence toward early surgery. *J Am Coll Cardiol.* 2006;47:1012-1017.
9. Levin ER, Gardner DG, Samson WK. Natriuretic peptides. *N Engl J Med.* 1998;339:321-328.
10. Omland T, Aakvaag A, Bonarjee VV, et al. Plasma brain natriuretic peptide as an indicator of left ventricular systolic function and long-term survival after acute myocardial infarction: comparison with plasma atrial natriuretic peptide and N-terminal proatrial natriuretic peptide. *Circulation.* 1996;93:1963-1969.
11. Weber M, Bazzino O, Navarro Estrada JL, et al. N-terminal B-type natriuretic peptide assessment provides incremental prognostic information in patients with acute coronary syndromes and normal troponin T values upon admission. *J Am Coll Cardiol.* 2008;51:1188-1195.

The Impact of Renin-Angiotensin-Aldosterone System Blockade on Heart Failure Outcomes and Mortality in Patients Identified to Have Aortic Regurgitation: A Large Population Cohort Study

Elder DHJ, Wei L, Szwejkowski BR, et al (Ninewells Hosp and Med School, Dundee, UK; Univ of Dundee, UK; et al)
J Am Coll Cardiol 58:2084-2091, 2011

Objectives.—The aim of this study was to investigate the effect of renin-angiotensin system blockade on outcomes in patients with aortic regurgitation (AR).

Background.—Angiotensin-converting enzyme (ACE) inhibitors have the potential to reduce afterload, blunt left ventricular wall stress, and limit left ventricular dilation and hypertrophy. However, long-term studies have yielded inconsistent results, and very few have assessed clinical outcomes.

Methods.—The Health Informatics Centre dispensed prescription and morbidity and mortality database for the population of Tayside, Scotland, was linked through a unique patient identifier to the Tayside echocardiography database. Patients diagnosed with at least moderate AR from 1993 to 2008 were identified. Cox regression analysis was used to assess differences in all-cause mortality and cardiovascular (CV) and AR events (heart failure hospitalizations, heart failure deaths, or aortic valve replacement) between those treated with and without ACE inhibitors or angiotensin receptor blockers (ARBs).

Results.—A total of 2,266 subjects with AR (median age 74 years; interquartile range: 64 to 81 years) were studied, with a mean follow-up period of 4.4 ± 3.7 years. Seven hundred and five patients (31%) received ACE inhibitor or ARB therapy. There were 582 all-cause deaths (25.7%). Patients treated with ACE inhibitors or ARBs had significantly lower all-cause mortality and fewer CV and AR events, with adjusted hazard ratios of 0.56 (95% confidence interval [CI]: 0.64 to 0.89; p < 0.01) for all-cause mortality, 0.77 (95% CI: 0.67 to 0.89; p < 0.01) for CV events, and 0.68 (95% CI: 0.54 to 0.87; p < 0.01) for AR events.

Conclusions.—This large retrospective study shows that the prescription of ACE inhibitors or ARBs in patients with moderate to severe AR was associated with significantly reduced all-cause mortality and CV and AR events. These data need to be confirmed by a prospective randomized controlled outcome trial (Fig 1).

▶ Chronic aortic regurgitation (AR) is a common valve abnormality resulting from a large number of etiologies and affecting up to 10% of the middle age and older population undergoing echocardiography.[1] The pathophysiology of AR involves chronic increased left ventricular (LV) volume overload with eccentric hypertrophy and a normal LV filling pressure that allows for an increased LV stroke volume so that the effective or forward stroke volume remains normal and the patients asymptomatic.[2-4] Eventually, the LV afterload increase results in further LV hypertrophy and inevitable LV myocardial systolic dysfunction. This occurs at an annual rate of about 6% of patients with moderate-severe AR, and in these patients, there is an annual mortality rate of 10%.[5] Vasodilators have been shown in short-term studies to reduce the progression of LV end-systolic and end-diastolic volumes and improve LV hemodynamic parameters, but there have been no studies of vasodilator impact on survival.[6-10] Animal studies have shown that there is abnormal activation of the renin-angiotensin system in severe AR and that angiotensin-blocking drugs are more effective than nifedipine in slowing LV remodeling and preserving LV function, decreasing brain natriuretic peptides, and decreasing the expression of fibrosis-related molecules, such as collagens I and III.[11,12] This study sought to investigate the potential survival benefits of angiotensin-converting enzyme inhibitors (ACEI) or angiotensin receptor blocking (ARBs) drugs in a large retrospective observational registry of patients with moderate to severe AR by echocardiography. Using data from

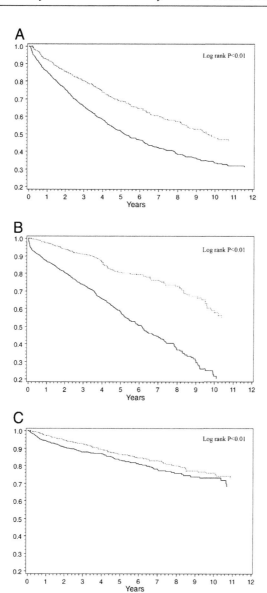

FIGURE 1.—Events and Survival by ACE Inhibitor or ARB Therapy. Kaplan-Meier curves illustrating the survival benefits in angiotensin-converting enzyme (ACE) inhibitor or angiotensin receptor blocker (ARB) users (**dotted lines**), compared with nonusers (**solid lines**), on (**A**) cardiovascular (CV) events (CV hospitalization or death), (**B**) all-cause mortality, and (**C**) aortic regurgitation (AR) events (aortic valve replacement, heart failure hospitalization, or heart failure death). (Reprinted from the Journal of the American College of Cardiology, Elder DHJ, Wei L, Szwejkowski BR, et al. The impact of renin-angiotensin-aldosterone system blockade on heart failure outcomes and mortality in patients identified to have aortic regurgitation: a large population cohort study. *J Am Coll Cardiol.* 2011;58:2084-2091. Copyright 2011, with permission from the American College of Cardiology.)

a very large echocardiographic database, patients with moderate to severe AR were linked with a database of detailed prescribing information on greater than 400 000 people[13] and other clinical databases. Of 2266 AR elderly patients, 876 (39%) were treated with ACEI or ARBs. After a mean follow-up period of 4.4 years, using a Cox regression analysis, the adjusted hazard ratio (HR) with the use of ACEI or ARBs for all-cause mortality was 0.56. The time-dependent analysis showed an HR of 0.45 for cardiovascular (CV) events, and 0.18 for CV mortality compared with those not treated with ACEI or ARBs. To minimize potential bias, a propensity score-matched cohort analysis was done with similar results. Due to conflicting evidence of randomized studies for the use of vasodilators in asymptomatic patients with moderate to severe AR,[14,15] the American College of Cardiology/American Heart Association guidelines no longer recommend vasodilators for the medical treatment of asymptomatic patients with AR and normal LV function, only for patients with severe AR and hypertension to reduce systolic blood pressure.[16] This retrospective, large study demands a randomized prospective study of ACEI or ARBs in asymptomatic patients with moderate to severe AR with normal LV systolic function to change the guidelines' recommendations.

M. D. Cheitlin, MD

References

1. Lebowitz NE, Bella JN, Roman MJ, et al. Prevalence and correlates of aortic regurgitation in American Indians: the Strong Heart Study. *J Am Coll Cardiol.* 2000;36:461-467.
2. Zoghbi WA, Enriquez-Sarano M, Foster E, et al. Recommendations for evaluation of the severity of native valvular regurgitation with two-dimensional and Doppler echocardiography. *J Am Soc Echocardiogr.* 2003;16:777-802.
3. Tornos MP, Olona M, Permanyer-Miralda G, et al. Clinical outcome of severe asymptomatic chronic aortic regurgitation: a long-term prospective follow-up study. *Am Heart J.* 1995;130:333-339.
4. Wisenbaugh T, Spann JF, Carabello BA. Differences in myocardial performance and load between patients with similar amounts of chronic aortic versus chronic mitral regurgitation. *J Am Coll Cardiol.* 1984;3:916-923.
5. Bonow RO, Lakatos E, Maron BJ, Epstein SE. Serial long-term assessment of the natural history of asymptomatic patients with chronic aortic regurgitation and normal left ventricular systolic function. *Circulation.* 1991;84:1625-1635.
6. Scognamiglio R, Fasoli G, Ponchia A, Dalla-Volta S. Long-term nifedipine unloading therapy in asymptomatic patients with chronic severe aortic regurgitation. *J Am Coll Cardiol.* 1990;16:424-429.
7. Søndergaard L, Aldershvile J, Hildebrandt P, Kelbaek H, Ståhlberg F, Thomsen C. Vasodilatation with felodipine in chronic asymptomatic aortic regurgitation. *Am Heart J.* 2000;139:667-674.
8. Greenberg BH, DeMots H, Murphy E, Rahimtoola S. Beneficial effects of hydralazine on rest and exercise hemodynamics in patients with chronic severe aortic insufficiency. *Circulation.* 1980;62:49-55.
9. Fioretti P, Benussi B, Scardi S, Klugmann S, Brower RW, Camerini F. Afterload reduction with nifedipine in aortic insufficiency. *Am J Cardiol.* 1982;49:1728-1732.
10. Lin M, Chiang HT, Lin SL, et al. Vasodilator therapy in chronic asymptomatic aortic regurgitation: enalapril versus hydralazine therapy. *J Am Coll Cardiol.* 1994;24:1046-1053.
11. Plante E, Gaudreau M, Lachance D, et al. Angiotensin-converting enzyme inhibitor captopril prevents volume overload cardiomyopathy in experimental chronic aortic valve regurgitation. *Can J Physiol Pharmacol.* 2004;82:191-199.

12. Plante E, Lachance D, Beaudoin J, et al. Comparative study of vasodilators in an animal model of chronic volume overload caused by severe aortic regurgitation. *Circ Heart Fail.* 2009;2:25-32.

13. Nadir MA, Wei L, Elder DH, et al. Impact of renin-angiotensin system blockade therapy on outcome in aortic stenosis. *J Am Coll Cardiol.* 2011;58:570-576.

14. Evangelista A, Tornos P, Sambola A, Permanyer-Miralda G, Soler-Soler J. Long-term vasodilator therapy in patients with severe aortic regurgitation. *N Engl J Med.* 2005;353:1342-1349.

15. Scognamiglio R, Rahimtoola SH, Fasoli G, Nistri S, Dalla Volta S. Nifedipine in asymptomatic patients with severe aortic regurgitation and normal left ventricular function. *N Engl J Med.* 1994;331:689-694.

16. American College of Cardiology; American Heart Association Task Force on Practice Guidelines (Writing Committee to revise the 1998 guidelines for the management of patients with valvular heart disease); Society of Cardiovascular Anesthesiologists, Bonow RO, Carabello BA, Chatterjee K, et al. ACC/AHA 2006 guidelines for the management of patients with valvular heart disease: a report of the American College of Cardiology/American Heart Association Task Force on Practice Guidelines (writing Committee to Revise the 1998 guidelines for the management of patients with valvular heart disease) developed in collaboration with the Society of Cardiovascular Anesthesiologists endorsed by the Society for Cardiovascular Angiography and Interventions and the Society of Thoracic Surgeons. *J Am Coll Cardiol.* 2006;48:e1-148.

Transcatheter Aortic-Valve Implantation for Aortic Stenosis in Patients Who Cannot Undergo Surgery

Leon MB, for the PARTNER Trial Investigators (Columbia Univ Med Ctr/NewYork—Presbyterian Hosp; et al)

N Engl J Med 363:1597-1607, 2010

Background.—Many patients with severe aortic stenosis and coexisting conditions are not candidates for surgical replacement of the aortic valve. Recently, transcatheter aortic-valve implantation (TAVI) has been suggested as a less invasive treatment for high-risk patients with aortic stenosis.

Methods.—We randomly assigned patients with severe aortic stenosis, whom surgeons considered not to be suitable candidates for surgery, to standard therapy (including balloon aortic valvuloplasty) or transfemoral transcatheter implantation of a balloon-expandable bovine pericardial valve. The primary end point was the rate of death from any cause.

Results.—A total of 358 patients with aortic stenosis who were not considered to be suitable candidates for surgery underwent randomization at 21 centers (17 in the United States). At 1 year, the rate of death from any cause (Kaplan—Meier analysis) was 30.7% with TAVI, as compared with 50.7% with standard therapy (hazard ratio with TAVI, 0.55; 95% confidence interval [CI], 0.40 to 0.74; P<0.001). The rate of the composite end point of death from any cause or repeat hospitalization was 42.5% with TAVI as compared with 71.6% with standard therapy (hazard ratio, 0.46; 95% CI, 0.35 to 0.59; P<0.001). Among survivors at 1 year, the rate of cardiac symptoms (New York Heart Association class III or IV) was lower among patients who had undergone TAVI than among those who had received standard therapy (25.2% vs. 58.0%, P<0.001).

At 30 days, TAVI, as compared with standard therapy, was associated with a higher incidence of major strokes (5.0% vs. 1.1%, P=0.06) and major vascular complications (16.2% vs. 1.1%, P<0.001). In the year after TAVI, there was no deterioration in the functioning of the bioprosthetic valve, as assessed by evidence of stenosis or regurgitation on an echocardiogram.

Conclusions.—In patients with severe aortic stenosis who were not suitable candidates for surgery, TAVI, as compared with standard therapy, significantly reduced the rates of death from any cause, the composite end point of death from any cause or repeat hospitalization, and cardiac symptoms, despite the higher incidence of major strokes and major vascular events. (Funded by Edwards Lifesciences; ClinicalTrials.gov number, NCT00530894.)

▶ Calcific aortic stenosis (AS) is the commonest valve lesion requiring surgical replacement, increasing in frequency with increasing age.[1,2] When symptoms develop, mean survival is 2 to 3 years,[3,4] and aortic valve replacement (AVR) at a low operative mortality even in elderly patients is indicated.[5] Surgery is also recommended even in asymptomatic patients when there is a decrease in left ventricular function or when other surgery such as coronary bypass surgery is contemplated.[4] The exception to these recommendations is the patient deemed too high a surgical risk, in which coexisting conditions that would be associated with a predicted probability of 50% or more of either perioperative death or a serious irreversible condition[6]; in these cases, medical management that has never shown an increase in survival is recommended. The Placement of Aortic Transcatheter Valves (PARTNER) trial has 2 groups of patients with severe AS: cohort A in which symptomatic patients with severe AS, considered high risk, with an estimated risk of death within 30 days after surgery of 15% or higher, were randomized to receive either transcatheter aortic valve implantation (TAVI) or conventional surgical AVR; and cohort B, in which patients with severe AS deemed to high risk for surgical AVR were randomized to receive either TAVI or conventional medical therapy, including balloon aortic valvuloplasty in 64%. This article is the report of the results of cohort B only (those of the sickest patients with AS) and is published prematurely because cohort A is still not published but was presented at the April 2011 American College of Cardiology (ACC) meeting. The results of the Cohort B group of the PARTNER trial are that these patients with severe AS deemed too high risk for AVR have a better survival rate and better symptom relief than those treated medically, at the expense of a higher incidence of bleeding, mainly arterial injury, and stroke. With changes in the transcatheter aortic valve technology, including newer stent frame geometry constructed from a thinner cobalt alloy and a lower profile catheter (18- to 19-French delivery system instead of a 22- to 24-French sheath), the incidence of arterial injury and bleeding should be reduced. The reported results at the ACC meeting of the cohort A group (high-risk AS but randomized to TAVI or AVR) were that similar mortality and symptom relief benefits of TAVI over AVR were seen in this less severely ill group of AS patients. This study is powerful evidence that the standard of care in high-risk AS patients should be TAVI when expertise in performing this procedure is available. In the future, trials of TAVI versus AVR will be reported in lower risk patients with severe AS.

M. D. Cheitlin, MD

References

1. Lindroos M, Kupari M, Heikkilä J, Tilvis R. Prevalence of aortic valve abnormalities in the elderly: an echocardiographic study of a random population sample. *J Am Coll Cardiol.* 1993;21:1220-1225.
2. Tunick PA, Freedberg RS, Kronzon I. Cardiac findings in the very elderly: analysis of echocardiography in fifty-eight nonagenarians. *Gerontology.* 1990;36:206-211.
3. Kelly TA, Rothbart RM, Cooper CM, Kaiser DL, Smucker ML, Gibson RS. Comparison of outcome of asymptomatic to symptomatic patients older than 20 years of age with valvular aortic stenosis. *Am J Cardiol.* 1988;61:123-130.
4. Bonow RO, Carabello BA, Chatterjee K, et al. 2008 Focused update incorporated Into the ACC/AHA 2006 guidelines for the management of patients with valvular heart disease: a report of the American College of Cardiology/American Heart Association Task Force on Practice Guidelines (Writing Committee to Revise the 1998 Guidelines for the Management of Patients With Valvular Heart Disease): endorsed by the Society of Cardiovascular Anesthesiologists, Society for Cardiovascular Angiography and Interventions, and Society of Thoracic Surgeons. *Circulation.* 2008;118:e523-e661.
5. O'Brien SM, Shahian DM, Filardo G, et al. The Society of Thoracic Surgeons 2008 cardiac surgery risk models: part 2—isolated valve surgery. *Ann Thorac Surg.* 2009;88:S23-S42.
6. Shroyer AL, Coombs LP, Peterson ED, et al. The Society of Thoracic Surgeons: 30-day operative mortality and morbidity risk models. *Ann Thorac Surg.* 2003; 75:1856-1864.

Miscellaneous

Cardiac Magnetic Resonance Imaging Pericardial Late Gadolinium Enhancement and Elevated Inflammatory Markers Can Predict the Reversibility of Constrictive Pericarditis After Antiinflammatory Medical Therapy: A Pilot Study

Feng DL, Glockner J, Kim K, et al (Metropolitan Heart and Vascular Inst, Minneapolis, MN; Mayo Clinic, Rochester, MN)
Circulation 124:1830-1837, 2011

Background.—Constrictive pericarditis (CP) is a disabling disease, and usually requires pericardiectomy to relieve heart failure. Reversible CP has been described, but there is no known method to predict the reversibility. Pericardial inflammation may be a marker for reversibility. As a pilot study, we assessed whether cardiac magnetic resonance imaging pericardial late gadolinium enhancement (LGE) and inflammatory biomarkers could predict the reversibility of CP after antiinflammatory therapy.

Method and Results.—Twenty-nine CP patients received antiinflammatory medications after cardiac magnetic resonance imaging. Fourteen patients had resolution of CP, whereas 15 patients had persistent CP after 13 months of follow-up. Baseline LGE pericardial thickness was greater in the group with reversible CP than in the persistent CP group (4 ± 1 versus 2 ± 1 mm, $P = 0.001$). Qualitative intensity of pericardial LGE was moderate or severe in 93% of the group with reversible CP and in 33% of the persistent CP group ($P = 0.002$). Cardiac magnetic resonance imaging LGE pericardial thickness ≥ 3 mm had 86% sensitivity and 80% specificity to predict CP reversibility. The group with reversible CP also had higher baseline C-reactive protein and erythrocyte sedimentation rate than the persistent CP group (59 ± 52 versus 12 ± 14 mg/L, $P = 0.04$ and 49 ± 25 versus 15 ± 16 mm/h, $P = 0.04$, respectively). Antiinflammatory therapy was associated with a reduction in C-reactive protein, erythrocyte sedimentation rate, and pericardial LGE in the group with reversible CP but not in the persistent CP group.

Conclusions.—Reversible CP was associated with pericardial and systemic inflammation. Antiinflammatory therapy was associated with a reduction in pericardial and systemic inflammation and LGE pericardial thickness, with resolution of CP physiology and symptoms. Further studies in a larger number of patients are needed.

▶ The development of constrictive pericarditis (CP) results in hemodynamic pathophysiologic changes that usually require surgical pericardiectomy. However, resolution of constrictive pericarditis without surgery has been reported.[1,2] One possibility is that in these patients, the constrictive pathophysiology resulted from inflammatory changes with edema and pericardial thickening that resolved resulting in the loss of cardiac compression.[3] The present study uses the observation that cardiac magnetic resonance (CMR) imaging with late gadolinium enhancement (LGE) accurately identifies pericardial inflammation.[4] In this study, contrast-enhanced CMR was done in 288 patients for pericardial enhancement, with 89 having a diagnosis of CP. Of these, 29 received anti-inflammatory medications (IM), and 60 received no IM. On follow-up of approximately 1 year, of those receiving IM, 48% resolved their CP. Of the 60 patients without IM, 65% had pericardiectomy, and the rest did not resolve their CP. Predictive of resolution of the CP was the presence of moderate to severe LGE compared with no or lesser degrees of LGE (93% vs 33%; $P = .002$). Furthermore, maximal thickness of pericardium measured on LGE was greater in those patients who resolved than in those that persisted with CP. Also patients who resolved had had more baseline systemic inflammation as manifested by higher C-reactive protein and erythrocyte sedimentation rate levels than those with persistent CP. The systemic inflammatory markers correlated with the severity of the LGE and IM was associated with significant reduction in systemic inflammatory markers and echocardiographic evidence of the pathophysiologic hemodynamics of CP. The problems with the study include possible difficulty in imaging the thickness of the LGE. Because this was a small, retrospective, observational study with a relatively short follow-up, it is unknown whether the patients with resolved CP will have a durable long-term resolution. Finally, because the number of patients was too small, it is not clear what the incremental value of severity of LGE is over simply the increased inflammatory markers in predicting reversibility. This was only a pilot study and will need a larger controlled study to validate these findings.

M. D. Cheitlin, MD

References

1. Sagristà-Sauleda J, Permanyer-Miralda G, Candell-Riera J, Angel J, Soler-Soler J. Transient cardiac constriction: an unrecognized pattern of evolution in effusive acute idiopathic pericarditis. *Am J Cardiol.* 1987;59:961-966.
2. Oh JK, Hatle LK, Mulvagh SL, Tajik AJ. Transient constrictive pericarditis: diagnosis by two-dimensional Doppler echocardiography. *Mayo Clin Proc.* 1993;68:1158-1164.
3. Haley JH, Tajik AJ, Danielson GK, Schaff HV, Mulvagh SL, Oh JK. Transient constrictive pericarditis: causes and natural history. *J Am Coll Cardiol.* 2004;43:271-275.
4. Taylor AM, Dymarkowski S, Verbeken EK, Bogaert J. Detection of pericardial inflammation with late-enhancement cardiac magnetic resonance imaging: initial results. *Eur Radiol.* 2006;16:569-574.

Colchicine prevents early postoperative pericardial and pleural effusions

Imazio M, Brucato A, Rovere ME, et al (Maria Vittoria Hosp, Torino, Italy; Ospedali Riuniti, Bergamo, Italy; Ospedale Mauriziano, Torino, Italy; et al)
Am Heart J 162:527-532.e1, 2011

Background.—No preventive pharmacologic strategies have been proven efficacious for the prevention of postoperative effusions after cardiac surgery. Colchicine is safe and efficacious for the prevention of pericarditis. On this basis, we realized a substudy of the COPPS trial to assess the efficacy and safety of colchicine for the prevention of postoperative pericardial and pleural effusions.

Methods.—The COPPS is a multicenter, double-blind, randomized trial, where 360 consecutive patients (mean age 65.7 ± 12.3 years, 66% men), 180 in each treatment arm, were randomized on the third postoperative day to receive placebo or colchicine for 1 month (1.0 mg twice daily for the first day, followed by a maintenance dose of 0.5 mg twice daily in patients ≥70 kg, and halved doses for patients <70 kg). The incidence of postoperative effusions was evaluated in each study group.

Results.—Despite similar baseline features, colchicine significantly reduced the incidence of postoperative pericardial (12.8% vs 22.8%, $P = .019$, relative risk reduction 43.9%, no. of patients needed to treat 10) and pleural effusions (12.2% vs 25.6%, $P = .002$, relative risk reduction 52.3%, no. of patients needed to treat 8). The rate of side effects (only gastrointestinal intolerance) and drug withdrawal was similar in the study groups with a trend toward an increased rate of both events for colchicine. In multivariable analysis, female gender (hazard ratio 1.76, 95% CI 1.03-3.03, $P = .040$) and pleura incision (hazard ratio 2.58, 95% CI 1.53-4.53, $P < .001$) were risk factors for postoperative effusions.

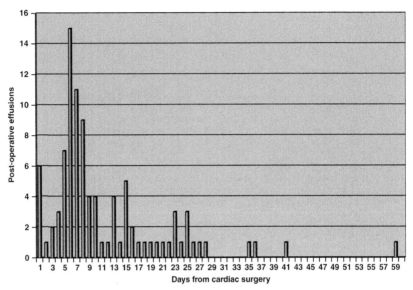

FIGURE 1.—Time course of postoperative effusions after cardiac surgery. (Reprinted from the American Heart Journal, Imazio M, Brucato A, Rovere ME, et al. Colchicine prevents early postoperative pericardial and pleural effusions. *Am Heart J.* 2011;162:527-532.e1. Copyright 2011, with permission from Elsevier.)

Conclusions.—Colchicine is safe and efficacious for the primary prevention of postoperative effusions after cardiac surgery (Figs 1 and 2).

▶ Postoperative pericardial and pleural effusions are common after cardiac surgery, and no pharmacologic strategies have been efficacious in prevention.[1,2] The incidence is variable and ranges from 2% to 64% of patients but is usually between 20% and 30%.[3,4] Although the effusions caused by the surgery itself frequently run a benign course,[5,6] the effusions that occur after several days but within a month from the surgery may indicate cardiac injury, be recurrent and increase time in the hospital,[7,8] or be caused by heart failure or pulmonary embolism. Symptomatic effusions due to postoperative pericarditis may require prolonged nonsteroidal anti-inflammatory drugs or corticosteroids and even require paracentesis. Colchicine may be of potential use here in that it has been shown to be safe and effective in prevention of pericarditis[9,10] and postpericardiotomy syndrome.[11] The current study, a substudy of the COPPS (Colchicine for the Prevention of the Post-pericardiotomy Syndrome) trial, found that colchicine prevented pericardial effusions (Relative Risk Reduction [RRR], 44%) and pleural effusions (RRR, 52%) without significant side effects.[11] The mechanism by which colchicine reduces the incidence of effusions is unknown but probably results from its inhibition of the process of microtubule formation inhibiting the movement of intercellular granules,

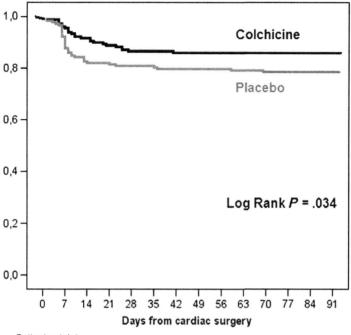

Patients at risk:
Colchicine:
    180 172 163 157 153 153 152 152   152 151 150   150 150 150
Placebo:
    180 163 144 143 141 141 139 138   138 137 135   135 135 134

FIGURE 2.—Kaplan-Meier postoperative pericardial effusion—free survival curve according to study groups (placebo/colchicine) in the first 90 days after cardiac surgery. (Reprinted from the American Heart Journal, Imazio M, Brucato A, Rovere ME, et al. Colchicine prevents early postoperative pericardial and pleural effusions. *Am Heart J.* 2011;162:527-532.e1. Copyright 2011, with permission from Elsevier.)

leukocyte function, and inflammation.[12] Reduction in postoperative effusions will decrease time in the hospital for some patients and improve their quality of life.

M. D. Cheitlin, MD

References

1. Meurin P, Tabet JY, Thabut G, et al; French Society of Cardiology. Nonsteroidal anti-inflammatory drug treatment for postoperative pericardial effusion: a multi-center randomized, double-blind trial. *Ann Intern Med.* 2010;152:137-143.
2. Imazio M. Asymptomatic postoperative pericardial effusions: against the routine use of anti-inflammatory drug therapy. *Ann Intern Med.* 2010;152:186-187.
3. Ashikhmina EA, Schaff HV, Sinak LJ, et al. Pericardial effusion after cardiac surgery: risk factors, patient profiles, and contemporary management. *Ann Thorac Surg.* 2010;89:112-118.
4. Pepi M, Muratori M, Barbier P, et al. Pericardial effusion after cardiac surgery: incidence, site, size, and haemodynamic consequences. *Br Heart J.* 1994;72:327-331.

5. Heidecker J, Sahn SA. The spectrum of pleural effusions after coronary artery bypass grafting surgery. *Clin Chest Med.* 2006;27:267-283.
6. Weitzman LB, Tinker WP, Kronzon I, Cohen ML, Glassman E, Spencer FC. The incidence and natural history of pericardial effusion after cardiac surgery—an echocardiographic study. *Circulation.* 1984;69:506-511.
7. Prince SE, Cunha BA. Postpericardiotomy syndrome. *Heart Lung.* 1997;26: 165-168.
8. Hoit BD. Pericardial and postpericardial injury syndromes. In: Rose BD, ed. *UptoDate.* Wellesley, MA: Uptodate online; 2010.
9. Imazio M, Bobbio M, Cecchi E, et al. Colchicine as first-choice therapy for recurrent pericarditis: results of the CORE (COlchicine for REcurrent pericarditis) trial. *Arch Intern Med.* 2005;165:1987-1991.
10. Imazio M, Brucato A, Trinchero R, et al. Colchicine for pericarditis: hype or hope. *Eur Heart J.* 2009;30:532-539.
11. Imazio M, Trinchero R, Brucato A, et al; COPPS Investigators. COlchicine for the Prevention of the Post-pericardiotomy Syndrome (COPPS): a multicentre, randomized, double-blind, placebo-controlled trial. *Eur Heart J.* 2010;31: 2749-2754.
12. Molad Y. Update on colchicine and its mechanism of action. *Curr Rheumatol Rep.* 2002;3:252-256.

Effect of short-term NSAID use on echocardiographic parameters in elderly people: a population-based cohort study

van den Hondel KE, Eijgelsheim M, Ruiter R, et al (Erasmus Med Ctr, Rotterdam, The Netherlands)
Heart 97:540-543, 2011

Background.—Non-steroidal anti-inflammatory drugs (NSAIDs) are associated with an increased risk of heart failure. NSAIDs inhibit the synthesis of renal prostaglandin, which results in a higher total blood volume, cardiac output and preload. The association between recent start of NSAIDs in elderly people and echocardiographic parameters was investigated.

Methods.—In the Rotterdam Study, a population-based cohort study, the effect of NSAIDs on left ventricular end-systolic dimension, left ventricular end-diastolic dimension, fractional shortening and left ventricular systolic function was studied in all participants for whom an echocardiogram was available (n=5307). NSAID use was categorised as current NSAID use on the date of echocardiography, past use and never used before echocardiography during the study period. Current use was divided into short-term NSAID use (≤ 14 days) and long-term NSAID use (>14 days). Associations between drug exposure and echocardiographic measurements were assessed using linear and logistic regression analyses.

Results.—Current NSAID use for <14 days was associated with a significantly higher left ventricular end-systolic dimension (+1.74 mm, 95% CI 0.20 to 3.28), left ventricular end-diastolic dimension (+3.69 mm, 95% CI 1.08 to 6.31) and significantly lower fractional shortening (−6.03%, 95% CI −9.81% to −2.26%) compared with non-users. Current NSAID use for >14 days was associated with a higher left end-diastolic dimension

(+1.96 mm, 95% CI 0.82 to 3.11) but there was no change in the other echocardiographic parameters.

Conclusion.—This study is the first to investigate the association between NSAIDs and echocardiographic parameters and suggests that there is a transient effect of short-term use of NSAIDs on the left ventricular dimension and function of the heart.

▶ Nonsteroidal anti-inflammatory drugs (NSAIDS) have been associated with the initiation or exacerbation of heart failure.[1,2] The elderly are at most risk from heart failure, and the incidence and prevalence are increasing in this age group.[3] NSAIDS inhibit renal prostaglandins, resulting in a lower renal blood flow and subsequent increased sodium reabsorption and water retention.[4] Additionally, prostaglandin inhibition stimulates the vasopressin effect in collecting tubules resulting in free water retention.[5,6] These effects increase blood volume and in susceptible individuals can precipitate heart failure. Since NSAIDS are used in the elderly, the potential to increase heart failure is of particular importance. The present population-based study in subjects 55 years or older shows that short-term use of NSAIDS increase end-diastolic and end-systolic diameters and decrease fractional shortening. Longer use of NSAIDS showed increase only in end-diastolic diameter consistent with the explanation that the heart was able to compensate through the Frank-Starling mechanism by increasing stroke volume, returning end-systolic diameter, and fractional shortening to baseline.

Most of the population studied was normal without heart disease, and no conclusion about the long-term effect of NSAIDS, especially in patients with cardiac disease, can be drawn from this study. The consequence of increasing blood volume and decreasing fractional shortening in patients with heart disease or even compensated heart failure is precipitating or worsening heart failure. Since this was a retrospective study with a single echocardiogram, to fully evaluate the danger of NSAIDS precipitating heart failure will require a placebo-controlled trial with echocardiograms at baseline and after a given exposure to NSAIDS. There are also hypertensive and prothrombotic effects of NSAIDS,[7-9] all of which make the use of NSAIDS in patients with heart disease questionable.

M. D. Cheitlin, MD

References

1. Page J, Henry D. Consumption of NSAIDs and the development of congestive heart failure in elderly patients: an underrecognized public health problem. *Arch Intern Med.* 2000;160:777-784.
2. Feenstra J, Heerdink ER, Grobbee DE, Stricker BH. Association of nonsteroidal anti-inflammatory drugs with first occurrence of heart failure and with relapsing heart failure: the Rotterdam Study. *Arch Intern Med.* 2002;162:265-270.
3. Kannel WB. Incidence and epidemiology of heart failure. *Heart Fail Rev.* 2000;5:167-173.
4. Delmas PD. Non-steroidal anti-inflammatory drugs and renal function. *Br J Rheumatol.* 1995;34:25-28.
5. Whelton A. Renal and related cardiovascular effects of conventional and COX-2-specific NSAIDs and non-NSAID analgesics. *Am J Ther.* 2000;7:63-74.

6. Bennett WM, Henrich WL, Stoff JS. The renal effects of nonsteroidal anti-inflammatory drugs: summary and recommendations. *Am J Kidney Dis.* 1996; 28:S56-S62.
7. Johnson AG, Nguyen TV, Day RO. Do nonsteroidal anti-inflammatory drugs affect blood pressure? A meta-analysis. *Ann Intern Med.* 1994;121:289-300.
8. Zhang J, Ding EL, Song Y. Adverse effects of cyclooxygenase 2 inhibitors on renal and arrhythmia events: meta-analysis of randomized trials. *JAMA.* 2006;296: 1619-1632.
9. Crofford LJ, Breyer MD, Strand CV, et al. Cardiovascular effects of selective COX-2 inhibition: is there a class effect? The International COX-2 Study Group. *J Rheumatol.* 2006;33:1403-1408.

Efficacy and Safety of *Bosentan* for Pulmonary Arterial Hypertension in Adults With Congenital Heart Disease

Monfredi O, Griffiths L, Clarke B, et al (Univ of Manchester, UK; Manchester Royal Infirmary, UK)

Am J Cardiol 108:1483-1488, 2011

The dual endothelin receptor antagonist, bosentan, has been shown to be well tolerated and effective in improving pulmonary arterial hypertension (PAH) symptoms in patients with Eisenmenger syndrome but data from longer-term studies are lacking. The aim of this study was to retrospectively analyze the long-term efficacy and safety of bosentan in adults with PAH secondary to congenital heart disease (PAH-CHD). Prospectively collected data from adult patients with PAH-CHD (with and without Down syndrome) initiated on bosentan from October 2007 through June 2010 were analyzed. Parameters measured before bosentan initiation (62.5 mg 2 times/day for 4 weeks titrated to 125 mg 2 times/day) and at each follow-up (1 month and 3, 6, 9, 12, 18, and 24 months) included exercise capacity (6-minute walk distance [6MWD]), pretest oxygen saturation, liver enzymes, and hemoglobin. Data were analyzed from 39 patients with PAH-CHD (10 with Down syndrome) who had received ≥1 dose of bosentan (mean duration of therapy 2.1 ± 1.5 years). A significant (p <0.0001) average improvement in 6MWD of 54 m over a 2-year period in patients with PAH-CHD without Down syndrome was observed. Men patients had a 6MWD of 33 m greater than women (p <0.01). In all patients, oxygen saturation, liver enzymes, and hemoglobin levels remained stable. There were no discontinuations from bosentan owing to adverse events. In conclusion, patients with PAH-CHD without Down syndrome gain long-term symptomatic benefits in exercise capacity after bosentan treatment. Men seem to benefit more on bosentan treatment. Bosentan appears to be well tolerated in patients with PAH-CHD with or without Down syndrome (Fig 1).

▶ Eisenmenger syndrome in patients with congenital heart disease until recently has lacked effective treatment. With the prostacyclin drugs and the endothelin antagonists, decrease in pulmonary artery pressure and pulmonary vascular resistance have been reported. The Bosentan Randomized Trial of Endothelin

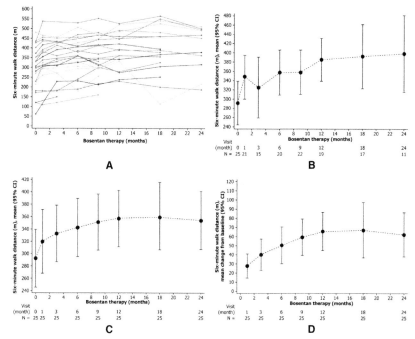

FIGURE 1.—Six-minute distance for patients without Down syndrome treated for up to 24 months with bosentan. (*A*) Absolute values for all patients. (*B*) Absolute values (mean ± SD) for all patients with no imputation for missing values. (*C*) Absolute values (mean ± SD) for all patients with last observation carried forward imputation to account for missing values. (*D*) Change from baseline values (mean ± SD) for all patients with last observation carried forward imputation to account for missing values. CI = confidence interval. (Reprinted from the American Journal of Cardiology, Monfredi O, Griffiths L, Clarke B, et al. Efficacy and safety of *bosentan* for pulmonary arterial hypertension in adults with congenital heart disease. *Am J Cardiol.* 2011;108:1483-1488. Copyright 2011, with permission from Elsevier.)

Antagonist Therapy-5 (BREATHE-5) study showed that bosentan, a dual endothelin receptor antagonist that blocks endothelin A and B receptors, improved exercise capacity and pulmonary hemodynamics in patients with Eisenmenger syndrome.[1] This is a study from a tertiary adult congenital cardiac center that reports the medium-term follow-up on 39 adult patients with congenital heart problems and Eisenmenger syndrome, 10 with Down syndrome, treated with bosentan as monotherapy with 2 patients also on sildenafil. The 6-minute walking distance (6MWD) improved impressively for up to 2 years follow-up, and the arterial O_2 saturation remained stable. The bosentan was well tolerated in the patients both with and without Down syndrome. This is consistent with 2 other retrospective studies that also showed improvement in exercise capacity with endothelin receptor antagonists over a similar follow-up time.[2,3] Recently there has been evidence that advanced therapy for Eisenmenger syndrome has increased survival compared with untreated patients.[4] Considering the earlier belief that patients with congenital heart disease—related severe pulmonary hypertension may have fewer terminal pulmonary vessels, and that the vascular obstruction was irreversible and therefore incapable of improvement with any type of therapy, these recent findings are more hopeful. One possibility is that the obstructed pulmonary vessels with therapy may remodel with luminal expansion. All these patients were on multiple drugs in addition to bosentan, and it is not possible to conclude that endothelin receptor antagonism alone was responsible for the improvement in exercise tolerance. The outlook for patients with Eisenmenger syndrome has gradually gotten brighter.

M. D. Cheitlin, MD

References

1. Galiè N, Beghetti M, Gatzoulis MA, et al; Bosentan Randomized Trial of Endothelin Antagonist Therapy-5 (BREATHE-5) Investigators. Bosentan therapy in patients with Eisenmenger syndrome: a multicenter, double-blind, randomized, placebo-controlled study. *Circulation.* 2006;114:48-54.
2. Diller GP, Dimopoulos K, Kaya MG, et al. Long-term safety, tolerability and efficacy of bosentan in adults with pulmonary arterial hypertension associated with congenital heart disease. *Heart.* 2007;93:974-976.
3. Kermeen FD, Franks C, O'Brien K, et al. Endothelin receptor antagonists are an effective long term treatment option in pulmonary arterial hypertension associated with congenital heart disease with or without trisomy 21. *Heart Lung Circ.* 2010; 19:595-600.
4. Dimopoulos K, Inuzuka R, Goletto S, et al. Improved survival among patients with Eisenmenger syndrome receiving advanced therapy for pulmonary arterial hypertension. *Circulation.* 2010;121:20-25.

Percutaneous Versus Surgical Revascularization in Patients With Ischemic Mitral Regurgitation

Kang D-H, Sun BJ, Kim D-H, et al (Univ of Ulsan, Seoul, Korea)
Circulation 124:S156-S162, 2011

Background.—The proper way of revascularization remains controversial in patients with ischemic mitral regurgitation (IMR). We sought to compare the long-term results of percutaneous coronary intervention (PCI) and surgical revascularization in IMR.

Methods and Results.—From 1996 to 2008, 185 consecutive patients (132 men; age, 63 ± 9 years) with significant IMR underwent PCI (PCI group) (n=66) or coronary artery bypass graft surgery (OP group) (n=119). In the OP group, 68 (57%) patients also underwent concomitant mitral annuloplasty. Significant IMR was defined as functional MR occurring >1 week after myocardial infarction with an effective regurgitant orifice area ≥ 0.2 cm^2. During a median follow-up of 54 months, there were 2 operative mortalities, 26 cardiac deaths, and 11 heart failure hospitalizations in the OP group and 22 cardiac deaths and 10 heart failure hospitalizations in the PCI group. The survival and cardiac mortality rates were not significantly different between the 2 groups, but event-free survival rates were significantly higher in the OP group. For the 45 propensity score-matched pairs, the risk of cardiac events was significantly lower in the OP group than in the PCI group (hazard ratio, 0.499; 95% CI, 0.251 to 0.990; $P = 0.043$). Compared with patients who underwent coronary artery bypass graft surgery alone, event-free survival rates were significantly higher in those who underwent additional mitral annuloplasty.

Conclusions.—Compared with PCI, surgical revascularization is associated with an improved long-term event-free survival, and concomitant mitral annuloplasty should be considered in patients with significant IMR.

▶ Ischemic mitral regurgitation (IMR) is frequently seen in the acute and chronic stages of myocardial infarction and is associated with an adverse prognosis, worse with increasing severity of the IMR.[1-3] Revascularization, both surgical and percutaneous (percutaneous coronary intervention [PCI]), has been shown to improve survival compared with medical management in patients with IMR,[3,4] but surgical revascularization has the advantage of a more complete revascularization and of improving the degree of MR by the addition of a mitral valve procedure. The down side of surgery is a higher procedural risk compared with PCI and the lack of proof that the reduction of the severity of the IMR adds to the benefit of revascularization.[5,6] This study, using a prospectively collected registry of patients with IMR, compares the long-term outcomes of PCI with surgical revascularization and evaluates the value of additional mitral annuloplasty. The patients had left ventricular (LV) systolic dysfunction, severe IMR defined by an effective orifice area ≥ 0.2 cm^2 more than 1 week after a myocardial infarction, and no evidence of primary valve disease. The method of revascularization and mitral valve repair was at the discretion of the patient's physician. A propensity score analysis was done on 45 matched pairs of patients after a follow-up period of almost 4.5 years. The primary clinical endpoint was the composite of in-hospital death, cardiac death, and hospitalization due to heart failure on follow-up. The study demonstrated that in patients with significant IMR and surgical revascularization with mitral annuloplasty, there is a higher event-free survival through improving IMR and LV function more effectively compared with PCI. Further, the greater the degree of IMR, the higher was the follow-up mortality, findings consistent with those of other studies.[2,7] In comparing surgical revascularization alone (coronary artery bypass grafting [CABG]) with revascularization and annuloplasty (mitral valve [MV] repair), on follow-up there was symptom improvement from baseline in both groups, greater in the MV repair group, and the functional status at 6 months after surgery was significantly better in the MV repair group. During follow-up, the event-free survival rates were significantly lower in the MV repair patients, but survival alone was no different. The problem with this study is that it was an observational study, and the decision for surgery alone versus with MV repair was not randomized. Also, it is not clear what should be done with patients who have only moderate IMR.

M. D. Cheitlin, MD

References

1. Lamas GA, Mitchell GF, Flaker GC, et al. Clinical significance of mitral regurgitation after acute myocardial infarction. Survival and ventricular enlargement investigators. *Circulation*. 1997;96:827-833.
2. Grigioni F, Enriquez-Sarano M, Zehr KJ, Bailey KR, Tajik AJ. Ischemic mitral regurgitation: long-term outcome and prognostic implications with quantitative Doppler assessment. *Circulation*. 2001;103:1759-1764.

3. Hickey MS, Smith LR, Muhlbaier L, et al. Current prognosis of ischemic mitral regurgitation. Implications for future management. *Circulation.* 1988;78:I51-I59.
4. Trichon BH, Glower DD, Shaw LK, et al. Survival after coronary revascularization, with and without mitral valve surgery, in patients with ischemic mitral regurgitation. *Circulation.* 2003;108:II103-II110.
5. Wu AH, Aaronson KD, Bolling SF, Pagani FD, Welch K, Koelling TM. Impact of mitral valve annuloplasty on mortality risk in patients with mitral regurgitation and left ventricular systolic dysfunction. *J Am Coll Cardiol.* 2005;45:381-387.
6. Mihaljevic T, Lam BK, Rajeswaran J, et al. Impact of mitral valve annuloplasty combined with revascularization in patients with functional ischemic mitral regurgitation. *J Am Coll Cardiol.* 2007;49:2191-2201.
7. Bursi F, Enriquez-Sarano M, Nkomo VT, et al. Heart failure and death after myocardial infarction in the community: the emerging role of mitral regurgitation. *Circulation.* 2005;111:295-301.

Benefit of atrial septal defect closure in adults: impact of age

Humenberger M, Rosenhek R, Gabriel H, et al (Med Univ of Vienna, Austria; et al)
Eur Heart J 32:553-560, 2011

Aims.—To evaluate the effect of age on the clinical benefit of atrial septal defect (ASD) closure in adults.

Methods and Results.—Functional status, the presence of arrhythmias, right ventricular (RV) remodelling, and pulmonary artery pressure (PAP) were studied in 236 consecutive patients undergoing transcatheter ASD closure [164 females, mean age of 49 ± 18 years, 78 younger than 40 years (Group A), 84 between 40 and 60 years (Group B) and 74 older than 60 years (Group C)]. Defect size [median 22 mm (inter-quartile range, 19, 26 mm)] and shunt ratio [Qp:Qs 2.2 (1.7, 2.9)] did not differ among age groups. Older patients had, however, more advanced symptoms and both, PAP ($r = 0.65$, $P < 0.0001$) and RV size ($r = 0.28$, $P < 0.0001$), were significantly related to age. Post-interventionally, RV size decreased from 41 ± 7, 43 ± 7, and 45 ± 6 mm to 32 ± 5, 34 ± 5, and 37 ± 5 mm for Groups A, B, and C, respectively ($P < 0.0001$), and PAP decreased from 31 ± 7, 37 ± 10, and 53 ± 17 mmHg to 26 ± 5, 30 ± 6, and 43 ± 14 mmHg ($P < 0.0001$), respectively. Absolute changes in RV size ($P = 0.80$) and PAP ($P = 0.24$) did not significantly differ among groups. Symptoms were present in 13, 49, and 83% of the patients before and in 3, 11, and 34% after intervention in Groups A, B, and C. Functional status was related to PAP.

Conclusions.—At any age, ASD closure is followed by symptomatic improvement and regression of PAP and RV size. However, the best outcome is achieved in patients with less functional impairment and less elevated PAP. Considering the continuous increase in symptoms, RV remodelling, and PAP with age, ASD closure must be recommended irrespective of symptoms early after diagnosis even in adults of advanced age (Figs 1-4).

▶ Patients with seconded atrial septal defects (ASD) with left-to-right shunts large enough to increase right atrial and right ventricular size, commonly with

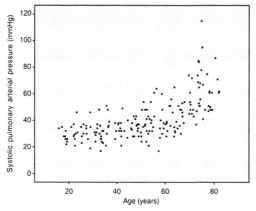

FIGURE 1.—Correlation between systolic pulmonary artery pressure and age ($r = 0.65$, $P < 0.0001$). (Reprinted from Humenberger M, Rosenhek R, Gabriel H, et al. Benefit of atrial septal defect closure in adults: impact of age. *Eur Heart J.* 2011;32:553-560, by permission of The European Society of Cardiology.)

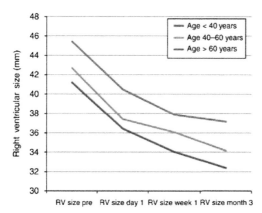

FIGURE 2.—Right ventricular (RV) size before, 1 day, 1 week, and 3 months after atrial septal defect closure for patients younger than 40 years (green line), patients aged 40–60 years (orange line), and patients older than 60 years (red line). For interpretation of the references to color in this figure legend, the reader is referred to web version of this article. (Reprinted from Humenberger M, Rosenhek R, Gabriel H, et al. Benefit of atrial septal defect closure in adults: impact of age. *Eur Heart J.* 2011;32:553-560, by permission of The European Society of Cardiology.)

a pulmonary blood flow/subcutaneous blood flow > 1.5, are recommended to undergo closure at any age.[1] Although there have been small series of short duration showing reduction in symptoms and decrease in right ventricular size in the older population after ASD closure,[2-4] the 1 randomized study in patients older than 40 years found reduced morbidity but not reduced mortality after closure.[5] Therefore, the benefits of ASD closure in adults, especially those over age 65, remain uncertain.[6-8] Transcatheter closure has become the procedure of choice when there are no contraindications and when experienced interventionists are available, and it appears to be safer for older patients with

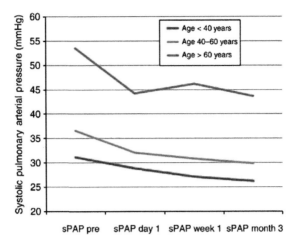

FIGURE 3.—Systolic pulmonary artery pressure (sPAP) before, 1 day, 1 week, and 3 months after atrial septal defect closure for patients younger than 40 years (green line), patients aged 40–60 years (orange line), and patients older than 60 years (red line). For interpretation of the references to color in this figure legend, the reader is referred to web version of this article. (Reprinted from Humenberger M, Rosenhek R, Gabriel H, et al. Benefit of atrial septal defect closure in adults: impact of age. *Eur Heart J*. 2011;32:553-560, by permission of The European Society of Cardiology.)

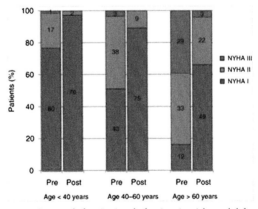

FIGURE 4.—Symptomatic status before (pre) and after (post) atrial septal defect closure for patients younger than 40 years, patients aged 40–60 years, and patients older than 60 years. (Reprinted from Humenberger M, Rosenhek R, Gabriel H, et al. Benefit of atrial septal defect closure in adults: impact of age. *Eur Heart J*. 2011;32:553-560, by permission of The European Society of Cardiology.)

comorbidities. This observational study on 236 consecutive patients with ASD (158 ≥ 40 years of age) is the largest study of consecutive adult patients with a comprehensive evaluation of the impact of age on the long-term effect of ASD closure on symptoms, atrial fibrillation (AF), right ventricular size, and pulmonary artery pressure (PAP). There were 16% of patients in whom transcatheter closure was contraindicated, and the ASD was closed surgically. The remaining 84% of defects were closed by transcatheter techniques, 99.6% successfully. There were no deaths, and there was 1 thromboembolism after the closure device had been placed. There were 3 other cerebrovascular events, 1 of which was minor cerebellar bleeding caused by anticoagulants for AF. The results showed a decrease in symptoms, in PAP and in right ventricular size similarly in each age group. With transcatheter closure, 6% of the patients developed AF within 3 months of the procedure, all of whom had sinus rhythm restored. Therefore, transcatheter closure may trigger transient AF, chronic AF is unlikely to be affected, and paroxysmal AF may improve, although that likely decreases with increasing age.[9] The problems with this study are its observational design, although the effect on survival can only be surmised because it would be unethical to do a randomized study. This study gives support to the ACC/AHA guideline recommendation for closure of significant ASD at any age.

M. D. Cheitlin, MD

References

1. Warnes CA, Williams RG, Bashore TM, et al. ACC/AHA 2008 guidelines for the management of adults with congenital heart disease: a report of the American College of Cardiology/American Heart Association Task Force on Practice Guidelines (writing committee to develop guidelines on the management of adults with congenital heart disease). *Circulation.* 2008;118:e714-e833.
2. Swan L, Varma C, Yip J, et al. Transcatheter device closure of atrial septal defects in the elderly: technical considerations and short-term outcomes. *Int J Cardiol.* 2006;107:207-210.
3. Elshershari H, Cao QL, Hijazi ZM. Transcatheter device closure of atrial septal defects in patients older than 60 years of age: immediate and follow-up results. *J Invasive Cardiol.* 2008;20:173-176.
4. Yalonetsky S, Lorber A. Comparative changes of pulmonary artery pressure values and tricuspid valve regurgitation following transcatheter atrial septal defect closure in adults and the elderly. *Congenit Heart Dis.* 2009;4:17-20.
5. Attie F, Rosas M, Granados N, Zabal C, Buendía A, Calderón J. Surgical treatment for secundum atrial septal defects in patients >40 years old. A randomized clinical trial. *J Am Coll Cardiol.* 2001;38:2035-2042.
6. Gatzoulis MA, Redington AN, Somerville J, Shore DF. Should atrial septal defects in adults be closed? *Ann Thorac Surg.* 1996;61:657-659.
7. Ward C. Secundum atrial septal defect: routine surgical treatment is not of proven benefit. *Br Heart J.* 1994;71:219-223.
8. Webb G. Do patients over 40 years of age benefit from closure of an atrial septal defect? *Heart.* 2001;85:249-250.
9. Spies C, Khandelwal A, Timmermanns I, Schräder R. Incidence of atrial fibrillation following transcatheter closure of atrial septal defects in adults. *Am J Cardiol.* 2008;102:902-906.

Left Ventricular Function in Adult Patients With Atrial Septal Defect: Implication for Development of Heart Failure After Transcatheter Closure

Masutani S, Senzaki H (Saitama Med Univ, Hidaka, Japan)
J Card Fail 17:957-963, 2011

Despite advances in device closure for atrial septal defect (ASD), post-closure heart failure observed in adult patients remains a clinical problem. Although right heart volume overload is the fundamental pathophysiology in ASD, the post-closure heart failure characterized by acute pulmonary congestion is likely because of age-related left ventricular diastolic dysfunction, which is manifested by acute volume loading with ASD closure. Aging also appears to play important roles in the pathophysiology of heart failure through several mechanisms other than diastolic dysfunction, including ventricular systolic and vascular stiffening and increased incidence of comorbidities that significantly affect cardiovascular function. Recent studies suggested that accurate assessment of preclosure diastolic function, such as test ASD occlusion, may help identify high-risk patients for post-closure heart failure. Anti-heart failure therapy before device closure or the use of fenestrated device appears to be effective in preventing post-closure heart failure in the high-risk patients. However, the long-term outcome of such patients remains to be elucidated. Future studies are warranted to construct an algorithm to identify and treat patients at high risk for heart failure after device closure of ASD (Figs 1 and 2).

▶ Device closure of secundum atrial septal defects (ASD) has become, when possible, the procedure of choice even in adults in institutions with experience in this technique.[1] Compared with surgery, device closure is associated with fewer complications and faster hemodynamic adaptation.[2,3] However, especially in the older adult, there are increasing reports of the development of heart failure (HF), manifested by pulmonary congestion, in patients with ASD device closure.[4-6] In some patients the presence of a large left-to-right shunt not only volume loads the right heart but may volume underload the left ventricle. These long-duration hemodynamics and age-related changes may occur in older patients with ASD and be responsible for the HF seen after sudden closure of the defect. The mechanism by which the pulmonary congestion occurs is probably related to the observation that in patients with ASD and large left-to-right shunts, the filling capacity of the left ventricle (LV) is

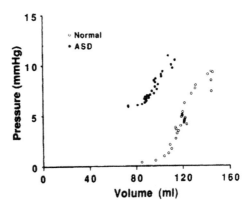

FIGURE 1.—Representative examples of left ventricular pressure-volume relationships during diastole of 1 cardiac cycle in a normal control and atrial septal defect (ASD) patient with pulmonary-to-systemic output ratio >3. Note the upward and leftward displacement of the pressure-volume relationship in the ASD patient. Reprinted with permission from Satoh et al.[13] *Editor's Note*: Please refer to original journal article for full references. (Reprinted from the Journal of Cardiac Failure, Masutani S, Senzaki H. Left ventricular function in adult patients with atrial septal defect: implication for development of heart failure after transcatheter closure. *J Card Fail*. 2011;17:957-963. Copyright 2011 with permission from Elsevier.)

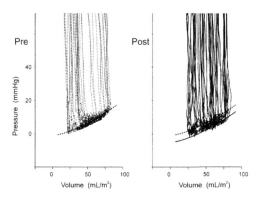

FIGURE 2.—End-diastolic pressure-volume relationships during inferior vena cava occlusion before (*left*) and after (*right*) device closure of atrial septal defect (ASD) in a 9-year-old patient with ASD. The end-diastolic pressure-volume relationship before the closure is reproduced in the right panel (*dashed line*) to assist comparison. End-diastolic pressure-volume relationship showed parallel downward shift immediately after ASD closure. (Reprinted from the Journal of Cardiac Failure, Masutani S, Senzaki H. Left ventricular function in adult patients with atrial septal defect: implication for development of heart failure after transcatheter closure. *J Card Fail.* 2011;17:957-963. Copyright 2011 with permission from Elsevier.)

diminished, suggested by observed comparable or greater LV end-diastolic pressure than seen in normal subjects.[7-9] Also, this stiffer diastolic LV was seen in studies showing a leftward and upward shift in the LV diastolic pressure-volume relationship.[7-9] With sudden closure of the ASD, there may be increased LV volume, thereby increasing suddenly the LV filling pressure and causing pulmonary congestion. This article reviews the current knowledge concerning LV mechanics both before and after ASD closure and explores in depth the possible factors responsible for the development of postclosure HF. Also discussed is how this knowledge is factored into clinical decision making when considering ASD closure, particularly focusing on the identification of patients at high risk of developing HF on closure.

M. D. Cheitlin, MD

References

1. Thanopoulos BD, Laskari CV, Tsaousis GS, Zarayelyan A, Vekiou A, Papadopoulos GS. Closure of atrial septal defects with the Amplatzer occlusion device: preliminary results. *J Am Coll Cardiol.* 1998;31:1110-1116.
2. Thomson JD, Aburawi EH, Watterson KG, Van Doorn C, Gibbs JL. Surgical and transcatheter (Amplatzer) closure of atrial septal defects: a prospective comparison of results and cost. *Heart.* 2002;87:466-469.
3. Du ZD, Hijazi ZM, Kleinman CS, Silverman NH, Larntz K. Comparison between transcatheter and surgical closure of secundum atrial septal defect in children and adults: results of a multicenter nonrandomized trial. *J Am Coll Cardiol.* 2002;39: 1836-1844.
4. Masutani S, Taketazu M, Mihara C, et al. Usefulness of early diastolic mitral annular velocity to predict plasma levels of brain natriuretic peptide and transient heart failure development after device closure of atrial septal defect. *Am J Cardiol.* 2009;104:1732-1736.
5. Ewert P, Berger F, Nagdyman N, et al. Masked left ventricular restriction in elderly patients with atrial septal defects: a contraindication for closure? *Catheter Cardiovasc Interv.* 2001;52:177-180.

424 / Cardiology

6. Holzer R, Cao QL, Hijazi ZM. Closure of a moderately large atrial septal defect with a self-fabricated fenestrated Amplatzer septal occluder in an 85-year-old patient with reduced diastolic elasticity of the left ventricle. *Catheter Cardiovasc Interv.* 2005;64:513-518.
7. Booth DC, Wisenbaugh T, Smith M, DeMaria AN. Left ventricular distensibility and passive elastic stiffness in atrial septal defect. *J Am Coll Cardiol.* 1988;12: 1231-1236.
8. Popio KA, Gorlin R, Teichholz LE, Cohn PF, Bechtel D, Herman MV. Abnormalities of left ventricular function and geometry in adults with an atrial septal defect. Ventriculographic, hemodynamic and echocardiographic studies. *Am J Cardiol.* 1975;36:302-308.
9. Satoh A, Katayama K, Hiro T, et al. Effect of right ventricular volume overload on left ventricular diastolic function in patients with atrial septal defect. *Jpn Circ J.* 1996;60:758-766.

Long-Term Follow-Up of Participants With Heart Failure in the Antihypertensive and Lipid-Lowering Treatment to Prevent Heart Attack Trial (ALLHAT)

Piller LB, for the ALLHAT Collaborative Research Group (Univ of Texas School of Public Health, Houston; et al)
Circulation 124:1811-1818, 2011

Background.—In the Antihypertensive and Lipid-Lowering Treatment to Prevent Heart Attack Trial (ALLHAT), a randomized, double-blind, practice-based, active-control, comparative effectiveness trial in high-risk hypertensive participants, risk of new-onset heart failure (HF) was higher in the amlodipine (2.5–10 mg/d) and lisinopril (10–40 mg/d) arms compared with the chlorthalidone (12.5–25 mg/d) arm. Similar to other studies, mortality rates following new-onset HF were very high (≥ 50% at 5 years), and were similar across randomized treatment arms. After the randomized phase of the trial ended in 2002, outcomes were determined from administrative databases.

Methods and Results.—With the use of national databases, posttrial follow-up mortality through 2006 was obtained on participants who developed new-onset HF during the randomized (in-trial) phase of ALLHAT. Mean follow-up for the entire period was 8.9 years. Of 1761 participants with incident HF in-trial, 1348 died. Post-HF all-cause mortality was similar across treatment groups, with adjusted hazard ratios (95% confidence intervals) of 0.95 (0.81–1.12) and 1.05 (0.89–1.25), respectively, for amlodipine and lisinopril compared with chlorthalidone, and 10-year adjusted rates of 86%, 87%, and 83%, respectively. All-cause mortality rates were also similar among those with reduced ejection fractions (84%) and preserved ejection fractions (81%), with no significant differences by randomized treatment arm.

Conclusions.—Once HF develops, risk of death is high and consistent across randomized treatment groups. Measures to prevent the development of HF, especially blood pressure control, must be a priority if mortality associated with the development of HF is to be addressed.

Clinical Trial Registration.—http://www.clinicaltrials.gov. Unique identifier: NCT00000542 (Fig 2).

▶ More than 5.8 million people in the United States have heart failure (HF), more than 670 000 new cases occur each year, and it is the most frequent reason for hospitalization in older patients.[1-3] Hypertension is a major cause of HF, and treatment with long-acting thiazide-type diuretics reduces the incidence of HF by 49% to 64%.[4-6] Other drugs such as beta-blockers, alpha-blockers, calcium channel blockers, and angiotensin converting enzyme inhibitors (ACEI) are also effective in treating hypertension and reducing HF and other hypertensive morbidity.[7,8] The Antihypertensive and Lipid-Lowering Treatment to Prevent Heart Attack Trial (ALLHAT) data are used here to look at the patients who had developed HF requiring hospitalization during the duration of the randomized, in-trial phase of the study. The patients were high-risk elderly patients with hypertension and 1 or more additional risk factors for heart attack. In a follow-up of mean 8.9 years, of those who developed HF, 77% died, and the all-cause mortality, whether attributed to any cause, was similar in the patients treated with amlodipine, lisinopril, and chlorthalidone. The 10-year mortality was high, and similar in those with preserved systolic dysfunction HF across treatment groups (83%–87%) and those with preserved systolic function HF (81%–89%). New-onset HF is a common complication of hypertension and

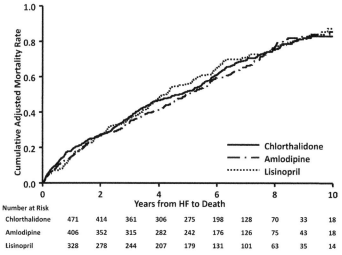

FIGURE 2.—Kaplan-Meier curves by treatment group for all-cause mortality of participants with hospitalized heart failure adjusted for baseline characteristics of age, race, gender, smoking, education, treatment of hypertension, systolic blood pressure, diastolic blood pressure, pulse, type II diabetes, left ventricular hypertrophy by ECG, history of coronary heart disease, body mass index, estimated glomerular filtration rate, and time to heart failure. Approximately 92% of participants with hospitalized (including hospitalized fatal) heart failure events during ALLHAT were part of the Heart Failure Validation Study (HFVS). This figure reflects only those participants with events meeting the ALLHAT HF definition in the HFVS[17,18] and eligible for extension. *Editor's Note:* Please refer to original journal article for full references. (Reprinted from Piller LB, for the ALLHAT Collaborative Research Group. Long-term follow-up of participants with heart failure in the antihypertensive and lipid-lowering treatment to prevent heart attack trial (ALLHAT). *Circulation.* 2011;124:1811-1818. © American Heart Association, Inc.)

has a very high subsequent mortality despite continued treatment of the hypertension.[3,9-11] There is no certainty that the results of this study would be the same in a lower-risk hypertensive population. Another problem with this study is that after the randomized trial period, medication data on the HF participants is lacking during the follow-up period. Finally, other posttrial therapies such as revascularization, implantable devices, and HF treatment were determined by the patient's physician and could have modified the outcome in these patients. This study is powerful evidence that it is imperative that patients with hypertension be treated vigorously to prevent the development of HF.

M. D. Cheitlin, MD

References

1. Lloyd-Jones D, Adams R, Carnethon M, et al; American Heart Association Statistics Committee and Stroke Statistics Subcommittee. Heart disease and stroke statistics—2009 update: a report from the American Heart Association Statistics Committee and Stroke Statistics Subcommittee. *Circulation.* 2009;119:e21-e181.
2. Haldeman GA, Croft JB, Giles WH, Rashidee A. Hospitalization of patients with heart failure: National Hospital Discharge Survey, 1985 to 1995. *Am Heart J.* 1999;137:352-360.
3. Levy D, Kenchaiah S, Larson MG, et al. Long-term trends in the incidence of and survival with heart failure. *N Engl J Med.* 2002;347:1397-1402.
4. Kostis JB, Davis BR, Cutler J, et al. Prevention of heart failure by antihypertensive drug treatment in older persons with isolated systolic hypertension. SHEP Cooperative Research Group. *JAMA.* 1997;278:212-216.
5. Beckett NS, Peters R, Fletcher AE, et al; HYVET Study Group. Treatment of hypertension in patients 80 years of age or older. *N Engl J Med.* 2008;358: 1887-1898.
6. Yip GW, Fung JW, Tan YT, Sanderson JE. Hypertension and heart failure: a dysfunction of systole, diastole or both? *J Hum Hypertens.* 2009;23:295-306.
7. Yusuf S, Sleight P, Pogue J, Bosch J, Davies R, Dagenais G. Effects of an angiotensin-converting-enzyme inhibitor, ramipril, on cardiovascular events in high-risk patients. The Heart Outcomes Prevention Evaluation Study Investigators. *N Engl J Med.* 2000;342:145-153.
8. Braunwald E, Domanski MJ, Fowler SE, et al; PEACE Trial Investigators. Angiotensin-converting-enzyme inhibition in stable coronary artery disease. *N Engl J Med.* 2004;351:2058-2068.
9. Ho KK, Anderson KM, Kannel WB, Grossman W, Levy D. Survival after the onset of congestive heart failure in Framingham Heart Study subjects. *Circulation.* 1993; 88:107-115.
10. Dahlöf B, Lindholm LH, Hansson L, Scherstén B, Ekbom T, Wester PO. Morbidity and mortality in the Swedish Trial in Old Patients with Hypertension (STOP-Hypertension). *Lancet.* 1991;338:1281-1285.
11. Shafazand M, Schaufelberger M, Lappas G, et al. Survival trends in men and women with heart failure of ischaemic and non-ischaemic origin: data for the period 1987–2003 from the Swedish Hospital Discharge Registry. *Eur Heart J.* 2009;30:671-678.

6 Cardiac Arrhythmias, Conduction Disturbances, and Electrophysiology

Atrial Fibrillation

Apixaban versus Warfarin in Patients with Atrial Fibrillation

Granger CB, for the ARISTOTLE Committees and Investigators (Duke Univ Med Ctr, Durham, NC; et al)
N Engl J Med 365:981-992, 2011

Background.—Vitamin K antagonists are highly effective in preventing stroke in patients with atrial fibrillation but have several limitations. Apixaban is a novel oral direct factor Xa inhibitor that has been shown to reduce the risk of stroke in a similar population in comparison with aspirin.

Methods.—In this randomized, double-blind trial, we compared apixaban (at a dose of 5 mg twice daily) with warfarin (target international normalized ratio, 2.0 to 3.0) in 18,201 patients with atrial fibrillation and at least one additional risk factor for stroke. The primary outcome was ischemic or hemorrhagic stroke or systemic embolism. The trial was designed to test for noninferiority, with key secondary objectives of testing for superiority with respect to the primary outcome and to the rates of major bleeding and death from any cause.

Results.—The median duration of follow-up was 1.8 years. The rate of the primary outcome was 1.27% per year in the apixaban group, as compared with 1.60% per year in the warfarin group (hazard ratio with apixaban, 0.79; 95% confidence interval [CI], 0.66 to 0.95; $P < 0.001$ for noninferiority; $P = 0.01$ for superiority). The rate of major bleeding was 2.13% per year in the apixaban group, as compared with 3.09% per year in the warfarin group (hazard ratio, 0.69; 95% CI, 0.60 to 0.80; $P < 0.001$), and the rates of death from any cause were 3.52% and 3.94%, respectively (hazard ratio, 0.89; 95% CI, 0.80 to 0.99; $P = 0.047$). The rate of hemorrhagic stroke was 0.24% per year in the apixaban group, as compared with 0.47% per year in the warfarin group (hazard ratio, 0.51; 95% CI, 0.35 to 0.75; $P < 0.001$), and the rate of ischemic or uncertain type of stroke was 0.97% per year in the apixaban group and 1.05% per year in the warfarin group (hazard ratio, 0.92; 95% CI, 0.74 to 1.13; $P = 0.42$).

Conclusions.—In patients with atrial fibrillation, apixaban was superior to warfarin in preventing stroke or systemic embolism, caused less bleeding, and resulted in lower mortality. (Funded by Bristol-Myers Squibb and Pfizer; ARISTOTLE ClinicalTrials.gov number, NCT00412984.)

▶ Prevention of thromboembolism is an important component of the treatment for patients with atrial fibrillation (AF). Stable therapeutic anticoagulation with warfarin requires strict diet control and frequent laboratory monitoring and can be difficult to manage in even the most closely monitored patients, such as those in clinical trials. Such challenges have led to multiple efforts to develop oral anticoagulants that can effectively prevent stroke and limit bleeding complications without requiring strict diet control or laboratory monitoring. One such agent was tested in the ARISTOTLE trial, which compares a novel oral anticoagulant, apixaban, to warfarin in high-risk patients with AF. ARISTOTLE was a randomized, double-blind trial in 18 201 patients with AF comparing apixaban 5 mg twice daily to dose-adjusted warfarin with a target international normalized ratio of 2 to 3. The primary outcome was ischemic or hemorrhagic stroke or systemic embolism. The trial had a noninferiority design with respect to the primary outcome. Secondary endpoints included superiority with respect to the primary endpoint and to the rates of major bleeding and death. Over a median follow-up period of 1.8 years, the rate of the primary outcome was 1.27% per year in the apixaban group, compared with 1.6% per year in the warfarin group (hazard ratio [HR] 0.79; 95% confidence interval [CI] 0.66–0.95; $P < .001$ for noninferiority and $P = .01$ for superiority). The rate of major bleeding was 2.13% per year in the apixaban group compared with 3.09% per year in the warfarin group (HR, 0.69; 95% CI, 0.60–0.80; $P < .001$). The rate of death from any cause was 3.52% in the apixaban group compared with 3.94% in the warfarin group (HR, 0.89; 95% CI, 0.8–0.99; $P = .047$). This trial demonstrated the ability of apixaban to reduce the risk of stroke while also reducing the risk of major bleeding (Fig 1 in the original article). The twice-daily dosing schedule is similar to dabigatran, another recently developed warfarin alternative. However, although the currently approved dose of dabigatran was shown in the RE-LY trial to be superior to warfarin in stroke prevention, it had a similar bleeding risk. Therefore, apixaban may have the added advantage of simultaneously improving efficacy while decreasing bleeding. However, such comparisons between studies should be done with caution because entry criteria, study design, and the groups studies had some differences. Although other factors such as cost and drug intolerance will affect the distribution and use of these new anticoagulants, apixaban appears to be a safe and effective alternative to warfarin.

C. P. Rowley, MD

Cost-Effectiveness of Dabigatran for Stroke Prophylaxis in Atrial Fibrillation

Shah SV, Gage BF (Washington Univ in St. Louis, MO)
Circulation 123:2562-2570, 2011

Background.—Recent studies have investigated alternatives to warfarin for stroke prophylaxis in patients with atrial fibrillation (AF), but whether these alternatives are cost-effective is unknown.

Methods and Results.—On the basis of the results from Randomized Evaluation of Long Term Anticoagulation Therapy (RE-LY) and other trials, we developed a decision-analysis model to compare the cost and quality-adjusted survival of various antithrombotic therapies. We ran our Markov model in a hypothetical cohort of 70-year-old patients with AF using a cost-effectiveness threshold of $50 000/quality-adjusted life-year. We estimated the cost of dabigatran as US $9 a day. For a patient with an average risk of major hemorrhage ($\approx 3\%$/y), the most cost-effective therapy depended on stroke risk. For patients with the lowest stroke rate (CHADS$_2$

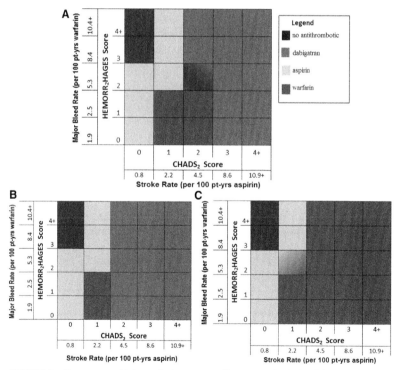

FIGURE 3.—Two-way sensitivity analysis at a cost-effectiveness threshold of $50 000 per quality-adjusted life-year. Cost-effectiveness depended on risks of stroke, bleeding, and total time in the therapeutic international normalized ratio range. In two-toned cells either therapy would be cost-effective. A, Base-case scenario. B, Time in the therapeutic range <57.1%. C, Time in the therapeutic range >72.6%. (Reprinted from Shah SV, Gage BF. Cost-effectiveness of dabigatran for stroke prophylaxis in atrial fibrillation. *Circulation.* 2011;123:2562-2570. © American Heart Association, Inc.)

stroke score of 0), only aspirin was cost-effective. For patients with a moderate stroke rate (CHADS$_2$ score of 1 or 2), warfarin was cost-effective unless the risk of hemorrhage was high or quality of international normalized ratio control was poor (time in the therapeutic range <57.1%). For patients with a high stroke risk (CHADS$_2$ stroke score ≥3), dabigatran 150 mg (twice daily) was cost-effective unless international normalized ratio control was excellent (time in the therapeutic range >72.6%). Neither dabigatran 110 mg nor dual therapy (aspirin and clopidogrel) was cost-effective.

Conclusions.—Dabigatran 150 mg (twice daily) was cost-effective in AF populations at high risk of hemorrhage or high risk of stroke unless international normalized ratio control with warfarin was excellent. Warfarin was cost-effective in moderate-risk AF populations unless international normalized ratio control was poor (Fig 3).

▶ Novel anticoagulants have demonstrated effectiveness in stroke prevention in patients with nonvalvular atrial fibrillation (NVAF). These medications may be superior to warfarin with respect to both efficacy and safety, and additionally, they do not require routine monitoring. They are, however, much more expensive than standard warfarin therapy. However, these costs may be offset by the costs of monitoring and treating complications. Using the results from RE-LY and other major trials, Shah et al have used a Markov model to estimate the cost-effectiveness of dabigatran and other therapies for stroke prevention in NVAF. Fig 3 demonstrates that dabigatran at 150 mg twice daily was cost-effective only in the patient populations at the highest risk of hemorrhage or at higher risk of stroke with poor international normalized ratio (INR) control. Health care providers may need to take into consideration stroke, bleeding risk, and INR control when deciding on the most clinically and cost-effective anticoagulation therapy in patients with NVAF.

F. Cuoco, MD, MBA

Prevention of stroke and systemic embolism with rivaroxaban compared with warfarin in patients with non-valvular atrial fibrillation and moderate renal impairment

Fox KAA, Piccini JP, Wojdyla D, et al (Univ of Edinburgh, UK)
Eur Heart J 32:2387-2394, 2011

Aims.—Patients with non-valvular atrial fibrillation (AF) and renal insufficiency are at increased risk for ischaemic stroke and bleeding during anticoagulation. Rivaroxaban, an oral, direct factor Xa inhibitor metabolized predominantly by the liver, preserves the benefit of warfarin for stroke prevention while causing fewer intracranial and fatal haemorrhages.

Methods and Results.—We randomized 14 264 patients with AF in a double-blind trial to rivaroxaban 20 mg/day [15 mg/day if creatinine clearance (CrCl) 30—49 mL/min] or dose-adjusted warfarin (target international normalized ratio 2.0—3.0). Compared with patients with CrCl >50 mL/min (mean age 73 years), the 2950 (20.7%) patients with CrCl 30—49 mL/min were older (79 years) and had higher event rates irrespective of study treatment. Among those with CrCl 30—49 mL/min, the primary endpoint of stroke or systemic embolism occurred in 2.32 per 100 patient-years with rivaroxaban 15 mg/day vs. 2.77 per 100 patient-years with warfarin [hazard ratio (HR) 0.84; 95% confidence interval (CI) 0.57—1.23] in the per-protocol population. Intention-to-treat analysis yielded similar results (HR 0.86; 95% CI 0.63—1.17) to the per-protocol results. Rates of the principal safety endpoint (major and clinically relevant non-major bleeding: 17.82 vs. 18.28 per 100 patient-years; $P = 0.76$) and intracranial bleeding (0.71 vs. 0.88 per 100 patient-years; $P = 0.54$) were similar with rivaroxaban or warfarin. Fatal bleeding (0.28 vs. 0.74% per 100 patient-years; $P = 0.047$) occurred less often with rivaroxaban.

Conclusion.—Patients with AF and moderate renal insufficiency have higher rates of stroke and bleeding than those with normal renal function. There was no evidence of heterogeneity in treatment effect across dosing groups. Dose adjustment in ROCKET-AF yielded results consistent with the overall trial in comparison with dose-adjusted warfarin (Fig 1, Table 3).

▶ Rivaroxaban is a novel oral direct factor Xa inhibitor that has been shown in Rivaroxaban Once-daily, oral, direct factor Xa inhibition compared with vitamin K antagonism for prevention of stroke and Embolism Trial in Atrial Fibrillation (ROCKET-AF) to be noninferior to warfarin with respect to stroke prevention in high-risk patients with AF. Due to the pharmocokinetic properties of rivaroxaban, there is a 25% to 30% increase in maximal serum concentration in patients with moderate renal dysfunction (CrCl 30—49 mL/min). Accordingly, such patients in ROCKET-AF were given dose-reduced rivaroxaban 15 mg daily rather than the standard 20 mg daily dose. In this analysis, the authors sought to determine whether dose-reduced rivaroxaban was effective for stroke reduction in patients with renal impairment. Of the 14 264 patients with AF randomized in

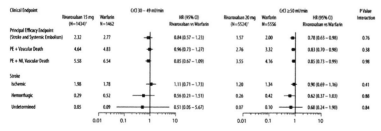

* The primary analysis was pre-specified to be performed in the per-protocol population on treatment, which included all patients who received at least 1 dose of study drug, did not have major protocol violations, and were followed for events while on study drug or within 2 days of last dose.
† Event rates per 100 pt/yrs of follow-up

FIGURE 1.—Efficacy events in the per-protocol (on-treatment) population. (Reprinted from Fox KAA, Piccini JP, Wojdyla D, et al. Prevention of stroke and systemic embolism with rivaroxaban compared with warfarin in patients with non-valvular atrial fibrillation and moderate renal impairment. *Eur Heart J.* 2011;32:2387-2394, by permission of The European Society of Cardiology.)

TABLE 3.—Bleeding Rates by Treatment Group Rivaroxaban vs. Warfarin

Clinical Endpoint	CrCl 30–49 mL/min			CrCl ≥50 mL/min			P-Value for Interaction
	Rivaroxaban 15 mg (n = 1474)[a]	Warfarin (n = 1476)[a]	Hazard Ratio (95% CI), Rivaroxaban vs. Warfarin	Rivaroxaban 20 mg (n = 5637)[a]	Warfarin (n = 5640)[a]	Hazard Ratio (95% CI), Rivaroxaban vs. Warfarin	
Primary safety endpoint	17.82	18.28	0.98 (0.84–1.14)	14.24	13.67	1.04 (0.96–1.13)	0.4496
Major bleeding	4.49	4.70	0.95 (0.72–1.26)	3.39	3.17	1.07 (0.91–1.26)	0.4800
Hb drop	3.76	3.28	1.14 (0.83–1.58)	2.54	2.03	1.25 (1.03–1.52)	0.6456
Transfusion	2.34	2.00	1.17 (0.77–1.76)	1.49	1.16	1.28 (0.99–1.65)	0.7066
Clinical organ	0.76	1.39	0.55 (0.30–1.00)	0.83	1.13	0.74 (0.55–0.99)	0.3866
Fatal bleeding	0.28	0.74	0.39 (0.15–0.99)	0.23	0.43	0.55 (0.32–0.93)	0.5302
Intracranial haemorrhage	0.71	0.88	0.81 (0.41–1.60)	0.44	0.71	0.62 (0.42–0.92)	0.5065

[a]Event rates per 100 patient-years of follow-up.

ROCKET-AF there were 2950 (20.7%) patients with CrCl 30 to 49 mL/min. Of those 2950 patients, 1474 received dose-reduced rivaroxaban, and 1476 received dose-adjusted warfarin with target international normalized ratio 2 to 3. In the per-protocol analysis, the primary endpoint of stroke or systemic embolism occurred in 2.32 per 100 patient-years in the rivaroxaban group compared with 2.77 per 100 patient-years in the warfarin group (hazard ratio, 0.84; 95% confidence interval, 0.57–1.23, Fig 1). Results were similar in the intention-to-treat analysis. The primary safety endpoint of major and clinically relevant nonmajor bleeding occurred in 17.82 versus 18.28 per 100 patient-years in the rivaroxaban and warfarin groups, respectively (Table 3). Fatal bleeding occurred in fewer patients in the rivaroxaban group compared with the warfarin group (0.28% vs 0.74% per 100 patient-years, respectively, $P = .047$). This substudy indicates that patients with impaired renal function had a higher risk of stroke as well as bleeding compared with patients with normal renal function, an observation that is consistent with those of prior studies. Additionally, it provides clinical evidence for safe and effective use of renally adjusted rivaroxaban for stroke prevention in patients with moderate renal impairment.

C. P. Rowley, MD

Synergistic Effect of the Combination of Ranolazine and Dronedarone to Suppress Atrial Fibrillation

Burashnikov A, Sicouri S, Di Diego JM, et al (Masonic Med Res Laboratory, Utica, NY; Gilead Sciences, Palo Alto, CA)
J Am Coll Cardiol 56:1216-1224, 2010

Objectives.—The aim of this study was to evaluate the effectiveness of a combination of dronedarone and ranolazine in suppression of atrial fibrillation (AF).

Background.—Safe and effective pharmacological management of AF remains one of the greatest unmet medical needs.

Methods.—The electrophysiological effects of dronedarone (10 μmol/l) and a relatively low concentration of ranolazine (5 μmol/l) separately and in combination were evaluated in canine isolated coronary-perfused right and left atrial and left ventricular preparations as well as in pulmonary vein preparations.

Results.—Ranolazine caused moderate atrial-selective prolongation of action potential duration and atrial-selective depression of sodium channel–mediated parameters, including maximal rate of rise of the action potential upstroke, leading to the development of atrial-specific post-repolarization refractoriness. Dronedarone caused little or no change in electrophysiological parameters in both atrial and ventricular preparations. The combination of dronedarone and ranolazine caused little change in action potential duration in either chamber but induced potent use-dependent atrial-selective depression of the sodium channel–mediated parameters (maximal rate of rise of the action potential upstroke, diastolic threshold of excitation, and the shortest cycle length permitting a 1:1 response) and considerable post-repolarization refractoriness. Separately, dronedarone or a low concentration of ranolazine prevented the induction of AF in 17% and 29% of preparations, respectively. In combination, the 2 drugs suppressed AF and triggered activity and prevented the induction of AF in 9 of 10 preparations (90%).

Conclusions.—Low concentrations of ranolazine and dronedarone produce relatively weak electrophysiological effects and weak suppression of AF when used separately but when combined exert potent synergistic effects, resulting in atrial-selective depression of sodium channel–dependent parameters and effective suppression of AF (Fig 3).

▶ Pharmacological therapy for atrial fibrillation (AF) is limited by poor efficacy and potential proarrhythmic toxicity of available drugs. Dronedarone has recently

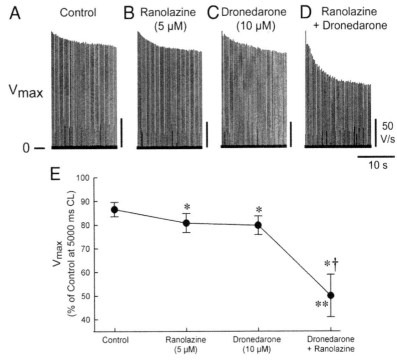

FIGURE 3.—Synergistic Effect of Ranolazine and Dronedarone to Depress V_{max} in PV. Synergistic effect of the combination of ranolazine and dronedarone on maximal rate of rise of the action potential upstroke (V_{max}) after an abrupt change in rate in pulmonary vein (PV) sleeve preparations. (A) V_{max} traces recorded after a change in cycle length (CL) from 5,000 to 300 ms. (B) Graph displaying composite data of V_{max} changes after acceleration of pacing rate from a CL of 5,000 to 300 ms (n = 4 to 8). *p < 0.05 versus control. †p < 0.05 versus ranolazine or dronedarone alone. **p < 0.05, change in V_{max} induced by combination ranolazine plus dronedarone (from washout) versus the sum of changes caused by ranolazine and dronedarone independently (both from washout). (Reprinted from the Journal of the American College of Cardiology, Burashnikov A, Sicouri S, Di Diego JM, et al. Synergistic effect of the combination of ranolazine and dronedarone to suppress atrial fibrillation. *J Am Coll Cardiol.* 2010;56:1216-1224. Copyright 2010, with permission from the American College of Cardiology.)

been shown to be safe and relatively effective in suppressing AF. Ranolazine was developed as an antianginal agent but has also been shown to have antiarrhythmic properties that are relatively more specific in atrial than ventricular myocardium. This atrial specificity of ranolazine becomes theoretically important in decreasing the risk of ventricular proarrhythmia. The present study demonstrates that superfusion of dronedarone and ranolazine in combination over atrial and ventricular myocardium in vitro had greater electrophysiologic effects than either drug individually. Specifically, dronedarone and ranolazine resulted in little change in the action potential duration but marked increase in effective refractory period, creating a marked increase in postrepolarization refractoriness (ie, inability to stimulate the myocardium even though the action potential has return to baseline resting potential). In addition, Vmax (the maximum rise in the action potential) was depressed more with combination therapy than either drug individually (Fig 3). Both the changes in refractoriness and Vmax were greater in atrial than ventricular myocardial preparation in concentration, similar to those achieved clinically. The combined atrial electrophysiologic effects of dronedarone and ranolazine resulted in increased termination of acetylcholine-induced AF, decreased inducibility of AF, and suppression of delayed after potentials in the pulmonary vein musculature to a much greater degree than with either drug alone. Although this in vitro study suggests that combination therapy may be effective and safe for treatment of AF, caution needs to be expressed in extrapolating this to the clinical arena. First, this is in vitro data. Second, the effects of antiarrhythmic drugs on acetylcholine-induced AF may not correlate well with efficacy of treatment in clinical AF. Third, the acute effects of dronedarone do not correlate with the effects of dronedarone given orally at steady state, and chronic data on ranolazine electrophysiologic effects are not available. Lastly, there is no assessment of ventricular proarrhythmic risk in this in vitro study, since such risk clinically is accrued over time under changing clinical conditions (eg, ischemic, heart failure, addition of other drugs). Until the results of an ongoing clinical trial assessing the efficacy and safety of dronedarone and ranolazine versus dronedarone alone are available, combination therapy cannot be recommended. Indeed, patients who are felt to need ranolazine and dronedarone concomitantly for the currently approved indications should be followed closely for possible proarrhythmic interactions.

J. M. Warton, MD

The Effect of Rate Control on Quality of Life in Patients With Permanent Atrial Fibrillation: Data From the RACE II (Rate Control Efficacy in Permanent Atrial Fibrillation II) Study
Groenveld HF, for the RACE II Investigators (Univ of Groningen, the Netherlands; et al)
J Am Coll Cardiol 58:1795-1803, 2011

Objectives.—The aim of this study was to investigate the influence of rate control on quality of life (QOL).

Background.—The RACE II (Rate Control Efficacy in Permanent Atrial Fibrillation II) trial showed that lenient rate control is not inferior to strict rate control in terms of cardiovascular morbidity and mortality. The influence of stringency of rate control on QOL is unknown.

Methods.—In RACE II, a total of 614 patients with permanent atrial fibrillation (AF) were randomized to lenient (resting heart rate [HR] <110 beats/min) or strict (resting HR <80 beats/min, HR during moderate exercise <110 beats/min) rate control. QOL was assessed in 437 patients using the Medical Outcomes Study 36-item Short-Form Health Survey (SF-36) questionnaire, AF severity scale, and Multidimensional Fatigue Inventory-20 (MFI-20) at baseline, 1 year, and end of study. QOL changes were related to patient characteristics.

Results.—Median follow-up was 3 years. Mean age was 68 ± 8 years, and 66% were males. At the end of follow-up, all SF-36 subscales were comparable between both groups. The AF severity scale was similar at baseline and end of study. At baseline and at end of study there were no differences in the MFI-20 subscales between the 2 groups. Symptoms at baseline, younger age, and less severe underlying disease, rather than assigned therapy or heart rate, were associated with QOL improvements. Female sex and cardiovascular endpoints during the study were associated with worsening of QOL.

Conclusions.—Stringency of heart rate control does not influence QOL. Instead, symptoms, sex, age, and severity of the underlying disease influence QOL (Fig 1).

▶ Several studies have shown that rhythm control with antiarrhythmic drugs is not superior to rate control in asymptomatic or mildly symptomatic patients. When a rate control strategy is adopted, the optimal heart rate goal remains

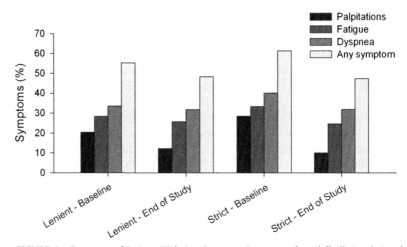

FIGURE 1.—Percentage of Patients With Any Symptom. Symptoms of atrial fibrillation during the study, displayed by randomization strategy at baseline and end of study. (Reprinted from the Journal of the American College of Cardiology, Groenveld HF, for the RACE II Investigators, The effect of rate control on quality of life in patients with permanent atrial fibrillation: data from the RACE II (Rate Control Efficacy in Permanent Atrial Fibrillation II) study. *J Am Coll Cardiol.* 2011;58:1795-1803. Copyright 2011, with permission from the American College of Cardiology.)

controversial. In the Rate Control Efficacy in Permanent Atrial Fibrillation II study (RACE II), mortality and morbidity were not influenced by strict versus lenient rate control in long-standing persistent atrial fibrillation patients. This substudy of RACE II addressed the effects of rate control strategies on quality of life (QOL). Using the SF-36 AF severity scale and MFI-20 metrics at baseline, 1 year, and at the end of the study, there was no demonstrated difference in QOL in strict and lenient rate control groups (Fig 1). Age, female sex, symptom severity and comorbid conditions were associated with worse QOL. Side effects of rate control agents were speculated to offset the benefit of better rate control. Additionally, more than 40% of patients were asymptomatic, which may have masked the outcome. Those with strict rate control experienced slightly more symptoms compared with lenient control. This report suggests that strict rate control has no measurable benefit in QOL for patients with long-standing persistent atrial fibrillation.

M. L. Bernard, MD, PhD

Complications arising from catheter ablation of atrial fibrillation: Temporal trends and predictors

Hoyt H, Bhonsale A, Chilukuri K, et al (Department of Medicine, School of Medicine, Johns Hopkins University, Baltimore, MD)
Heart Rhythm 8:1869-1874, 2011

Background.—The reported complication rate of catheter ablation of atrial fibrillation (AF) varies.

Objective.—Our goal was to assess temporal trends and the effect of both institutional and individual operators' experience on the incidence of complications.

Methods.—All patients undergoing AF ablation at Johns Hopkins Hospital between February 2001 and December 2010 were prospectively enrolled in a database. Major complications were defined as those that were life-threatening, resulted in permanent harm, required intervention, or significantly prolonged hospitalization.

Results.—Fifty-six major complications occurred in 1190 procedures (4.7%). The majority of complications were vascular (18; 1.5%), followed by pericardial tamponade (13; 1.1%) and cerebrovascular accident (12; 1.1%). No cases of death or atrioesophageal fistula occurred. The overall complication rate decreased from 11.1% in 2002 to 1.6% in 2010 ($P < .05$). On univariate analysis, demographic and clinical factors associated with the increased risk of complications were CHADS$_2$ score of ≥ 2 (hazard ratio [HR] = 2.5; 95% confidence interval [CI] = 1.4−4.4; $P = .002$), female gender (HR = 2.0; 95% CI = 1.2−3.5; $P = .014$), and age (HR = 1.03; 95% CI = 1.0−1.1; $P = .042$). Gender and CHADS$_2$ score of ≥ 2 remained independent predictors of complication on multivariable analysis.

Conclusion.—The complication rate of catheter ablation of AF decreased with increased institutional experience. Female gender and CHADS$_2$ score of $\geq$2 are significant independent risk factors for complications and should be considered when referring patients for AF ablation.

▶ Atrial fibrillation ablation has emerged as the mainstay of therapy for drug-refractory nonpermanent atrial fibrillation. The technical aspects of the procedure have undergone a transformation, resulting in fewer periprocedural complications and improved outcomes. Hoyt et al report on a large series of atrial fibrillation ablation patients ($n = 1190$) spanning 10 years at a single center. Major complications decreased from 11.1% to 1.6% over the span of the study, which was largely driven by reduction in catheter-related injury and increased operator experience. Most common complications were vascular injury, pericardial tamponade, and cerebrovascular accident (CVA). Vascular complications were reduced when warfarin was uninterrupted at the time of procedure compared with bridging with heparin. CVA rates were unchanged throughout the time period. Age, female sex, and CHADS$_2$ score 2 or greater were associated with increased complications. This report will serve as an important benchmark for complications associated with atrial fibrillation.

M. L. Bernard, MD, PhD

New-Onset Postoperative Atrial Fibrillation Predicts Late Mortality After Mitral Valve Surgery

Bramer S, van Straten AHM, Soliman Hamad MA, et al (Catharina Hosp, Eindhoven, The Netherlands; Tilburg Univ, The Netherlands; Maastricht Univ Med Ctr — MUMC, The Netherlands)
Ann Thorac Surg 92:2091-2096, 2011

Background.—New-onset postoperative atrial fibrillation (POAF) is a common rhythm disturbance after mitral valve surgery. In this study we investigated the independent effect of POAF on early and late mortality after mitral valve surgery.

Methods.—Data of patients who consecutively underwent mitral valve surgery with or without concomitant coronary or tricuspid valve surgery between January 2003 and June 2010 were prospectively collected. The study included 856 patients with preoperative sinus rhythm, and no history of atrial fibrillation. Logistic regression and Cox proportional hazard analyses were performed to investigate independent predictors of early and late mortality. Propensity score adjustment was performed to reduce the effect of confounders.

Results.—The median follow-up was 3.1 years (range, 0 to 7.4 years). The POAF was documented in 361 patients (42%). Early mortality did not differ in patients with and without POAF ($p = 0.93$). Postoperative atrial fibrillation was not identified as predictor for early mortality. Late survival was worse in patients with POAF (log-rank, $p < 0.001$). Multivariate and propensity score adjusted Cox proportional hazard analyses demonstrated that POAF was an independent predictor for late mortality with hazard ratios of 2.09 and 1.61 ($p = 0.001$ and $p = 0.033$, respectively).

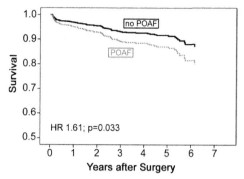

FIGURE 3.—Adjusted cumulative late survival after mitral valve surgery ($n = 780$) using propensity score. (HR = hazard ratio; POAF = postoperative atrial fibrillation.) (This article was published in The Annals of Thoracic Surgery, Bramer S, van Straten AHM, Soliman Hamad MA, et al. New-onset postoperative atrial fibrillation predicts late mortality after mitral valve surgery. *Ann Thorac Surg.* 2011;92:2091-2096. © The Society of Thoracic Surgeons 2011.)

Conclusions.—Postoperative atrial fibrillation is an independent predictor for late all-cause mortality after mitral valve surgery but not for early all-cause mortality (Fig 3).

▶ This is a retrospective study of 856 patients who underwent mitral valve surgery. The purpose was to assess the impact of atrial fibrillation (AF) on early and late survival. Those with AF or a history thereof were excluded. Concomitant procedure included coronary artery bypass graft and tricuspid repair. Patients were monitored continuously for at least 48 hours then 3 times daily until discharge. Multivariable logistic regression and propensity matching were used to minimize confounding factors.

All patients were in sinus rhythm at the time of surgery. The incidence of AF after surgery was 42%. Early mortality was no different between those who did and did not experience AF (6.9% vs 7.1%, $P = .93$). Using multivariable analysis, perioperative AF did predict mortality with a hazard ratio of 2.09. Using propensity matching, this effect persisted with a lower hazard ratio of 1.61 (Fig 3).

While interesting, the retrospective nature of this study requires the results to be interpreted with caution. Many important factors were unavailable including the rhythm at the time of discharge and the duration of AF. Follow-up data were not available. The number of patients who went into AF after discharge is unknown. It is unclear if AF is the cause or a marker of reduced survival in patients after mitral valve surgery. The authors conclude prospective randomized trials are needed to determine if prophylactic pharmacologic or even surgical intervention might decrease the incidence of postoperative AF and thereby improve survival.

J. M. Toole, MD

Postablation asymptomatic cerebral lesions: Long-term follow-up using magnetic resonance imaging

Deneke T, Shin D-I, Balta O, et al (Academic Heart Ctr Cologne-Porz, Germany; et al)

Heart Rhythm 8:1705-1711, 2011

Background.—Catheter ablation of atrial fibrillation (AF) is complicated by cerebral emboli resulting in acute ischemia. Recently, cerebral ischemic microlesions have been identified with diffusion-weighted magnet resonance imaging (MRI).

Objective.—The clinical course and longer-term characteristics of these lesions are not known and were investigated in this study.

Methods.—Of 86 patients, 33 (38%) had new asymptomatic cerebral lesions documented on MRI after catheter ablation for AF; 14 of these 33 (42%) underwent repeat MRI at different time intervals (2 weeks to 1 year) during follow-up, and clinical symptoms as well as size and number of residual lesions were documented.

Results.—In postablation cerebral MRI, 50 new lesions were identified (3.6 lesions/patient) in 14 patients. No patient presented any neurological symptoms. Distribution of the lesions was predominantly in the left hemisphere (60%) and the cerebellum (26%); 52% of the lesions were small (≤3 mm maximum diameter), 42% were medium (4 to 10 mm) and 3 lesions (6%) had a maximum diameter >10 mm. Follow-up MRI after a median of 3 months revealed 3 residual lesions in 3 of 14 patients corresponding to the large acute postablation lesions (>10 mm). The remaining 47 of 50 (94%) of the small or medium-sized lesions were not detectable at follow-up evaluation.

Conclusions.—Most asymptomatic cerebral lesions observed acutely after AF ablation procedures were ≤10 mm in diameter. 94% of all lesions healed without scarring at follow-up >2 weeks after ablation. The larger acute lesions produced chronic glial scars. Neither chronic nor acute lesions were associated with neurological symptoms.

▶ Evidence of asymptomatic cerebral embolism after atrial fibrillation (AF) has been reported to occur in between 10% and 40% of patients in small clinical series. In this study, using predominantly multipolar catheters with phased RF application, a technology suggested to have a higher risk of embolic events, there was a 38% incidence of new lesions on follow-up magnetic resonance imaging (MRI) 1 to 2 days after ablation with an average of 3.6 lesions per patient with lesions. Phased RF technology was used in 91% of these patients, again raising the concern about this technology. Late follow-up MRI was performed in only 14 of the 33 patients with new lesions and demonstrated complete resolution of small or medium-size lesions in all cases, but persistence of large lesions greater than 10 mm with some resolution was seen in 3 patients. Although no neurologic abnormalities could be found on physical examination, detailed neuropsychiatric testing was not performed to assess the impact, if any, of these lesions. This and other studies indicate the need for meticulous attention to anticoagulation prior to, during, and after ablation as well as care to prevent air and fibrin emboli from sheaths and catheters during ablation. It also suggests the need for monitoring silent cerebral emboli during new technology assessments.

J. M. Warton, MD

Radiofrequency Ablation of Atrial Fibrillation in Patients With Mechanical Mitral Valve Prostheses: Safety, Feasibility, Electrophysiologic Findings, and Outcomes
Hussein AA, Wazni OM, Harb S, et al (Cleveland Clinic, OH; et al)
J Am Coll Cardiol 58:596-602, 2011

Objectives.—The purpose of this study was to evaluate the feasibility, safety, and outcomes of radiofrequency ablation of atrial fibrillation (AF) in patients with mechanical mitral valve replacement (MVR).

Background.—The role of ablative therapy in patients with MVR is not yet established, with safety concerns and very few outcome data.

Methods.—Between January 2003 and December 2008, we followed up 81 patients with MVR undergoing first-time AF ablation (compared with 162 age- and sex-matched controls). Arrhythmia recurrences were identified by symptoms with documentation, event monitoring, Holter monitoring, and electrocardiograms.

Results.—All MVR and control patients underwent ablation under therapeutic international normalized ratio. No entrapment of catheters or stroke occurred. There were no differences in terms of procedure-related complications between the groups (p = NS). Patients with MVR had larger atria (p < 0.0001), lower left ventricular ejection fractions (p = 0.0001), and more concomitant atrial flutter at baseline (p < 0.0001). Over a 24-month follow-up, they had higher recurrence rates compared with controls (49.4% vs. 27.7% after a single ablation, p = 0.0006). The creation of flutter lines significantly reduced recurrences in patients with any history of atrial flutter (16.7% vs. 60.9%, p = 0.009). At last follow-up, 82.7% of MVR patients had their arrhythmia controlled (69.1% not receiving antiarrhythmic drugs).

Conclusions.—Radiofrequency ablation is feasible and safe for patients with MVR. It allowed restoration of sinus rhythm in a substantial proportion of patients undergoing ablation. An abnormal atrial substrate underlies recurrences in these patients. The ablation procedure needs to be further refined with a focus on extra pulmonary vein triggers and concomitant flutters to improve outcomes.

▶ This study is the largest study to date assessing the utility of atrial fibrillation (AF) ablation in patients with prior mitral valve replacement (MVR). Using an age- and gender-matched cohort for comparison for the study period between 2003 and 2008, this study shows the efficacy was less after either single or multiple ablations in patients with prior MVR. Some previous studies have found similar efficacy in the MVR group compared with controls, but all studies show longer procedure and fluoroscopy times due to the greater complexity of ablation in patients with prior MVR. In particular, macroreentrant atrial tachycardias (ATs) created by disease- or surgically related scarring complicate the procedure and increase the need for repeat ablations. Thus, close attention to ablation or prevention of ATs, including insuring bidirectional block of linear lesions for this purpose, during initial ablation may improve overall success. In this study, the relatively high rate of concomitant surgical maze procedure at the time of MVR may have further compounded the scarring and creation of ATs. Nonetheless, this and other studies indicate that catheter ablation of AF in patients with prior MVR is still a reasonable therapeutic option in patients with medically refractory AF.

J. M. Warton, MD

Cardiac resynchronization therapy in patients undergoing atrioventricular junction ablation for permanent atrial fibrillation: a randomized trial
Brignole M, Botto G, Mont L, et al (Ospedali del Tigullio, Lavagna, Italy; Ospedale S. Anna, Como, Italy; Univ of Barcelona, Spain; et al)
Eur Heart J 32:2420-2429, 2011

Aims.—On the basis of the current knowledge, cardiac resynchronization therapy (CRT) cannot be recommended as a first-line treatment for patients with severely symptomatic permanent atrial fibrillation undergoing atrioventricular (AV) junction ablation. We examined whether CRT was superior to conventional right ventricular (RV) pacing in reducing heart failure (HF) events.

Methods and Results.—In this prospective, multi-centre study, we randomly assigned 186 patients, in whom AV junction ablation and CRT device implantation had been successfully performed, to receive optimized echo-guided CRT (97 patients) or RV apical pacing (89 patients). The data were analysed according to the intention-to-treat principle. During a median follow-up of 20 months (interquartile range 11−24), the primary composite endpoint of death from HF, hospitalization due to HF, or worsening HF occurred in 11 (11) patients in the CRT group and 23 (26) patients in the RV group [CRT vs. RV group: sub-hazard ratio (SHR) 0.37 (95 CI 0.18−0.73), $P = 0.005$]. In the CRT group, compared with the RV group, fewer patients had worsening HF [SHR 0.27 (95 CI 0.12−0.58), $P = 0.001$] and hospitalizations for HF [SHR 0.20 (95 CI 0.06−0.72), $P = 0.013$]. Total mortality was similar in both groups [hazard ratio (HR) 1.57 (95 CI 0.58−4.27), $P = 0.372$]. The beneficial effects of CRT were consistent in patients who had ejection fraction ≤ 35, New York Heart Association Class $\geq III$ and QRS width ≥ 120 and in those who did not. At multi-variable Cox regression, only CRT mode remained an independent predictor of absence of clinical failure during the follow-up [HR = 0.23 (95 CI 0.08−0.66), $P = 0.007$].

Conclusions.—In patients undergoing 'Ablate and Pace' therapy for severely symptomatic permanent atrial fibrillation, CRT is superior to RV

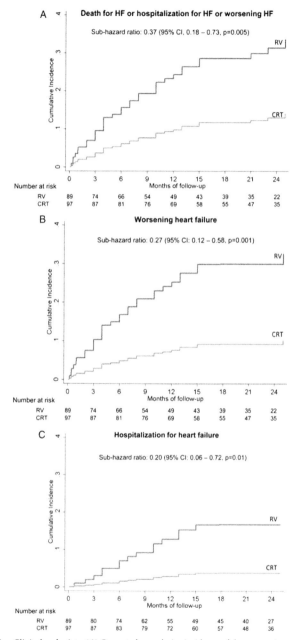

FIGURE 1.—Clinical endpoints. (*A*) Corrected cumulative incidence of the composite outcome of death from heart failure, hospitalization due to heart failure, or worsening heart failure ('clinical failure') (primary outcome). (*B*) Corrected cumulative incidence of worsening heart failure. (*C*) Corrected cumulative incidence of hospitalization for heart failure. HF, heart failure. (Reprinted from Brignole M, Botto G, Mont L, et al. Cardiac resynchronization therapy in patients undergoing atrioventricular junction ablation for permanent atrial fibrillation: a randomized trial. *Eur Heart J.* 2011;32:2420-2429, by permission of The European Society of Cardiology.)

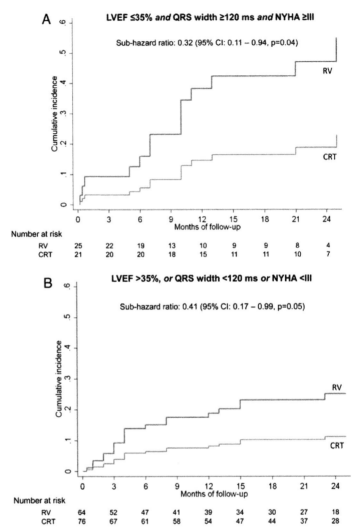

FIGURE 3.—Risk of clinical failure (primary composite endpoint), according to the indications for cardiac resynchronization therapy of the most recent guidelines. (*A*) Patients meeting the criteria of the recommendations of the guidelines. (*B*) Patients not meeting the recommendations of the guidelines. (Reprinted from Brignole M, Botto G, Mont L, et al. Cardiac resynchronization therapy in patients undergoing atrioventricular junction ablation for permanent atrial fibrillation: a randomized trial. *Eur Heart J.* 2011;32:2420-2429, by permission of The European Society of Cardiology.)

apical pacing in reducing the clinical manifestations of HF. (ClinicalTrials. gov number: NCT00111527) (Figs 1 and 3).

▶ The large landmark studies of cardiac resynchronization therapy (CRT) excluded patients who were pacemaker dependent. Accordingly, there is a paucity of data on this subject. This study was a prospective, randomized trial comparing

CRT and right ventricular (RV) pacing in patients with chronic atrial fibrillation and a reduced left ventricular ejection fraction undergoing atrioventricular (AV) node ablation. Fig 1 shows statistical improvement in all parameters addressed by CRT therapy. Fig 3 compares those patients that were eligible for CRT therapy with those that were not eligible via the guidelines based primarily on QRS duration preablation. Clearly, one of the advantages of pacing and ablating is true control of the ventricular rate, which often is inadequate on drug therapy, as well as regularization of R to R intervals, which is only partially controlled by adequate drug therapy. Interestingly, only two-thirds of the patients who had ejection fractions of less than 35% received implantable cardiac defibrillator therapy. However, there was only sudden death in the whole group for these 20 months of follow-up. Both groups reported an increase in ejection fraction after ablation, whether it was RV or CRT pacing. The CRT group had the greatest overall improvement. However, in the group who satisfied guidelines for CRT therapy, the improvement of ejection fraction by a CRT was less than that with RV pacing, which is surprising. Although the control group used obligatory RV pacing, which is known to have deleterious long-term effects, this study suggests that if complete heart block is present or AV node ablation is planned in the presence of LV dysfunction, then CRT is superior to RV pacing.

R. B. Leman, MD

Cardiac Resynchronization Therapy Reduces Left Atrial Volume and the Risk of Atrial Tachyarrhythmias in MADIT-CRT (Multicenter Automatic Defibrillator Implantation Trial with Cardiac Resynchronization Therapy)

Brenyo A, Link MS, Barsheshet A, et al (Univ of Rochester Med Ctr, NY; Tufts New England Med Ctr, Boston, MA; et al)
J Am Coll Cardiol 58:1682-1689, 2011

Objectives.—We hypothesized that reductions in left atrial volume (LAV) with a cardiac resynchronization therapy-defibrillator (CRT-D) would translate into a subsequent reduction in the risk of atrial tachyarrhythmias (AT).

Background.—There is limited information regarding the effect of CRT-D on the risk of AT.

Methods.—Percent reduction in LAV at 1 year following CRT-D implantation (pre-specified as low [lowest quartile: <20% reduction in LAV] and high [≥20% reduction in LAV] response to CRT-D) were related to the risk of subsequent AT (comprising atrial fibrillation, atrial flutter, atrial tachycardia, and supraventricular tachyarrhythmias) among patients enrolled in MADIT-CRT (Multicenter Automatic Defibrillator Implantation Trial with Cardiac Resynchronization Therapy).

Results.—The cumulative probability of AT 2.5 years after assessment of echocardiographic response was lowest among high LAV responders to CRT-D (3%) and significantly higher among both low LAV responders to CRT-D (9%) and implantable cardioverter-defibrillator—only patients (7%; p = 0.03 for the difference among the 3 groups). Consistently, multivariate

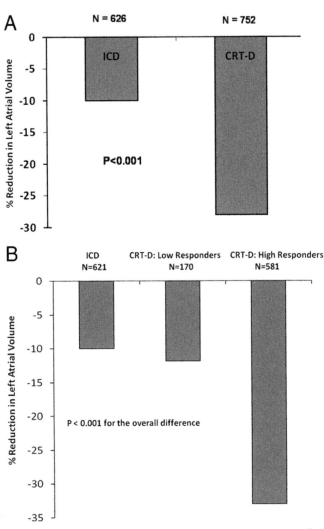

FIGURE 1.—Mean Percent Reductions in LAV. (A) The 2 treatment arms. (B) The implantable cardioverter-defibrillator (ICD) arm and low and high responders to cardiac resynchronization therapy-defibrillator (CRT-D). Percent reductions in left atrial volumes (LAVs) were calculated as the difference between 1-year volume and baseline volume, divided by baseline volume, among the 1,372 patients with available paired baseline and 1-year echocardiograms. (Reprinted from the Journal of the American College of Cardiology, Brenyo A, Link MS, Barsheshet A, et al. Cardiac resynchronization therapy reduces left atrial volume and the risk of atrial tachyarrhythmias in MADIT-CRT (Multicenter Automatic Defibrillator Implantation Trial with Cardiac Resynchronization Therapy). J Am Coll Cardiol. 2011;58:1682-1689. Copyright 2011, with permission from the American College of Cardiology.)

analysis showed that high LAV responders to CRT-D experienced a significant 53% (p = 0.01) reduction in the risk of subsequent AT as compared with implantable cardioverter-defibrillator—only patients, whereas low LAV responders did not derive a significant risk reduction with CRT-D therapy

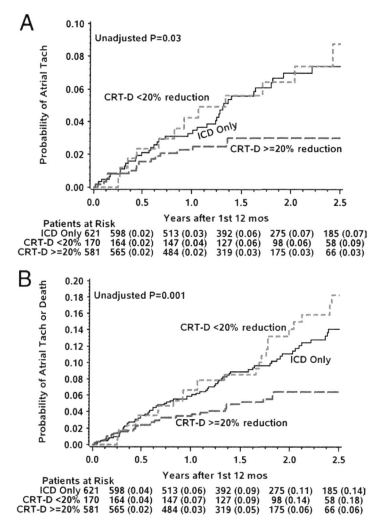

FIGURE 3.—Kaplan-Meier Estimates of the Cumulative Probability of AT and AT or Death. (A) Atrial tachyarrhythmias (ATs) and (B) AT or death by LAV response (≥20% vs. <20%) to CRT-D therapy and in ICD-only patients. Follow-up time beginning after the 1-year echocardiographic assessment of LAV response. Abbreviations as in Figure 1. (Reprinted from the Journal of the American College of Cardiology, Brenyo A, Link MS, Barsheshet A, et al. Cardiac resynchronization therapy reduces left atrial volume and the risk of atrial tachyarrhythmias in MADIT-CRT (Multicenter Automatic Defibrillator Implantation Trial with Cardiac Resynchronization Therapy). *J Am Coll Cardiol.* 2011;58:1682-1689. Copyright 2011, with permission from the American College of Cardiology.)

(hazard ratio [HR]: 1.05 [95% confidence interval (CI): 0.54 to 2.00]; p = 0.89). Patients who developed in-trial AT experienced significant increases in the risk for both the combined endpoint of heart failure or death (HR: 2.28 [95% CI: 1.45 to 3.59]; p < 0.001) and the separate occurrence of all-cause mortality (HR: 1.89 [95% CI: 1.08 to 3.62]; p = 0.01).

Conclusions.—In the MADIT-CRT study, favorable reverse remodeling of the left atrium with CRT-D therapy was associated with a significant reduction in risk of subsequent AT. (Multicenter Automatic Defibrillator Implantation Trial with Cardiac Resynchronization Therapy [MADIT-CRT]; NCT00180271) (Figs 1 and 3).

▶ Cardiac resynchronization therapy (CRT) results in a reduction of mitral regurgitation and left ventricular filling pressures. Accordingly, it is postulated that these changes should cause left atrial remodeling and fewer atrial tachyarrhythmias. However, previous retrospective studies have provided conflicting data on the impact of CRT on atrial fibrillation and other atrial arrhythmias. In this substudy of MADIT-CRT, the most comprehensive analysis of this problem is reported. The authors show that CRT is associated with significant reverse remodeling, as evidenced by changes in left atrial volumes (Fig 1). Moreover, CRT is also associated with a reduction in atrial arrhythmias. A significant reduction of left atrial size is a strong predictor of freedom from atrial arrhythmias (Fig 3). These results parallel studies from REVERSE and MADIT-CRT in mild heart failure patients showing that left ventricular reverse remodeling is associated with fewer ventricular arrhythmias. The reduction of arrhythmias associated with structural improvements with CRT is likely one of the important mechanisms for improved outcome with this therapy.

M. R. Gold, MD, PhD

Continuous biatrial pacing to prevent early recurrence of atrial fibrillation after the Maze procedure
Wang W, Buehler D, Feng XD, et al (Scripps Memorial Hosp, San Diego, CA; Shanxi Cardiovascular Hosp, Taiyuan, China)
J Thorac Cardiovasc Surg 142:989-994, 2011

Objective.—It has been suggested that overdrive biatrial pacing may prevent the recurrence of atrial fibrillation after the Maze procedure. To further evaluate this hypothesis, we performed a randomized prospective study in 100 patients undergoing valve surgery concomitant with a full Maze procedure to determine the effectiveness of biatrial pacing in the postoperative period to reduce early recurrence of atrial fibrillation.

Method.—Between January 2002 and December 2008, 100 patients undergoing mitral valve ± tricuspid valve surgery concomitant with the Maze procedure were randomized into 2 equal groups: the study group using overdrive biatrial pacing and a control group without pacing. One pacing wire was attached to the crista terminalis area of the right atrium, and the other pacing wire was attached to the Bachmann's bundle area located in the roof of the left atrium. The atria were paced continuously in AAI mode at a rate of 80 pulses per minute or 10 pulses above the underlying rate for 5 days. The end points were the onset of recurrent atrial fibrillation or discharge.

Results.—The incidence of recurrent postoperative atrial fibrillation was significantly less in the study group, with 6 of 50 patients (12%) incurring atrial fibrillation compared with 18 of 50 patients (36%) in the control group ($P < .01$). The length of hospital stay was significantly reduced in the study group ($P < .01$), and the mean costs of hospital stay were significantly lower in the control group ($P < .05$).

Conclusions.—Biatrial overdrive pacing is well tolerated and more effective in preventing the early recurrence of atrial fibrillation after the Maze procedure. This therapy also results in shortened hospital stays and decreased hospital costs. However, the impacts of the long-term results in the Maze procedure require further study.

▶ Atrial fibrillation (AF) is a common problem after cardiac surgery. Patients who experience this rhythm have longer hospital stays, higher hospital costs, and higher risk of morbidities such as stroke, congestive heart failure, and anticoagulation-related complications. The authors report the results of a prospective, randomized trial of continuous biatrial pacing in 100 patients after Maze procedure. The experimental group had pacing wires placed on the crista terminalis and the dome of the left atrium in the vicinity of Bachmann bundle and were paced at 80 beats per minute or 10 beats faster than their native rhythm for 5 days.

The experimental group had a lower incidence of AF (12% vs 36%, $P = .01$), shorter hospital stay (6.1 vs 8.7 days, $P = .01$), and reduced cost (14% reduction). The strength of this study is its prospective and randomized design. The weaknesses are the lack of longer-term follow-up and relatively unique patient population. It is unclear whether postoperative atrial pacing offers long-term benefits nor is it clear that it will be beneficial for patients undergoing procedures other than Maze.

This study supports the use of the simple, near risk-free, and inexpensive technique of biatrial continuous pacing after valve/Maze procedures.

J. M. Toole, MD

Incidence and Predictors of Pacemaker Placement After Surgical Ablation for Atrial Fibrillation

Worku B, Pak S-W, Cheema F, et al (Columbia Univ College of Physicians and Surgeons/New York Presbyterian Hosp)
Ann Thorac Surg 92:2085-2090, 2011

Background.—Bradyarrhythmia requiring pacemaker placement is a relatively common complication after surgical ablation for atrial fibrillation (AF). We report our experience with surgical ablation procedures using various energy modalities and lesion sets in an attempt to identify the risk factors associated with postoperative pacemaker requirement.

Methods.—Intraoperative data were collected prospectively, and preoperative and postoperative data were collected retrospectively. Energy modality and lesion sets used were dependent on availability on the date of the procedure and surgeon preference.

Results.—From October 1999 to October 2009, 701 patients underwent surgical ablation for AF at our institution. Forty-five patients (7.6%) required early postoperative pacemaker placement. There were no significant differences in baseline characteristics or associated procedures between patients who required pacemaker placement and those who did not. Ninety-day mortality was greater in patients requiring pacemaker placement (15.6% versus 6.6%; $p = 0.025$). In multivariable analysis, a pacemaker requirement was more likely with the use of microwave energy (odds ratio [OR] 2.87; confidence interval [CI], 1.41 to 5.84; $p = 0.004$) and a right atrial lesion set (OR, 2.82; CI, 1.07 to 7.45; $p = 0.036$).

Conclusions.—In conclusion, over our 10-year experience with surgical AF ablations, the incidence of pacemaker requirement was much lower than that reported in series of classic "cut and sew" Maze procedures, even among patients undergoing full biatrial ablations. Although biatrial ablation is currently our favored approach to patients with long-standing or persistent AF, right atrial lesion sets increase the risk of this complication and should be used judiciously.

▶ The authors examine their extensive experience with surgical atrial fibrillation (AF) ablation techniques to identify the incidence and risk factors for permanent pacemaker placement. They retrospectively reviewed 701 cases done over a 10-year period at a single institution. A permanent pacemaker was required in 45 (7.6%) patients. Ninety-day mortality was significantly higher in those requiring a pacemaker (15.6% vs 6.6%, $P = .025$) although Kaplan-Meier survival was equivalent. On multivariable analysis, right atrial lesion sets and the use of microwave as an energy source were both found to be independent predictors of pacemaker placement.

The strengths of this study are the large sample size and the subsequent ability to compare each AF ablation technique. The weaknesses include its retrospective design and inherent bias. Specifically, the authors acknowledge their preference for biatrial lesion sets in the setting of long-standing or persistent AF. This degree of AF may be related to more advanced electrophysiologic or structural heart disease, which might account for the observed higher 90-day mortality in pacer recipients. The higher observed incidence of pacer requirement associated with the use of microwave energy is not as easily explained. While direct cause cannot be determined from this retrospective review, thermal spread from the energy source may be greater with this technology and lead to less discrete lesions and more collateral tissue damage.

The incidence of permanent pacemaker requirement after AF ablation is low. Consideration should be given to the risks and benefits of this procedure when selecting patient, energy source, and lesion set.

J. M. Toole, MD

Independent Susceptibility Markers for Atrial Fibrillation on Chromosome 4q25

Lubitz SA, Sinner MF, Lunetta KL, et al (Massachusetts General Hosp, Charlestown; Univ Hosp Grosshadern and Inst of Med Informatics, Munich, Germany; Natl Heart, Lung, and Blood Inst's Framingham Heart Study, MA; et al)
Circulation 122:976-984, 2010

Background.—Genetic variants on chromosome 4q25 are associated with atrial fibrillation (AF). We sought to determine whether there is more than 1 susceptibility signal at this locus.

Methods and Results.—Thirty-four haplotype-tagging single-nucleotide polymorphisms (SNPs) at the 4q25 locus were genotyped in 790 case and 1177 control subjects from Massachusetts General Hospital and tested for association with AF. We replicated SNPs associated with AF after adjustment for the most significantly associated SNP in 5066 case and 30 661 referent subjects from the German Competence Network for Atrial Fibrillation, Atherosclerosis Risk In Communities Study, Cleveland Clinic Lone AF Study, Cardiovascular Health Study, and Rotterdam Study. All subjects were of European ancestry. A multimarker risk score composed of SNPs that tagged distinct AF susceptibility signals was constructed and tested for association with AF, and all results were subjected to meta-analysis. The previously reported SNP, rs2200733, was most significantly associated with AF (minor allele odds ratio 1.80, 95% confidence interval 1.50 to 2.15, $P=1.2\times10^{-20}$) in the discovery sample. Adjustment for rs2200733 genotype revealed 2 additional susceptibility signals marked by rs17570669 and rs3853445. A graded risk of AF was observed with an increasing number of AF risk alleles at SNPs that tagged these 3 susceptibility signals.

Conclusions.—We identified 2 novel AF susceptibility signals on chromosome 4q25. Consideration of multiple susceptibility signals at chromosome 4q25 identifies individuals with an increased risk of AF and may localize regulatory elements at the locus with biological relevance in the pathogenesis of AF.

▶ The genetic basis for atrial fibrillation (AF) is poorly understood, although several chromosome abnormalities have been shown to be associated with AF, such as loci on the long arms of chromosome 10 and 6. This study further evaluates the long arm of the fourth chromosome at locus 25 (4q25), which has previously been shown to potentially contain the single nucleotide polymorphism labeled rs2200733. The present study identified 2 other susceptibility signals, labeled rf17570699 and rs3853445, that were also associated with an increased risk of AF. Interestingly, there was increasing risk of AF with the addition of each of the sites in combination. Although preliminary work suggests some role of 4q25 in genetic regulation, it is not known how mutations in the 4q25 region cause AF. Nonetheless, studies such as this may lead to stronger means of risk stratification and may lead to novel pharmacogenetic means of treating AF.

J. M. Warton, MD

Devices

Biventricular pacing is superior to right ventricular pacing in bradycardia patients with preserved systolic function: 2-year results of the PACE trial

Chan JY-S, Fang F, Zhang Q, et al (The Chinese Univ of Hong Kong, UK; et al)
Eur Heart J 32:2533-2540, 2011

Aims.—The Pacing to Avoid Cardiac Enlargement (PACE) trial is a prospective, double-blinded, randomized, multicentre study that reported the superiority of biventricular (BiV) pacing to right ventricular apical (RVA) pacing in the prevention of left ventricular (LV) adverse remodelling and deterioration of systolic function at 1 year. In the current analysis, we report the results at extended 2-year follow-up for changes in LV function and remodelling.

Methods and Results.—Patients ($n = 177$) with bradycardia and preserved LV ejection fraction (EF $\geq 45\%$) were randomized to receive RVA or BiV pacing. The co-primary endpoints were LVEF and LV end-systolic volume (LVESV).

Eighty-one (92%) of 88 in the RVA pacing group and 82 (92%) of 89 patients in the BiV pacing group completed 2-year follow-up with a valid echocardiography. In the RVA pacing group, LVEF further decreased from the first to the second year, but it remained unchanged in the BiV pacing group, leading to a significant difference of 9.9 percentage points between groups at 2-year follow-up ($P < 0.001$). Similarly, LVESV continues to enlarge from the first to the second year in the RVA pacing group, leading to a difference of 13.0 mL ($P < 0.001$) between groups. Predefined subgroup analysis showed consistent results with the whole study population for both co-primary endpoints, which included patients with pre-existing LV diastolic dysfunction. Eighteen patients in the BiV pacing group (20.2%) and 55 in the RVA pacing group (62.5%) had a significant reduction of LVEF (of $\geq 5\%$, $P < 0.001$).

Conclusion.—Left ventricular adverse remodelling and deterioration of systolic function continues at the second year after RVA pacing. This deterioration is prevented by BiV pacing (Fig 1).

▶ Cardiac resynchronization therapy (CRT) with biventricular pacing is well-established therapy for the treatment of advanced heart failure in the setting of left ventricular systolic dysfunction and QRS prolongation. More recent studies have found that CRT is also very effective among patients with mild heart failure, a reduced ejection fraction (EF), and QRS prolongation, primarily left bundle branch block (LBBB). One of the less well-studied aspects of CRT is its application for patients with frequent right ventricular (RV) pacing. This mimics an LBBB and is a class II indication for CRT among patients with a reduced EF based on several studies, including Pacing to Avoid Cardiac Enlargement (PACE). In this study, a prospective, randomized comparison of RV and biventricular pacing was performed in patients with preserved EF (> 45%). The PACE trial showed that more than 2 years of RV pacing is associated with a deterioration of left

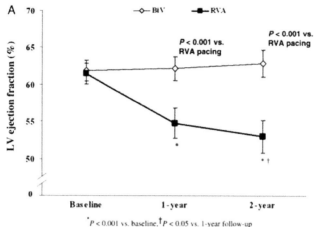

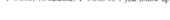

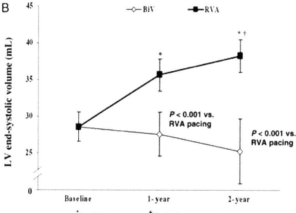

FIGURE 1.—Comparison of co-primary endpoints between biventricular pacing (BiV) and right ventricular apical pacing (RVA) at 24 months. An open diamond denotesmean values for the right ventricular apical pacing group and a filled box denotes the mean values for the biventricular pacing group. The repeated measure ANOVA showed a significant decrease in the left ventricular ejection fraction in the right ventricular apical group (A), whereas the left ventricular end-systolic volume was increased (B). The bars indicate 95% confidence intervals. Intra-group analysis showed a significant difference for both endpoints among the three time intervals for the right ventricular apical group: *$P < 0.001$ vs. baseline and †$P < 0.05$ vs. 1 year in the same pacing group. (Reprinted from Chan JY-S, Fang F, Zhang Q, et al. Biventricular pacing is superior to right ventricular pacing in bradycardia patients with preserved systolic function: 2-year results of the PACE trial. *Eur Heart J.* 2011;32:2533-2540, by permission of The European Society of Cardiology.)

ventricular (LV) function with a reduction of EF from 61% to 55%. However, this was not associated with any clinical differences between groups. Although the differences noted were statistically significant, they may not be clinically meaningful, at least over the mid-term results studies. Accordingly, routine placement of CRT devices in patients with obligatory ventricular pacing and preserved LV function is not warranted at this time, given the increased costs and complications associated with this approach in the absence of proven clinical benefit.

M. R. Gold, MD, PhD

Cardiac Resynchronization Therapy as a Therapeutic Option in Patients With Moderate-Severe Functional Mitral Regurgitation and High Operative Risk
van Bommel RJ, Marsan NA, Delgado V, et al (Leiden Univ Med Ctr, the Netherlands)
Circulation 124:912-919, 2011

Background.—Functional mitral regurgitation (MR) is a common finding in heart failure patients with dilated cardiomyopathy and has important prognostic implications. However, the increased operative risk of these patients may result in low referral or high denial rate for mitral valve surgery. Cardiac resynchronization therapy (CRT) has been shown to have a favorable effect on MR. Aims of this study were to (1) evaluate CRT as a therapeutic option in heart failure patients with functional MR and high operative risk and (2) investigate the effect of MR improvement after CRT on prognosis.

Methods and Results.—A total of 98 consecutive patients with moderate-severe functional MR and high operative risk underwent CRT according to current guidelines. Echocardiography was performed at baseline and 6-month follow-up; severity of MR was graded according to a multiparametric approach. Significant improvement of MR was defined as a reduction ≥ 1 grade. All-cause mortality was assessed during follow-up (median 32 [range 6.0 to 116] months). Thirteen patients (13%) died before 6-months follow-up. In the remaining 85 patients, significant reduction in MR was observed in all evaluated parameters. In particular, 42 patients (49%) improved ≥ 1 grade of MR and were considered MR improvers. Survival was superior in MR improvers compared to MR nonimprovers (log rank $P<0.001$). Mitral regurgitation improvement was an independent prognostic factor for survival (hazard ratio 0.35, confidence interval 0.13 to 0.94; $P=0.043$).

Conclusions.—Cardiac resynchronization therapy is a potential therapeutic option in heart failure patients with moderate-severe functional MR and high risk for surgery. Improvement in MR results in superior survival after CRT (Fig 3, Table 3).

▶ Functional mitral regurgitation (MR) is a common finding with prognostic implications in heart failure patients with dilated cardiomyopathy. An increased operative risk and controversy of the benefits of surgical correction result in low referral and high denial rates for mitral valve surgery. Cardiac resynchronization therapy (CRT) has been found to have a favorable effect on MR, so this study was aimed to evaluate CRT as a therapeutic option in high-risk heart failure patients with functional MR. There were 98 consecutive patients (74% male, 63% ischemic) with moderate to severe functional MR and high operative risk evaluated who underwent CRT according to current guidelines. Echocardiography was performed at baseline and 6-month follow-up, and all-cause mortality

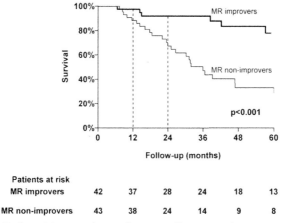

Patients at risk

MR improvers	42	37	28	24	18	13
MR non-improvers	43	38	24	14	9	8

FIGURE 3.—Kaplan–Meier survival curves for time to all-cause mortality in MR improvers versus MR nonimprovers. During long-term follow-up, survival was superior in MR improvers compared with MR nonimprovers; log rank $P<0.001$. Respective 1- and 2-year survival rates were 97% and 92% in MR improvers compared with 88% and 67% in MR nonimprovers. MR indicates mitral regurgitation. (Reprinted from van Bommel RJ, Marsan NA, Delgado V, et al. Cardiac resynchronization therapy as a therapeutic option in patients with moderate-severe functional mitral regurgitation and high operative risk. *Circulation*. 2011;124:912-919. © American Heart Association, Inc.)

TABLE 3.—Changes in Clinical and Echocardiographic Characteristics of MR Improvers and Nonimprovers at 6-Month Follow-Up

Variable	MR Improvers (n=42)		MR Nonimprovers (n=43)		P Between Groups	P Interaction Group and Time
	Baseline	Follow-Up	Baseline	Follow-Up		
NYHA class	3.0±0.2	1.9±0.7‡	3.2±0.4	2.3±0.6‡	0.005	0.117
6 MWT, m	299±113	407±121*	266±105	329±106‡	0.022	0.061
QoL score	35±17	19±16*	42±18	28±17*	0.019	0.783
LVEDV, mL	255±84	214±78‡	267±93	252±81*	0.174	0.004
LVESV, mL	201±80	146±69‡	208±83	187±70†	0.151	<0.001
LVEF, %	23±7	33±10‡	23±6	27±7†	0.039	<0.001
VCW, cm	0.73±0.14	0.44±0.16†	0.74±0.17	0.73±0.13	<0.001	<0.001
EROA, cm²	0.51±0.16	0.31±0.12*	0.52±0.16	0.54±0.16	0.002	<0.001
TA, cm²	7.1±2.1	5.5±1.7‡	7.4±1.9	7.1±2.0*	0.033	<0.001
LA volume, mL	102±43	78±27‡	104±32	104±32	0.050	<0.001
Jet area/LA area, %	51±14	29±15*	52±14	53±13	<0.001	<0.001
SPAP, mm Hg	34±10	25±6*	37±9	38±9	<0.001	<0.001
MR grade	3.3±0.5	1.8±0.6*	3.3±0.5	3.4±0.6	<0.001	<0.001

MR indicates mitral regurgitation; NYHA, New York Heart Association; 6 MWT, 6-minute walk test; QoL, quality of life; LVEDV, left ventricular end-diastolic volume; LVESV, left ventricular end-systolic volume; LVEF, left ventricular ejection fraction; VCW, vena contracta width; EROA, effective regurgitant orifice area; TA, tenting area; LA, left atrium; and SPAP, systolic pulmonary artery pressure.
*$P<0.05$, baseline vs follow-up.
†$P=0.001$, baseline vs follow-up.
‡$P<0.001$, baseline vs follow-up.

was assessed during follow-up (median, 32 months [6.0–116]). In the 85 patients that survived to the 6-month follow-up, 42 patients (49%) were noted to have MR improvement (reduction ≥1 grade). Both the MR improvers and nonimprovers had an improvement in clinical characteristics as displayed in Table 3, although the improvements were more pronounced in the subgroup with improved MR. Fig 3 shows survival was superior in terms of all-cause mortality in the MR-improved subgroup (P < .001). One- and 2-year survival rates were 97% and 92% in the MR improved group compared with 88% and 67% in MR nonimproved, respectively (log rank, P = .117 at 1 year; log rank, P = .13 at 2 years). MR improvement was also found to be a strong independent predictor of survival after CRT with a corrected hazard ratio of 0.35 (95% confidence interval, 0.13 to 0.94, P = .043). The current findings are consistent with those of prior studies that have found improvement in MR with CRT, although this study shows superior survival with MR improvement (reduction ≥1 grade) independent of other variables. As further benefits of CRT continue to be described and indications continue to expand, the predictors of a reduction in significant MR should be studied further.

P. C. Netzler, MD

Cost-effectiveness of cardiac resynchronization therapy in patients with asymptomatic to mild heart failure: insights from the European cohort of the REVERSE (Resynchronization Reverses remodeling in Systolic Left Ventricular Dysfunction)

Linde C, on behalf of the REVERSE study group (Univ Hosp, Stockholm, Sweden; et al)
Eur Heart J 32:1631-1639, 2011

Aims.—To assess the cost-effectiveness of cardiac resynchronization therapy (CRT) compared with optimal medical therapy in patients with New York Heart Association (NYHA) II heart failure (HF) or NYHA I with previous HF symptoms.

Methods and Results.—A proportion in state model with Monte Carlo simulation was developed to assess the costs, life years and quality-adjusted life year (QALYs) associated with CRT-ON and -OFF over a 10 year time period. Data from 262 patients in the European cohort of the REVERSE clinical trial (QRS ≥ 120 ms, left ventricular ejection fraction ≤ 40, CRT-ON, $n = 180$, CRT-OFF, $n = 82$) were used to model all-cause mortality, change in NYHA class and resource use. EQ-5D preference weights were taken from a previous cost-effectiveness model of CRT and unit costs from national UK databases. Costs and benefits were discounted at 3.5% p.a. Extensive deterministic and probabilistic sensitivity analyses were performed. Compared with CRT-OFF, 0.94 life years or 0.80 QALYs were gained in the CRT ON group at an additional cost of €11 455, yielding an incremental cost-effectiveness ratio of €14 278 per quality-adjusted life year (QALY) gained. At a threshold of €33 000 (£30 000) per QALY gained, the probability that CRT is cost-effective is 79.6%. Cardiac resynchronization therapy becomes cost effective after ~4.5 years. Cardiac resynchronization therapy needs only to demonstrate a modest impact on all cause mortality (hazard

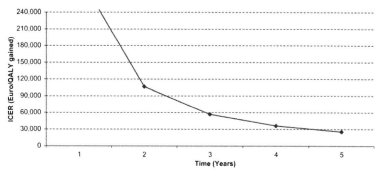

FIGURE 4.—Impact of alternative time horizons on the cost-effectiveness of cardiac resynchronization therapy. (Reprinted from Linde C, on behalf of the REVERSE study group. Cost-effectiveness of cardiac resynchronization therapy in patients with asymptomatic to mild heart failure: insights from the European cohort of the REVERSE (Resynchronization Reverses remodeling in Systolic Left Ventricular Dysfunction). *Eur Heart J.* 2011;32:1631-1639, by permission of The European Society of Cardiology.)

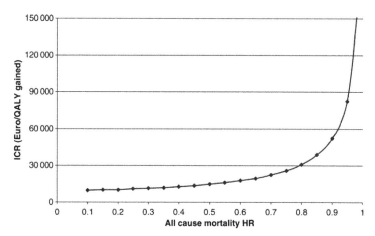

FIGURE 5.—Impact of changes in mortality treatment effect on the cost-effectiveness of cardiac resynchronization therapy. (Reprinted from Linde C, on behalf of the REVERSE study group. Cost-effectiveness of cardiac resynchronization therapy in patients with asymptomatic to mild heart failure: insights from the European cohort of the REVERSE (Resynchronization Reverses remodeling in Systolic Left Ventricular Dysfunction). *Eur Heart J.* 2011;32:1631-1639, by permission of The European Society of Cardiology.)

ratio=0.82) in order to demonstrate cost-effectiveness. The results are robust to changes in all other parameters.

Conclusion.—Cardiac resynchronization therapy is a cost-effective intervention for patients with mildly symptomatic HF and for asymptomatic patients with left ventricular dysfunction and previous HF symptoms (Figs 4 and 5).

▶ Much of the dramatic reductions in cardiovascular mortality observed over the last 40 years can be attributed to the application of effective therapies earlier in the disease course or even for primary prevention. Such examples include β-blockers, statins and implantable cardiac defibrillators (ICDs). Cardiac resynchronization therapy (CRT) with biventricular pacing is a well-proven therapy in patients with advanced heart failure, left ventricular dysfunction, and QRS prolongation, particularly left bundle branch block (LBBB). More recently, 3 studies were completed applying CRT to mild heart failure: REVERSE, MADIT-CRT, and RAFT. In the first cost-effectiveness analysis performed on the European cohort of REVERSE, it is shown that this is a very cost effective approach, assuming a long duration of therapy (Fig 4) and modest mortality benefit (Fig 5). Interestingly, the larger and longer-duration studies of CRT in mild heart failure showed a mortality benefit in class II patients (RAFT) or those with LBBB (MADIT-CRT). These data indicate that CRT will be cost effective if appropriately used in class I or II heart failure patients with LV dysfunction and LBBB.

M. R. Gold, MD, PhD

Driving restrictions after implantable cardioverter defibrillator implantation: an evidence-based approach
Thijssen J, Borleffs CJW, van Rees JB, et al (Leiden Univ Med Ctr, The Netherlands)
Eur Heart J 32:2678-2687, 2011

Aims.—Little evidence is available regarding restrictions from driving following implantable cardioverter defibrillator (ICD) implantation or following first appropriate or inappropriate shock. The purpose of the current analysis was to provide evidence for driving restrictions based on real-world incidences of shocks (appropriate and inappropriate).

Methods and Results.—A total of 2786 primary and secondary prevention ICD patients were included. The occurrence of shocks was noted during a median follow-up of 996 days (inter-quartile range, 428–1833 days). With the risk of harm (RH) formula, using the incidence of sudden cardiac incapacitation, the annual RH to others posed by a driver with an ICD was calculated. Based on Canadian data, the annual RH to others of 5 in 100 000 (0.005) was used as a cut-off value. In both primary and secondary prevention ICD patients with private driving habits, no restrictions to drive directly following implantation, or an inappropriate shock are warranted. However, following an appropriate shock, these patients are at an increased risk to cause harm to other road users and therefore should be restricted to drive for a period of 2 and 4 months, respectively. In addition, all ICD patients with professional driving habits have a substantial elevated risk to cause harm to other road users during the complete follow-up after both implantation and shock and should therefore be restricted to drive permanently.

Conclusion.—The current analysis provides a clinically applicable tool for guideline committees to establish evidence-based driving restrictions (Fig 5).

▶ Guidelines are lacking for driving motor vehicles following implantable cardioverter defibrillator (ICD) placement. This study included 2786 patients following

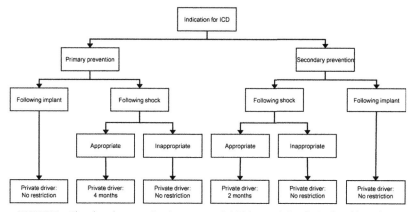

FIGURE 5.—Flowchart demonstrating the recommended driving restrictions for implantable cardioverter defibrillator patients with private driving habits. Based on the current analysis, implantable cardioverter defibrillator patients with professional driving habits should be restricted to drive in all circumstances and therefore are not in the figure. (Reprinted from Thijssen J, Borleffs CJW, van Rees JB, et al. Driving restrictions after implantable cardioverter defibrillator implantation: an evidence-based approach. *Eur Heart J.* 2011;32:2678-2687, by permission of The European Society of Cardiology.)

ICD. The median time for follow-up in primary prevention (1718) patients was 2 years and was 4 years for secondary prevention (1068) patients. A risk harm formula was used based on Canadian data to try to determine whether restrictions for driving should be obtained for appropriate and inappropriate shocks. Only first and second shocks were used in the data. Assessment of risk harm was developed from a formula to quantify the risk of people driving with ICDs based on the Canadian Cardiovascular Society Consensus Conference. It was assumed that 31% of the patients may experience syncope or near syncope during an appropriate shock. The assumption that inappropriate shocks had the same instance of syncope would overestimate the need to limit driving in this population, but it did not. The true incidence of syncope while driving is unknown. It is assumed that injury to others at ≤5 in 100 000 would be acceptable to allow people to drive. By using risk assessment guidance, the group developed (Fig 5) a flow chart to determine when driving restrictions should be applied. As expected, those with primary prevention had fewer initial shocks (10%) than those in secondary prevention (17%). Surprisingly, the mean time for initial shock in primary prevention was shorter (417 days) than for and secondary prevention patients (509 days). An earlier resumption of driving for secondary prevention would be indicated by this study. The limitations of this study are the changes in device therapy since 1996, lack of antitachycardia pacing therapy, and the assumption of true syncope or near syncope as a percentage of both appropriate and inappropriate shocks. Nevertheless, this study comes to a reasonable mathematical conclusion on these observational data (Fig 5) and adds important data to formulate future guidelines for driving.

B. Leman, MD

Complete removal as a routine treatment for any cardiovascular implantable electronic device—associated infection

Pichlmaier M, Knigina L, Kutschka I, et al (Hannover Med School, Germany)
J Thorac Cardiovasc Surg 142:1482-1490, 2011

Objective.—Pacemaker and implantable cardioverter defibrillator lead endocarditis mandates removal of all foreign material. In supposedly limited (pocket) infections, such a radical approach is still controversial. Thus, some patients are potentially exposed to persistent and recurrent infection because of retained material. Procedural risks and the success of eradicating infection were examined if involvement of the complete system was assumed in any cardiovascular implantable electronic device infection and complete removal was thus mandatory.

Methods.—A 12-year experience with 192 consecutive cases of bacterial pacemaker (152) or defibrillator (40) infections is presented. Complete removal of all prosthetic material was always aimed for. This was followed by antibiotic treatment for 4 to 6 weeks under temporary pacing if required, and then the new system was implanted. A total of 104 parameters concerning patient characteristics and operative and postoperative treatment were examined for their influence on outcome.

Results.—Infection was eradicated in 92.8% of patients. Recurrence was predominantly caused by failure to remove all prosthetic material ($P < .001$). If the protocol was strictly followed, infection was eradicated in 97.4% of patients. Conversely, 71.4% of patients with retained material showed recurrence. Further risk factors were poor dental hygiene and evidence of chronic subclinical infection. Morbidity and mortality of the interventional and open procedures were low. Open lead extraction was performed primarily in 34 patients (17.7%) and secondarily in 3 patients (1.9%). Temporary pacing and long-term antibiotic treatment were well tolerated.

Conclusions.—Complete removal of prosthetic material in any cardiovascular implantable electronic device infection is safe and associated with low morbidity and mortality. Success of eradicating infection is high if all system components are removed. Temporary pacing in dependent patients may be performed safely on an outpatient basis (Fig 3).

▶ The authors summarize their 12-year experience with treatment of 192 infected pacemakers or defibrillators. While removal of all components of the device is recognized as the standard of care for lead endocarditis or sepsis, the treatment for isolated pocket infection is less clear. The authors have adopted the strategy of complete removal of all components for any infection and report their excellent results.

The overall success rate for eradication of the infection was 92.8%. When considering those patients from whom all hardware was removed, the success rate was 97.4%. In those with retained hardware, 71.4% experienced a recurrence (Fig 3). This study reinforces the basic surgical principle of clearing all foreign material from an infected site. Of note, all extractions were performed in the operating room by a cardiovascular surgeon allowing for prompt treatment of rare but

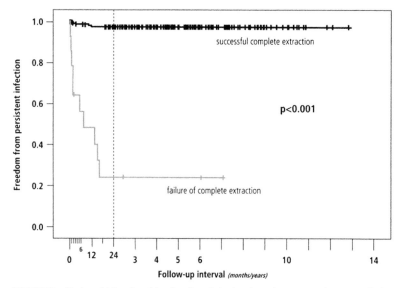

FIGURE 3.—Kaplan—Meier plot of freedom from infection dependent on complete removal of prosthetic material. Note nonlinear time axis stressing the initial 24 months after surgery. (Reprinted from the Journal of Thoracic and Cardiovascular Surgery, Pichlmaier M, Knigina L, Kutschka I, et al. Complete removal as a routine treatment for any cardiovascular implantable electronic device—associated infection. *J Thorac Cardiovasc Surg.* 2011;142:1482-1490. Copyright 2011, with permission from The American Association for Thoracic Surgery.)

potentially lethal complications, such as mediastinal vascular or cardiac injuries. Techniques used included stylets, locking stylets, and sheaths.

This important article demonstrates that the total eradication of infection is dependent on complete removal of all hardware regardless of lead involvement. Retained hardware leads to alarmingly high rates of recurrent infection. In addition to the aforementioned techniques, laser sheath extraction has proven to be a safe and effective adjunctive technique and may decrease the incidence of retained hardware.[1] While not specifically addressed in this study, the results reinforce other observations that these procedures should be performed by experienced operators (surgeons or cardiologists) at sufficiently high volume centers to maximize outcomes.

J. M. Toole, MD

Reference

1. Kratz JM, Toole JM. Pacemaker and internal cardioverter defibrillator lead extraction: a safe and effective surgical approach. *Ann Thorac Surg.* 2010;90:1411-1417.

Dual-Chamber Implantable Cardioverter-Defibrillator Selection Is Associated With Increased Complication Rates and Mortality Among Patients Enrolled in the NCDR Implantable Cardioverter-Defibrillator Registry

Dewland TA, Pellegrini CN, Wang Y, et al (Univ of California, San Francisco; Yale Univ, New Haven, CT; et al)
J Am Coll Cardiol 58:1007-1013, 2011

Objectives.—The aim of this study was to compare single- versus dual-chamber implantable cardioverter-defibrillator (ICD) implantation and complication rates in a large, real-world population.

Background.—The majority of patients enrolled in ICD efficacy trials received single-chamber devices. Although dual-chamber ICDs offer theoretical advantages over single-chamber defibrillators, the clinical superiority of dual-chamber models has not been conclusively proven, and they may increase complications.

Methods.—The National Cardiovascular Data Registry ICD Registry was used to examine the association between baseline characteristics and device selection in 104,049 patients receiving single- and dual-chamber ICDs between January 1, 2006, and December 31, 2007. A longitudinal cohort design was then used to determine in-hospital complication rates.

Results.—Dual-chamber devices were implanted in 64,489 patients (62%). Adverse events were more frequent with dual-chamber than with single-chamber device implantation (3.17% vs. 2.11%, $p < 0.001$), as was the rate of in-hospital mortality (0.40% vs. 0.23%, $p < 0.001$). After adjusting for demographics, medical comorbidities, diagnostic test data, and ICD indication, the odds of any complication (odds ratio: 1.40; 95% confidence interval: 1.28 to 1.52; $p < 0.001$) and in-hospital mortality (odds ratio: 1.45; 95% confidence interval: 1.20 to 1.74; $p < 0.001$) were increased with dual-chamber versus single-chamber ICD implantation.

Conclusions.—In this large, multicenter cohort of patients, dual-chamber ICD use was common. Dual-chamber device implantation was associated with increases in periprocedural complications and in-hospital mortality compared with single-chamber defibrillator selection (Tables 3 and 4).

▶ Despite the fact that patients in implantable cardioverter-defibrillator (ICD) efficacy trials predominantly received single-chamber devices, dual-chamber devices have been implanted in the majority (> 60%) of patients registered in the National Cardiovascular Data Registry (NCDR) ICD registry. While dual-chamber devices may offer theoretical advantages over single-chamber ICDs, such as atrial rate support and improved discrimination, their clinical superiority has not been demonstrated in randomized trials. Additionally, they may be associated with more complications. This study used NCDR ICD registry data to compare complication and mortality rates between single-chamber and dual-chamber ICDs. Table 3 summarizes the complications associated with ICD implantations, and Table 4 demonstrates the increased complication rates (unadjusted odds ratio [OR], 1.49) and in-hospital mortality rates (unadjusted OR, 1.69) associated with dual-chamber ICD implants. Although this study is observational and does

TABLE 3.—Single-Versus Dual-Chamber ICD Implantation Complication Rates

| Adverse Event | ICD Type | | p Value |
	Single Chamber	Dual Chamber	
Cardiac arrest	91 (0.23%)	203 (0.31%)	0.01
Drug reaction	33 (0.08%)	69 (0.11%)	0.24
Cardiac perforation	22 (0.06%)	42 (0.07%)	0.55
Cardiac valve injury	0 (0.00%)	1 (<0.01%)	0.43
Conduction block	7 (0.02%)	22 (0.03%)	0.12
Coronary venous dissection	4 (0.01%)	76 (0.12%)	<0.001
Hematoma	282 (0.71%)	593 (0.92%)	<0.001
Lead dislodgement	198 (0.50%)	565 (0.88%)	<0.001
Hemothorax	22 (0.06%)	52 (0.08%)	0.14
Pneumothorax	144 (0.36%)	339 (0.53%)	<0.001
Peripheral nerve injury	2 (0.01%)	3 (<0.01%)	0.93
Peripheral embolus	7 (0.02%)	21 (0.03%)	0.16
Phlebitis (superficial)	10 (0.03%)	40 (0.06%)	0.009
Phlebitis (deep)	6 (0.02%)	17 (0.03%)	0.24
Transient ischemic attack	3 (0.01%)	13 (0.02%)	0.11
Stroke	21 (0.05%)	41 (0.06%)	0.50
Myocardial infarction	6 (0.02%)	23 (0.04%)	0.05
Pericardial tamponade	19 (0.05%)	59 (0.09%)	0.01
Arteriovenous fistula	0 (0.00%)	5 (0.01%)	0.08
Infection related to device	12 (0.03%)	18 (0.03%)	0.82
Any adverse event	833 (2.11%)	2,047 (3.17%)	<0.001
All-cause mortality	91 (0.23%)	259 (0.40%)	<0.001
Cardiovascular cause	56 (0.14%)	181 (0.28%)	<0.001
Noncardiovascular cause	35 (0.09%)	78 (0.12%)	0.12
Death in laboratory	6 (0.02%)	17 (0.03%)	0.24

Values are n (%).
ICD = implantable cardioverter-defibrillator.

TABLE 4.—Odds of Adverse Events Associated With Dual-Chamber ICD Implantation

	Unadjusted OR	95% CI	p Value	Multivariate OR	95% CI	p Value
Any complication	1.49	1.37−1.61	<0.001	1.40	1.28−1.52	<0.001
In-hospital mortality	1.69	1.42−2.01	<0.001	1.45	1.20−1.74	<0.001

CI = confidence interval; ICD = implantable cardioverter-defibrillator; OR = odds ratio.

not preclude direct causality, the routine use of dual chamber devices should be scrutinized. Clinicians should carefully consider the indications for, as well as the risks and benefits of, implanting dual- versus single-chamber ICDs. Because atrial support pacing in the absence of bradycardia has not been found to be useful and dual-chamber discrimination algorithms are not superior to single chamber, it appears that dual-chamber ICDs are overused.

F. Cuoco, MD

Impact of Implanted Recalled Sprint Fidelis Lead on Patient Mortality

Morrison TB, Friedman PA, Kallinen LM, et al (Mayo Clinic, Rochester, MN; Minneapolis Heart Inst, MN; et al)
J Am Coll Cardiol 58:278-283, 2011

Objectives.—This study sought to compare all-cause mortality in patients with Fidelis leads (Medtronic, Minneapolis, Minnesota) to those with a non-advisory lead.

Background.—Although Fidelis leads are prone to fracture, and rare deaths due to lead failure have been reported, it is unclear whether the presence of a Fidelis lead is associated with increased mortality. This study compares all-cause mortality in a large cohort of patients with Fidelis and Quattro implantable cardioverter-defibrillator (ICD) leads.

Methods.—All patients with Fidelis (Medtronic models 6931, 6948, and 6949) and Quattro (Medtronic model 6947) leads followed at 3 tertiary care centers were identified from the medical records (implant dates: November 19, 2001, to December 23, 2008). Clinical and device-specific data were collected into a common database. Deaths were identified from medical records and the Social Security Death Index. Survival was estimated using the Kaplan-Meier method.

Results.—A total of 2,671 patients (1,030 Fidelis and 1,641 Quattro) were identified. There were 398 deaths: 147 in the Fidelis group (mean follow-up: 34.4 months) and 251 in the Quattro group (mean follow-up: 39.9 months). No deaths were associated with 85 Fidelis and 23 Quattro failures. At 4 years, survival was diminished in patients with Fidelis compared with Quattro leads (80.7% vs. 83.9%, p = 0.025). After adjustment for factors associated with mortality, survival was similar between groups. One hundred percent pacing was not associated with mortality. Elective removal of nonfailed leads was performed in 5.1% of Fidelis and 0.9% of Quattro patients.

Conclusions.—In a conservatively managed cohort, in whom observation was predominantly utilized, adjusted survival is similar between patients with Fidelis and Quattro ICD leads (Table 3).

▶ Fidelis lead fractures are a major cause of inappropriate implantable cardioverter defibrillator (ICD) shocks and have a lead failure rate of 5% to 10% within 48 months. This study examines mortality associated with Medtronic Fidelis and Quattro leads in a retrospective analysis of 2671 patients. Fidelis leads were associated with increased mortality in univariate, but not multivariate, analysis (Table 3). There were no cases of mortality linked with lead failure. Lead failures occurred in 85 of 1030 and 23 of 1641 Fidelis and Quattro leads, respectively. Lead failure presented with inappropriate shock in 38 of 85 (45%) of Fidelis lead patients. For pacemaker-dependent patients, there was no excess mortality in this cohort associated with lead failures. Furthermore, leads that did not fail were more likely to be removed in dependent patients. This large retrospective analysis of patients with Fidelis and Quattro finds that Fidelis leads are at increased risk for lead failure and inappropriate shocks but not for increased

TABLE 3.—Multivariate Predictors of Mortality

	Hazard Ratio (95% CI)	p Value
Lead type (Fidelis vs. Quattro)	1.056 (0.84−1.33)	0.6353
ICD indication (secondary vs. primary)	1.380 (1.08−1.76)	0.0097
Atrial lead	1.409 (1.10−1.81)	0.0077
Heart failure	1.611 (1.21−2.14)	0.001
Number of generator replacements	0.310 (0.24−0.41)	<0.0001
Age (per 1-yr increase)	1.036 (1.026−1.05)	<0.0001
History of peripheral arterial disease	1.529 (1.18−1.99)	0.0016
Ejection fraction (per 1% increase)	0.978 (0.968−0.99)	<0.0001
Atrial fibrillation	1.609 (1.31−1.98)	<0.0001
Chronic dialysis	3.298 (2.19−4.97)	<0.0001
Chronic obstructive pulmonary disease	1.372 (1.08−1.75)	0.0108

mortality. Thus, aggressive prophylactic lead extraction of patients with Fidelis leads is not warranted at this time. However, it remains unresolved as to which patients should receive new leads or lead extraction at the time of pulse generator replacement.

M. L. Bernard, MD, PhD

Left Ventricular Versus Simultaneous Biventricular Pacing in Patients With Heart Failure and a QRS Complex ≥120 Milliseconds

Thibault B, for the Evaluation of Resynchronization Therapy for Heart Failure (GREATER-EARTH) Investigators (Montreal Heart Institute and Université de Montréal, Québec, Canada; et al)

Circulation 124:2874-2881, 2011

Background.—Left ventricular (LV) pacing alone may theoretically avoid deleterious effects of right ventricular pacing.

Methods and Results.—In a multicenter, double-blind, crossover trial, we compared the effects of LV and biventricular (BiV) pacing on exercise tolerance and LV remodeling in patients with an LV ejection fraction ≤35%, QRS ≥120 milliseconds, and symptoms of heart failure. A total of 211 patients were recruited from 11 centers. After a run-in period of 2 to 8 weeks, 121 qualifying patients were randomized to LV followed by BiV pacing or vice versa for consecutive 6-month periods. The greatest improvement in New York Heart Association class and 6-minute walk test occurred during the run-in phase before randomization. Exercise duration at 75% of peak Vo_2 (primary outcome) increased from 9.3 ± 6.4 to 14.0 ± 11.9 and 14.3 ± 12.5 minutes with LV and BiV pacing, respectively, with no difference between groups ($P = 0.4327$). LV ejection fraction improved from $24.4 \pm 6.3\%$ to $31.9 \pm 10.8\%$ and $30.9 \pm 9.8\%$ with LV and BiV pacing, respectively, with no difference between groups ($P = 0.4530$). Reductions in LV end-systolic volume were likewise similar ($P = 0.6788$). The proportion of clinical responders (≥20% increase in exercise duration) to LV and BiV

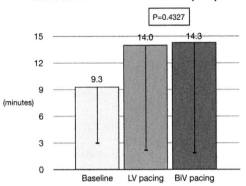

FIGURE 2.—Submaximal exercise duration at baseline and according to pacing mode. LV denotes left ventricular; CRT, cardiac resynchronization therapy; and BiV, biventricular. (Reprinted from Thibault B, for the Evaluation of Resynchronization Therapy for Heart Failure (GREATER-EARTH) Investigators. Left ventricular versus simultaneous biventricular pacing in patients with heart failure and a QRS complex ≥120 milliseconds. *Circulation*. 2011;124:2874-2881. © American Heart Association, Inc.)

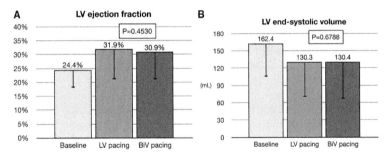

FIGURE 3.—Echocardiographic assessment of left ventricular (LV) function. LV ejection fraction (A) and LV end-systolic volume (B) are depicted at baseline and according to pacing modality. CRT denotes cardiac resynchronization therapy; BiV, biventricular. (Reprinted from Thibault B, for the Evaluation of Resynchronization Therapy for Heart Failure (GREATER-EARTH) Investigators. Left ventricular versus simultaneous biventricular pacing in patients with heart failure and a QRS complex ≥120 milliseconds. *Circulation*. 2011;124:2874-2881. © American Heart Association, Inc.)

pacing was 48.0% and 55.1% ($P = 0.1615$). Positive remodeling responses (≥15% reduction in LV end-systolic volume) were observed in 46.7% and 55.4% ($P = 0.0881$). Overall, 30.6% of LV nonresponders improved with BiV and 17.1% of BiV nonresponders improved with LV pacing.

Conclusion.—LV pacing is not superior to BiV pacing. However, nonresponders to BiV pacing may respond favorably to LV pacing, suggesting a potential role as tiered therapy.

Clinical Trial Registration.—URL: http://www.clinicaltrials.gov. Unique identifier: NCT00901212 (Figs 2 and 3).

▶ Cardiac resynchronization therapy (CRT) has proven benefits in patients with reduced left ventricular (LV) ejection fraction, interventricular conduction delay, and heart failure symptoms. Clinical response rates, however, are not uniform and vary greatly among patients. Thibault et al conducted a multicenter, randomized, controlled crossover trial comparing the effects of single-site LV pacing versus biventricular pacing in 121 patients with typical indications for resynchronization therapy. After device implantation and a run-in period during which heart failure medications were adjusted, patients were randomized to biventricular pacing versus LV-only pacing at an AV delay determined by surface electrocardiogram to maximize left ventricular activation. Patients were randomized in a crossover fashion to 6-month periods in each pacing mode. Outcomes were analyzed with gas exchange analysis, submaximal exercise testing, Short Form-36 Minnesota Living with Heart Failure Questionnaire, pro-B type natriuretic peptide levels, and echocardiography at the end of each 6-month period. At study completion, there were no significant differences in patient outcomes with respect to any of the predetermined outcomes (Figs 2 and 3). There were similar improvements in both patient groups with respect to exercise capacity, LV size and function, as well as quality of life score. This study suggests that lone left ventricular pacing is not superior to biventricular pacing in patients with typical indications for cardiac resynchronization therapy. However, it also suggests that RV pacing is unlikely to have a significant effect on CRT response, so right ventricular lead position is likely not critical, and LV only can be considered when simple pacing is needed in the absence of defibrillation backup.

J. L. Sturdivant, MD

Response to preventive cardiac resynchronization therapy in patients with ischaemic and nonischaemic cardiomyopathy in MADIT-CRT

Barsheshet A, Goldenberg I, Moss AJ, et al (Univ of Rochester Med Ctr, NY; et al)

Eur Heart J 32:1622-1630, 2011

Aims.—There are no data regarding the differential response to cardiac resynchronization therapy with defibrillator (CRT-D) by the aetiology of cardiomyopathy in mildly symptomatic patients. We evaluated the outcome of patients enrolled in MADIT-CRT by ischaemic and non-ischaemic aetiology of cardiomyopathy (ICM and non-ICM, respectively).

Methods and Results.—The clinical response to CRT-D was assessed among ICM ($n = 1046$) and non-ICM ($n = 774$) patients enrolled in MADIT-CRT during an average follow-up of 2.4 years, and echocardiographic response was assessed at 1 year. Cardiac resynchronization therapy with defibrillator vs. ICD therapy was associated with respective 34% ($P = 0.001$) and 44% ($P = 0.002$) reductions in the risk of heart failure or death among ICM and non-ICM patients (P for interaction $= 0.455$). In the ICM group, CRT-D was associated with mean ($\pm$SD) 29 $\pm$ 14% and 18 $\pm$ 10% reductions in left ventricular end-systolic volume (LVESV) and left ventricular end-diastolic volume (LVEDV), respectively. In the non-ICM group, CRT-D was associated with significantly greater volume reductions compared with the ICM group [37 $\pm$ 16% and 24 $\pm$ 12% reductions

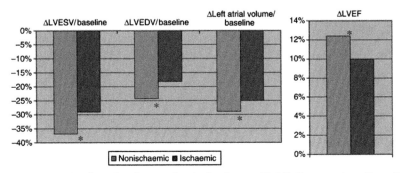

FIGURE 2.—The effects of cardiac resynchronization therapy with defibrillator on echocardiographic measures in ischaemic and non-ischaemic cardiomyopathy patients. *P < 0.001. The bars represent median values. △LVEF = 1 year LVEF (%) − baseline LVEF (%). △ Volume/baseline = (1 year volume − baseline volume)/baseline volume. LVEF, left ventricle ejection fraction; LVEDV, left ventricle end-diastolic volume; LVESV, left ventricle end-systolic volume. (Reprinted from Barsheshet A, Goldenberg I, Moss AJ, et al. Response to preventive cardiac resynchronization therapy in patients with ischaemic and nonischaemic cardiomyopathy in MADIT-CRT. *Eur Heart J.* 2011;32:1622-1630, by permission of The European Society of Cardiology.)

in LVESV and LVEDV, respectively (*P* < 0.001 for all)]. Risk subsets in the ICM group that showed a favourable clinical response to CRT-D included patients with QRS ≥150 ms, systolic blood pressure <115 mmHg, and left bundle branch block (LBBB), whereas in the non-ICM group females, patients with diabetes mellitus, and LBBB, displayed a favourable clinical response.

Conclusion.—Mildly symptomatic ICM and non-ICM patients show significant differences in the echocardiographic response to CRT-D and in the clinical benefit within risk subsets suggesting that risk assessment for CRT-D in this population should be aetiology-specific (Fig 2, Table 2).

▶ Cardiac resynchronization therapy (CRT) is effective therapy to improve functional status, reduce hospitalization and mortality, and improve cardiac function (reverse remodeling). Studies of advanced heart failure subjects have found that the greatest benefit is observed among subjects with left bundle branch block and very prolonged QRS duration (> 150 msec). In general, patients with dilated cardiomyopathy show a greater remodeling response, although the clinical benefit is similar. In this study, these observations are extended to milder heart failure in the MADIT-CRT trial. The clinical response was similar in the ischemic and nonischemic groups (Table 2). However, the magnitude of reverse remodeling was greater in nonischemic patients (Fig 2). These results parallel those noted in severe heart failure and indicate that a smaller remodeling response will produce equivalent clinical benefit in higher-risk (ischemic) patients. Thus, different criteria should be used to assess echo responses to CRT in ischemic versus nonischemic subjects. This study further extends the general observations that the response to CRT is independent of heart failure severity with similar predictors of response, magnitude of benefit, and sustained effects.

M. R. Gold, MD, PhD

TABLE 2.—Clinical Effect of Cardiac Resynchronization Therapy with Defibrillator vs. ICD by Ischaemic Aetiology

	All Ischaemic (n = 1046)		Ischaemic NYHA II (n = 781)		Non-Ischaemic (n = 774)		P for Interaction*
	Adjusted HR (95% CI)	P-Value	Adjusted HR (95% CI)	P-Value	Adjusted HR (95% CI)	P-Value	
HF or death	0.66 (0.52–0.85)	0.001	0.62 (0.47–0.83)	0.001	0.56 (0.39–0.80)	0.002	0.455
HF event	0.58 (0.45–0.77)	<0.001	0.57 (0.41–0.77)	<0.001	0.50 (0.35–0.75)	0.001	0.562
Death	0.99 (0.65–1.52)	0.984	0.96 (0.59–1.55)	0.854	0.87 (0.45–1.67)	0.669	0.728

Adjusted HR = CRT-D:ICD hazard ratio adjusted for gender, age ≥65 years, diabetes mellitus, QRS ≥150 ms, EF <25%, eGFR <60 mL/min/1.73 m², and systolic blood pressure <115 mmHg.
*P for treatment-by-aetiology (all ischaemic vs. non-ischaemic) interaction.

The relationship between ventricular electrical delay and left ventricular remodelling with cardiac resynchronization therapy

Gold MR, Birgersdotter-Green U, Singh JP, et al (Med Univ of South Carolina, Charleston; Univ of California San Diego; Massachusetts General Hosp, Boston; et al)
Eur Heart J 32:2516-2524, 2011

Aims.—The aim of the present study was to evaluate the relationship between left ventricular (LV) electrical delay, as measured by the QLV interval, and outcomes in a prospectively designed substudy of the SMART-AV Trial.

Methods and Results.—This was a multicentre study of patients with advanced heart failure undergoing cardiac resynchronization therapy (CRT) defibrillator implantation. In 426 subjects, QLV was measured as the interval from the onset of the QRS from the surface ECG to the first large peak of the LV electrogram. Left ventricular volumes were measured by echocardiography at baseline and after 6 months of CRT by a blinded core laboratory. Quality of life (QOL) was assessed by a standardized questionnaire. When separated by quartiles based on QLV duration, reverse remodelling response rates (>15% reduction in LV end systolic volume) increased progressively from 38.7 to 68.4% and QOL response rate (>10

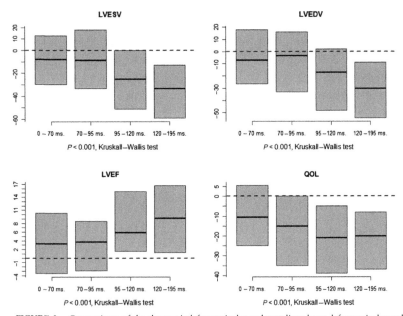

FIGURE 3.—Comparisons of the changes in left ventricular end-systolic volume, left ventricular end-diastolic volume, ejection fraction, and quality of life from implant baseline to 6 months for the QLV quartiles. The data were presented as median ± inter-quartile range (box). (Reprinted from Gold MR, Birgersdotter-Green U, Singh JP, et al. The relationship between ventricular electrical delay and left ventricular remodelling with cardiac resynchronization therapy. *Eur Heart J*. 2011;32:2516-2524, by permission of The European Society of Cardiology.)

TABLE 2.—Relationship of QLV with Clinical Outcomes

	Q1: 0–70 ms (%)	Q2: 70–95 ms (%)	Q3: 95–120 ms (%)	Q4: 120–195 ms (%)	Total (%)	Overall P-value	Q4 Vs. Q1 P-Value
			QLV Quartiles				
Patients with HF events	15 (12.1)	7 (7.1)	7 (6.4)	6 (6.3)	35 (8.2)	0.37	0.17
NYHA							
Improved	89 (73.0)	79 (80.6)	76 (71.0)	77 (83.7)	321 (76.6)	0.04	0.04
No change	33 (27.1)	16 (16.3)	30 (28.0)	14 (15.2)	93 (22.2)		
Worsened	0 (0.0)	3 (3.1)	1 (0.9)	1 (1.1)	5 (1.2)		
Six minute walk delta	52±118	68±91	50±104	70±93	59±103	0.36	0.13

points reduction) increased from 50 to 72%. Patients in the highest quartile of QLV had a 3.21-fold increase (1.58–6.50, $P = 0.001$) in their odds of a reverse remodelling response after correcting for QRS duration, bundle branch block type, and clinical characteristics by multivariate logistic regression analysis.

Conclusion.—Electrical dyssynchrony, as measured by QLV, was strongly and independently associated with reverse remodelling and QOL with CRT. Acute measurements of QLV may be useful to guide LV lead placement (Fig 3, Table 2).

▶ The benefits of cardiac resynchronization therapy (CRT) in patients with significant left ventricular (LV) dysfunction and electrical dyssynchrony (particularly with left bundle branch block (LBBB) and QRS duration ≥150 ms) is well established; however, identifying predictors of clinical response has been difficult. QLV is a measure of electrical dyssynchrony and is calculated as the delay from QRS onset to the electrical activity measured at the LV lead location. As a substudy of the SMART-AV trial, QLV was evaluated for the first time in a large trial with blinded adjudication of endpoints. This study demonstrated that increased QLV duration is associated with increased reverse remodeling response rates as well as improved QOL scores (see Fig 3 and Table 2). QLV remained a significant predictor of reverse remodeling response in multivariate analysis after correcting for well-known predictors of response including QRS duration, LBBB morphology, and other clinical characteristics. QLV may be a promising tool for predicting CRT response and optimizing LV lead placement and should be evaluated formally in a randomized controlled clinical trial.

F. Cuoco, MD

Efficacy and Safety of Celivarone, With Amiodarone as Calibrator, in Patients With an Implantable Cardioverter-Defibrillator for Prevention of Implantable Cardioverter-Defibrillator Interventions or Death: The ALPHEE Study

Kowey PR, on behalf of the ALPHEE Study Investigators (Lankenau Hosp and Inst of Med Res, Wynnewood, PA; et al)

Circulation 124:2649-2660, 2011

Background.—Celivarone is a new antiarrhythmic agent developed for the treatment of ventricular arrhythmias. This study investigated the efficacy and safety of celivarone in preventing implantable cardioverter-defibrillator (ICD) interventions or death.

Methods and Results.—Celivarone (50, 100, or 300 mg/d) was assessed compared with placebo in this randomized, double-blind, placebo-controlled, parallel-group study. Amiodarone (200 mg/d after loading dose of 600 mg/d for 10 days) was used as a calibrator. A total of 486 patients with a left ventricular ejection fraction ≤40% and at least 1 ICD intervention for ventricular tachycardia or ventricular fibrillation in the previous month or ICD implantation in the previous month for documented ventricular tachycardia/ventricular fibrillation were randomized. Median treatment duration was 9 months. The primary efficacy end point was occurrence of ventricular tachycardia/ventricular fibrillation-triggered ICD interventions (shocks or antitachycardia pacing) or sudden death. The proportion of patients experiencing an appropriate ICD intervention or sudden death was 61.5% in the placebo group; 67.0%, 58.8%, and 54.9% in the celivarone 50-, 100-, and 300-mg groups, respectively; and 45.3% in the amiodarone group. Hazard ratios versus placebo for the primary end point ranged from 0.860 for celivarone 300 mg to 1.199 for celivarone 50 mg. None of the comparisons versus placebo were statistically significant. Celivarone had an acceptable safety profile.

Conclusions.—Celivarone was not effective for the prevention of ICD interventions or sudden death.

Clinical Trial Registration.—http://www.clinicaltrials.gov. Unique identifier: NCT00993382 (Fig 3).

▶ Amiodarone is widely considered to be the most efficacious antiarrhythmic drug, but its use is limited by serious long-term risks. Accordingly, several new drugs have been developed that are structurally related to amiodarone but presumably with less toxicity. One such drug is celivarone, which was evaluated in the ALPHEE study. A total of 486 patients with an appropriate implantable cardioverter defibrillator (ICD) intervention in the preceding month were entered in this study comparing celivarone 50, 100, or 300 mg/d versus placebo. An interesting part of the study is using amiodarone as a calibrator. The concept of a calibrator arm was to obtain evidence of efficacy in a group versus placebo to validate the study design. Fig 3 shows that amiodarone was effective in reduction of shocks; however, unexpectedly it increased all-cause mortality. Celivarone did not decrease the number of shocks or arrhythmias. Although the calibrator amiodarone was again effective as an antiarrhythmic agent, it did not reduce sudden

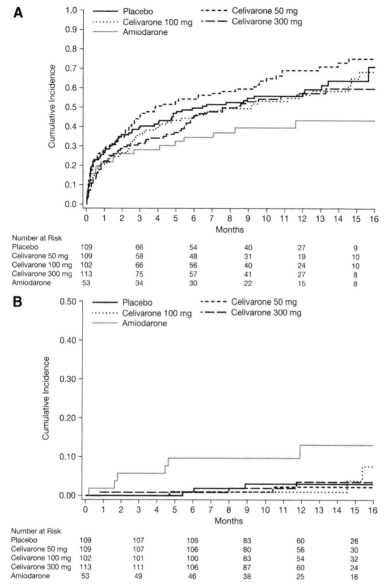

FIGURE 3.—Kaplan-Meier cumulative incidence curves from randomization to the first episode of each component of the primary end point (intention-to-treat population). **A,** Ventricular tachycardia/ ventricular fibrillation—triggered implantable cardioverter-defibrillator intervention. **B,** Sudden death. (Reprinted from Kowey PR, on behalf of the ALPHEE Study Investigators. Efficacy and safety of celivarone, with amiodarone as calibrator, in patients with an implantable cardioverter-defibrillator for prevention of implantable cardioverter-defibrillator interventions or death: the ALPHEE study. *Circulation.* 2011;124:2649-2660. © American Heart Association, Inc.)

death or mortality in the calibrator arm. Clearly, amiodarone has been shown to reduce shock and decrease arrhythmias but has not improved survival in patients. Unfortunately, the multichannel congener of amiodarone, celivarone, was shown not to be effective in controlling arrhythmias, which will likely halt further development of this agent.

R. B. Leman, MD

Sudden Cardiac Death

Adherence to a Low-Risk, Healthy Lifestyle and Risk of Sudden Cardiac Death Among Women
Chiuve SE, Fung TT, Rexrode KM, et al (Brigham and Women's Hosp and Harvard Med School, Boston, MA)
JAMA 306:62-69, 2011

Context.—Sudden cardiac death (SCD) accounts for more than half of all cardiac deaths; the majority of SCD events occur as the first manifestation of heart disease, especially among women. Primary preventive strategies are needed to reduce SCD incidence.

Objective.—To estimate the degree to which adherence to a healthy lifestyle may lower the risk of SCD among women.

Design, Setting, and Participants.—A prospective cohort study of 81 722 US women in the Nurses' Health Study from June 1984 to June 2010. Lifestyle factors were assessed via questionnaires every 2 to 4 years. A low-risk lifestyle was defined as not smoking, body mass index of less than 25, exercise duration of 30 minutes/day or longer, and top 40% of the alternate Mediterranean diet score, which emphasizes high intake of vegetables, fruits, nuts, legumes, whole grains, and fish and moderate intake of alcohol.

Main Outcome Measure.—Sudden cardiac death (defined as death occurring within 1 hour after symptom onset without evidence of circulatory collapse).

Results.—There were 321 cases of SCD during 26 years of follow-up. Women were a mean age of 72 years at the time of the SCD event. All 4 low-risk lifestyle factors were significantly and independently associated with a lower risk of SCD. The absolute risks of SCD were 22 cases/100 000 person-years among women with 0 low-risk factors, 17 cases/100 000 person-years with 1 low-risk factor, 18 cases/100 000 person-years with 2 low-risk factors, 13 cases/100 000 person-years with 3 low-risk factors, and 16 cases/100 000 person-years with 4 low-risk factors. Compared with women with 0 low-risk factors, the multivariable relative risk of SCD was 0.54 (95% confidence interval [CI], 0.34-0.86) for women with 1 low-risk factor, 0.41 (95% CI, 0.25-0.65) for 2 low-risk factors, 0.33 (95% CI, 0.20-0.54) for 3 low-risk factors, and 0.08 (95% CI, 0.03-0.23) for 4 low-risk factors. The proportion of SCD attributable to smoking, inactivity, overweight, and poor diet was 81%(95% CI, 52%-93%). Among women without clinically diagnosed coronary heart disease, the percentage of population attributable risk was 79% (95% CI, 40%-93%).

Conclusion.—Adherence to a low-risk lifestyle is associated with a low risk of SCD.

▶ Current practice for sudden cardiac death (SCD) risk management focuses on identification of those at highest risk and providing optimal medical and, in select cases, device-based therapy. Unfortunately, SCD most often affects those who would otherwise be deemed relatively low to moderate risk, limiting the impact of these interventions on mortality from SCD at the population level. Although it is well known that lifestyle factors affect risk of cardiovascular disease (CVD), and as a result, SCD, the effect of modification of these risk factors on SCD is less well established. However, if lifestyle modification can attenuate SCD risk, the potential benefit to the general, unselected population could be significant. Given the inherent difficulties in performing a randomized, controlled trial to test this hypothesis, Chiuve et al instead report their observational data on the risk of SCD in 81 722 participants in the Nurses' Health Study. Over a 26-year period, they regularly collected detailed information on active medical conditions and lifestyle, including tobacco use, exercise, dietary habits, and body mass index (BMI). These 4 lifestyle factors were examined as both dichotomous (low vs high risk) and continuous variables in multivariable analyses of SCD risk in this population. In both analyses, healthy habits in each of these categories were independently and significantly associated with lower risk of SCD. Furthermore, the effect was cumulative, with each additional low-risk feature conferring a lower risk of SCD (Fig in the original article). They estimated the population attributable risk (the proportion of SCD that would not have occurred if all women were low risk) to be 81% for the entire cohort. The observational nature of this study clearly introduces the possibility of confounding the analysis. However, it would be exceedingly difficult to perform a randomized trial of sufficient size to demonstrate a significant reduction in SCD risk with lifestyle modification. The participants of the Nurses' Health Study were also predominantly white women, and caution should be exercised before generalizing these associations to more diverse populations. Despite these limitations, Chiuve et al provide compelling evidence that a lifestyle of nonsmoking, regular exercise, healthy diet, and low BMI are associated with a lower risk of SCD. Low-risk interventions that focus on these factors could have a significant impact on the incidence of SCD in the future.

W. W. Brabham, MD

Impact of Onsite or Dispatched Automated External Defibrillator Use on Survival After Out-of-Hospital Cardiac Arrest
Berdowski J, Blom MT, Bardai A, et al (Academic Med Ctr—Univ of Amsterdam, the Netherlands)
Circulation 124:2225-2232, 2011

Background.—There have been few studies on the effectiveness of bystander automated external defibrillator (AED) use in out-of-hospital cardiac arrest. The objective of this study was to determine whether actual use of onsite or dispatched AED reduces the time to first shock compared with no AED use and thereby improves survival.

Methods and Results.—We performed a population-based cohort study of 2833 consecutive patients with a nontraumatic out-of-hospital cardiac arrest before emergency medical system arrival between 2006 and 2009. The primary outcome, neurologically intact survival to discharge, was compared by use of multivariable logistic regression analysis. An onsite AED had been applied in 128 of the 2833 cases, a dispatched AED in 478, and no AED in 2227. Onsite AED use reduced the time to first shock from 11 to 4.1 minute. Neurologically intact survival was 49.6% for patients treated with an onsite AED compared with 14.3% without an AED (unadjusted odds ratio, 5.63; 95% confidence interval, 3.91−8.10). The odds ratio remained statistically significant after adjustment for confounding (odds ratio, 2.72; 95% confidence interval, 1.77−4.18). Dispatched AED use reduced the time from call to first shock to 8.5 minutes. Neurologically intact survival was 17.2% for patients treated with a dispatched AED (unadjusted odds ratio, 1.07; 95% confidence interval, 0.82−1.39). Every year, onsite AEDs saved 3.6 lives per 1 million inhabitants; dispatched AEDs saved 1.2 lives.

Conclusions.—The use of an onsite AED leads to a doubling of neurologically intact survival. In our system, the survival benefit of dispatched AED use was much smaller than that of onsite AED use (Table 5).

▶ Survival from cardiac arrest is critically and inversely related to time to defibrillation. The automated external defibrillator (AED) is an effective tool to improve access to defibrillation, as it can be safely used by both health care professionals and bystanders with minimal or no training. In the out-of-hospital setting, AEDs have been shown to improve time to defibrillation and survival when placed in casinos, airports, airplanes, and in other strategic public locations. Several studies of AED use by first responders have also demonstrated improvements in response times, time to defibrillation, and survival. Fixed placement of AEDs and equipping

TABLE 5.—Observed and Expected Neurologically Intact Survival by Automated External Defibrillator Treatment Received

	Treated With an Onsite AED (n=128)	Treated With a Dispatched AED (n=478)	Not Treated With an AED (n=2227)
Observed survival, % (n)	49.6 (63)	17.2 (82)	14.3 (319)
Expected survival* without AED use, mean %	27.5	16.1	14.4
Lives saved by AED use per year[†]	8.7	1.6	NA
Lives saved by AED use per 1 million inhabitants[‡] per year	3.6	1.2	

AED indicates automated external defibrillator.
*The expected survival was calculated from a multivariable logistic regression model with the variables AED use, age, location of the collapse, witnessed collapse, and shockable initial rhythm by setting the indicator for AED use to 0. The shown expected survival percentage was the average of the individual expected survival percentage.
[†]The total time of the study was 3.25 years.
[‡]The study population is 2.4 million.

first responders with these devices represent 2 different strategies of AED implementation for management of out-of-hospital cardiac arrest. Previous studies have typically compared these basic strategies with control arms consisting of traditional emergency medical systems (EMS). The study by Berdowski et al provides a unique comparison of onsite AED use, dispatched (first-responder) AED use, and traditional EMS through an analysis of the prospective Amsterdam Resuscitation Study (ARREST) registry. Treatment with an onsite AED clearly reduced time to defibrillation in comparison with both dispatched AED and traditional EMS, which correlated with significantly higher survival rates. Odds of survival remained significantly higher with onsite AEDs relative to traditional EMS after multivariable logistic regression analysis and within subgroups of arrests in public locations (not in the home), arrests treated with bystander cardiopulmonary resuscitation, and those with shockable rhythms. Dispatched AED use was associated with shorter time to defibrillation compared with traditional EMS (8.5 vs 11 minutes), but this did not result in a significant difference in survival rates. Significantly higher odds of survival with dispatched AED use was observed in the subgroup of arrests occurring in public locations. Importantly, all strategies were equal in the subgroup of patients presenting with nonshockable rhythms. The authors estimated that onsite AED use almost doubled survival compared with no AED (Table 5). While these results suggest superiority of a strategy of onsite AEDs compared with first responders, there are several limitations that should be recognized. As an observational cohort study, potential confounding cannot be completely eliminated with statistical adjustment. Second, the first responder system in this cohort resulted in only marginal improvements in response time and time to first shock. In other settings with a higher first responder-to-EMS ratio, these differences could be significantly larger. Finally, public access AED programs are costly, and effective distribution of AEDs continues to be a challenge. Onsite AEDs will always be preferable given the clear benefit in survival, but in many health care systems, first responder AEDs will continue to be a reasonable alternative.

W. W. Brabham, MD

High-Density Substrate Mapping in Brugada Syndrome: Combined Role of Conduction and Repolarization Heterogeneities in Arrhythmogenesis

Lambiase PD, Ahmed AK, Ciaccio EJ, et al (Univ College London, UK; Columbia Univ, NY; et al)

Circulation 120:106-117, 2009

Background.—Two principal mechanisms are thought to be responsible for Brugada syndrome (BS): (1) right ventricular (RV) conduction delay and (2) RV subepicardial action potential shortening. This in vivo high-density mapping study evaluated the conduction and repolarization properties of the RV in BS subjects.

Methods and Results.—A noncontact mapping array was positioned in the RV of 18 BS patients and 20 controls. Using a standard S_1-S_2 protocol, restitution curves of local activation time and activation recovery interval were constructed to determine local maximal restitution slopes. Significant regional conduction delays in the anterolateral free wall of the RV outflow tract of BS patients were identified. The mean increase in delay was 3-fold greater in this region than in control ($P = 0 < 0.001$). Local activation gradient was also maximally reduced in this area: 0.33 ± 0.1 (mean ± SD) mm/ms in BS patients versus 0.51 ± 0.15 mm/ms in controls ($P < 0.0005$). The uniformity of wavefront propagation as measured by the square of the correlation coefficient, r^2, was greater in BS patients versus controls (0.94 ± 0.04 versus 0.89 ± 0.09 [mean ± SD]; $P < 0.05$). The odds ratio of BS hearts having any RV segment with maximal restitution slope >1 was 3.86 versus controls. Five episodes of provoked ventricular tachycardia arose from wave breaks originating from RV outflow tract slow-conduction zones in 5 BS patients.

Conclusions.—Marked regional endocardial conduction delay and heterogeneities in repolarization exist in BS. Wave break in areas of maximal conduction delay appears to be critical in the initiation and maintenance of ventricular tachycardia. These data indicate that further studies of mapping BS to identify slow-conduction zones should be considered to determine their role in spontaneous ventricular arrhythmias.

▶ Brugada syndrome is a genetic abnormality that results in the electrocardiographic finding of either a complete or incomplete right bundle branch block pattern with anterior precordial ST elevation and is associated with an increased risk of sudden death. Using high-density noncontact mapping, this study shows delayed and slowed conduction into the right ventricular outflow track (RVOT) of patients with Brugada syndrome. This RVOT conduction delay explains the electrocardiographic appearance of a right bundle branch block pattern in this syndrome. Programmed stimulation resulted in progressive conduction delay, development of fractionated electrograms, and in some patients, conduction block and reentry to initiate ventricular tachycardia or fibrillation. Additionally, repolarization was shorter in the RVOT and demonstrated altered restitution compared with other RV sites, which results in potentially greater dispersion of refractoriness. This interesting study provides data to support the pathophysiologic basis for the arrhythmogenic changes in Brugada syndrome.

J. M. Warton, MD

Incidence and Predictors of Implantable Cardioverter-Defibrillator Therapy in Patients With Arrhythmogenic Right Ventricular Dysplasia/Cardiomyopathy Undergoing Implantable Cardioverter-Defibrillator Implantation for Primary Prevention

Bhonsale A, James CA, Tichnell C, et al (The Johns Hopkins Univ School of Medicine, Baltimore, MD)
J Am Coll Cardiol 58:1485-1496, 2011

Objectives.—The purpose of this study was to define the incidence and predictors of implantable cardioverter-defibrillator (ICD) therapy in patients

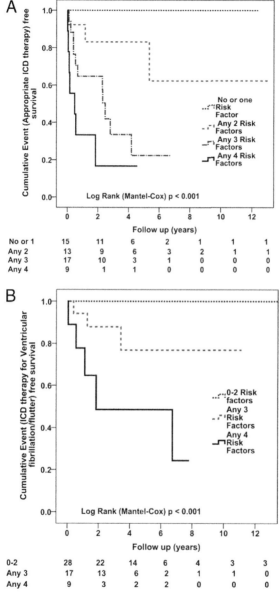

FIGURE 5.—Incremental Risk of Appropriate ICD Therapy With Multiple Risk Factors. Cumulative survival free of appropriate implantable cardioverter-defibrillator (ICD) therapy (**A**) and ICD therapy for VF/VFL (**B**) stratified by the number of risk factors (the risk factors considered are inducibility at electrophysiologic study, the presence of nonsustained ventricular tachycardia, Holter premature ventricular complex count >1,000/24 h, and proband status). (Reprinted from the Journal of the American College of Cardiology, Bhonsale A, James CA, Tichnell C, et al. Incidence and predictors of implantable cardioverter-defibrillator therapy in patients with arrhythmogenic right ventricular dysplasia/cardiomyopathy undergoing implantable cardioverter-defibrillator implantation for primary prevention. *J Am Coll Cardiol.* 2011;58:1485-1496. Copyright 2011, with permission from the American College of Cardiology.)

with arrhythmogenic right ventricular dysplasia/cardiomyopathy (ARVD/C) after placement of an ICD for primary prevention.

Background.—Patients with a diagnosis of ARVD/C often receive an ICD for prevention of sudden cardiac death.

Methods.—Patients (n = 84) from the Johns Hopkins registry with definite or probable ARVD/C who underwent ICD implantation for primary prevention were studied. Detailed phenotypic, genotype, and ICD event information was obtained and appropriate ICD therapies were adjudicated based on intracardiac electrograms.

Results.—Over a mean follow-up of 4.7 ± 3.4 years, appropriate ICD therapy was seen in 40 patients (48%), of whom 16 (19%) received interventions for potentially fatal ventricular fibrillation/flutter episodes. Proband status ($p < 0.001$), inducibility at electrophysiologic study ($p = 0.005$), presence of nonsustained ventricular tachycardia ($p < 0.001$), and Holter premature ventricular complex count $>1,000/24$ h ($p = 0.024$) were identified as significant predictors of appropriate ICD therapy. The 5-year survival free of appropriate ICD therapy for patients with 1, 2, 3, and 4 risk factors was 100%, 83%, 21%, and 15%, respectively. Inducibility at electrophysiologic study (hazard ratio: 4.5, 95% confidence interval: 1.4 to 15, $p = 0.013$) and nonsustained ventricular tachycardia (hazard ratio: 10.5, 95% confidence interval: 2.4 to 46.2, $p = 0.002$) remained as significant predictors on multivariable analysis.

Conclusions.—Nearly one-half of the ARVD/C patients with primary prevention ICD implantation experience appropriate ICD interventions. Inducibility at electrophysiologic study and nonsustained ventricular tachycardia are independent strong predictors of appropriate ICD therapy. An increase in ventricular ectopy burden was associated with progressively lower event-free (appropriate ICD interventions) survival. Incremental risk of ventricular arrhythmias and ICD therapy was observed with the presence of multiple risk factors (Fig 5).

▶ Arrhythmogenic right ventricular dysplasia/cardiomyopathy (ARVD/C) is a relatively uncommon disorder that is associated with an increased risk for ventricular arrhythmias and sudden cardiac death (SCD). The predictors of appropriate implantable cardioverter-defibrillator (ICD) therapy in this population implanted for primary prevention is not well established. Accordingly, this study included patients from the Johns Hopkins ARVD/C registry. There were 4 major risk factors for appropriate ICD therapy identified: proband status, indelibility at electrophysiology study, nonsustained ventricular tachycardia, and frequent premature ventricular complex count (> 1000/24 h) on Holter monitor. Fig 5 illustrates Kaplan-Meier Curves demonstrating the increased risk of appropriate ICD therapy with multiple risk factors. Almost one-half of patients with ARVD/C implanted for primary prevention received appropriate ICD therapy over a mean follow-up of 5 years, confirming that this is a very high-risk patient population. Moreover, this risk stratification scheme helps identify patients at highest risk for ventricular tachycardia.

F. Cuoco, MD

The value of a family history of sudden death in patients with diagnostic type I Brugada ECG pattern

Sarkozy A, Sorgente A, Boussy T, et al (UZ Brussel—VUB, Belgium; et al)
Eur Heart J 32:2153-2160, 2011

Aims.—We sought to investigate the value of a family history of sudden death (SD) in Brugada syndrome (BS).

Methods and Results.—Two hundred and eighty consecutive patients (mean age: 41 ± 18 years, 168 males) with diagnostic type I Brugada ECG pattern were included. Sudden death occurred in 69 (43) of 157 families. One hundred and ten SDs were analysed. During follow-up VF (ventricular fibrillation) or SD-free survival rate was not different between patients with or without a family history of SD of a first-degree relative, between patients with or without a family history of multiple SD of a first-degree relative at any age and between patients with or without a family history of SD in first-degree relatives ≤35 years. One patient had family history of SD of two first-degree relative ≤35 years with arrhythmic event during follow-up. In univariate analysis male gender ($P = 0.01$), aborted SD ($P < 0.001$), syncope ($P = 0.04$), spontaneous type I ECG ($P < 0.001$), and inducibility during electrophysiological (EP) study ($P < 0.001$) were associated with worse prognosis. The absence of syncope, aborted SD, spontaneous type I ECG, and inducibility during EP study was associated with a significantly better prognosis ($P < 0.001$).

Conclusion.—Family history of SD is not predictive for future arrhythmic events even if considering only SD in first-degree relatives or SD in first-degree relatives at a young age. The absence of syncope, aborted SD, spontaneous type I ECG, and inducibility during EP study is associated with a good five-year prognosis (Table 1).

▶ The Brugada syndrome (BS) is a genetic disease caused by mutations in cardiac ion channel genes and is associated with an increased risk of arrhythmic sudden death (SD). Consensus reports have defined both diagnostic criteria and a risk stratification scheme for management of the BS. It is advised that for asymptomatic patients without spontaneous electrocardiogram (ECG) abnormality in the presence of family history of SD suspected due to BS, an electrophysiology (EP) study should be used for risk stratification. Multiple studies have evaluated the role of family history of SD in BS; however, this study was the first to evaluate the importance of the degree of relation, the age at time of SD, and the role of multiple SDs in 1 family. Two hundred eight consecutive patients with diagnostic type I Brugada ECG were included with SD occurring in 69 of 157 families. During follow-up, ventricular fibrillation (VF) or SD-free survival rate was not different between patients with or without a family history of SD of a first-degree relative, between patients with or without a family history of multiple SD of a first-degree relative at any age, and between patients with or without a family history of SD in first-degree relatives ≤35 years. Univariate analysis (Table 1) showed that male gender, aborted SD, syncope, spontaneous type I ECG, and inducibility during EP study were associated with worse prognosis.

TABLE 1.—Clinical Characteristics of the Study Population

Clinical Characteristics	All Patients, n (%)	Patients Without Arrhythmic Events, n (%)	Patients with Arrhythmic Events, n (%)	P-Value
Number of patients	280	262	18	
Age (mean±SD, years)	41 ± 18	41 ± 18	37 ± 19	0.3
Gender, Male	168 (60)	152 (58)	16 (89)	0.01
Proband	157 (56)	141 (54)	16 (89)	0.003
Family history of SD	149 (53)	141 (54)	8 (44)	0.5
Clinical presentation				
Asymptomatic	169 (60)	165 (63)	4 (22)	0.001
Presyncope, palpitation[a]	44 (16)	41 (16)	3 (17)	1
Syncope[a]	68 (24)	60 (23)	8 (44)	0.05
Aborted SD[a]	14 (5)	7 (3)	7 (39)	<0.001
Baseline ECG				
Type I	65 (23)	53 (20)	12 (66)	<0.001
Type II	49 (18)	47 (18)	2 (11)	0.8
Type III	15 (5)	15 (6)	0	0.6
Normal	151 (54)	149 (57)	4 (22)	0.006
EPS inducible VT/VF[b] (238 patients)	61 (26)	49 (19)	12 (66)	<0.001

[a]Categories are not mutually exclusive.
[b]EPS, electrophysiological study; VT/VF, ventricular tachycardia/ventricular fibrillation.

Despite the limitations of relatively short follow-up, this study provides further evidence that family history of SD is not predictive for future arrhythmic events even if considering only SD in first-degree relatives or SD in family members at a young age. Therefore, one should use other patient-specific clinical data other than just family history to decide when to perform an EP study that will risk stratifying asymptomatic individuals without spontaneous type I ECG changes.

P. C. Netzler, MD

Sports-Related Sudden Death in the General Population

Marijon E, Tafflet M, Celermajer DS, et al (Paris Cardiovascular Res Ctr PARCC, France; Univ of Sydney, Australia; et al)

Circulation 124:672-681, 2011

Background.—Although such data are available for young competitive athletes, the prevalence, characteristics, and outcome of sports-related sudden death have not been assessed previously in the general population.

Methods and Results.—A prospective and comprehensive national survey was performed throughout France from 2005 to 2010, involving subjects 10 to 75 years of age. Case detection for sports-related sudden death, including resuscitated cardiac arrest, was undertaken via national ambulance service reporting and Web-based screening of media releases. The overall burden of sports-related sudden death was 4.6 cases per million population per year, with 6% of cases occurring in young competitive athletes. Sensitivity analyses used to address suspected underreporting demonstrated an incidence ranging from 5 to 17 new cases per million population per year. More than 90% of cases occurred in the context of recreational sports. The age of subjects was relatively young (mean ± SD 46 ± 15 years), with a predominance of men (95%). Although most cases were witnessed (93%), bystander cardiopulmonary resuscitation was only commenced in 30.7% of cases. Bystander cardiopulmonary resuscitation (odds ratio 3.73, 95% confidence interval 2.19 to 6.39, *P*<0.0001) and initial use of cardiac defibrillation (odds ratio 3.71, 95% confidence interval 2.07 to 6.64, *P*<0.0001) were the strongest independent predictors for survival to hospital discharge (15.7%, 95% confidence interval 13.2% to 18.2%).

Conclusions.—Sports-related sudden death in the general population is considerably more common than previously suspected. Most cases are witnessed, yet bystander cardiopulmonary resuscitation was only initiated in one third of cases. Given the often predictable setting of sports-related sudden death and that prompt interventions were significantly associated with improved survival, these data have implications for health services planning (Table 3).

▶ Sudden cardiac death (SCD) occurring in young athletes is a high visibility but infrequent event. It has been largely studied as it relates to inherited

TABLE 3.—Univariate Analysis for Survival to Hospital Discharge

Predictors of Survival: Variables	OR	95% CI	*P*
Women vs men	1.59	0.76−3.32	0.21
Age, y			
10−30	1.00		<0.0001
31−50	0.60	0.36−0.99	
51−75	0.26	0.15−0.44	
Known CVD vs others	0.56	0.28−1.12	0.10
Seasons			
Winter	1.00		0.18
Spring	1.61	0.92−2.84	
Summer	1.13	0.62−2.04	
Autumn	1.64	0.89−3.00	
Weekend	1.60	1.10−2.32	0.01
Team sports	0.98	0.66−1.45	0.92
Intensity of exercise			
Light	1.00		0.002
Moderate	1.70	0.40−7.51	
Vigorous	3.36	0.78−14.5	
Sport facilities vs others	2.83	1.88−4.25	<0.0001
Competitive vs recreational setting	1.32	0.83−2.12	0.24
Young competitive athlete	1.62	0.82−3.18	0.16
Presence of witness	6.73	1.62−27.8	0.009
Bystander CPR	9.83	6.42−15.04	<0.0001
Collapse to start of CPR delay, min			
0−2	1.00		<0.0001
3−4	0.44	0.22−0.91	
5−10	0.13	0.06−0.28	
11−20	0.10	0.05−0.23	
Initial shockable rhythm	9.60	5.88−15.70	<0.0001

OR indicates odds ratio; CI, confidence interval; CVD, cardiovascular disease; and CPR, cardiopulmonary resuscitation.

disorders predisposing one to sudden death. However, sports-related SCD in the general population has not been systematically studied and is likely to have a different risk profile than that of the young competitive athlete. This study prospectively evaluated sports-related sudden death in France in subjects 10 to 75 years old who died during sport or within 1 hour of cessation of sports activity. Using surveys of emergency medical personnel as well as media reports of sports-related sudden death, the circumstances of sudden death events and patient characteristics were recorded and analyzed. After 5 years of observation 820 sports-related sudden deaths were recorded, translating to an estimated 4.6 per million population per year. The mean age was 46 ± 15 years, 95% were male, and 86% of subjects performed regular sports or training. A known history of cardiovascular disease was present in 11.7% of cases, and 12.7% had chest pain in the days preceding the event. Activities that were most associated with SD were cycling (30.6%), running (21.3%), and soccer (13.0%), which likely reflect the most common activities in France. Approximately one-half of sudden deaths occurred in public sports facilities. Bystander cardiopulmonary resuscitation (CPR) was initiated in only 30.7% of cases, although 93% were witnessed. The overall survival rate to hospital discharge was 15.7%, with the following factors independently associated with survival to hospital discharge: bystander CPR, time from collapse to start of CPR, and initial use of an external cardioverter defibrillator (Table 3). Although there are limitations of such a widespread observational study including the lack of autopsy data identifying etiology of sudden death, these data indicate that sports-related SCD is more common than may have been previously appreciated. Importantly, this study also identifies factors associated with favorable outcomes including bystander CPR and early defibrillation, which is consistent with other studies of out-of-hospital cardiac arrest in non-sports–related populations. These results may have implications for public health campaigns including importance of CPR education and availability of AEDs during participation in recreational sports.

C. P. Rowley, MD

Miscellaneous

Colchicine Reduces Postoperative Atrial Fibrillation: Results of the Colchicine for the Prevention of the Postpericardiotomy Syndrome (COPPS) Atrial Fibrillation Substudy

Imazio M, for the COPPS Investigators (Maria Vittoria Hosp, Torino, Italy; et al)
Circulation 124:2290-2295, 2011

Background.—Inflammation and pericarditis may be contributing factors for postoperative atrial fibrillation (POAF), and both are potentially affected by antiinflammatory drugs and colchicine, which has been shown to be safe and efficacious for the prevention of pericarditis and the postpericardiotomy syndrome (PPS). The aim of the Colchicine for the Prevention of the Post-Pericardiotomy Syndrome (COPPS) POAF substudy was to test the efficacy and safety of colchicine for the prevention of POAF after cardiac surgery.

Methods and Results.—The COPPS POAF substudy included 336 patients (mean age, 65.7 ± 12.3 years; 69% male) of the COPPS trial, a multicenter, double-blind, randomized trial. Substudy patients were in sinus rhythm before starting the intervention (placebo/colchicine 1.0 mg twice daily starting on postoperative day 3 followed by a maintenance dose of 0.5 mg twice daily for 1 month in patients ≥70 kg, halved doses for patients <70 kg or intolerant to the highest dose). The substudy primary end point was the incidence of POAF on intervention at 1 month. Despite well-balanced baseline characteristics, patients on colchicine had a reduced incidence of POAF (12.0% versus 22.0%, respectively; $P = 0.021$; relative risk reduction, 45%; number needed to treat, 11) with a shorter in-hospital stay (9.4 ± 3.7 versus 10.3 ± 4.3 days; $P = 0.040$) and rehabilitation stay (12.1 ± 6.1 versus 13.9 ± 6.5 days; $P = 0.009$). Side effects were similar in the study groups.

Conclusion.—Colchicine seems safe and efficacious in the reduction of POAF with the potentiality of halving the complication and reducing the hospital stay.

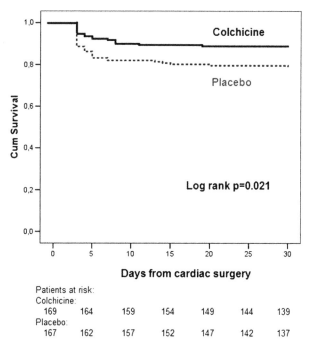

FIGURE 2.—Kaplan-Meier postoperative atrial fibrillation—free survival after postoperative day 3 according to treatment groups. Intervention with placebo/colchicine was started on postoperative day 3. (Reprinted from Imazio M, for the COPPS Investigators, Colchicine reduces postoperative atrial fibrillation: results of the Colchicine for the Prevention of the Postpericardiotomy Syndrome (COPPS) atrial fibrillation substudy. *Circulation.* 2011;124:2290-2295. © American Heart Association, Inc.)

Clinical Trial Registration.—URL: http://www.clinicaltrials.gov. Unique identifier: NCT00128427 (Fig 2).

▶ Atrial fibrillation (AF) is very common following cardiac surgery. In contrast to AF in the general population, which is typically due to enhanced automaticity from the pulmonary veins, postoperative AF is more commonly associated with inflammation. Accordingly, this study was part of a prospective, multicenter, randomized trial of colchicine following cardiac surgery in 6 Italian centers. The authors show that colchicine was well tolerated and associated with about a 45% relative reduction in postoperative AF (Fig 2). Hospitalization was also shortened in the colchicine group, although hospital durations were long in both groups compared with US standards. Beta-blockers are well documented to reduce postoperative AF and were underused in this trial. However, colchicine remains an independent predictor of AF of similar magnitude to β-blockers. These findings indicate that colchicine may be a safe and important additional agent to reduce postoperative AF. Further study is needed to confirm these results and to identify the role of colchicine in combination with other pharmacologic agents in this population.

M. R. Gold, MD, PhD

Reversal of outflow tract ventricular premature depolarization–induced cardiomyopathy with ablation: Effect of residual arrhythmia burden and preexisting cardiomyopathy on outcome

Mountantonakis SE, Frankel DS, Gerstenfeld EP, et al (Hosp of the Univ of Pennsylvania, Philadelphia)
Heart Rhythm 8:1608-1614, 2011

Background.—Outflow tract ventricular premature depolarizations (VPDs) can be associated with reversible left ventricular cardiomyopathy (LVCM). Limited data exist regarding the outcome after ablation of outflow tract VPDs from the LV and the impact of residual VPDs or preexisting LVCM prior to the diagnosis of VPDs on recovery of LV function.

Objective.—To examine the safety, efficacy, and long-term effect of radiofrequency ablation on LV function in patients with LVCM and frequent outflow tract VPDs and examine the effect of ablation in patients with LVCM known to precede the onset of VPDs and the impact of residual VPD frequency on recovery of LV function.

Methods.—Sixty-nine patients (43 men; age 51 ± 16 years) with nonischemic LVCM (left ventricular ejection fraction [LVEF] 35% ± 9%, left ventricular diastolic diameter [LVDD] 5.8 ± 0.7 cm) were referred for ablation of frequent outflow tract VPDs (29% ± 13%).

Results.—VPDs originated in the right ventricular outflow tract in 27 (39%) patients and the left ventricular outflow tract in 42 (61%) patients. After follow-up of 11 ± 6 months, 44 (66%) patients had rare (<2%) VPDs, 15 (22%) had decreased VPD burden (>80% reduction and always

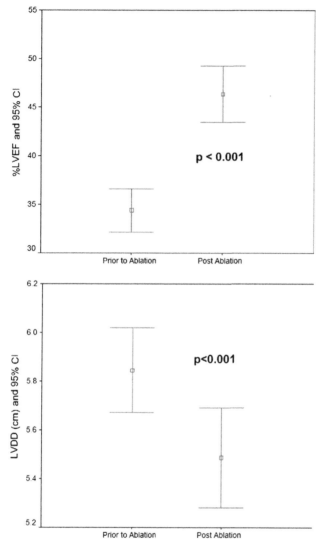

FIGURE 2.—Improvement in left ventricular ejection fraction (LVEF) and left ventricular end-diastolic diameter (LVDD) after ablation among the entire cohort. (Reprinted from Heart Rhythm, Mountantonakis SE, Frankel DS, Gerstenfeld EP, et al. Reversal of outflow tract ventricular premature depolarization—induced cardiomyopathy with ablation: Effect of residual arrhythmia burden and preexisting cardiomyopathy on outcome. *Heart Rhythm*. 2011;8:1608-1614. Copyright 2011, with permission from Heart Rhythm Society.)

<5000 VPDs), and 8 (12%) had no clinical improvement with persistent (5 patients) or recurrent (3 patients) VPDs. Only patients with either rare or decreased VPD burden had a significant improvement in LVEF (ΔLVEF 14% ± 9% vs 13% ± 7% vs −3% ± 6%, respectively, $P < .001$) and

LVDD (ΔLVDD -4 ± 5 vs -2 ± 4 vs 0 ± 4, respectively, $P = .038$), regardless of chamber of origin. The magnitude of LVEF improvement correlated with the decline in residual VPD burden ($r = 0.475$, $P = .007$). Patients with preexisting LVCM had a more modest but still significant improvement in LV function compared to patients without preexisting LVCM (ΔLVEF 8% vs 13%, $P = .046$). Multivariate analysis revealed ablation outcome, higher LVEF, and absence of preexisting LVCM were independently associated with LVEF improvement.

Conclusion.—Frequent outflow tract VPDs are associated with LVCM regardless of ventricle of origin. Significant (>80%) reduction in VPD burden has comparable improvement in LV function to complete VPD elimination. Successful VPD ablation may be beneficial even in patients with preexisting LVCM (Fig 2).

▶ Premature ventricular contraction (PVC) cardiomyopathy is a relatively rare but potentially reversible cause of nonischemic left ventricular (LV) cardiomyopathy and heart failure. Traditionally, it is believed that 20% or more beats need to be PVCs to lead to decreased LV function. In this study, the authors evaluated their large experience including all patients with at least 5000 PVCs per day. They demonstrate that success rates for ablation of ventricular premature depolarizations (VPDs) is high (> 90%) and that successful ablation is associated with improvement in LV function and reduction in LV chamber size (see Fig 2). Patients improved similarly with complete VPD elimination and significant reduction in VPD burden (> 80% decrease). Additionally, patients with preexisting cardiomyopathy also improved after successful PVC ablation, albeit to a lesser magnitude than patients without prior LV dysfunction. Catheter ablation has potentially high success rates and can result in significant clinical improvements in patients with suspected PVC cardiomyopathy and should be considered early if medical therapy fails.

F. Cuoco, MD, MBA

Ablation of atrioventricular nodal reentrant tachycardia in the elderly: results from the German Ablation Registry

Hoffmann BA, Brachmann J, Andresen D, et al (Univ Heart Ctr, Hamburg, Germany; Hosp Coburg, Germany; Vivantes Hosp, Berlin; et al)
Heart Rhythm 8:981-987, 2011

Background.—Catheter ablation (CA) is considered the treatment of choice for patients with atrioventricular nodal reentrant tachycardia (AVNRT). However, there is a tendency to avoid CA in the elderly because of a presumed increased risk of periprocedural atrioventricular (AV) nodal block.

Objective.—The purpose of this prospective registry was to assess age-related differences in the efficacy and safety of CA within a large population with AVNRT.

Methods.—A total of 3,234 consecutive patients from 48 German trial centers who underwent CA of AVNRT between March 2007 and May 2010 were enrolled in this study. The cohort was divided into three age groups: <50 years (group 1, n = 1,268 [39.2%]; median age = 40 [30.0–45.0] years, 74.1% women), 50–75 years old (group 2, n = 1,707 [52.8%]; 63.0 [58.0–69.0] years, 63.0% women), and >75 years old (group 3, n = 259 [8.0%]; 79.0 [77.0–82.0] years, 50.6% women).

Results.—CA was performed with radiofrequency current (RFC) in 97.7% and cryoablation technology in 2.3% of all cases. No differences were observed among the three groups with regard to primary CA success rate (98.7% vs. 98.8 % vs. 98.5%; *P* =.92) and overall procedure duration (75.0 minutes [50.0–105.0]; *P* =.93). Hemodynamically stable pericardial effusion occurred in five group 2 (0.3%) and two group 3 (0.8%) patients but in none of the group 1 (*P* <.05) patients. Complete AV block requiring permanent pacemaker implantation occurred in two patients in group 1 (0.2%) and six patients in group 2 (0.4%) but none in group 3 (*P* = 0.41). During a median follow-up period of 511.5 days (396.0–771.0), AVNRT recurrence occurred in 5.7% of all patients. Patients >75 years (group 3) had a significantly longer hospital stay (3.0 days [2.0–5.0]) compared with group 1 (2.0 days [1.0–2.0]) or group 2 (2.0 days [1.0–3.0]) patients (*P* <.0001).

Conclusion.—CA of AVNRT is highly effective and safe and does not pose an increased risk for complete AV block in patients over 75 years of age, despite a higher prevalence of structural heart disease. Antiarrhythmic drug therapy is often ineffective in this age group; thus, CA for AVNRT should be considered the preferred treatment even in elderly patients (Table 3).

▶ Catheter ablation of typical atrioventricular nodal reentrant tachycardia (AVNRT) is now generally considered first-line therapy in symptomatic patients. Complication rates for this procedure are documented to be low, and long-term success rates are exceptional (> 95%). The alternative treatment of antiarrhythmic drug therapy is complicated by significant side effects and low efficacy. Despite these observations, there continues to be age bias in treatment. Older patients are frequently denied therapy because of perceived increased risk of high-grade heart block, vascular complication, or necessity for pacemaker implantation. To

TABLE 3.—Procedural Complications

	Total, %	Group 1, % (<50 Years Old)	Group 2, % (50–75 Years Old)	Group 3, % (>75 Years Old)	*P*
Death (n)	0.03 (1)	0	0	0.4 (1)	<.01
Acute myocardial infarction (n)	0.03 (1)	0	0	0.4 (1)	<.01
Cerebral stroke (n)	0	0	0	0	—
Pericardial effusion (n)	0.2 (7)	0	0.3 (5)	0.8 (2)	<.05
Pneumothorax (n)	0.1 (2)	0.2 (2)	0	0	.21
Major hemorrhage (n)	0.03 (1)	0	0.06 (1)	0	.64
Cardiac surgery (n)	0	0	0	0	—

address this issue, this study was a multicenter analysis of more than 3000 consecutive patients who underwent ablation for AVNRT. Patients were retrospectively partitioned into age groups consisting of age younger than 50, age 50 to 75, and older than 75 years. The vast majority of patients received typical therapy with radiofrequency ablation. Patients in excess of 75 years of age represented 8.2% of the cohort. After analysis, there were no significant differences in complications (Table 3), including the incidence of high-grade atrioventricular block, vascular complication, or long-term success rate between any of the cohorts. This study further demonstrates the safety and efficacy of routine radiofrequency catheter ablation of typical AVNRT and indicates that age should not be a barrier to this treatment modality.

J. L. Sturdivant, MD

Rivaroxaban versus Warfarin in Nonvalvular Atrial Fibrillation
Patel MR, the ROCKET AF Steering Committee, for the ROCKET AF Investigators (Duke Univ Med Ctr, Durham, NC; et al)
N Engl J Med 365:883-891, 2011

Background.—The use of warfarin reduces the rate of ischemic stroke in patients with atrial fibrillation but requires frequent monitoring and dose adjustment. Rivaroxaban, an oral factor Xa inhibitor, may provide more consistent and predictable anticoagulation than warfarin.

Methods.—In a double-blind trial, we randomly assigned 14,264 patients with nonvalvular atrial fibrillation who were at increased risk for stroke to receive either rivaroxaban (at a daily dose of 20 mg) or dose-adjusted warfarin. The per-protocol, as-treated primary analysis was designed to determine whether rivaroxaban was noninferior to warfarin for the primary end point of stroke or systemic embolism.

Results.—In the primary analysis, the primary end point occurred in 188 patients in the rivaroxaban group (1.7% per year) and in 241 in the warfarin group (2.2% per year) (hazard ratio in the rivaroxaban group, 0.79; 95% confidence interval [CI], 0.66 to 0.96; P<0.001 for noninferiority). In the intention-to-treat analysis, the primary end point occurred in 269 patients in the rivaroxaban group (2.1% per year) and in 306 patients in the warfarin group (2.4% per year) (hazard ratio, 0.88; 95% CI, 0.74 to 1.03; P<0.001 for noninferiority; P=0.12 for superiority). Major and nonmajor clinically relevant bleeding occurred in 1475 patients in the rivaroxaban group (14.9% per year) and in 1449 in the warfarin group (14.5% per year) (hazard ratio, 1.03; 95% CI, 0.96 to 1.11; P=0.44), with significant reductions in intracranial hemorrhage (0.5% vs. 0.7%, P=0.02) and fatal bleeding (0.2% vs. 0.5%, P=0.003) in the rivaroxaban group.

Conclusions.—In patients with atrial fibrillation, rivaroxaban was noninferior to warfarin for the prevention of stroke or systemic embolism. There was no significant between-group difference in the risk of major bleeding, although intracranial and fatal bleeding occurred less frequently

TABLE 2.—Primary End Point of Stroke or Systemic Embolism*

| Study Population | Rivaroxaban | | | Warfarin | | | Hazard Ratio (95% CI)[†] | P Value | |
	No. of Patients	No. of Events	Event Rate no./100 patient-yr	No. of Patients	No. of Events	Event Rate no./100 patient-yr		Noninferiority	Superiority
Per-protocol, as-treated population[‡]	6958	188	1.7	7004	241	2.2	0.79 (0.66–0.96)	<0.001	
Safety, as-treated population	7061	189	1.7	7082	243	2.2	0.79 (0.65–0.95)		0.02
Intention-to-treat population[§]	7081	269	2.1	7090	306	2.4	0.88 (0.75–1.03)	<0.001	0.12
During treatment		188	1.7		240	2.2	0.79 (0.66–0.96)		0.02
After discontinuation		81	4.7		66	4.3	1.10 (0.79–1.52)		0.58

*The median follow-up period was 590 days for the per-protocol, as-treated population during treatment; 590 days for the safety, as-treated population during treatment; and 707 days for the intention-to-treat population.
[†]Hazard ratios are for the rivaroxaban group as compared with the warfarin group.
[‡]The primary analysis was performed in the as-treated, per-protocol population during treatment.
[§]Follow-up in the intention-to-treat population continued until notification of study termination.

in the rivaroxaban group. (Funded by Johnson & Johnson and Bayer; ROCKET AF ClinicalTrials.gov number, NCT00403767.) (Table 2).

▶ Atrial fibrillation (AF) is associated with an increased risk of thromboembolic stroke. Warfarin reduces the rate of strokes in patients with nonvalvular atrial fibrillation; however, food and drug interactions necessitate frequent monitoring and dosage changes, making the drug less than ideal. Rivaroxaban, a once-daily oral factor Xa inhibitor is believed to provide more consistent and predictable anticoagulation. To compare the efficacy of warfarin and rivaroxaban in AF, ROCKET AF, a multicenter, randomized, double-blind, double-dummy, event-driven trial was conducted in 1178 sites in 45 countries. A total of 14 264 patients with moderate-to-high risk of stroke, with mean and median CHADS2 scores of 3.5 and 3.0, respectively, were randomly assigned to daily rivaroxaban or adjusted dose warfarin with goal international normalized ratio (INR) of 2.0 to 3.0. The median duration of treatment was 590 days, and the median follow-up period was 707 days with the primary efficacy endpoint of stroke or systemic embolism. Table 2 displays that in patients both in the per-protocol population and in the intention-to-treat analysis, rivaroxaban was found to be noninferior to warfarin with regard to the primary endpoint. During treatment in the intention-to-treat population, patients in the rivaroxaban group had a lower rate of stroke or systemic embolism (188 events, 1.7% per year) than in the warfarin group (240 events, 2.2% per year) ($P = .02$). The principal safety endpoint was a composite of major and nonmajor clinically relevant bleeding events and was similar in the 2 groups (3.6% and 3.4%, respectively, $P = .58$). Major bleeding from a gastrointestinal site was more common in the rivaroxaban group (3.2% compared with 2.2% with warfarin, $P < .001$), whereas rates of intracranial hemorrhage were significantly higher in the warfarin group (0.7% vs 0.5% per year, $P = .02$). Of note, the proportion of time the patients in the warfarin group had a therapeutic INR was only 55%, which is lower than in prior studies of new anticoagulants. However, this also illustrates one of the clinical problems with warfarin: the instability of the therapeutic dose. Because of this study, rivaroxaban will likely be a popular alternative to warfarin, as it provides noninferior prevention of strokes or systemic embolism with similar rates of bleeding in a once-daily dosing. The more predictable pharmacokinetics and the reduced intracranial bleeding seem to be a common difference between newer anticoagulants (factor Xa or direct thrombin inhibitors) and warfarin. In clinical practice, this is offset by the higher costs of the drug and concerns about the lack of reversal agents when bleeding does occur.

P. C. Netzler, MD

Article Index

Chapter 1: Hypertension

NICE clinical guideline 127: Hypertension: Clinical management of primary hypertension in adults   1

Relative effectiveness of clinic and home blood pressure monitoring compared with ambulatory blood pressure monitoring in diagnosis of hypertension: systematic review   4

ACCF/AHA 2011 Expert Consensus Document on Hypertension in the Elderly: A Report of the American College of Cardiology Foundation Task Force on Clinical Expert Consensus Documents Developed in Collaboration With the American Academy of Neurology, American Geriatrics Society, American Society for Preventive Cardiology, American Society of Hypertension, American Society of Nephrology, Association of Black Cardiologists, and European Society of Hypertension   6

Systematic Review: Blood Pressure Target in Chronic Kidney Disease and Proteinuria as an Effect Modifier   9

Antihypertensive Treatment and Secondary Prevention of Cardiovascular Disease Events Among Persons Without Hypertension: A Meta-Analysis   11

The effects of blood pressure reduction and of different blood pressure-lowering regimens on major cardiovascular events according to baseline blood pressure: meta-analysis of randomized trials   13

National, regional, and global trends in systolic blood pressure since 1980: systematic analysis of health examination surveys and epidemiological studies with 786 country-years and 5·4 million participants   15

Effects of telmisartan, irbesartan, valsartan, candesartan, and losartan on cancers in 15 trials enrolling 138 769 individuals   18

Angiotensin receptor blockers and risk of myocardial infarction: meta-analyses and trial sequential analyses of 147 020 patients from randomised trials   20

Antihypertensive drugs and risk of cancer: network meta-analyses and trial sequential analyses of 324 168 participants from randomised trials   22

The cost-effectiveness of interventions designed to reduce sodium intake   24

Antihypertensive Efficacy of Hydrochlorothiazide as Evaluated by Ambulatory Blood Pressure Monitoring: A Meta-Analysis of Randomized Trials   26

Effect of Renin-Angiotensin System Blockade on Calcium Channel Blocker-Associated Peripheral Edema   28

Presence of baseline prehypertension and risk of incident stroke: A meta-analysis   31

Baseline predictors of resistant hypertension in the Anglo-Scandinavian Cardiac Outcome Trial (ASCOT): a risk score to identify those at high-risk   33

Fatal and Nonfatal Outcomes, Incidence of Hypertension, and Blood Pressure Changes in Relation to Urinary Sodium Excretion   35

Sodium and Potassium Intake and Mortality Among US Adults: Prospective Data From the Third National Health and Nutrition Examination Survey   38

Effect of pay for performance on the management and outcomes of hypertension in the United Kingdom: interrupted time series study   40

Maternal exposure to angiotensin converting enzyme inhibitors in the first trimester and risk of malformations in offspring: a retrospective cohort study 43

Long-term follow-up of 111 patients with angiotensin-converting enzyme inhibitor-related angioedema 45

Chlorthalidone Reduces Cardiovascular Events Compared With Hydrochlorothiazide: A Retrospective Cohort Analysis 47

Long-Term Effects of Chlorthalidone Versus Hydrochlorothiazide on Electrocardiographic Left Ventricular Hypertrophy in the Multiple Risk Factor Intervention Trial 49

Association of blood pressure in late adolescence with subsequent mortality: cohort study of Swedish male conscripts 51

Blood Pressure Targets Recommended by Guidelines and Incidence of Cardiovascular and Renal Events in the Ongoing Telmisartan Alone and in Combination With Ramipril Global Endpoint Trial (ONTARGET) 53

Better compliance to antihypertensive medications reduces cardiovascular risk 55

Effects of intensive blood pressure reduction on myocardial infarction and stroke in diabetes: a meta-analysis in 73 913 patients 57

Prevalence of Resistant Hypertension in the United States, 2003−2008 59

Uncontrolled and Apparent Treatment Resistant Hypertension in the United States, 1988 to 2008 61

Clinical features of 8295 patients with resistant hypertension classified on the basis of ambulatory blood pressure monitoring 63

Urinary Sodium and Potassium Excretion and Risk of Cardiovascular Events 65

Cardiovascular Outcomes in Framingham Participants With Diabetes: The Importance of Blood Pressure 68

Heterogeneity in antihypertensive treatment discontinuation between drugs belonging to the same class 69

Measuring blood pressure for decision making and quality reporting: where and how many measures? 72

Level of Systolic Blood Pressure Within the Normal Range and Risk of Recurrent Stroke 74

Prognostic role of ambulatory blood pressure measurement in patients with nondialysis chronic kidney disease 76

Association Between Chlorthalidone Treatment of Systolic Hypertension and Long-term Survival 78

Genetic variants in novel pathways influence blood pressure and cardiovascular disease risk 81

Reliability of palpation of the radial artery compared with auscultation of the brachial artery in measuring SBP 82

Determinants of masked hypertension in the general population: the Finn-Home study 85

Cost-effectiveness of options for the diagnosis of high blood pressure in primary care: a modelling study 87

The angiotensin-receptor blocker candesartan for treatment of acute stroke (SCAST): a randomised, placebo-controlled, double-blind trial   89

Moderate dietary sodium restriction added to angiotensin converting enzyme inhibition compared with dual blockade in lowering proteinuria and blood pressure: randomised controlled trial   92

A double-blind, randomized study comparing the antihypertensive effect of eplerenone and spironolactone in patients with hypertension and evidence of primary aldosteronism   94

Is a systolic blood pressure target <140 mmHg indicated in all hypertensives? Subgroup analyses of findings from the randomized FEVER trial   96

Effects of Manidipine and Delapril in Hypertensive Patients With Type 2 Diabetes Mellitus: The Delapril and Manidipine for Nephroprotection in Diabetes (DEMAND) Randomized Clinical Trial   99

Aliskiren and the calcium channel blocker amlodipine combination as an initial treatment strategy for hypertension control (ACCELERATE): a randomised, parallel-group trial   101

Conventional versus automated measurement of blood pressure in primary care patients with systolic hypertension: randomised parallel design controlled trial   104

Home Blood Pressure Management and Improved Blood Pressure Control: Results From a Randomized Controlled Trial   106

Culturally Appropriate Storytelling to Improve Blood Pressure: A Randomized Trial   108

Chapter 2: Pediatric Cardiovascular Disease

The evolving role of intraoperative balloon pulmonary valvuloplasty in valve-sparing repair of tetralogy of Fallot   111

Late Repair of the Native Pulmonary Valve in Patients With Pulmonary Insufficiency After Surgery for Tetralogy of Fallot   112

Long-term results of pulmonary artery rehabilitation in patients with pulmonary atresia, ventricular septal defect, pulmonary artery hypoplasia, and major aortopulmonary collaterals   113

Pulmonary Atresia, Ventricular Septal Defect, and Major Aortopulmonary Collaterals: Neonatal Pulmonary Artery Rehabilitation Without Unifocalization   114

Pulmonary valve replacement in chronic pulmonary regurgitation in adults with congenital heart disease: Impact of preoperative QRS-duration and NT-proBNP levels on postoperative right ventricular function   115

Long term outcome of mechanical valve prosthesis in the pulmonary position   116

Anatomic repair for congenitally corrected transposition of the great arteries: A single-institution 19-year experience   117

Congenitally Corrected Transposition of the Great Arteries: Ventricular Function at the Time of Systemic Atrioventricular Valve Replacement Predicts Long-Term Ventricular Function   118

A Multicenter, Randomized Trial Comparing Heparin/Warfarin and Acetylsalicylic Acid as Primary Thromboprophylaxis for 2 Years After the Fontan Procedure in Children   119

Cavopulmonary pathway modification in patients with heterotaxy and newly diagnosed or persistent pulmonary arteriovenous malformations after a modified Fontan operation — 120

Center Variation in Patient Age and Weight at Fontan Operation and Impact on Postoperative Outcomes — 121

Clinical outcomes of prophylactic Damus-Kaye-Stansel anastomosis concomitant with bidirectional Glenn procedure — 122

Early Results of the "Clamp and Sew" Fontan Procedure Without the Use of Circulatory Support — 123

Impact of the Evolution of the Fontan Operation on Early and Late Mortality: A Single-Center Experience of 405 Patients Over 3 Decades — 124

Comparison of risk factors and outcomes for pediatric patients listed for heart transplantation after bidirectional Glenn and after Fontan: An analysis from the Pediatric Heart Transplant Study — 125

A Comparison of the Modified Blalock-Taussig Shunt With the Right Ventricle-to-Pulmonary Artery Conduit — 126

Changes of Right Ventricular Function and Longitudinal Deformation in Children with Hypoplastic Left Heart Syndrome Before and After the Norwood Operation — 127

Comprehensive evaluation of right ventricular function in children with different anatomical subtypes of hypoplastic left heart syndrome after Fontan surgery — 128

Regional Myocardial Dysfunction following Norwood with Right Ventricle to Pulmonary Artery Conduit in Patients with Hypoplastic Left Heart Syndrome — 129

New approach to interstage care for palliated high-risk patients with congenital heart disease — 130

Pulmonary Artery and Conduit Reintervention Rates After Norwood Using a Right Ventricle to Pulmonary Artery Conduit — 131

Interstage attrition between bidirectional Glenn and Fontan palliation in children with hypoplastic left heart syndrome — 132

Concomitant stenting of the patent ductus arteriosus and radiofrequency valvotomy in pulmonary atresia with intact ventricular septum and intermediate right ventricle: Early in-hospital and medium-term outcomes — 134

Surgical Interventions for Atrioventricular Septal Defect Subtypes: The Pediatric Heart Network Experience — 135

Adolescents With d-Transposition of the Great Arteries Corrected With the Arterial Switch Procedure: Neuropsychological Assessment and Structural Brain Imaging — 136

Anomalous Aortic Origin of a Coronary Artery: Medium-Term Results After Surgical Repair in 50 Patients — 137

Best Practices in Managing Transition to Adulthood for Adolescents With Congenital Heart Disease: The Transition Process and Medical and Psychosocial Issues: A Scientific Statement From the American Heart Association — 138

Comprehensive Use of Cardiopulmonary Exercise Testing Identifies Adults With Congenital Heart Disease at Increased Mortality Risk in the Medium Term — 139

Geriatric Congenital Heart Disease: Burden of Disease and Predictors of Mortality — 140

Cardiovascular changes after transcatheter endovascular stenting of adult aortic coarctation — 141

Comparison of Risk of Hypertensive Complications of Pregnancy Among Women With Versus Without Coarctation of the Aorta — 142

Alternative approach for selected severe pulmonary hypertension of congenital heart defect without initial correction — Palliative surgical treatment — 143

Cardiac resynchronization therapy in paediatric and congenital heart disease patients — 144

Left Ventricular Function After Left Ventriculotomy for Surgical Treatment of Multiple Muscular Ventricular Septal Defects — 145

Coronary Artery Disease in Adult Congenital Heart Disease: Outcome After Coronary Artery Bypass Grafting — 146

Evaluation of image quality and radiation dose at prospective ECG-triggered axial 256-slice multi-detector CT in infants with congenital heart disease — 147

Left Ventricular Function in Adult Patients With Atrial Septal Defect: Implication for Development of Heart Failure After Transcatheter Closure — 148

Costs of Prenatal Detection of Congenital Heart Disease — 149

Generalised muscle weakness in young adults with congenital heart disease — 149

Erosion of an Amplatzer Septal Occluder Device Into the Aortic Root — 150

A genetic contribution to risk for postoperative junctional ectopic tachycardia in children undergoing surgery for congenital heart disease — 151

Cardiovascular Screening with Electrocardiography and Echocardiography in Collegiate Athletes — 152

Chapter 3: Cardiac Surgery

2011 ACCF/AHA guideline for coronary artery bypass graft surgery: Executive summary: A report of the American College of Cardiology Foundation/American Heart Association Task Force on Practice Guidelines — 155

Coronary-Artery Bypass Surgery in Patients with Left Ventricular Dysfunction — 158

Long-Term Outcomes of Endoscopic Vein Harvesting After Coronary Artery Bypass Grafting — 159

Quality of Life after PCI with Drug-Eluting Stents or Coronary-Artery Bypass Surgery — 161

Randomized Comparison of Percutaneous Coronary Intervention With Sirolimus-Eluting Stents Versus Coronary Artery Bypass Grafting in Unprotected Left Main Stem Stenosis — 162

Elevated parathyroid hormone predicts mortality in dialysis patients undergoing valve surgery — 164

Percutaneous Repair or Surgery for Mitral Regurgitation — 165

Valve Configuration Determines Long-Term Results After Repair of the Bicuspid Aortic Valve — 167

Continuous Flow Left Ventricular Assist Device Outcomes in Commercial Use Compared With the Prior Clinical Trial — 169

Inhaled nitric oxide after left ventricular assist device implantation: A prospective, randomized, double-blind, multicenter, placebo-controlled trial — 170

Changing outcomes in patients bridged to heart transplantation with continuous-versus pulsatile-flow ventricular assist devices: An analysis of the registry of the International Society for Heart and Lung Transplantation   171

Mitral valve repair in heart failure: Five-year follow-up from the mitral valve replacement stratum of the Acorn randomized trial   172

Bypass Versus Drug-Eluting Stents at Three Years in SYNTAX Patients With Diabetes Mellitus or Metabolic Syndrome   174

Cardiac stem cells in patients with ischaemic cardiomyopathy (SCIPIO): initial results of a randomised phase 1 trial   175

Effect of Everolimus Introduction on Cardiac Allograft Vasculopathy—Results of a Randomized, Multicenter Trial   177

Transcatheter versus Surgical Aortic-Valve Replacement in High-Risk Patients   178

Chapter 4: Coronary Heart Disease

30-Year Trends in Heart Failure in Patients Hospitalized With Acute Myocardial Infarction   181

Acute coronary syndrome and cocaine use: 8-year prevalence and inhospital outcomes   183

Association Between Adoption of Evidence-Based Treatment and Survival for Patients With ST-Elevation Myocardial Infarction   185

Association of Door-In to Door-Out Time With Reperfusion Delays and Outcomes Among Patients Transferred for Primary Percutaneous Coronary Intervention   187

Association of Mortality With Years of Education in Patients With ST-Segment Elevation Myocardial Infarction Treated With Fibrinolysis   188

Composition of Coronary Thrombus in Acute Myocardial Infarction   190

Causes of Delay and Associated Mortality in Patients Transferred With ST-Segment—Elevation Myocardial Infarction   193

Effect of upstream clopidogrel treatment in patients with ST-segment elevation myocardial infarction undergoing primary percutaneous coronary intervention   194

Heparin plus a glycoprotein IIb/IIIa inhibitor versus bivalirudin monotherapy and paclitaxel-eluting stents versus bare-metal stents in acute myocardial infarction (HORIZONS-AMI): final 3-year results from a multicentre, randomised controlled trial   197

Primary angioplasty vs. fibrinolysis in very old patients with acute myocardial infarction: TRIANA (TRatamiento del Infarto Agudo de miocardio eN Ancianos) randomized trial and pooled analysis with previous studies   199

Randomized Comparison of Pre-Hospital—Initiated Facilitated Percutaneous Coronary Intervention Versus Primary Percutaneous Coronary Intervention in Acute Myocardial Infarction Very Early After Symptom Onset: The LIPSIA-STEMI Trial (Leipzig Immediate Prehospital Facilitated Angioplasty in ST-Segment Myocardial Infarction)   201

Sex Differences in Patient-Reported Symptoms Associated With Myocardial Infarction (from the Population-Based MONICA/KORA Myocardial Infarction Registry)   204

The Occluded Artery Trial (OAT) Viability Ancillary Study (OAT-NUC): Influence of infarct zone viability on left ventricular remodeling after percutaneous coronary intervention versus optimal medical therapy alone   206

Ticagrelor Compared With Clopidogrel by Geographic Region in the Platelet Inhibition and Patient Outcomes (PLATO) Trial   208

Functional SYNTAX Score for Risk Assessment in Multivessel Coronary Artery Disease   210

Intra-aortic Balloon Counterpulsation and Infarct Size in Patients With Acute Anterior Myocardial Infarction Without Shock: The CRISP AMI Randomized Trial   212

Intramyocardial, Autologous CD34+ Cell Therapy for Refractory Angina   214

Appropriateness of Percutaneous Coronary Intervention   216

Aspirin Plus Clopidogrel Versus Aspirin Alone After Coronary Artery Bypass Grafting: The Clopidogrel After Surgery for Coronary Artery Disease (CASCADE) Trial   219

Comparison of coronary bypass surgery with drug-eluting stenting for the treatment of left main and/or three-vessel disease: 3-year follow-up of the SYNTAX trial   221

Effect of Timing of Chronic Preoperative Aspirin Discontinuation on Morbidity and Mortality in Coronary Artery Bypass Surgery   223

Effects of Optimal Medical Treatment With or Without Coronary Revascularization on Angina and Subsequent Revascularizations in Patients With Type 2 Diabetes Mellitus and Stable Ischemic Heart Disease   226

Impact of Angiographic Complete Revascularization After Drug-Eluting Stent Implantation or Coronary Artery Bypass Graft Surgery for Multivessel Coronary Artery Disease   229

Long-Term Comparison of Drug-Eluting Stents and Coronary Artery Bypass Grafting for Multivessel Coronary Revascularization: 5-Year Outcomes From the Asan Medical Center-Multivessel Revascularization Registry   231

Radial Artery Grafts vs Saphenous Vein Grafts in Coronary Artery Bypass Surgery: A Randomized Trial   233

Radial versus femoral access for coronary angiography and intervention in patients with acute coronary syndromes (RIVAL): a randomised, parallel group, multicentre trial   235

Recent Changes in Practice of Elective Percutaneous Coronary Intervention for Stable Angina   238

Secondary Prevention After Coronary Artery Bypass Graft Surgery: Findings of a National Randomized Controlled Trial and Sustained Society-Led Incorporation Into Practice   240

Trends in Coronary Revascularization in the United States From 2001 to 2009: Recent Declines in Percutaneous Coronary Intervention Volumes   242

Adolescent BMI Trajectory and Risk of Diabetes versus Coronary Disease   245

Global Variation in the Relative Burden of Stroke and Ischemic Heart Disease   247

Incidence of Cardiovascular Risk Factors in an Indian Urban Cohort: Results From the New Delhi Birth Cohort   249

National, regional, and global trends in body-mass index since 1980: systematic analysis of health examination surveys and epidemiological studies with 960 country-years and 9·1 million participants — 252

Nationwide Cohort Study of Risk of Ischemic Heart Disease in Patients With Celiac Disease — 255

Public health importance of triggers of myocardial infarction: a comparative risk assessment — 257

Using Additional Information on Working Hours to Predict Coronary Heart Disease: A Cohort Study — 258

Clinical Events as a Function of Proton Pump Inhibitor Use, Clopidogrel Use, and Cytochrome P450 2C19 Genotype in a Large Nationwide Cohort of Acute Myocardial Infarction: Results From the French Registry of Acute ST-Elevation and Non–ST-Elevation Myocardial Infarction (FAST-MI) Registry — 261

Absolute and Attributable Risks of Atrial Fibrillation in Relation to Optimal and Borderline Risk Factors: The Atherosclerosis Risk in Communities (ARIC) Study — 262

Atherosclerosis in Ancient Egyptian Mummies: The Horus Study — 265

C-reactive protein concentration and the vascular benefits of statin therapy: an analysis of 20 536 patients in the Heart Protection Study — 267

Development and Validation of a Risk Calculator for Prediction of Cardiac Risk After Surgery — 269

Dose Response Between Physical Activity and Risk of Coronary Heart Disease: A Meta-Analysis — 271

Isolated Coronary Artery Bypass Graft Combined With Bone Marrow Mononuclear Cells Delivered Through a Graft Vessel for Patients With Previous Myocardial Infarction and Chronic Heart Failure: A Single-Center, Randomized, Double-Blind, Placebo-Controlled Clinical Trial — 273

Positron Emission Tomography Measurement of Periodontal ^{18}F-Fluorodeoxyglucose Uptake Is Associated With Histologically Determined Carotid Plaque Inflammation — 275

Predictors of Coronary Heart Disease Events Among Asymptomatic Persons With Low Low-Density Lipoprotein Cholesterol: MESA (Multi-Ethnic Study of Atherosclerosis) — 278

Prevalence and Predictors of Concomitant Carotid and Coronary Artery Atherosclerotic Disease — 280

Use of Herbal Products and Potential Interactions in Patients With Cardiovascular Diseases — 282

3-Year Follow-Up of Patients With Coronary Artery Spasm as Cause of Acute Coronary Syndrome: The CASPAR (Coronary Artery Spasm in Patients With Acute Coronary Syndrome) Study Follow-Up — 284

Optimal timing of coronary angiography and potential intervention in non-ST-elevation acute coronary syndromes — 287

Chapter 5: Non-Coronary Heart Disease in Adults

Dose-dependent augmentation of cardiac systolic function with the selective cardiac myosin activator, omecamtiv mecarbil: a first-in-man study — 291

Cardiac Resynchronization Therapy as a Therapeutic Option in Patients With Moderate-Severe Functional Mitral Regurgitation and High Operative Risk — 295

Cardiac resynchronization therapy in patients with left ventricular systolic dysfunction and right bundle branch block: A systematic review — 296

Defining potential to benefit from implantable cardioverter defibrillator therapy: the role of biomarkers — 299

Mortality Reduction of Cardiac Resynchronization and Implantable Cardioverter-Defibrillator Therapy in Heart Failure: An Updated Meta-Analysis. Does Recent Evidence Change the Standard of Care? — 303

Prognostic value of cardiac troponin T in patients with moderate to severe heart failure scheduled for cardiac resynchronization therapy — 306

Relationship between improvement in left ventricular dyssynchrony and contractile function and clinical outcome with cardiac resynchronization therapy: the MADIT-CRT trial — 309

Impact of Remote Telemedical Management on Mortality and Hospitalizations in Ambulatory Patients With Chronic Heart Failure: The Telemedical Interventional Monitoring in Heart Failure Study — 312

Clinical Strategies and Outcomes in Advanced Heart Failure Patients Older Than 70 Years of Age Receiving the HeartMate II Left Ventricular Assist Device: A Community Hospital Experience — 315

Isolated Coronary Artery Bypass Graft Combined With Bone Marrow Mononuclear Cells Delivered Through a Graft Vessel for Patients With Previous Myocardial Infarction and Chronic Heart Failure: A Single-Center, Randomized, Double-Blind, Placebo-Controlled Clinical Trial — 319

Factors associated with improvement in ejection fraction in clinical practice among patients with heart failure: Findings from IMPROVE HF — 321

Intensive glycemic control has no impact on the risk of heart failure in type 2 diabetic patients: Evidence from a 37,229 patient meta-analysis — 323

Effects of selective heart rate reduction with ivabradine on left ventricular remodelling and function: results from the SHIFT echocardiography substudy — 327

Efficacy of statin therapy in chronic systolic cardiac insufficiency: A meta-analysis — 330

Eplerenone Survival Benefits in Heart Failure Patients Post-Myocardial Infarction Are Independent From its Diuretic and Potassium-Sparing Effects: Insights From an EPHESUS (Eplerenone Post-Acute Myocardial Infarction Heart Failure Efficacy and Survival Study) Substudy — 333

Erythropoietin as a treatment of anemia in heart failure: Systematic review of randomized trials — 336

Pulmonary Hypertension in Heart Failure With Preserved Ejection Fraction: A Target of Phosphodiesterase-5 Inhibition in a 1-Year Study — 340

Cardiac resynchronisation therapy in patients with heart failure and a normal QRS duration: the RESPOND study — 342

Comparison of Mortality and Morbidity in Patients With Atrial Fibrillation and Heart Failure With Preserved Versus Decreased Left Ventricular Ejection Fraction — 345

Disordered Iron Homeostasis in Chronic Heart Failure: Prevalence, Predictors, and Relation to Anemia, Exercise Capacity, and Survival — 349

Mortality and Readmission of Patients With Heart Failure, Atrial Fibrillation, or Coronary Artery Disease Undergoing Noncardiac Surgery: An Analysis of 38 047 Patients — 353

Prognostic value of serial measurements of highly sensitive cardiac troponin I in stable outpatients with nonischemic chronic heart failure — 355

Long-Term Survival in Patients With Resting Obstructive Hypertrophic Cardiomyopathy: Comparison of Conservative Versus Invasive Treatment — 358

Comparison of Prevalence, Clinical Course, and Pathological Findings of Left Ventricular Systolic Impairment Versus Normal Systolic Function in Patients With Hypertrophic Cardiomyopathy — 362

Alcohol Septal Ablation for the Treatment of Hypertrophic Obstructive Cardiomyopathy: A Multicenter North American Registry — 365

Chemical Cardiomyopathies: The Negative Effects of Medications and Nonprescribed Drugs on the Heart — 367

Clinical Characteristics and Cardiovascular Magnetic Resonance Findings in Stress (Takotsubo) Cardiomyopathy — 370

Isolated Noncompaction of the Left Ventricular Myocardium in Adults: A Systematic Overview — 372

Anticoagulant therapy in pregnant women with mechanical prosthetic heart valves: no easy option — 375

Changes in mitral regurgitation and left ventricular geometry during exercise affect exercise capacity in patients with systolic heart failure — 377

Do statins improve outcomes and delay the progression of non-rheumatic calcific aortic stenosis? — 380

Independent prognostic value of functional mitral regurgitation in patients with heart failure. A quantitative analysis of 1256 patients with ischaemic and non-ischaemic dilated cardiomyopathy — 382

Internal and external validation of a model to predict adverse outcomes in patients with left-sided infective endocarditis — 386

Long-term outcome of combined valve repair and maze procedure for nonrheumatic mitral regurgitation — 389

Midwall Fibrosis Is an Independent Predictor of Mortality in Patients With Aortic Stenosis — 392

Percutaneous Repair or Surgery for Mitral Regurgitation — 395

Prospective Validation of the Prognostic Usefulness of B-Type Natriuretic Peptide in Asymptomatic Patients With Chronic Severe Aortic Regurgitation — 398

The Impact of Renin-Angiotensin-Aldosterone System Blockade on Heart Failure Outcomes and Mortality in Patients Identified to Have Aortic Regurgitation: A Large Population Cohort Study — 401

Transcatheter Aortic-Valve Implantation for Aortic Stenosis in Patients Who Cannot Undergo Surgery — 405

Cardiac Magnetic Resonance Imaging Pericardial Late Gadolinium Enhancement and Elevated Inflammatory Markers Can Predict the Reversibility of Constrictive Pericarditis After Antiinflammatory Medical Therapy: A Pilot Study — 407

Colchicine prevents early postoperative pericardial and pleural effusions — 409

Effect of short-term NSAID use on echocardiographic parameters in elderly people: a population-based cohort study — 412

Efficacy and Safety of *Bosentan* for Pulmonary Arterial Hypertension in Adults With Congenital Heart Disease   414

Percutaneous Versus Surgical Revascularization in Patients With Ischemic Mitral Regurgitation   416

Benefit of atrial septal defect closure in adults: impact of age   418

Left Ventricular Function in Adult Patients With Atrial Septal Defect: Implication for Development of Heart Failure After Transcatheter Closure   421

Long-Term Follow-Up of Participants With Heart Failure in the Antihypertensive and Lipid-Lowering Treatment to Prevent Heart Attack Trial (ALLHAT)   424

Chapter 6: Cardiac Arrhythmias, Conduction Disturbances, and Electrophysiology

Apixaban versus Warfarin in Patients with Atrial Fibrillation   427

Cost-Effectiveness of Dabigatran for Stroke Prophylaxis in Atrial Fibrillation   429

Prevention of stroke and systemic embolism with rivaroxaban compared with warfarin in patients with non-valvular atrial fibrillation and moderate renal impairment   430

Synergistic Effect of the Combination of Ranolazine and Dronedarone to Suppress Atrial Fibrillation   433

The Effect of Rate Control on Quality of Life in Patients With Permanent Atrial Fibrillation: Data From the RACE II (Rate Control Efficacy in Permanent Atrial Fibrillation II) Study   435

Complications arising from catheter ablation of atrial fibrillation: Temporal trends and predictors   437

New-Onset Postoperative Atrial Fibrillation Predicts Late Mortality After Mitral Valve Surgery   438

Postablation asymptomatic cerebral lesions: Long-term follow-up using magnetic resonance imaging   440

Radiofrequency Ablation of Atrial Fibrillation in Patients With Mechanical Mitral Valve Prostheses: Safety, Feasibility, Electrophysiologic Findings, and Outcomes   441

Cardiac resynchronization therapy in patients undergoing atrioventricular junction ablation for permanent atrial fibrillation: a randomized trial   442

Cardiac Resynchronization Therapy Reduces Left Atrial Volume and the Risk of Atrial Tachyarrhythmias in MADIT-CRT (Multicenter Automatic Defibrillator Implantation Trial with Cardiac Resynchronization Therapy)   445

Continuous biatrial pacing to prevent early recurrence of atrial fibrillation after the Maze procedure   448

Incidence and Predictors of Pacemaker Placement After Surgical Ablation for Atrial Fibrillation   449

Independent Susceptibility Markers for Atrial Fibrillation on Chromosome 4q25   451

Biventricular pacing is superior to right ventricular pacing in bradycardia patients with preserved systolic function: 2-year results of the PACE trial   452

Cardiac Resynchronization Therapy as a Therapeutic Option in Patients With Moderate-Severe Functional Mitral Regurgitation and High Operative Risk   454

Cost-effectiveness of cardiac resynchronization therapy in patients with asymptomatic to mild heart failure: insights from the European cohort of the REVERSE (Resynchronization Reverses remodeling in Systolic Left Ventricular Dysfunction) — 456

Driving restrictions after implantable cardioverter defibrillator implantation: an evidence-based approach — 458

Complete removal as a routine treatment for any cardiovascular implantable electronic device—associated infection — 460

Dual-Chamber Implantable Cardioverter-Defibrillator Selection Is Associated With Increased Complication Rates and Mortality Among Patients Enrolled in the NCDR Implantable Cardioverter-Defibrillator Registry — 462

Impact of Implanted Recalled Sprint Fidelis Lead on Patient Mortality — 464

Left Ventricular Versus Simultaneous Biventricular Pacing in Patients With Heart Failure and a QRS Complex ≥120 Milliseconds — 465

Response to preventive cardiac resynchronization therapy in patients with ischaemic and nonischaemic cardiomyopathy in MADIT-CRT — 467

The relationship between ventricular electrical delay and left ventricular remodelling with cardiac resynchronization therapy — 470

Efficacy and Safety of Celivarone, With Amiodarone as Calibrator, in Patients With an Implantable Cardioverter-Defibrillator for Prevention of Implantable Cardioverter-Defibrillator Interventions or Death: The ALPHEE Study — 472

Adherence to a Low-Risk, Healthy Lifestyle and Risk of Sudden Cardiac Death Among Women — 474

Impact of Onsite or Dispatched Automated External Defibrillator Use on Survival After Out-of-Hospital Cardiac Arrest — 475

High-Density Substrate Mapping in Brugada Syndrome: Combined Role of Conduction and Repolarization Heterogeneities in Arrhythmogenesis — 477

Incidence and Predictors of Implantable Cardioverter-Defibrillator Therapy in Patients With Arrhythmogenic Right Ventricular Dysplasia/Cardiomyopathy Undergoing Implantable Cardioverter-Defibrillator Implantation for Primary Prevention — 478

The value of a family history of sudden death in patients with diagnostic type I Brugada ECG pattern — 481

Sports-Related Sudden Death in the General Population — 482

Colchicine Reduces Postoperative Atrial Fibrillation: Results of the Colchicine for the Prevention of the Postpericardiotomy Syndrome (COPPS) Atrial Fibrillation Substudy — 484

Reversal of outflow tract ventricular premature depolarization—induced cardiomyopathy with ablation: Effect of residual arrhythmia burden and preexisting cardiomyopathy on outcome — 486

Ablation of atrioventricular nodal reentrant tachycardia in the elderly: results from the German Ablation Registry — 488

Rivaroxaban versus Warfarin in Nonvalvular Atrial Fibrillation — 490

Author Index

A

Aakhus S, 306
Aarones M, 306
Abou Issa O, 167
Acker MA, 172
Adamson RM, 315
Afek A, 245
Afilalo J, 140
Agarwal R, 76
Ahmed AK, 477
Ahmed B, 238
Aicher D, 167
Allam AH, 265
Allison JJ, 108
Alwi M, 134
Anagnostopoulos PV, 123
Anderson JL, 155
Andrade S, 43
Andresen D, 488
Angeli F, 57
Arbel Y, 280
Arena R, 340
Aronow WS, 6
Arora S, 177
Askling J, 255
Athanasiadis A, 284
Avery AJ, 40
Axon RN, 61

B

Babu-Narayan SV, 141
Badheka AO, 345
Baird-Gunning J, 323
Bakal JA, 353
Ball W, 358
Balta O, 440
Banegas JR, 63
Bangalore S, 20, 22, 28
Banning AP, 174
Bardai A, 475
Barron DJ, 117
Barsheshet A, 445, 467
Barton P, 87
Batsos C, 149
Batty GD, 258
Bazzino OO, 398
Bellinger DC, 136
Beltrami L, 45
Benjo A, 26
Berdowski J, 475
Bernhardt P, 370
Bertoldi EG, 303

Bhatia NL, 372
Bhonsale A, 437, 478
Birgersdotter-Green U, 470
Blackstone E, 223
Blankstein R, 278
Blom MT, 475
Blom NA, 144
Bolli R, 175
Bolling SF, 172
Borgia F, 139
Borgman KY, 151
Borgulya G, 284
Borleffs CJW, 458
Borrelli S, 76
Bosworth HB, 106
Botto G, 442
Boudriot E, 162
Boussy T, 481
Brachmann J, 488
Bramer S, 438
Brenyo A, 445
Breymann T, 115
Brignole M, 442
Brizard CP, 114
Brown DW, 111
Brown MJ, 101
Brucato A, 409
Budoff MJ, 278
Buehler D, 448
Bueno H, 199
Burashnikov A, 433
Burkhart HM, 146

C

Cabrera J, 78
Cannell TM, 141
Carberry KE, 132
Carlo WF, 132
Carrillo X, 183
Casabé JH, 362
Casper TC, 129
Castagno D, 323
Cavallotti L, 380
Celermajer DS, 482
Chan JY-S, 452
Chan PS, 216
Chang B, 31
Cheema F, 449
Chen G, 68
Chen Y-S, 143
Cheng JQ, 78
Chillcott S, 315
Chilukuri K, 437

Chinali M, 181
Chiuve SE, 474
Choo K-K, 134
Chugh AR, 175
Ciaccio EJ, 477
Clarke B, 414
Clarke CP, 291
Cohen DJ, 161
Collet J-P, 190
Connolly HM, 118
Corrao G, 55
Cunha V, 303
Curós A, 183
Czernichow S, 13

D

Dacey LJ, 159
Dagenais GR, 226
D'Amario D, 175
Danaei G, 15
Dawes M, 104
de la Sierra A, 63
Dearani JA, 118, 146
Delgado V, 144, 295, 454
Deneke T, 440
Dewland TA, 462
Di Diego JM, 433
Diller G-P, 139
Ding EL, 271
Dini FL, 382
Dobrolet NC, 130
Don CW, 242
Dorsch MP, 47
Dos L, 116
Dragulescu A, 113
Drakos SG, 171
Duval S, 193
Dweck MR, 392

E

Earley A, 9
Economy KE, 142
Egan BM, 61
Eijgelsheim M, 412
Eitel I, 370
Elder DHJ, 401
Entjes R, 210
Erickson SR, 47
Ernst ME, 49
Eshelbrenner CL, 11

F

Faggiano P, 382
Fang F, 452
Fay R, 333
Feldman T, 165, 395
Feldman TE, 221
Feng DL, 407
Feng XD, 448
Fernández A, 362
Fernández-Hidalgo N, 386
Fifer KM, 275
Figueredo VM, 367
Finucane MM, 252
Fiore AC, 126
Fleg JL, 6
Foley PWX, 342
Folsom AR, 262
Fonarow GC, 321
Fouilloux V, 113
Fox KAA, 430
Frankel DS, 486
Friedman PA, 464
Fujita T, 389
Fung TT, 474
Furck A, 127

G

Gabriel H, 418
Gage BF, 429
Gentile G, 57
Gerstenfeld EP, 486
Gilard M, 261
Gillespie BW, 47
Girke S, 115
Glockner J, 407
Godwin M, 104
Gold MR, 470
Goldenberg I, 467
Goldman S, 233
Granger CB, 427
Greutmann M, 149
Griffiths L, 414
Groenveld HF, 435
Groves BM, 365
Guazzi M, 340
Gullestad L, 306
Gupta AK, 33
Gupta H, 269
Gupta PK, 269

H

Ha AC, 296
Hamer M, 258
Hänninen M-RA, 85
Harb S, 441
Haynes SM, 9
Heier M, 204
Heinle JS, 132
Hillis LD, 155
Hoashi T, 122
Hodgkinson J, 4
Hoffmann BA, 488
Hoffmann U, 128
Holman W, 233
Houston TK, 108
Hoyt H, 437
Hu S, 273, 319
Hu T, 11
Huang M-P, 147
Huang S-C, 143
Huffman MD, 249
Humenberger M, 418
Hussein AA, 441
Huxley RR, 262

I

Imazio M, 409, 484
Inuzuka R, 139
Irwin N, 342
Ivanov J, 358
Izumo M, 377

J

Jacob M, 223
Jaggers J, 121
Jahangir A, 282
James CA, 478
James S, 255
Jegatheeswaran A, 149
Jernberg T, 185
Jessup M, 172
Jhang WK, 145
Jhund PS, 323
John R, 169
Johnson NC, 123
Johnston SC, 247
Jolly SS, 235

Joshi S, 392
Jowett S, 87
Jureidini S, 126

K

Kagisaki K, 122, 124
Kallinen LM, 464
Kammache I, 113
Kamouh A, 150
Kang D-H, 416
Kappetein AP, 221
Kastrati A, 287
Katritsis DG, 287
Kawahara C, 355
Kaza AK, 135
Keren A, 296
Kim AS, 247
Kim D-H, 416
Kim K, 407
Kim Y-H, 229, 231
Kimmelstiel CD, 206
Kirchberger I, 204
Kivimäki M, 258
Kizilbash MA, 345
Kjeldsen SE, 22
Klein LW, 216
Knigina L, 460
Kobayashi J, 389
Koehler F, 312
Konstantinov IE, 114
Kostis JB, 78
Kotecha D, 336
Koul S, 194
Kovach JR, 125
Kowey PR, 472
Krieger EV, 142
Krumholz HM, 187
Kuch B, 204
Kucheryavaya AY, 171
Kuklina EV, 38
Kulik A, 219
Kumar S, 20, 22
Kunihara T, 167
Künzli N, 257
Kutschka I, 460

L

Labarthe D, 24
Lambiase PD, 477

Landzberg MJ, 142
LaPar DJ, 131
Le May MR, 219
Le TL, 149
Lee J-Y, 229
Lee M, 31
Leon MB, 405
Li D-K, 43
Li JS, 121
Liang C-H, 147
Liava'a M, 114
Lin M-T, 143
Linde C, 456
Link MS, 445
Liu S, 273, 319
Liu T, 38
Lopez FL, 262
López J, 386
Losordo DW, 214
Lovibond K, 87
Lubitz SA, 451
Ludvigsson JF, 255
Lunetta KL, 451

M

Mack MJ, 174
MacK MJ, 221
Magalski A, 152
Mahaffey KW, 208
Mainwaring RD, 112, 137
Makani H, 26, 28
Mancia G, 53, 69
Mandal AKJ, 349
Mangiacapra F, 210
Mant J, 4
Maria V, 282
Marijon E, 482
Marsan NA, 295, 454
Marshall AC, 120
Martin U, 4
Marx GR, 120
Masutani S, 148, 421
McAlister FA, 68, 353
McCoy M, 152
McElhinney DB, 120
McInnes GT, 101
McLintock C, 375
McManus DD, 181
Mehta RH, 188
Ménard J, 94, 333
Mendez AB, 116
Menon SC, 129
Mente A, 65
Merlino L, 69

Mery CM, 131
Messerli FH, 26
Meyer D, 170
Miedema MD, 193
Minich LL, 129
Minutolo R, 76
Missouris CG, 349
Miyazaki A, 124
Mohiaddin RH, 141
Möller P, 128
Monagle P, 119
Monfredi O, 414
Mongeon F-P, 118
Mont L, 442
Moonen M, 377
Morrison TB, 464
Moss AJ, 467
Mountantonakis SE, 486
Muga R, 183
Muñoz-Guijosa C, 116
Murigu T, 392
Murtuza B, 117
Myers MG, 104

N

Naftel DC, 125
Nagaswami C, 190
Nagueh SF, 365
Naka Y, 169
Nallamothu BK, 187
Nam C-W, 210
Nativi JN, 171
Nawrot TS, 257
Neovius M, 51
Nery PB, 296
Newell MC, 193
Ng LL, 299
Ngo K, 336
Nicotra F, 55
Nieves JA, 130
Niiranen TJ, 85

O

Oberti PF, 398
O'Donnell MJ, 65
Ohuchi H, 124
Okonko DO, 349
Oliveira C, 149
Olsen MK, 72, 106
Ong P, 284
O'Shea JC, 188
Osman MN, 150

Ovbiagele B, 74
Owen JP, 151

P

Pak S-W, 449
Papst CC, 101
Park D-W, 229, 231
Park J-J, 145
Parodi A, 55, 69
Parolari A, 380
Parthasarathy HK, 94
Patel K, 342
Patel MR, 212, 216, 490
Pearce FB, 125
Pearte CA, 206
Pellegrini CN, 462
Pepine CJ, 6
Perez L, 257
Persell SD, 59
Pertman J, 271
Petko C, 127, 128
Piccini JP, 430
Pichlmaier M, 460
Piller LB, 424
Pilote L, 140
Pirolli T, 112
Pizarro R, 398
Polanczyk CA, 303
Potapov E, 170
Pouleur A-C, 309
Powell W, 242
Powers BJ, 72, 106
Punn R, 112
Puukka PJ, 85

Q

Qadir S, 275

R

Radzi NAM, 134
Rakowski H, 358
Rathod A, 345
Rathod RH, 111
Reboldi G, 57
Reddy VM, 137
Redon J, 53
Reinhartz O, 137
Revilla A, 386
Rexrode KM, 474
Riley RF, 242

Rivkin MJ, 136
Robinson JD, 111
Romero J, 28
Rosenhek R, 418
Rosenthal N, 150
Ross-Degnan D, 40
Rossi A, 382
Rossignol P, 333
Rovere ME, 409
Ruggenenti P, 99
Ruiter R, 412

S

Sable C, 138
Saczynski JS, 181
Sadeh B, 280
Saikali KG, 291
Sakai H, 355
Sandset EC, 89
Sarkozy A, 481
Sattelmair J, 271
Saver JL, 31
Scherstén F, 194
Schumacher H, 53
Schwartz L, 365
Scott PA, 299
Seckeler MD, 131
Segura J, 63
Senzaki H, 148, 421
Serruys PW, 174
Serumaga B, 40
Sethi GK, 233
Shah SV, 429
Shai I, 245
Sharma J, 164
Shaw LJ, 278
Shimada M, 122
Shin D-I, 440
Shin HJ, 145
Shinkawa T, 123
Sicouri S, 433
Silvain J, 190
Simon T, 261
Singh JP, 470
Sinner MF, 451
Siontis GCM, 287
Slagman MCJ, 92
Smalling RW, 212
Smedira N, 223
Smedira NG, 169
Smith AH, 151
Smith CR, 178
Smith JG, 194

Smith PK, 155
Smith VA, 72
Soliman Hamad MA, 438
Song H-G, 231
Sorgente A, 481
Stahovich M, 315
Stebbins AL, 188
Steg PG, 261
Steinvil A, 280
Stolarz-Skrzypek K, 35
Stone GW, 197
Stulak JM, 146
Stumper O, 117
Subramanian S, 275
Sun A, 330
Sun BJ, 416
Sundaram A, 269
Sundström J, 51
Sussman M, 108
Suzuki K, 377
Swaminathan M, 170
Szwejkowski BR, 401

T

Tachjian A, 282
Tafflet M, 482
Tajik AJ, 372
Tardif J-C, 327
Teerlink JR, 291
Therrien J, 140
Thibault B, 465
Thiele H, 162, 201, 212
Thijssen J, 458
Thompson AM, 11
Thompson RC, 265
Tichnell C, 478
Tirosh A, 245
Tobin C, 126
Tobler D, 149
Toda K, 389
Townsend PA, 299
Tremoli E, 380
Tsutamoto T, 355
Tynelius P, 51

U

Udelson JE, 206
Uebing A, 127
Ueland T, 177
Upadhyay A, 9

V

van Bommel RJ, 295, 454
van den Born B-JH, 82
van den Hondel KE, 412
van der Hoeven NV, 82
van der Hulst AE, 144
van Diepen S, 353
van Montfrans GA, 82
van Rees JB, 458
van Straten AHM, 438
Velazquez EJ, 158
Vicenzi M, 340
Vigliano CA, 362
Voisine P, 219
von Knobelsdorff-Bren-
    kenhoff F, 370

W

Walker RL, 68
Wallace MC, 121
Walters JA, 336
Walther T, 162
Wang G, 24
Wang TY, 187
Wang W, 448
Wang Y, 462
Wann LS, 265
Wazni OM, 441
Weber CJ, 164
Wei L, 401
Welch EM, 130
Wennerblom B, 177
Westhoff-Bleck M, 115
Wetterslev J, 20
White WB, 94
Wilansky S, 372
Wilcox JE, 321
Williams B, 1
Williams JB, 240
Wojdyla D, 430
Worku B, 449
Wypij D, 136

Y

Yan H, 164
Yancy CW, 321
Yang C, 43
Yang Q, 38
Yusuf S, 65

Z

Zabel M, 152
Zanichelli A, 45

Zhang L, 330
Zhang Q, 452
Zhang S, 330
Zhang Y, 96

Zhao Y, 61
Zhao Z-J, 147
Zheng Z, 273, 319
Zingale L, 45

Printed and bound by CPI Group (UK) Ltd, Croydon, CR0 4YY

08/05/2025

01864678-0017